Understanding Mitochondrial Diseases

Understanding
Mitochondrial Diseases

Editor: Ronan Nixon

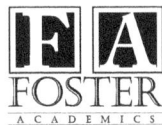

FA FOSTER
A C A D E M I C S

www.fosteracademics.com

www.fosteracademics.com

FA FOSTER ACADEMICS

Cataloging-in-Publication Data

Understanding mitochondrial diseases / edited by Ronan Nixon.
       p. cm.
Includes bibliographical references and index.
ISBN 978-1-63242-903-2
1. Mitochondrial pathology. 2. Mitochondrial membranes--Abnormalities. 3. Metabolism--Disorders.
4. Pathology, Cellular. I. Nixon, Ronan.
RB147.5 .U53 2020
616.07--dc23

Foster Academics,
118-35 Queens Blvd., Suite 400,
Forest Hills, NY 11375, USA

ISBN 978-1-63242-903-2 (Hardback)

Contents

Preface

This book aims to highlight the current researches and provides a platform to further the scope of innovations in this area. This book is a product of the combined efforts of many researchers and scientists, after going through thorough studies and analysis from different parts of the world. The objective of this book is to provide the readers with the latest information of the field.

Mitochondrial diseases refer to a group of disorders that are caused due to dysfunctional mitochondria. They may arise due to mutations in the mitochondrial DNA or in nuclear genes which code for mitochondrial components. Some of the conditions for which there exists evidence for the association of mitochondrial dysfunction are Huntington's disease, Alzheimer's disease, bipolar disorder, Parkinson's disease, schizophrenia, etc. When defective mitochondria occur in the muscles, nerves or cerebrum, they lead to debilitating conditions. The symptoms of mitochondrial disease are loss of muscle coordination, poor growth, muscle weakness, hearing and learning disabilities, visual difficulties, liver disease, heart disease, kidney disease, gastrointestinal disorders, etc. The most common diagnostic tests for the detection of mitochondrial diseases are PCR and specific mutation analysis, southern blot and sequencing. Spindle therapy, embryonic mitochondrial transplant and protofection are potential treatments for inherited mitochondrial diseases. This book includes some of the vital pieces of work being conducted across the world, on various topics related to mitochondrial diseases. It consists of contributions made by international experts. With state-of-the-art inputs by acclaimed experts of medical genetics, this book targets students and professionals.

I would like to express my sincere thanks to the authors for their dedicated efforts in the completion of this book. I acknowledge the efforts of the publisher for providing constant support. Lastly, I would like to thank my family for their support in all academic endeavors.

Editor

Degree of Glutathione Deficiency and Redox Imbalance Depend on Subtype of Mitochondrial Disease and Clinical Status

Gregory M. Enns[1]*, Tereza Moore[2], Anthony Le[2], Kondala Atkuri[3], Monisha K. Shah[1], Kristina Cusmano-Ozog[1¤], Anna-Kaisa Niemi[1], Tina M. Cowan[2]

1 Department of Pediatrics, Division of Medical Genetics, Lucile Packard Children's Hospital, Stanford University, Stanford, California, United States of America, 2 Department of Pathology, Stanford University, Stanford, California, United States of America, 3 Department of Genetics, Stanford University, Stanford, California, United States of America

Abstract

Mitochondrial disorders are associated with decreased energy production and redox imbalance. Glutathione plays a central role in redox signaling and protecting cells from oxidative damage. In order to understand the consequences of mitochondrial dysfunction on *in vivo* redox status, and to determine how this varies by mitochondrial disease subtype and clinical severity, we used a sensitive tandem mass spectrometry assay to precisely quantify whole blood reduced (GSH) and oxidized (GSSG) glutathione levels in a large cohort of mitochondrial disorder patients. Glutathione redox potential was calculated using the Nernst equation. Compared to healthy controls (n = 59), mitochondrial disease patients (n = 58) as a group showed significant redox imbalance (redox potential −251 mV±9.7, p<0.0001) with an increased level of oxidation by ~9 mV compared to controls (−260 mV±6.4). Underlying this abnormality were significantly lower whole blood GSH levels (p = 0.0008) and GSH/GSSG ratio (p = 0.0002), and significantly higher GSSG levels (p<0.0001) in mitochondrial disease patients compared to controls. Redox potential was significantly more oxidized in all mitochondrial disease subgroups including Leigh syndrome (n = 15), electron transport chain abnormalities (n = 10), mitochondrial encephalomyopathy, lactic acidosis and stroke-like episodes (n = 8), mtDNA deletion syndrome (n = 7), mtDNA depletion syndrome (n = 7), and miscellaneous other mitochondrial disorders (n = 11). Patients hospitalized in metabolic crisis (n = 7) showed the greatest degree of redox imbalance at −242 mV±7. Peripheral whole blood GSH and GSSG levels are promising biomarkers of mitochondrial dysfunction, and may give insights into the contribution of oxidative stress to the pathophysiology of the various mitochondrial disorders. In particular, evaluation of redox potential may be useful in monitoring of clinical status or response to redox-modulating therapies in clinical trials.

Editor: Feng Ling, RIKEN Advanced Science Institute, Japan

Funding: The project described in this publication was supported by the Stanford NIH/NCRR CTSA award number UL1 RR025744 and by the Lucile Packard Foundation for Children's Health. Michael and Ellen Michelson, Bobbie and Mike Wilsey, the United Mitochondrial Disease foundation, Help Mito Kids and Edison Pharmaceuticals, Inc. provided additional support for this research. The funders had no role in study design, data collection and analysis, decision to publish, or preparation of the manuscript.

Competing Interests: The authors have read the journal's policy and have the following competing interests: Dr. Enns has received unrestricted research funds from Edison Pharmaceuticals, Inc.

* E-mail: greg.enns@stanford.edu

¤ Current address: Departments of Genetics and Metabolism, Children's National Medical Center, Washington, DC, United States of America

Introduction

Inherited disorders of the mitochondrial respiratory chain can affect any organ system and are associated with significant morbidity and mortality [1]. These disorders are caused by a wide array of mutations in either the mitochondrial or nuclear genome, and encompass a broad range of molecular, biochemical and phenotypic features [1]. Collectively, they are relatively common compared with other inborn errors of metabolism, with an estimated prevalence of at least 1 in 5,000 individuals [2]. Despite this high prevalence, there are limited therapeutic options for patients; only a few controlled clinical trials have been performed and there are no FDA-approved therapies designed specifically for mitochondrial disorders [3,4]. This may in part be due to our incomplete understanding of disease pathophysiology, including possible differences in pathogenic mechanisms between the disease subtypes, as well as a paucity of reliable biomarkers with which to monitor disease progression and response to therapy [5].

Mitochondrial dysfunction leads to decreased energy production and increased production of free radicals including reactive oxygen and nitrogen species (RONS) [6–10], particularly by respiratory chain complexes I and III [11–14]. Although RONS are important products of the mitochondrial electron transport chain (ETC), serving as intracellular messengers and signals for a variety of cellular functions including mitochondrial biogenesis and apoptosis [15], abnormal increases in RONS production result in damage to cellular lipids, proteins and nucleic acids as intracellular antioxidant systems become overwhelmed [13,16].

Glutathione (L-γ-glutamyl-L-cysteinylglycine) is the most abundant intracellular thiol tripeptide and is present in all mammalian tissues, and plays a key role in cellular defense against oxidant damage [17]. Normal tissue levels range from approximately 0.1 mM to 10 mM, with the highest concentrations reported in liver, spleen, kidney, lens, erythrocytes and leukocytes [18]. Blood GSH levels have been considered to reflect the overall body GSH status, and hence are a potential indication of disease risk in humans [18–22]. Low glutathione concentrations are present in muscle samples obtained from individuals with primary mitochondrial disease [23]. Glutathione deficiency has also been reported in a variety of disorders associated with impaired mitochondrial function, including Friedreich ataxia [20], Leigh syndrome [21], organic acidemias [22,24], and neurological disorders such as Alzheimer disease [25], Parkinson disease [26] and amyotropic lateral sclerosis [27]. These studies support the idea that glutathione levels may be a useful indicator of overall redox balance, and that this metric may give insights into various types of mitochondrial dysfunction.

Using a high-dimensional fluorescence-activated cell sorter (Hi-D FACS) technique, we previously demonstrated decreased intracellular glutathione (iGSH) concentration in CD4 and CD8 lymphocytes derived from individuals with primary or secondary mitochondrial dysfunction [28]. To extend these findings, we recently reported a new liquid chromatography-tandem mass spectrometry (LC-MS/MS) method for the accurate and sensitive quantitation of reduced (GSH) and oxidized (GSSG) glutathione levels in whole blood [29]. Here we utilize this approach for the evaluation of glutathione redox status in a large cohort of patients with mitochondrial disease. In order to understand more clearly the *in vivo* consequences of ETC dysfunction, we now report the results of LC-MS/MS analysis of GSH and GSSG concentrations and redox potential in whole blood from individuals with different subtypes of primary mitochondrial disorders. We were particularly interested in determining 1) if such measurements hold promise as biomarkers in mitochondrial disorders as a whole; 2) if redox imbalance varies depending on the subtype of mitochondrial disease; and 3) if redox imbalance is a sensitive indicator of clinical status.

Materials and Methods

Subject Population

Blood samples (n = 87) from individuals with mitochondrial disease (n = 58) were obtained during routine clinic visits during periods of relative health (Tables S1 to S6). Seven additional samples were obtained from patients during hospital admission for management of metabolic crises (subjects 28, 37, 53, 59, 60, 61, and 62), including four patients not otherwise tested (Table S7). The total study population therefore consisted of 94 blood samples from 62 individuals. Only subjects with "definite" mitochondrial disease as defined by the modified Walker criteria [30] were studied, and included patients with Leigh syndrome (n = 15), electron transport chain (ETC) abnormalities (n = 10), mitochondrial encephalomyopathy, lactic acidosis and stroke-like episodes (MELAS) (n = 8), mtDNA deletion syndrome (n = 7), mtDNA depletion syndrome (n = 7), and miscellaneous other mitochondrial disorders (n = 11). The mtDNA deletion patients all carried a large mtDNA deletion and had either a Kearns-Sayre syndrome (n = 4) or Pearson syndrome (n = 3) phenotype. The Pearson syndrome patients did not have clinically significant anemia at the

time of blood sampling (Table S4). "Metabolic crisis" was defined as worsening clinical status associated with the need for hospitalization for management. Metabolic abnormalities, such as metabolic acidosis, lactic acidosis, and abnormalities including increasing blood transaminase, creatine kinase, or glucose levels were associated with the episodes (Table S7). The Stanford University Institutional Review Board (IRB) approved this study, and samples were collected only after obtaining written informed consent from participants or from the parents or legally authorized representatives of children or minors enrolled in this study. Whole blood GSH and GSSG concentrations from control subjects (residual blood samples from 59 healthy individuals [31 male, 28 female; age 1–87 years, mean 25 years]) have previously been published [29], and were used for comparisons in this study.

Assessment of Clinical and Antioxidant Status

Clinical status was determined using the Newcastle Paediatric Mitochondrial Disease Scale (NPMDS) [31], a measure comprised of objective assessments of current function, system-specific involvement and current clinical (sections I-III) as well as a quality of life questionnaire (section IV). NPMDS scores were determined for 23 patients during outpatient clinic visits and three patients during metabolic crises, and are presented as the sum of scores for sections I-III, the score for section IV, and the overall sum (Tables S1 to S7). In addition, three adults had clinical status determined using the Newcastle Mitochondrial Disease Adult Scale (NMDAS) (Tables S2, S3 and S6). Information regarding pharmacologic supplementation with antioxidants, including N-acetylcysteine, ascorbate, vitamin E, α-lipoic acid or coenzyme Q_{10}, was obtained by patient or parent report at the time of sample collection. Antioxidant supplementation was not standardized among patients.

Glutathione Measurements

Sample collection, preparation and analysis were carried out as previously described [29]. In brief, blood samples were refrigerated immediately following collection and processed within 24 hours by adding a precipitating solution of sulfosalicylic acid containing the derivatizing agent N-ethylmaleimide (NEM). Derivatized samples were stored at −80°C prior to analysis. Samples were analyzed by LC-MS/MS using stable-isotope internal standards of GSH (GSH-^{13}C,^{15}N) and GSSG (GSSG-^{13}C,^{15}N) (AnaSpec Inc., Fremont, CA) for quantitation. GSH-NEM and GSSG ions and fragments monitored in the positive mode using transitions m/z 433>304 and m/z 613>355, respectively. Stable-isotope internal standards were monitored as m/z 435>306 (GSH-^{13}C, ^{15}N-NEM) and m/z 617>359 (GSSG-^{13}C,^{15}N). Data from MS/MS were acquired with Analyst software, version 1.4 and calculations were performed with Chemoview application, version 1.2b9.

Calculation of Redox Potential

The Nernst equation, E_h (mV) = E_0+30log([GSSG]/[GSH]^2), was used to calculate whole blood redox potential [32], where GSH and GSSG are concentrations in moles/liter and E_0 is − 264 mV at pH 7.4 [33]. The value for E_0 at pH 7.4 is based on an adjustment of −5.9 mV for every 0.1 increase in pH, taking E_0 at pH 7.0 as −240 [32,33].

Statistical Analysis

Based on our previous experience with the measurement of intracellular GSH in mitochondrial disease patients [28], we expected to detect GSH deficiency in the current study population compared to controls. Therefore, sample size was calculated based on a mean difference of 20%, as has been reported in previous research [28], with a power of 0.80 and an alpha (α) of 0.05. A significant difference was determined at p<α. Analysis of variance (ANOVA) was used to determine group differences in mitochondrial disease subgroup (Leigh syndrome, ETC disorders, MELAS, mtDNA deletion syndrome, mtDNA depletion syndrome, and miscellaneous) and whole blood levels of GSH, GSSG, GSH/GSSSG ratio, and redox potential. Differences between mean whole blood levels of specific disease subgroup and mean whole blood levels of controls (one-to-one comparisons) were conducted using Student's t-test. Spearman's correlation was used to assess the correlation between disease severity (as measured by the NPMDS sections I to III combined, section IV, and sections I to IV combined), age, and mutant load with whole blood glutathione data. Multiple blood samples were available from 18 subjects (Tables S1 to S6). In order to decrease potential bias, in cases of multiple samples a mean value for each subject was used for data analysis. For analysis of NPMDS scores, the clinical status sections of the NPMDS or NMDAS (sections I to III) were initially combined and analyzed separately from section IV (quality of life questionnaire). NPMDS sections I to IV were also combined and analyzed in aggregate. Data were analyzed using SAS software, version 9.4 (SAS Institute Inc., Cary, NC, USA).

Results

Subject Population and Sample Collection

Subject demographics and diagnoses are shown in Table 1. In total, 94 samples from 62 subjects with definite mitochondrial disease according to the modified Walker criteria [30] were analyzed. The majority of samples were collected during routine clinic visits (n = 87 in 58 patients). Seven samples were collected from hospitalized patients; three patients contributed samples from both clinic visits and hospital stays, while four patients had samples collected only during hospitalization. Except where specifically noted, the analyses below relate to mitochondrial patients seen during clinic visits in relatively good health.

Control Samples

We previously reported the mean whole blood GSH concentration in a control population (n = 59) of 900 μM±141, and GSSG of 1.17 μM±0.43 [29]. Using these measurements, the GSH/GSSG ratio was calculated as 881±374; and redox potential as −260 mV±6.4 (Table 2).

Mitochondrial Disease Samples

When all samples (n = 87) from clinically stable mitochondrial disease patients (n = 58) were analyzed in aggregate, results showed a significantly more oxidized redox potential (p<0.0001) than controls, as well as lower GSH levels (p = 0.0008) and GSH/GSSG ratio (p = 0.0002) and higher levels of GSSG (p<0.0001) (Table 2, Figure 1). These differences were not explained by potential differences in hematocrit or hemoglobin concentration, which were determined in 47 samples at the same time as glutathione collection. Six samples were associated with hemoglobin concentration <10 g/dL and/or hematocrit <30. There was no correlation between GSH concentrations or redox potential between samples obtained from these anemic patients compared to those with normal hemoglobin and hematocrit values (n = 41). Among all patients with mitochondrial disease, no significant differences in redox potential or glutathione levels were found between males and females, or between patients taking antioxidant supplements (n = 34) versus those who were not (n = 24). Patients taking antioxidants had a lower mean GSH level compared to those not taking antioxidant supplements (754 μM±139 v. 885 μM±128; p = 0.0006).

Leigh Syndrome

Fifteen subjects with clinical and radiographic features consistent with Leigh syndrome were studied, including patients with a deficiency of complex I (n = 2), complex IV due to Surf1 deficiency (n = 3), complex V (n = 2), multiple ETC complexes (n = 3), or an unspecified biochemical abnormality (n = 5). A total of 17 blood samples collected during outpatient visits were analyzed (Table S1). The mean redox potential among Leigh syndrome patients was −250 mV±11.2, significantly more oxidized than in controls (p = 0.0046). In addition, whole blood GSH concentration in Leigh syndrome patients was significantly lower than controls (p< 0.0001), as well as patients with ETC disorders without Leigh syndrome (p = 0.0218) and patients with mtDNA deletions (p = 0.0472) (Table 2). Glutathione levels and redox potential between Leigh syndrome subgroups were also compared in order to ascertain whether differences could be detected on the basis of type of underlying ETC complex deficiency, and no significant differences were found.

ETC Disorders

Thirteen samples from 10 subjects with abnormalities of the mitochondrial ETC confirmed by enzymatic or molecular analyses were studied, including patients with an isolated deficiency of complex I (n = 4) or complex IV (n = 3), and those with combined deficiencies of complex I+III (n = 2) or complex I+IV (n = 1) (Table S2). The mean redox potential among all patients in this group (−251±11.3) was significantly more oxidized (p = 0.0447), although taken alone neither the GSH level nor GSSG level nor GSH/GSSG ratio achieved significance (Table 2). Because RONS production is especially associated with dysfunction of complexes I and III [11–14], data were also analyzed excluding the three subjects who did not have a deficiency of either of these complexes. No significant differences in redox potential, GSH, GSSG, or GSH/GSSG ratio were detected in this subset of mitochondrial disease patients (n = 7) compared to controls.

MELAS

All MELAS patients studied (n = 8) had the common A to G transition at mitochondrial nucleotide position 3243 (m.3243A> G). Mutant load in blood was determined for six of the subjects and ranged from 12–70%. A total of 16 blood samples from MELAS patients were tested, with a mean GSH redox potential of −255±4.2 (p = 0.0304). GSH and GSSG levels were not significantly different than controls, while the GSH/GSSG ratio did achieve significance (p = 0.0149) (Table 2). Among the six MELAS patients for whom blood mutant load was known (Table S3), there was no correlation between this and any of the studied glutathione indices.

mtDNA Deletions

A total of eleven blood samples from seven subjects with mtDNA deletion syndrome were analyzed. All patients had a large mtDNA deletion typically associated with Kearns-Sayre syndrome or Pearson syndrome, as well as consistent clinical features (Table S4). As a group, mtDNA deletion patients had a significantly more oxidized redox potential (p = 0.0420) and lower GSG/GSSG ratio (p = 0.0045) than controls, as well as higher levels of GSSG (p = 0.0052). GSH levels were only slightly lower than, but not statically different from, control values (Table 2). Blood mutant

Table 1. Patient demographics.

Diagnosis	Number of Subjects	Gender (M:F)	Age (years [range; mean±SD])
Leigh syndrome:	18	14:4	0.5–26.4; 6.4±5.8
Unknown defect (n = 6)			
Surf-1 deficiency (n = 4)			
Complex I deficiency (n = 3)			
Combined ETC defects (n = 3)			
Complex V deficiency (n = 2)			
ETC disorders:	10	5:5	1.6–27.8; 13.3±7.5
Complex I deficiency (n = 4)			
Complex I+III deficiency (n = 2)			
Complex I+IV deficiency (n = 1)			
Complex IV deficiency (n = 3)			
MELAS (m.3243G>C)	8	6:2	2.1–46.2; 20.6±15.5
mtDNA deletion syndrome:	7	5:2	1.6–50.3; 15.0±14.9
KSS (n = 4)			
PS (n = 3)			
mtDNA depletion sydrome:	8	2:6	0.5–27.0; 12.3±8.9
POLG1 (n = 4)			
dGK (n = 1)			
TK2 (n = 1)			
RRM2b (n = 1)			
Unknown defect (n = 1)			
Miscellaneous disorders:	11	1:10	1.5–43.5; 16.0±13.8
Friedreich ataxia (n = 3)			
Complex V deficiency (n = 2)			
PDH deficiency (n = 2)			
MLASA (n = 2)			
Coenzyme Q$_{10}$ deficiency (n = 1)			
Mitochondrial myopathy (n = 1)			
Total	62	33:29	0.5–50.3; 13.6±12.2

Demographics for all patients, combining those seen in routine clinic visits and those hospitalized for metabolic crises, are shown. Abbreviations: dGK = deoxyguanosine kinase deficiency; FA = Friedreich ataxia; KSS = Kearns-Sayre syndrome; MELAS = mitochondrial encephalomyopathy, lactic acidosis and stroke-like episodes; MLASA = mitochondrial myopathy, lactic acidosis and sideroblastic anemia; PDH = pyruvate dehydrogenase deficiency; POLG1 = polymerase γ deficiency; PS = Pearson syndrome; RRM2B = ribonucleotide reductase M2 B deficiency; SURF1 = surf-1 deficiency; TK2 = thymidine kinase deficiency.

load was quantified in only two mtDNA deletion patients, so we were unable to perform further correlation analysis in this group. In addition, patients with either a Kearns-Sayre syndrome (n = 4) or Pearson syndrome (n = 3) phenotype were compared to each other and no significant differences in redox parameters were detected.

mtDNA Depletion Syndrome

Blood samples (n = 15) from subjects (n = 7) with disorders causing mtDNA depletion were studied, including three patients with polymerase-γ deficiency, and one each with a deficiency of deoxyguanosine kinase, thymidine kinase 2 and ribonucleotide reductase M2B. The enzymatic diagnosis for one additional patient was unknown (Table S5). As a group, mtDNA depletion patients showed significantly oxidized redox potential (p = 0.0249) and higher GSSG levels (p = 0.0032) compared to controls, but GSH levels and GSH/GSSG were not significantly different (Table 2).

Miscellaneous Mitochondrial Disorders

An additional 15 samples from subjects (n = 11) with mitochondrial disorders that did not fit into the above categories were also analyzed. This group included three patients with Friedreich ataxia, two with complex V deficiency, two with mitochondrial myopathy and sideroblastic anemia (MLASA), two with pyruvate dehydrogenase deficiency, one with coenzyme Q$_{10}$ deficiency, and one with an unspecified mitochondrial myopathy (Table S6). Among these patients, redox potential was significantly more oxidized than controls (p = 0.0091), and GSH levels (p = 0.0025) and GSH/GSSG ratio (p = 0.0132) were significantly lower. No difference was noted in GSSG levels (Table 2).

Clinical Status and NPMDS Scores

Seven samples were obtained from mitochondrial patients who were admitted to the hospital in metabolic crisis (Table S7). Among these patients, the mean redox potential was − 242 mV±7.2, which was significantly more oxidized than all mitochondrial patients who were in relatively good health

Table 2. Comparison of Glutathione Redox Status by Mitochondrial Disease Category.

Mitochondrial Disease Category	GSH (µM)	P-Value*	GSSG (µM)	P-Value*	GSH/GSSG Ratio	P-Value*	Redox potential (mV)	P-Value*
Leigh syndrome (n=15)	735±125	<0.0001**	2.40±2.36	0.065	646±541	0.0516	−250±11.2	0.0046**
ETC disorders (n=10)	847±112	0.2648	2.53±2.29	0.0935	626±618	0.2324	−251±11.3	0.0447**
MELAS (n=8)	829±126	0.1807	1.66±0.82	0.1417	658±187	0.0149**	−255±4.2	0.0304**
mtDNA deletions (n=7)	885±208	0.7999	2.53±0.85	0.0052**	453±249	0.0045**	−249±10.8	0.0420**
mtDNA depletion (n=7)	870±190	0.6113	1.72±0.51	0.0032**	614±354	0.0773	−254±8.9	0.0249**
Miscellaneous (n=11)	758±115	0.0025**	2.23±2.27	0.1550	572±345	0.0132**	−250±10.9	0.0091**
Metabolic Crisis (n=7)	550±93	<0.0001**	1.76±1.00	0.5052	390±178	0.0306**	−242±7.2	0.0259**
Combined (n=58)	808±149	0.0008**	2.23±1.84	<0.0001**	596±424	0.0002**	−251±9.7	<0.0001**
Controls (n=59)	900±141		1.17±0.43		881±374		−260±6.4	

Glutathione indices for all mitochondrial disease patients combined, as well as for different subgroups of mitochondrial disease, are shown. The combined category excludes samples collected during times of metabolic crisis.
*comparing mitochondrial disease category to control, except for Metabolic Crisis category in which comparisons were made to mitochondrial disease patients not in crisis;
**significant at P<0.05.

(p = 0.0259). The mean concentrations of whole blood GSH (550 µM±93) and GSH/GSSG ratio (390±178) were significantly lower than controls (p<0.0001 and p = 0.0306 respectively), while the mean GSSG concentration (1.76 µM±1.00) was not significantly different from controls. NPMDS scores were evaluated for 29 patients (Tables S1 to S7), and were analyzed as the combined score from sections I to III (i.e., an overall objective clinical severity score), quality of life score (section IV) and total score (sections I to IV combined). Although there was a general trend of increasing NPMDS score with a more oxidized redox potential, a significant correlation was not observed between NPMDS score and any of the glutathione indices.

Discussion

Using a sensitive LC-MS/MS assay for measuring whole blood glutathione, we have demonstrated significant redox imbalance in a large cohort of patients with mitochondrial disease, with the greatest abnormality seen in patients who were acutely ill. This study represents the largest single collection of mitochondrial patients who have had redox status examined to date, and allowed for the further subdivision of patients by disease subgroup based on molecular etiology and/or clinical category. In addition, our robust analytical approach, consistently applied to all samples analyzed, was validated in the clinical setting and specifically controlled for artifacts of sample collection and handling including the autooxidation of GSH to GSSG [29]. This study extends our previous report of GSH deficiency in leukocytes from mitochondrial disease and organic acidemia patients as analyzed by Hi-D FACS [28], a semi-quantitative technique that measures intracellular GSH but not GSSG, and is not wholly amenable to the clinical setting.

Precise determinations of whole blood reduced and oxidized glutathione allowed us to calculate the glutathione redox potential using the Nernst equation, which accounts for both the intrinsic properties of the redox couple as well as their relative concentrations [32]. Because the glutathione system plays a critical role maintaining overall redox status of the body [34], the GSSG/2GSH redox couple can be taken as representative of the redox environment of a biological system [33]. Although absolute levels of GSH and GSSG varied substantially within and between patients and provided only a limited picture of redox status, the calculated redox potential was a more stable indicator and provided additional insights. Only a limited number of patients have undergone serial sampling; however, it is interesting to note that the two patients who were evaluated on four or more occasions (patients 29 and 45) had relatively stable redox potentials. Several patients (e.g. patients 3, 31, 34, 37 and 41) showed a moderate degree of variability in redox potential during the course of the study. In some instances, fluctuation was associated with changes in co-factor supplementation. Further longitudinal studies on a larger cohort are needed in order to determine both the degree and significance of any fluctuations in redox status in individual patients. Our calculated whole blood glutathione redox potentials are in good agreement with previously reported estimates of redox potential in tissues, which range between −260 mV and −185 mV [35,36]. Using this approach, we demonstrate that redox potential in mitochondrial disease patients shows significant redox imbalance, with an increased level of oxidation of approximately 9 mV over controls. Moreover, mitochondrial disease patients who were hospitalized for treatment of an acute metabolic crisis had lower GSH levels and more pronounced redox imbalance. In the hospitalized patients, other co-morbid conditions, such as intercurrent viral illness, exacerba-

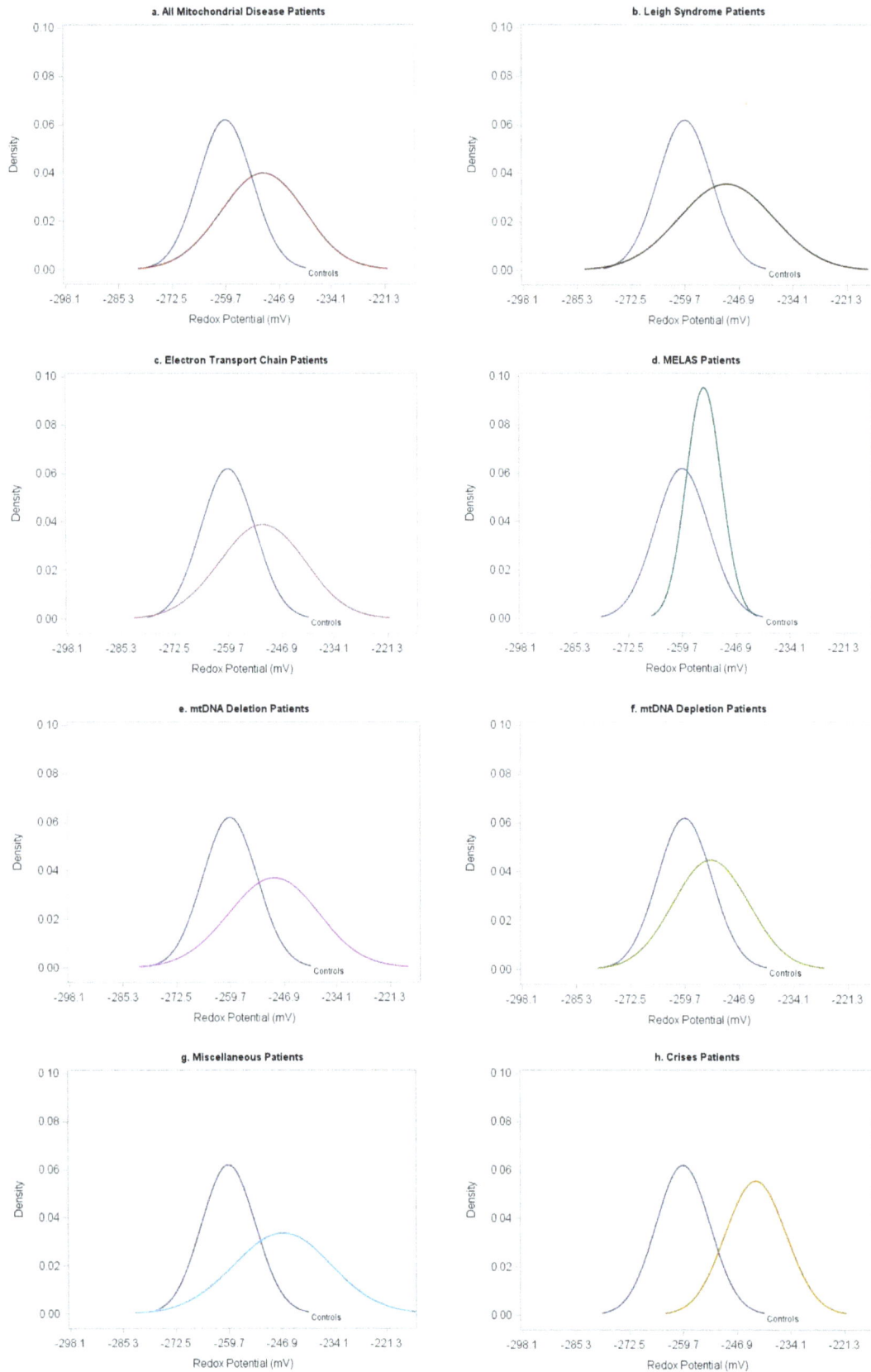

Figure 1. Glutathione redox potential distribution curves. The redox potential distribution curve for each mitochondrial disease subgroup is compared to the normal distribution of control redox potential in order to show how distribution of redox potential differs from the controls. a) Mitochondrial disease patients combined, excluding those in metabolic crisis; b) Leigh syndrome patients; c) Electron transport chain disorder

patients; d) Mitochondrial encephalomyopathy, lactic acidosis and stroke-like episode patients; e) mtDNA deletion patients; f) mtDNA depletion patients; g) Miscellaneous mitochondrial disease patients; g) Mitochondrial disease patients hospitalized in metabolic crisis. Normal distribution plots were created with SAS 9.4. The density of the normal distribution is the height for a given value on the x-axis.

tion of seizures, hyperglycemia, or metabolic acidosis, may have contributed to the baseline mitochondrial stress inherent in these disorders. In addition, although further studies on a larger number of hospitalized patients are needed, our preliminary findings suggest that the severity of the co-morbid condition may also play a role in determining ultimate redox status. For example, one patient in status epilepticus had a redox potential of -232 mV compared to a potential of -247 mV in another patient admitted with seizure exacerbation who was not in status epilepticus at the time of blood sampling (Table S7). In short, mitochondrial disease patients as a whole appear to have a more oxidized redox status at baseline compared to controls, and redox status becomes more oxidized in times of crisis.

In contrast to previous studies combining mitochondrial patients into a single, heterogeneous group [28], our population size allowed us to classify patients into subgroups based on phenotype and biochemical or molecular pathology (Tables S1 to S7) in order to evaluate whether redox status varies depending on the underlying phenotype, biochemical defect, or both. While abnormalities in glutathione levels and redox potential were observed in all subgroups of mitochondrial disease, our results indicate that there may be differences in levels of GSH, GSSG and the redox potential even between subgroups (Table 2). Interestingly, whole blood GSH levels were significantly lower in Leigh syndrome and miscellaneous categories of mitochondrial disease, but not in other subgroups.

Although we were able to classify patients into subgroups, considerable heterogeneity related to underlying molecular and biochemical features was still present within each category of mitochondrial disease. For example, the Leigh syndrome cohort, although sharing a classic mitochondrial disease clinical phenotype, was characterized by biochemical or molecular defects that affected a variety of respiratory chain subunits. Nevertheless, as a group, the Leigh syndrome patients demonstrated clear redox abnormalities. Interestingly, a recent open-label study using EPI-743, a novel redox-modulating drug, to treat a heterogeneous group of 10 Leigh syndrome patients demonstrated clinical improvement in all patients, despite the presence of multiple underlying molecular etiologies [37]. Such a therapeutic response across multiple genetic causes suggests that a common pathway related to pathogenesis may exist in Leigh syndrome. Studies of additional patients are needed in order to more clearly elucidate differences between mitochondrial subgroups and the role of oxidative stress in the pathophysiology of mitochondrial dysfunction caused by different biochemical or molecular defects.

The relatively normal levels of whole blood GSH observed in patients with pathological mtDNA mutations or deletions may in part be due to *in vivo* selection. In tissues with a high turnover, such as the hematopoietic system, stem cells with relatively normal mtDNA content have a selective advantage and, subsequently, mutant load in blood may be low [38,39]. Heteroplasmy data were available for seven MELAS patients, and only two had >50% mutant load in blood (Table S3). Although all MELAS patients had evidence of neurological impairment, the peripheral blood mutant load may not have reflected the degree of heteroplasmy present in other parts of the body. Given these considerations, it is not surprising that we did not identify a direct relationship between blood mutant load and redox status in MELAS. A recent study in 14 Japanese MELAS patients detected evidence for peripheral redox imbalance by measuring diacron-reactive oxygen metabolites and biological antioxidant potential testing. Although mutant load was not reported, the patients studied had more severe clinical symptoms than our cohort [40]. Further studies in MELAS patients with more significant clinical disease and higher levels of mutant load in peripheral blood would be needed in order to study the potential relationship between mutant load and redox status in more detail. Only two of our mtDNA deletion patients had blood heteroplasmy analysis, so it was not possible to study the relationship between blood mutant load and redox status in this group.

The demonstration that redox abnormalities are present in mitochondrial disease patients even when relatively well, and further worsen during periods of acute illness (Table S7), is consistent with reports correlating changes in the half-cell reduction potential of the GSSG/2GSH with the biological status of the cell. These reports note the progression from proliferation to differentiation and, finally, cell death being associated with an increasingly oxidized redox state [33]. The degree of oxidation is related to the likelihood of cells undergoing apoptosis or necrosis; a moderate, but lethal oxidative stimulus causes apoptosis, whereas a severe stimulus results in necrosis [33,41–43]. This response may be mediated by redox-dependent interactions with downstream signaling pathways involving release of apoptogenic factors including cytochrome *c* and apoptosis inducing factor [44–46]. Decreased cellular GSH precedes the release of cytochrome *c* and, therefore, redox status may represent the major determinant of the apoptotic switch [33,43]. Redox status has also been closely linked to a number of other intracellular signaling cascades via redox-sensitive transcription factors, including activator protein-1, nuclear factor kappa B, NE-F2 related factor, and p53 [47–50]. Therefore, *in vivo* GSH deficiency and a relatively oxidized redox status in individuals with mitochondrial disorders are likely to be associated with significant perturbation of these signaling pathways, an observation which could potentially inform the development of new therapeutic approaches for these disorders.

Our earlier work using Hi-D FACS to study white blood cell subsets from patients with primary or secondary mitochondrial dysfunction showed that antioxidant supplements improved iGSH levels [28]. In contrast, mean whole blood GSH level was lower in patients taking antioxidants compared to those not taking supplements during the time of sample collection, and no significant differences were noted in GSSG, GSH/GSSG ratio or redox potential between these two groups. The lack of uniformity of antioxidant supplementation with respect to types of supplements used and dosing makes comparisons between those taking or not taking supplements problematic. Patients taking antioxidants may also have been doing so because of the presence of more severe disease, which could potentially explain the lower mean GSH level. Given the particularly low GSH levels in Leigh syndrome patients, it seems likely that disease severity among studied cohorts has played some role in these findings. The earlier study of 21 mitochondrial disease patients included only a single Leigh syndrome patient, while the majority had various ETC disorders or MELAS [28]. An open-label clinical trial using EPI-743, a novel *para*-benzoquinone analog with electron cycling capacity, in 10 Leigh syndrome patients who had a variety of underlying molecular or enzymatic defects showed a significant increase in GSH levels in lymphocytes following the start of therapy [21]. Similar to the whole blood findings reported in the current study, Pastore *et al.* detected a significant decrease in leukocyte GSH and increased oxidized forms of glutathione in the Leigh syndrome patients at baseline [21]. Therefore, it is also possible that white blood cells are more sensitive to changes related to antioxidant therapy, but further studies directly comparing measurement of redox status in different blood compartments in patients who have mitochondrial function caused by a variety of etiologies are needed to clarify this point.

In summary, we report significant differences in glutathione status and redox potential in patients with mitochondrial disorders compared to controls. These abnormalities were present even during times of relative health, but were exacerbated in times of metabolic crisis. The greatest degree of oxidation during periods of relative health was observed in patients with the most severe clinical manifestation of mitochondrial disease including Leigh syndrome, while even more severe redox imbalance was present in patients in the midst of a metabolic crisis. Although our findings are preliminary, the measurement of redox potential via the GSSG/2GSH couple holds promise as a biomarker for mitochondrial dysfunction, and may also yield further insights related to variation of oxidative metabolism between different subtypes of mitochondrial disease.

Supporting Information

Table S1   Leigh syndrome patients.

Table S2   Electron transport chain abnormality patients.

Table S3   Mitochondrial encephalomyopathy, lactic acidosis and stroke-like episodes (MELAS) patients.

Table S4   mtDNA deletion syndrome patients.

Table S5   mtDNA depletion syndrome patients.

Table S6   Miscellaneous mitochondrial disorders patients.

Table S7   Mitochondrial patients hospitalized for "metabolic crisis".

Author Contributions

Conceived and designed the experiments: GME TM AL KA KCO AKN TMC. Performed the experiments: GME TM AL KCO AKN TMC. Analyzed the data: GME TM AL KA MKS KCO AKN TMC. Contributed reagents/materials/analysis tools: MKS TMC. Contributed to the writing of the manuscript: GME MKS TMC.

References

1. DiMauro S, Schon EA (2003) Mitochondrial respiratory-chain diseases. N Engl J Med 348: 2656–2668.
2. Schaefer AM, Taylor RW, Turnbull DM, Chinnery PF (2004) The epidemiology of mitochondrial disorders–past, present and future. Biochim Biophys Acta 1659: 115–120.
3. Kerr DS (2010) Treatment of mitochondrial electron transport chain disorders: a review of clinical trials over the past decade. Mol Genet Metab 99: 246–255.
4. Stacpoole PW (2011) Why are there no proven therapies for genetic mitochondrial diseases? Mitochondrion 11: 679–685.
5. Kerr DS (2013) Review of clinical trials for mitochondrial disorders: 1997–2012. Neurotherapeutics 10: 307–319.
6. Pitkanen S, Robinson BH (1996) Mitochondrial complex I deficiency leads to increased production of superoxide radicals and induction of superoxide dismutase. J Clin Invest 98: 345–351.
7. Wallace DC (1999) Mitochondrial diseases in man and mouse. Science 283: 1482–1488.
8. Sandhu JK, Sodja C, McRae K, Li Y, Rippstein P, et al. (2005) Effects of nitric oxide donors on cybrids harbouring the mitochondrial myopathy, encephalopathy, lactic acidosis and stroke-like episodes (MELAS) A3243G mitochondrial DNA mutation. Biochem J 391: 191–202.
9. Iuso A, Scacco S, Piccoli C, Bellomo F, Petruzzella V, et al. (2006) Dysfunctions of cellular oxidative metabolism in patients with mutations in the NDUFS1 and NDUFS4 genes of complex I. J Biol Chem 281: 10374–10380.
10. Haun F, Nakamura T, Lipton SA (2013) Dysfunctional Mitochondrial Dynamics in the Pathophysiology of Neurodegenerative Diseases. J Cell Death 6: 27–35.
11. Chance B, Sies H, Boveris A (1979) Hydroperoxide metabolism in mammalian organs. Physiol Rev 59: 527–605.
12. Hansford RG, Hogue BA, Mildaziene V (1997) Dependence of H2O2 formation by rat heart mitochondria on substrate availability and donor age. J Bioenerg Biomembr 29: 89–95.
13. Wright AF, Jacobson SG, Cideciyan AV, Roman AJ, Shu X, et al. (2004) Lifespan and mitochondrial control of neurodegeneration. Nat Genet 36: 1153–1158.
14. St-Pierre J, Buckingham JA, Roebuck SJ, Brand MD (2002) Topology of superoxide production from different sites in the mitochondrial electron transport chain. J Biol Chem 277: 44784–44790.
15. Forman HJ, Dickinson DA (2003) Oxidative signaling and glutathione synthesis. Biofactors 17: 1–12.
16. Esposito LA, Melov S, Panov A, Cottrell BA, Wallace DC (1999) Mitochondrial disease in mouse results in increased oxidative stress. Proc Natl Acad Sci U S A 96: 4820–4825.
17. Cadenas E (2004) Mitochondrial free radical production and cell signaling. Mol Aspects Med 25: 17–26.
18. Pastore A, Federici G, Bertini E, Piemonte F (2003) Analysis of glutathione: implication in redox and detoxification. Clin Chim Acta 333: 19–39.
19. Pastore A, Piemonte F, Locatelli M, Lo Russo A, Gaeta LM, et al. (2001) Determination of blood total, reduced, and oxidized glutathione in pediatric subjects. Clin Chem 47: 1467–1469.
20. Piemonte F, Pastore A, Tozzi G, Tagliacozzi D, Santorelli FM, et al. (2001) Glutathione in blood of patients with Friedreich's ataxia. Eur J Clin Invest 31: 1007–1011.
21. Pastore A, Petrillo S, Tozzi G, Carrozzo R, Martinelli D, et al. (2013) Glutathione: a redox signature in monitoring EPI-743 therapy in children with mitochondrial encephalomyopathies. Mol Genet Metab 109: 208–214.
22. Pastore A, Martinelli D, Piemonte F, Tozzi G, Boenzi S, et al. (2014) Glutathione metabolism in cobalamin deficiency type C (cblC). J Inherit Metab Dis 37: 125–129.
23. Hargreaves IP, Sheena Y, Land JM, Heales SJ (2005) Glutathione deficiency in patients with mitochondrial disease: implications for pathogenesis and treatment. J Inherit Metab Dis 28: 81–88.
24. Salmi H, Leonard JV, Lapatto R (2012) Patients with organic acidaemias have an altered thiol status. Acta Paediatr 101: e505–508.
25. Ansari MA, Scheff SW (2010) Oxidative stress in the progression of Alzheimer disease in the frontal cortex. J Neuropathol Exp Neurol 69: 155–167.
26. Merad-Boudia M, Nicole A, Santiard-Baron D, Saille C, Ceballos-Picot I (1998) Mitochondrial impairment as an early event in the process of apoptosis induced by glutathione depletion in neuronal cells: relevance to Parkinson's disease. Biochem Pharmacol 56: 645–655.
27. Schulz JB, Lindenau J, Seyfried J, Dichgans J (2000) Glutathione, oxidative stress and neurodegeneration. Eur J Biochem 267: 4904–4911.
28. Atkuri KR, Cowan TM, Kwan T, Ng A, Herzenberg LA, et al. (2009) Inherited disorders affecting mitochondrial function are associated with glutathione deficiency and hypocitrullinemia. Proc Natl Acad Sci U S A 106: 3941–3945.
29. Moore T, Le A, Niemi AK, Kwan T, Cusmano-Ozog K, et al. (2013) A new LC-MS/MS method for the clinical determination of reduced and oxidized glutathione from whole blood. J Chromatogr B Analyt Technol Biomed Life Sci 929C: 51–55.
30. Bernier FP, Boneh A, Dennett X, Chow CW, Cleary MA, et al. (2002) Diagnostic criteria for respiratory chain disorders in adults and children. Neurology 59: 1406–1411.
31. Phoenix C, Schaefer AM, Elson JL, Morava E, Bugiani M, et al. (2006) A scale to monitor progression and treatment of mitochondrial disease in children. Neuromuscul Disord 16: 814–820.
32. Jones DP (2002) Redox potential of GSH/GSSG couple: assay and biological significance. Methods Enzymol 348: 93–112.
33. Schafer FQ, Buettner GR (2001) Redox environment of the cell as viewed through the redox state of the glutathione disulfide/glutathione couple. Free Radic Biol Med 30: 1191–1212.
34. Jones DP (2006) Redefining oxidative stress. Antioxid Redox Signal 8: 1865–1879.

35. Gilbert HF (1990) Molecular and cellular aspects of thiol-disulfide exchange. Adv Enzymol Relat Areas Mol Biol 63: 69–172.

36. Kirlin WG, Cai J, Thompson SA, Diaz D, Kavanagh TJ, et al. (1999) Glutathione redox potential in response to differentiation and enzyme inducers. Free Radic Biol Med 27: 1208–1218.

37. Martinelli D, Catteruccia M, Piemonte F, Pastore A, Tozzi G, et al. (2012) EPI-743 reverses the progression of the pediatric mitochondrial disease–genetically defined Leigh Syndrome. Mol Genet Metab 107: 383–388.

38. Rahman S, Poulton J, Marchington D, Suomalainen A (2001) Decrease of 3243 A–>G mtDNA mutation from blood in MELAS syndrome: a longitudinal study. Am J Hum Genet 68: 238–240.

39. Holt IJ, Harding AE, Morgan-Hughes JA (1988) Deletions of muscle mitochondrial DNA in patients with mitochondrial myopathies. Nature 331: 717–719.

40. Ikawa M, Arakawa K, Hamano T, Nagata M, Nakamoto Y, et al. (2012) Evaluation of systemic redox states in patients carrying the MELAS A3243G mutation in mitochondrial DNA. Eur Neurol 67: 232–237.

41. Lennon SV, Martin SJ, Cotter TG (1991) Dose-dependent induction of apoptosis in human tumour cell lines by widely diverging stimuli. Cell Prolif 24: 203–214.

42. Buttke TM, Sandstrom PA (1994) Oxidative stress as a mediator of apoptosis. Immunol Today 15: 7–10.

43. Cai J, Jones DP (1998) Superoxide in apoptosis. Mitochondrial generation triggered by cytochrome c loss. J Biol Chem 273: 11401–11404.

44. Ellerby LM, Ellerby HM, Park SM, Holleran AL, Murphy AN, et al. (1996) Shift of the cellular oxidation-reduction potential in neural cells expressing Bcl-2. J Neurochem 67: 1259–1267.

45. Zimmermann AK, Loucks FA, Schroeder EK, Bouchard RJ, Tyler KL, et al. (2007) Glutathione binding to the Bcl-2 homology-3 domain groove: a molecular basis for Bcl-2 antioxidant function at mitochondria. J Biol Chem 282: 29296–29304.

46. Circu ML, Aw TY (2012) Glutathione and modulation of cell apoptosis. Biochim Biophys Acta 1823: 1767–1777.

47. Makino Y, Yoshikawa N, Okamoto K, Hirota K, Yodoi J, et al. (1999) Direct association with thioredoxin allows redox regulation of glucocorticoid receptor function. J Biol Chem 274: 3182–3188.

48. Hansen JM, Watson WH, Jones DP (2004) Compartmentation of Nrf-2 redox control: regulation of cytoplasmic activation by glutathione and DNA binding by thioredoxin-1. Toxicol Sci 82: 308–317.

49. Go YM, Jones DP (2010) Redox control systems in the nucleus: mechanisms and functions. Antioxid Redox Signal 13: 489–509.

50. Zhang Z, Tsukikawa M, Peng M, Polyak E, Nakamaru-Ogiso E, et al. (2013) Primary respiratory chain disease causes tissue-specific dysregulation of the global transcriptome and nutrient-sensing signaling network. PLoS One 8: e69282.

2

Pilot, Randomized Study Assessing Safety, Tolerability and Efficacy of Simplified LPV/r Maintenance Therapy in HIV Patients on the 1st PI-Based Regimen

Pedro Cahn[1], Julio Montaner[2], Patrice Junod[3], Patricia Patterson[1], Alejandro Krolewiecki[1], Jaime Andrade-Villanueva[4], Isabel Cassetti[5], Juan Sierra-Madero[6], Arnaldo David Casiró[7], Raul Bortolozzi[8], Sergio Horacio Lupo[9], Nadia Longo[10], Emmanouil Rampakakis[10], Nabil Ackad[11], John S. Sampalis[10,12]*

1 Fundacion Huesped, Buenos Aires, Argentina, 2 University of British Columbia, Vancouver, Canada, 3 Clinique Médicale du Quartier Latin, Montréal, Canada, 4 Antiguo Hospital Civil de Guadalajara "Fray Antonio Alcalde", CUCS, Universidad de Guadalajara, Guadalajara, Jalisco, Mexico, 5 Helios Salud, Buenos Aires, Argentina, 6 Instituto Nacional de Ciencias Medicas y Nutricion, Mexico, Mexico, 7 Hospital General de Agudos Teodoro Alvarez, Buenos Aires, Argentina, 8 División Estudios Clínicos, Centro Diagnóstico Médico de Alta Complejidad S.A. (CIBIC), Santa Fé, Argentina, 9 Instituto CAICI, Santa Fé, Argentina, 10 JSS Medical Research, Westmount, Canada, 11 Abbott Laboratories, Montréal, Canada, 12 McGill University, Montréal, Canada

Abstract

Objectives: To compare the efficacy and safety of an individualized treatment-simplification strategy consisting of switching from a highly-active anti-retroviral treatment (HAART) with a ritonavir-boosted protease inhibitor (PI/r) and 2 nucleoside reverse-transcriptase inhibitors (NRTIs) to lopinavir/ritonavir (LPV/r) monotherapy, with intensification by 2 NRTIs if necessary, to that of continuing their HAART.

Methods: This is a one-year, randomized, open-label, multi-center study in virologically-suppressed HIV-1-infected adults on their first PI/r-containing treatment, randomized to either LPV/r-monotherapy or continue their current treatment. Treatment efficacy was determined by plasma HIV-1 RNA viral load (VL), time-to-virologic rebound, patient-reported outcomes (PROs) and CD4+T-cell-count changes. Safety was assessed with the incidence of treatment-emergent adverse events (AE).

Results: Forty-one patients were randomized to LPV/r and 39 to continue their HAART. No statistically-significant differences between the two study groups in demographics and baseline characteristics were observed. At day-360, 71(39:LPV/r;32:HAART) patients completed treatment, while 9(2:LPV/r;7:HAART) discontinued. In a Last Observation Carried Forward Intent-to-Treat analysis, 40(98%) patients on LPV/r and 37(95%) on HAART had VL<200copies/mL (P = 0.61). Time-to-virologic rebound, changes in PROs, CD4+ T-cell-count and VL from baseline, also exhibited no statistically-significant between-group differences. Most frequent AEs were diarrhea (19%), headache (18%) and influenza (16%). Four (10%) patients on LPV/r were intensified with 2 NRTIs, all regaining virologic control. Eight serious AEs were reported by 5(2:LPV/r;3:HAART) patients.

Conclusion: At day-360, virologic efficacy and safety of LPV/r appears comparable to that of a PI+2NRTIs HAART. These results suggest that our individualized, simplified maintenance strategy with LPV/r-monotherapy and protocol-mandated NRTI re-introduction upon viral rebound, in virologically-suppressed patients merits further prospective long-term evaluation.

Editor: Alan Landay, Rush University, United States of America

Funding: This study was supported by a grant-in-aid by Abbott Canada. The funder was involved in the conception and design of the experiment but had no role in data collection and analysis, decision to publish, or writing of the manuscript. JSS Medical Research, a CRO contracted by Abbott, analyzed the data and wrote the manuscript.

Competing Interests: NA is an Abbott employee, NL, ER and JSS are employees of JSS Medical Research, the CRO contracted by Abbott to conduct the study and perform the data analysis.

* E-mail: jsampalis@jssresearch.com

Introduction

The standard treatment approach in HIV-1 infection involves using a combination of at least three antiretroviral (ARV) drugs, designated highly active antiretroviral therapy (HAART) to fully suppress plasma HIV-1 RNA viral load (VL), in a sustainable fashion. Currently recommended first line antiretroviral regimens consist of two nucleoside (NRTI) or nucleotide (NtRTI) analog reverse transcriptase inhibitors and either a non-nucleoside reverse transcriptase inhibitor (NNRTI), an integrase strand transfer inhibitor (INSTI) or a ritonavir-boosted protease inhibitor (PI/r) [1]. While adherence to HAART regimens is essential to achieve and maintain long-term virological suppression [2,3,4,5], suboptimal adherence is often observed due to the complexity of the treatment regimens as well as their associated short- and long-term toxicities. The subsequent failure to adequately suppress viral replication permits the rapid selection of resistant mutations, viral rebound and resumption of disease progression [6,7].

A number of regimen simplification treatment approaches have been explored to improve adherence, reduce the risk of virologic failure and long-term toxicities, and enhance the patient's quality of life [8]. In induction/maintenance therapy, a standard three drug regimen is used to achieve virologic suppression, followed by the use of a simpler regimen to maintain viral control. Lopinavir (LPV) is a PI with potent *in vitro* activity against HIV [9] which has been clinically used in combination with ritonavir (r), a cytochrome P450 3A4 enzyme inhibitor, to enhance its pharmacokinetic properties. LPV/r-based combination ARV regimens have been shown to be effective in the treatment of ARV therapy (ART)-naive patients, both short-term and long-term [4,10,11]. However, when used as monotherapy LPV/r was found to achieve lower levels of virologic suppression as compared to LPV/r-based triple ART [12]. In contrast, in a more recent study, Arribas et al. demonstrated that maintenance LPV/r monotherapy was not inferior to triple therapy (LPV/r + 2 NRTIs) in its ability to maintain suppression of the VL among patients with prior stable virologic suppression [13].

The objective of this pilot study was to assess the efficacy and safety of a simplified strategy aimed to optimize the use of LPV/r monotherapy maintenance, whereby intensification with two NRTIs was allowed if VL in plasma became detectable, among patients stably suppressed on PI/r triple-combination therapy.

Methods

The protocol for this trial and supporting CONSORT checklist are available as supporting information; see Checklist S1 and Protocol S1.

Patients

Eligible patients were HIV-1 infected adults who: i) were on their first ART regimen, composed of any two NRTIs plus LPV/r or a PI/r combination; and ii) had been virologically suppressed with a HIV-1 RNA viral load of <50 copies/ml for at least 6 months prior to study entry and a CD4+ T-cell count ≥ 100 cells/mm^3. Patients were excluded if they were HBsAg+, had active tuberculosis or an opportunistic infection, active malignancy (except Kaposi's Sarcoma), elevated hepatic transaminases (ALT/AST >5x Upper Limit of Normal), or an uncontrolled substance abuse or psychiatric illness that could preclude compliance with the protocol. Patients were also excluded if they were pregnant or lactating, had received an investigational drug within 30 days prior to study initiation, or had modified their ART within three months of study entry or were intending to do so during the course of the study.

Study Design

This was a one-year pilot, prospective, open-label, randomized, comparative, multi-center study. The study was conducted according to the tenets of the Declaration of Helsinki and approved by an independent ethics review board (Ethica Clinical Research Inc., Montreal, Quebec). All participating patients provided written informed consent prior to study entry. Patients were recruited between January 2005 and July 2007 across 9 sites in Canada, Argentina, and Mexico, and were randomized to receive in a 1:1 ratio either monotherapy with LPV/r (IM) or the standard HAART regimen (ST). Randomization was centrally coordinated by a third-party data management center and was stratified by center. A sealed envelope containing the randomized allocation was sent by the data management center to the physician who was blinded for the randomization schedule, and was opened by the patient. The allocation document was subsequently signed by the physician and mailed back to the data management center. Patients randomized to the IM group were provided with co-formulated LPV/r 133.3/33.3 mg soft gel capsules and were instructed to take 3 capsules BID orally with food. Clinical assessments took place at Screening/Baseline (Day -1) and Days 15, 30, 60, 90, 120, 150, 180, 240, 300, and 360. Efficacy measures included plasma HIV-1 RNA levels and CD4+ T-cell counts. Safety was assessed with the incidence of treatment emergent adverse events (AE), vital signs, clinical laboratory data, including venous lactic acid and serum lipid levels.

Patients with HIV-1 RNA >50 copies/ml in one visit were retested between 7 and 30 days later. If the second viral load was <50 copies/ml the patients continued on their randomized therapy, while if it was >50 and <200 copies/mL the patients were followed on protocol and were retested until either <50 or >200 copies/ml was confirmed. If the second viral load was >200 copies/ml, patients in the ST arm were considered to have met the endpoint of virologic failure, and treatment was to be modified at the discretion of the investigator/treating physician. In the monotherapy arm, if the second viral load was >200 copies/ml, intensification with two NRTIs was allowed (either the same NRTIs as before randomization or different ones) and the patient was maintained on the randomized treatment starting the visit schedule from the beginning. Intensified patients who developed a viral load of >50 copies/ml and a subsequent viral load of >200 copies/ml were considered to have reached the study endpoint of virologic failure, and therapy was to be modified at the discretion of the investigator or the treating physician.

Outcome Measures

The primary efficacy endpoint was the percentage of patients with plasma HIV-1 RNA level <200 copies/ml at Day 360. Secondary efficacy measures were the percentage of patients with plasma HIV-1 RNA <50 copies/mL at Day 360 (as determined by the Roche AMPLICOR HIV-1 MONITOR Ultra-Sensitive Assay, version 1.5; lower limit of detection (LLOD) = 50 copies/mL), the time to confirmed virologic rebound (≥ 200 copies/ml and ≥ 50 copies/ml) or meeting the criteria for virologic failure as described above through Day 360, as well as the mean change in Viral Load and CD4+ T-cell count from baseline to final assessment.

The impact on patient-reported outcomes (PROs) was assessed using the Symptoms Distress Module (SDM) which was administered at each visit. This questionnaire was developed by the NIAID AIDS Clinical Trials group and consists of 20 questions evaluating the impact of specific symptoms, possibly related to the treatment, on the patient's life. The total score is calculated as the sum of the five point response to the 20 questions where 0 = symptom not reported, 1 = I have this symptom and it doesn't bother me, 2 = I have this symptom and it bothers me a little, 3 = I have this symptom and it bothers me, and 4 = I have this symptom and it bothers me a lot. The SDM score ranges from 0 to 80 and higher values indicate worse PROs.

Safety was determined by the incidence of treatment emergent adverse events (AE), changes in vital signs and clinical laboratory data, as well as the occurrence of metabolic toxicity as indicated by the venous lactic acid and fasting serum lipid levels. AE relationship to the study medication was based on the judgment of the treating physician.

Statistical Methods

Sample size calculations for the current study were based on the expected difference between the two treatment groups in the proportion of patients with virologic control defined as <200 copies/mL at Day 360. Previous studies have shown that at 48 weeks, approximately 90% of virologically suppressed patients treated with LPV/r remain virologically controlled [14]. In order to detect as statistically significant a relative risk for being virologically suppressed of 1.35 with 80% power and two tailed significance level of 5%, a total of 50 fully evaluable patients per group were required. The study was ended when 80 patients were enrolled due to low recruitment rate.

Between-group differences in the rates of virologic control (proportion of patients with viral load <200 copies/mL and <50 copies/mL at day 360) were assessed with the Chi-Square test. The odds ratio (OR) with 95% confidence intervals was used as the measure of treatment effect. In this analysis the Last Observation Carried Forward (LOCF) approach was used for patients that discontinued the study prior to the 360 day follow up. The time to first confirmed virologic rebound was estimated using the Kaplan Meier Survival function, and the maximum likelihood test was used to compare the two groups with respect to the rate of virologic rebound. The Student's t-test for independent samples was used to assess between group differences with respect to the change in CD4+ T-cell count, VL and SDM score from baseline to final assessment. Repeated Measures Analysis of variance with Mixed Effects to account for unequal follow up were used to assess the treatment effect on CD4+ T-cell count, VL and SDM over time. Paired Student's t-test was used to descriptively assess the change in CD4+ T-cell count, VL and SDM within the two treatment groups, while simple linear regression models were used to assess these changes over time within the two treatment groups. Safety was assessed by the incidence of adverse events. All analyses were performed using the intent-to-treat population, defined as all patients enrolled who had taken at least one dose of the study medications and had completed at least one follow up visit.

Results

A total of 80 patients were enrolled in the study, met the intent-to-treat (ITT) criteria and were randomly assigned to treatment, of which, 71 (89%) completed the study and 9 (11%) prematurely discontinued. Among these 9 discontinued patients, 7 belonged to the ST group and 2 to the IM group. Reasons for discontinuation and patient disposition are described in Figure 1.

As summarized in Table 1, demographics and baseline characteristics for the ITT population exhibited no statistically significant differences between groups. The mean (SD) age at screening was 39 (9.3) years. Patients were predominantly males (84%) and Caucasian (94%), with a mean (SD) duration since initial HIV diagnosis of 3.3 (3.0) years. At baseline, the mean (SD) CD4+ T-cell count and $\log_{10}$ HIV-1 RNA were 383 (195) cells/mm^3 and 1.68 (0.08) $\log_{10}$copies/ml, respectively. The most common ARV medications used prior to randomization, were: lamivudine 44 (55%), LPV/r 44 (55%), low dose ritonavir 34 (42%), zidovudine/lamivudine 31 (39%), and zidovudine 26 (33%). There were 23 patients on a LPV/r combination and 18 patients on a non-LPV/r regimen in the IM group, prior to randomization. Similarly, 23 patients in the ST group were on a LPV/r combination while 16 patients were on a non-LPV/r combination.

The primary outcome measure of the study was the proportion of patients with plasma HIV-1 RNA <200 copies/ml at 360 days. In an ITT analysis using the LOCF principle, 37 of the 39 patients (95%) in the ST group and 40 of the 41 patients (98%) in the IM group had plasma HIV-1 RNA <200 copies/ml (OR = 0.46; 95% CI: 0.04–5.31; P = 0.611). With respect to the proportion of

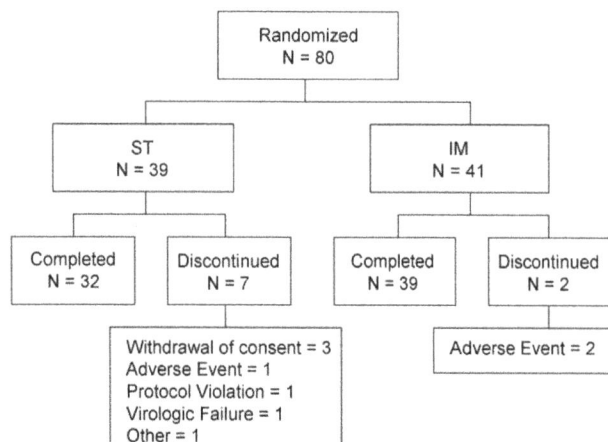

Figure 1. Patient Disposition. * *ST: Standard Treatment; IM: Induction/Maintenance.*

Table 1. Patient Demographics and Baseline Characteristics in the ITT population.

Parameter:	ST (N = 39)	IM (N = 41)	Total (N = 80)
Age (years)			
Mean (SD)	37.7 (8.51)	39.9 (9.89)	38.9 (9.25)
Median (Range)	37.0 (24.0 – 59.0)	39.0 (23.0 – 75.0)	38.0 (23.0 – 75.0)
Gender			
Male; N (%)	36 (92.3%)	31 (75.6%)	67 (83.8%)
Race: N (%)			
Caucasian	36 (92.3%)	39 (95.1%)	75 (93.8%)
American Indian/ Alaska Native	3 (7.7%)	2 (4.9%)	5 (6.2%)
Disease duration 2(years)			
N	26	27	53
Mean (SD)	3.4 (3.85)	3.1 (2.00)	3.3 (3.02)
Absolute CD4+ T-cell count (cell/mm³)			
N	39	41	80
Mean (SD)	401.2 (222.5)	364.6 (164.3)	382.5 (194.5)
Viral load (log₁₀ RNA copies/mL)			
N	39	41	80
Mean (SD)	1.689 (0.063)	1.680 (0.087)	1.684 (0.076)

(a): > 200 HIV-1 RNA copies / ml

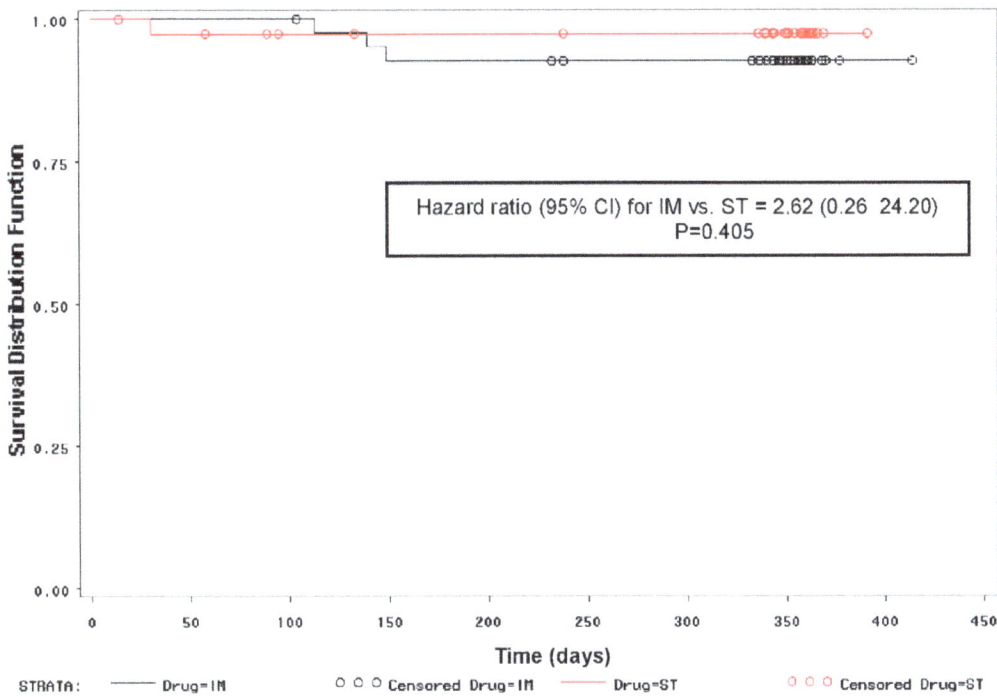

Hazard ratio (95% CI) for IM vs. ST = 2.62 (0.26 24.20)
P=0.405

(b): > 50 HIV-1 RNA copies / ml

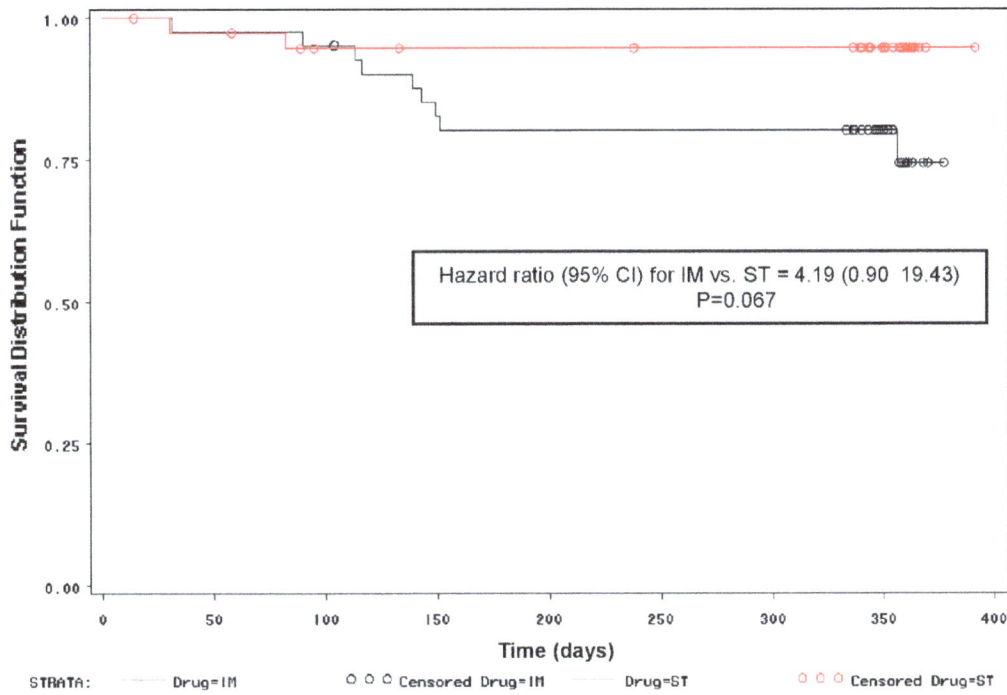

Hazard ratio (95% CI) for IM vs. ST = 4.19 (0.90 19.43)
P=0.067

* Censored observations represent patients who exited the study without experiencing virologic rebound

Figure 2. Kaplan Meier Analysis for time to confirmed virologic rebound. (a): >200 HIV-1 RNA copies / ml. (b): >50 HIV-1 RNA copies / ml.
* Censored observations represent patients who exited the study without experiencing virologic rebound.

patients with plasma HIV-1 RNA <50 copies/ml at 360 days, applying again the LOCF principle, there were 36 patients (92%) for the ST and 39 (95%) for the IM group (OR = 0.61; 95% CI: 0.097–3.897; P = 0.671). Four (10%) patients on LPV/r were intensified with 2 NRTIs and all of them regained virologic control, as demonstrated by achieving a plasma HIV-1 RNA <50 copies/mL following the intensification.

The Kaplan Meier estimates of the proportion of patients with sustained virologic response are shown in Figure 2. Applying the maximum likelihood analysis on these estimates for the time to first confirmed virologic rebound of ≥200 plasma HIV-1 RNA copies/ml, a hazard ratio (95% CI) of 2.62 (0.26–24.20) for IM versus ST was calculated, which was not statistically significant (P = 0.405) (Figure 2a). Similarly, the time to first confirmed virologic rebound of ≥50 HIV-1 RNA copies/ml was comparable in the two groups with an estimated hazard ratio (95% CI) of 4.19 (0.90–19.43), which only approached statistical significance (P = 0.067) (Figure 2b).

The results in Table 2 show that there were no significant between-group differences with respect to the mean changes in CD4+ T-cell counts (P = 0.463) and HIV-1 VL (P = 0.361) from baseline to final assessment. Furthermore, Repeated Measures Analysis of Variance with Mixed Effects indicate that the change in these parameters over time during the 360 day follow up period, was also similar between the two groups (P = 0.794 and P = 0.413, respectively).

Using the SDM to assess the PROs, it was determined that the patients in the IM group experienced a decline in the SDM from 31.7 at baseline to 26.2 at 360 days (P = 0.003), indicating a statistically significant improvement in the PROs. On the contrary, patients in the ST group experienced a statistically non-significant decline from 31.8 at baseline to 29.6 at 360 days (P = 0.094). Nevertheless, the difference in the change in SDM from baseline to 360 days of treatment between the two treatment groups was not statistically significant (P = 0.131). Similarly, linear regression analysis showed that the change in SDM over time was statistically significant for the IM group (P = 0.001), but not for the ST group (P = 0.949) (Figure 3). However, Repeated Measures Analysis of Variance again failed to detect a significant between-group difference with respect to the change in SDM over time (P = 0.189).

A total of 658 AEs were reported for 66 (83%) patients. Of these, 269 AEs were reported by 32 (82%) patients in the ST group while 389 AEs were reported by 34 (83%) patients in the IM group. Both the incidence and the profile of adverse events were comparable between the two groups, showing no apparent

differences. The most frequently reported adverse events were diarrhea (19%), headache (18%), influenza (16%), nasopharyngitis (13%), back pain (10%), hypertriglyceremia (8%) and insomnia (8%). Adverse events were predominantly mild in severity and judged unrelated to the study drug. There were three SAEs reported by two patients in the IM group (1 thrombocytopenia, 1 upper abdominal pain and 1 pneumonia) and five SAEs reported by three patients in the ST group, of which seven were considered severe and one in the IM group was moderate. All SAEs were considered unrelated to the study drug.

Discussion

The goal of this pilot, randomized clinical trial was to compare an individualized, simplified maintenance LPV/r-based strategy with reintroduction of two NRTIs upon viral rebound in plasma, to the standard continued triple-drug therapy with respect to sustained virologic response over 360 days, among virologically suppressed HIV-1-infected patients on their first PI/r-based HAART regimen. Our results demonstrate comparable safety, efficacy and tolerability for the induction/maintenance strategy and the continued standard HAART treatment. Overall, virologic success rates of over 90% and 95% were documented when using the 50 and 200 copies/mL plasma viral load thresholds, respectively. Importantly, intensification by NRTIs was required in only 10% of the patients randomized to LPV/r which, in all instances, resulted in regaining virologic control as defined by a sustained plasma HIV-1 RNA level of <50 copies/mL. Additional immunologic and virologic parameters including the change in the CD4-T-cell count and the viral load from baseline to final assessment, the rate of change in these two parameters over the 360 days, and time to virologic rebound defined as >200 HIV-1 RNA copies/ml, were also not statistically different between the two groups. With regards to the time to VL>50 HIV-1 RNA copies/ml, a trend towards the favor of the ST was observed, which was however not statistically significant. Previous studies have shown that ritonavir-boosted PI monotherapy is associated with low-level viremia (50–200 copies/mL), the clinical relevance of which is still not clear [15]. Changes in PROs, as measured by the SDM, favored the induction/maintenance group showing bigger improvement in the patients randomized to the simplified maintenance strategy.

The results of the current study are in agreement with those from the OK04 study [13,14], showing that 85% vs. 90% and 77% vs. 78% of patients on LPV/r monotherapy vs. patients on standard triple therapy group remained virologically suppressed

Table 2. Virologic and Immunologic Response.

Parameter	Visit	ST		IM		Total		P - Value [1]
		N	Mean (SD)	N	Mean (SD)	N	Mean (SD)	
Absolute CD4+ T-cell count	Baseline	39	401.2 (222.5)	41	364.6 (164.3)	80	382.5 (194.5)	0.404
	360 days	32	478.6 (246.4)	39	453.8 (249.4)	71	465.0 (246.6)	0.678
	Change	32	56.8 (168.93)	39	89.3 (196.18)	71	74.6 (183.84)	0.463
Viral load $\log_{10}$ RNA copies/ml	Baseline	39	1.689 (0.063)	41	1.680 (0.087)	80	1.684 (0.076)	0.592
	360 days	31	1.692 (0.079)	39	1.734 (0.249)	70	1.715 (0.193)	0.369
	Change	31	0.006 (0.032)	39	0.055 (0.245)	70	0.033 (0.184)	0.361

[1]Based on student's t-test for independent samples.

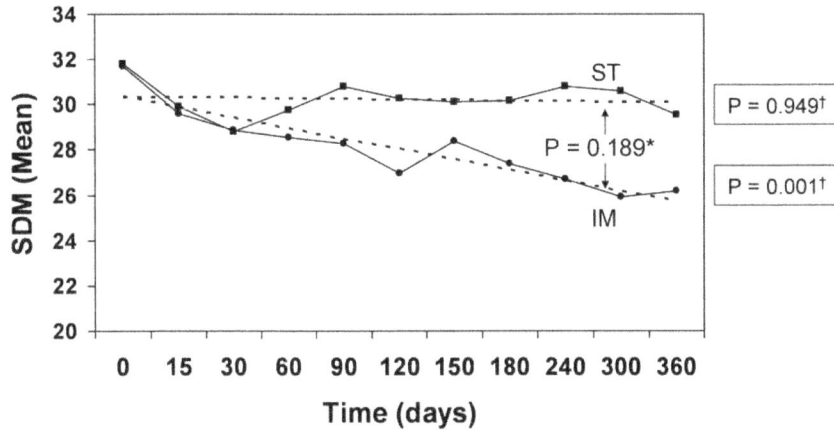

Figure 3. PROs by Treatment Group and Follow-Up Visits. [1] *Dotted lines represent the linear regression function based on the least squares method.* [2] *SDM, Symptoms Distress Module; ■, Standard Treatment; ♦, Induction/Maintenance. * P-value for between-group difference in change over time based on Repeated Measures Analysis of Variance* [†] *P-value for within-group change over time based on linear regression analysis.*

with HIV-1-RNA levels <50 copies/mL after 48 and 96 weeks, respectively. Furthermore, the longer studies by Pulido et al. [16], Cameron et al. [17] and Nunes et al. [18] also demonstrated comparable virological suppression defined as <50 copies/ml and <80 copies/ml, respectively, between the LPV/r monotherapy and combination therapy arms at 48 months and at later stages.

Use of class-sparing regimens, such as the one described in this study, offers the advantage of saving alternative ARV classes as a "back-up" option for new ARV combinations, in the case of ART failure. Furthermore, such regimens could help avoid the side effects associated with nucleoside analogue-containing regimens including renal or bone toxicity and high cardiovascular risk associated with tenofovir disoproxil fumarate and abacavir, respectively [19,20,21]. Mitochondrial toxicity with older NRTIs, currently used in resource-limited settings, was described by Brinkman and coworkers [22], and confirmed by other authors [23,24]. The clinical presentation of NRTI toxicities seen in HIV-infected individuals is dependent on the organ system affected, including lipoatrophy, lactic acidosis, peripheral neuropathy, hepatic steatosis, myopathy, cardiomyopathy, pancreatitis, bone marrow suppression, lactic acidosis, and the Fanconi syndrome. Hepatic failure with refractory lactic acidosis is the most serious disease complication related to mitochondrial dysfunction [22,25]. The prescribing information for all NRTIs includes a black-box warning of the potential risk of lactic acidosis, which is constantly updated [26]. Recently, the FDA released a new warning regarding treatment with didanosine (ddI) about a rare, but serious, complication: non-cirrhotic portal hypertension [27]. Stavudine [28,29] and less frequently zidovudine [30,31] have also been previously linked to severe lactic acidosis. Although the risk of developing lactic acidosis has fallen due to the dramatic decrease in the number of patients receiving stavudine in the developed world, stavudine continues to be used in developing countries, where cases of severe toxicity continue to be seen [32]. Therefore, the NRTI-sparing strategy might be of particular interest in resource-poor settings whereby, in addition to avoiding the above-mentioned toxicities, more affordable strategies could allow more efficient access to ART.

One of the possible limitations of the current study is the small sample size and the fact that the calculated sample size was not achieved due to low recruitment rate. However, the differences between the two groups with respect to virologic suppression and immunological changes were clinically non-important in addition to not being statistically significant. This observed similarity between the treatment groups provides evidence for the comparability of their effectiveness. Nevertheless, larger studies with longer follow up would be helpful in confirming these conclusions. The open label design of the study represents a methodological limitation. However, this design is in line with real-life practice while the objective and blinded ascertainment of virologic and immunologic parameters precludes the possibility of differential ascertainment bias.

In conclusion, our study reports encouraging preliminary safety and efficacy outcomes using an individualized, simplification maintenance strategy of LPV/r monotherapy with NRTI re-introduction upon viral rebound in plasma, among virologically suppressed patients on their first PI/r-based HAART. Based on these results, our strategy of simplified maintenance with LPV/r monotherapy merits further prospective long term evaluation of its safety and effectiveness in larger cohorts. Evaluation of the simplified strategy proposed here is particularly important as it provides a potentially simple and more affordable strategy for long term ART, that may be particularly relevant to the current global effort to expand access to HAART to millions in need.

Author Contributions

Conceived and designed the experiments: PC JM NA JSS. Performed the experiments: PC JM PJ PP AK JA-V IC JS-M ADC RB SHL. Analyzed the data: NL ER JSS. Contributed reagents/materials/analysis tools: PC JM PJ PP AK JA-V IC JS-M ADC RB SHL NA NL ER JSS. Wrote the paper: NL ER JSS. Manuscript Revision: PC JM PJ PP AK JA-V IC JS-M ADC RB SHL NL ER NA JSS. Obtained Funding: NA. Patient Recruitment: PC JM PJ PP AK JA-V IC JS-M ADC RB SHL.

References

1. Panel on Antiretroviral Guidelines for Adult and Adolescents. Guidelines for the use of antiretroviral agents in HIV-1-infected adults and adolescents Department of Health and Human Services. December 1. (2009) pp 1–161. Available: http://www.aidsinfo.nih.gov/ContentFiles/AdultandAdolescentGL.pdf. Accessed 2010 Mar 30.

2. Gallant JE, Staszewski S, Pozniak AL, DeJesus E, Suleiman JM, et al. (2004) Efficacy and safety of tenofovir DF vs stavudine in combination therapy in antiretroviral-naïve patients: a 3-year randomized trial. JAMA 292(2): 191–201.

3. Gulick RM, Meibohm A, Havlir D, Eron JJ, Mosley A, et al. (2003) Six-year follow-up of HIV-1-infected adults in a clinical trial of antiretroviral therapy with indinavir, zidovudine, and lamivudine. AIDS 17(16): 2345–9.

4. Hicks C, King MS, Gulick RM, White AC Jr., Eron JJ Jr., et al. (2004) Long-term safety and durable antiretroviral activity of lopinavir/ritonavir in treatment-naïve patients: 4 year follow-up study. AIDS 18(5): 775–9.

5. Murphy RL, da Silva BA, Hicks CB, Eron JJ, Gulick RM, et al. (2008) Seven-year efficacy of a lopinavir/ritonavir-based regimen in antiretroviral-naïve HIV-1-infected patients. HIV Clin Trials 9(1): 1–10.

6. Bangsberg DR, Porco TC, Kagay C, Charlebois ED, Deeks SG, et al. (2004) Modeling the HIV protease inhibitor adherence-resistance curve by use of empirically derived estimates. J Infect Dis 190(1): 162–5.

7. Braithwaite RS, Shechter S, Roberts MS, Schaefer A, Bangsberg DR, et al. (2006) Explaining variability in the relationship between antiretroviral adherence and HIV mutation accumulation. J Antimicrob Chemother 58(5): 1036–43.

8. McKinnon JE, Mellors JW, Swindells S (2009) Simplification strategies to reduce antiretroviral drug exposure: progress and prospects. Antivir Ther 14(1): 1–12.

9. Sham HL, Kempf DJ, Molla A, Marsh KC, Kumar GN, et al. (1998) ABT-378, a highly potent inhibitor of the human immunodeficiency virus protease. Antimicrob Agents Chemother 42(12): 3218–24.

10. Walmsley S, Bernstein B, King M, Arribas J, Beall G, et al. (2002) Lopinavir-ritonavir versus nelfinavir for the initial treatment of HIV infection. N Engl J Med 346(26): 2039–46.

11. Domingo P, Suárez-Lozano I, Torres F, Teira R, Lopez-Aldeguer J, et al. (2008) First-line antiretroviral therapy with efavirenz or lopinavir/ritonavir plus two nucleoside analogues: the SUSKA study, a non-randomized comparison from the VACH cohort. J Antimicrob Chemother 61(6): 1348–58.

12. Delfraissy JF, Flandre P, Delaugerre C, Ghosn J, Horban A, et al. (2008) Lopinavir/ritonavir monotherapy or plus zidovudine and lamivudine in antiretroviral-naive HIV-infected patients. AIDS 22(3): 385–93.

13. Arribas JR, Delgado R, Arranz A, Muñoz R, Portilla J, et al. (2009) Lopinavir-ritonavir monotherapy versus lopinavir-ritonavir and 2 nucleosides for maintenance therapy of HIV: 96-week analysis. J Acquir Immune Defic Syndr 51(2): 147–52.

14. Pulido F, Arribas JR, Delgado R, Cabrero E, González-García J, et al. (2008) OK04 Study Group. Lopinavir-ritonavir monotherapy versus lopinavir-ritonavir and two nucleosides for maintenance therapy of HIV. AIDS 22(2): F1–9.

15. Bierman WF, van Agtmael MA, Nijhuis M, Danner SA, Boucher CA (2009) HIV monotherapy with ritonavir-boosted protease inhibitors: a systematic review. AIDS Jan 28; 23(3): 279–91.

16. Pulido F, Delgado R, Pérez-Valero I, González-García J, Miralles P, et al. (2008) Long-term (4 years) efficacy of lopinavir / ritonavir monotherapy for maintenance of HIV suppression. J Antimicrob Chemother 61(6): 1359–61.

17. Cameron DW, da Silva BA, Arribas JR, Myers RA, Bellos NC http://www.ncbi.nlm.nih.gov/pubmed?term = %22King MS%22%5BAuthor%5Detal, A

18. Nunes EP, Santini de Oliveira M, Merçon M, Zajdenverg R, Faulhaber JC, et al. (2009) Monotherapy with Lopinavir/Ritonavir as maintenance after HIV-1 viral suppression: results of a 96-week randomized, controlled, open-label, pilot trial (KalMo study). HIV Clin Trials 10(6): 368–74.

19. Hall AM, Hendry BM, Nitsch D, Connolly JO (2011) Tenofovir-Associated Kidney Toxicity in HIV-Infected Patients: A Review of the Evidence. Am J Kidney Dis May; 57(5): 773–80.

20. Woodward CL, Hall AM, Williams IG, Madge S, Copas A, et al. (2009) Tenofovir-associated renal and bone toxicity. HIV Med Sep; 10(8): 482–7.

21. Choi AI, Vittinghoff E, Deeks SG, Weekley CC, Li Y, et al. (2011) Cardiovascular risks associated with abacavir and tenofovir exposure in HIV-infected persons. AIDS Jun 19; 25(10): 1289–98.

22. Brinkman K, ter Hofstede HJ, Burger DM, Smeitink JA, Koopmans PP (1998) Adverse effects of reverse transcriptase inhibitors: mitochondrial toxicity as common pathway. AIDS 12: 1735–1744.

23. Kakuda TN, Brundage RC, Anderson PL, Fletcher CV (1999) Nucleoside reverse transcriptase inhibitor-induced mitochondrial toxicity as an etiology for lipodystrophy. AIDS 13: 2311–2312.

24. Côté HC, Brumme ZL, Craib KJ, Alexander CS, Wynhoven B, et al. (2002) Changes in mitochondrial DNA as a marker of nucleoside toxicity in HIV-infected patients. N Engl J Med 346(11): 811–20.

25. Carr A, Morey A, Mallon P, Williams D, Thorburn DR (2001) Fatal portal hypertension, liver failure, and mitochondrial dysfunction after HIV-1 nucleoside analogue-induced hepatitis and lactic acidaemia. Lancet 357(9266): 1412–4.

26. Drug Safety Communication U.S. Food and Drug Administration, Available: http://www.fda.gov/Safety/MedWatch/SafetyInformation/SafetyAlertsforHumanMedicalProducts/default.htm..

27. Drug Safety Communication U.S. Food and Drug Administration, January 29, Available: http://www.fda.gov/Safety/MedWatch/SafetyInformation/SafetyAlertsforHumanMedicalProducts/ucm199343.htm. Accessed 2010 Feb 10.

28. Mokrzycki MH, Harris C, May H, Laut J, Palmisano J (2000) Lactic acidosis associated with stavudine administration: a report of five cases. Clin Infect Dis 30(1): 198–200.

29. Miller KD, Cameron M, Wood LV, Dalakas MC, Kovacs JA (2000) Lactic acidosis and hepatic steatosis associated with use of stavudine: report of four cases. Ann Intern Med 133(3): 192–6.

30. Stein DS (1994) A new syndrome of hepatomegaly with severe steatosis in HIV seropositive patients. AIDS Clin Care 6: 17–21.

31. Sundar K, Suarez M, Banogon PE, Shapiro JM (1997) Zidovudine-induced fatal lactic acidosis and hepatic failure in patients with acquired immunodeficiency syndrome: report of two patients and review of the literature. Crit Care Med 25(8): 1425–30.

32. Hill A, Ruxrungtham K, Hanvanich M, Katlama C, Wolf E, et al. (2007) Systematic review of clinical trials evaluating low doses of stavudine as part of antiretroviral treatment. Expert Opin Pharmacother 8(5): 679–88.

3

Regionalized Pathology Correlates with Augmentation of mtDNA Copy Numbers in a Patient with Myoclonic Epilepsy with Ragged-Red Fibers (MERRF-Syndrome)

Anja Brinckmann[1], Claudia Weiss[1], Friederike Wilbert[1,5], Arpad von Moers[2], Angelika Zwirner[1], Gisela Stoltenburg-Didinger[3], Ekkehard Wilichowski[4], Markus Schuelke[1,5]*

1 Department of Neuropediatrics, Charité University Medical School, Berlin, Germany, 2 DRK-Kliniken Westend, Berlin, Germany, 3 Department of Neuropathology, Charité University Medical School, Berlin, Germany, 4 Department of Pediatrics and Pediatric Neurology, Georg August University, Göttingen, Germany, 5 NeuroCure Clinical Research Center, Charité University Medical School, Berlin, Germany

Abstract

Human patients with myoclonic epilepsy with ragged-red fibers (MERRF) suffer from regionalized pathology caused by a mutation in the mitochondrial DNA (m.8344A→G). In MERRF-syndrome brain and skeletal muscles are predominantly affected, despite mtDNA being present in any tissue. In the past such tissue-specificity could not be explained by varying mtDNA mutation loads. In search for a region-specific pathology in human individuals we determined the mtDNA/nDNA ratios along with the mutation loads in 43 different *post mortem* tissue samples of a 16-year-old female MERRF patient and in four previously healthy victims of motor vehicle accidents. In brain and muscle we further determined the quantity of mitochondrial proteins (COX subunits II and IV), transcription factors (NRF1 and TFAM), and VDAC1 (Porin) as a marker for the mitochondrial mass. In the patient the mutation loads varied merely between 89–100%. However, mtDNA copy numbers were increased 3–7 fold in predominantly affected brain areas (e.g. hippocampus, cortex and putamen) and in skeletal muscle. Similar increases were absent in unaffected tissues (e.g. heart, lung, kidney, liver, and gastrointestinal organs). Such mtDNA copy number increase was not paralleled by an augmentation of mitochondrial mass in some investigated tissues, predominantly in the most affected tissue regions of the brain. We thus conclude that "futile" stimulation of mtDNA replication *per se* or a secondary failure to increase the mitochondrial mass may contribute to the regionalized pathology seen in MERRF-syndrome.

Editor: Iris Schrijver, Stanford University School of Medicine, United States of America

Funding: The project was funded by the Deutsche Forschungsgemeinschaft within the SFB 665 TP C4 "Developmental Disorders of the Nervous System" and the NeuroCure Cluster of Excellence (Exc 257) at the Charite, Berlin. M.S. is a member of the German network for mitochondrial disorders (mitoNET, 01GM0866), funded by the German ministry of education and research (BMBF, Bonn, Germany). The funders had no role in study design, data collection and analysis, decision to publish, or preparation of the manuscript.

Competing Interests: The authors have declared that no competing interests exist.

* E-mail: markus.schuelke@charite.de

Introduction

Mutations of the mitochondrial DNA (mtDNA) cause a variety of serious genetic disorders with maternal inheritance [1]. One example is the MERRF-syndrome (myoclonic epilepsy with ragged-red fibers, MIM 545000), which is characterized by myoclonic seizures, ataxia, dementia, muscle weakness and accumulations of structurally abnormal mitochondria in the skeletal muscle [2]. MERRF-syndrome is most frequently associated with the m.8344A→G mutation in the mitochondrial tRNA^{Lys} gene (*MTTK*) [3]. The mutation usually occurs in heteroplasmic state where wildtype and mutant mtDNA copies coexist. Generally, MERRF patients have a high percentage of mutant mtDNA (>90%) in blood and muscle and the degree of heteroplasmy (= mutation load) is evenly distributed between different organs [4–6], which stands in contrast to the MELAS-syndrome (MIM 540000), where more variation is found [7]. Cultured myotubes from MERRF patients show a biochemical defect only if their mutation load surpasses 85% and show a steep decline of COX-activity and mitochondrial translation rate beyond this threshold [8]. Even though mitochondria are present in every cell, MERRF-syndrome has a regionalized pathology, predominantly involving the brain (hippocampus, cerebral cortex and striatum) and the skeletal muscle, but often sparing the heart and other intestinal organs. In the past, researchers have tried to explain this phenomenon by differences of mutation load for the m.8344A→G mutation in the various organs. However, various studies did not confirm such an association [4–6,9]. Alternatively, it was hypothesized that the affected tissues had lower threshold levels for clinical manifestation than their unaffected counterparts. Other explanations were tissue specific mechanisms for the regulation of energy metabolism, potentially at the level of mtDNA replication, transcription or translation.

Here we studied the regionalized pathology of MERRF-syndrome on tissue and molecular level through investigation of 43 *post mortem* tissue-samples from different regions of a 16-year-old girl with MERRF-syndrome and of blood DNA samples from her family (Figure 1A).

Methods

Ethics statement

Written informed consent according to the Declaration of Helsinki was obtained from the involved persons and guardians.

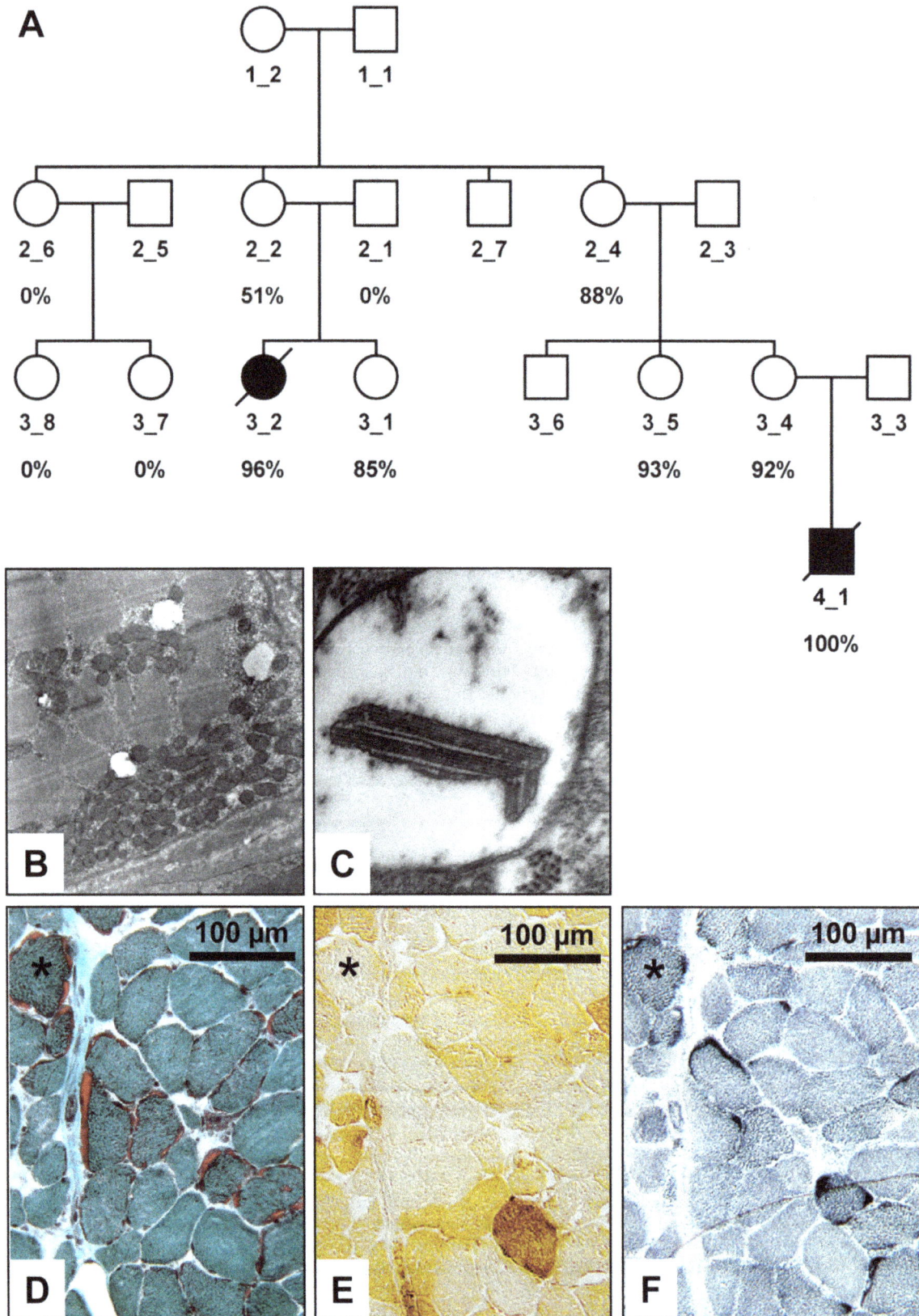

Figure 1. Analysis of the MERRF patient and her family members. (**A**) Pedigree of the family of the index patient (3_2). The mutation loads for the m.8344A→G mtDNA mutation, as determined by Pyrosequencing® are given below the pedigree symbols. The black symbols depict patients, who were clinically affected with MERRF-syndrome; however, even family members with 93% mutant mtDNA in blood cells did not report any MERRF-specific symptoms and their symbols thus remain white. (**B**) The electron microscopic image of the *iliopsoas* muscle (12,000×) shows massive subsarcolemmal accumulations of mitochondria, which represent the contents of a ragged-red fiber. (**C**) At higher magnification (85,000×) ballooned

mitochondria with paracrystalline inclusions can be seen. (**D**) Ragged-red fibers in the Gömöri trichrome stain of the *iliopsoas* muscle that are COX negative in (**E**), and show subsarcolemmal accumulations of enzyme activity in the SDH stain (**F**).

The study on human subjects was approved by the IRB of the Charité. Consent for the animal studies was obtained from the LaGeSo Berlin (O 0083/08) according to the animal welfare act.

Morphometric analysis

A tissue sample from the patient's insular cortex (Brodman area 43) including all neuronal layers and the white matter was fixed for >4 weeks in phosphate-buffered 4% formaldehyde, dehydrated and subsequently embedded in paraffin. Microtome sections of 5 μm were mounted on glass slides, deparaffinized, stained with anti-NeuN and subsequently with Cy3-labeled fluorescent secondary antibodies. The cell nuclei were counterstained with DAPI. An unbiased counting frame of 186.2×139.6 μm^2 was then systematically moved through the cortical layers of interest and photographs were taken on the UV and Cy3-channel through a 20× oil immersion objective (Leica Microsystems, Wetzlar, Germany) with a SPOT3 cooled CCD camera (Visitron, Puchheim, Germany). From each cortical layer we analyzed five such frames which thus represented 130,000 μm^2 of cross-sectional plane per respective cortical layer. The two images from the DAPI and the Cy3-channel were superimposed with false colors and on each frame we separately counted the total number of DAPI positive nuclei *versus* those nuclei that co-localized with a NeuN-signal representing neuronal cells that had been cut in the plane of the nucleus. All 2D-counts were corrected with the Abercrombie formula [10] taking into consideration the thickness of the section (5 μm) and the diameter of the cell nuclei. The Ferret's diameter of the nuclei was 14 ± 5 μm and had been determined in 50 random neuronal nuclei at their largest optical cross-sectional diameter with a 63× oil immersion objective. The Abercrombie-corrected cell densities were then compared to published reference values that had been obtained by the same staining and 2D-counting method [11,12]. The final results were then depicted as neurons/mm^2 and as glia/neuron ratio (Figure 2A,B).

Pyrosequencing® assay for determination of mutation load

DNA was isolated from blood cells and from tissues according to standard procedures using a 96-well tissue DNA extraction kit (Qiagen, Hilden, Germany). We amplified a 139 bp PCR-product of the mitochondrial tRNA^{Lys} gene with the primer pair 5'-CCC TAT AGC ACC CCC TCT AC-3' and 5'-Biotin-TGG GCC ATA CGG TAG TAT TT-3'. The PCR product was sequenced using the automated PSQ^{TM} HS 96A system with the primer 5'-TAA GTT AAA GAT TAA GAG A-3'. To correct for potential systematic errors of the assay, all data points of the samples were normalized to a calibration curve, generated with standardized mixtures of wildtype and mutant mtDNA ($R^2 = 0,9997$; Figure S3).

qPCR for determination of mtDNA copy numbers

The following primers and probes were used for amplification one gene encoded by the mtDNA and another single copy gene encoded by the nDNA: **MTND1** (= **mtDNA copy numbers**): (F) 5'-CTA CAA CCC TTC GCT GAC GC-3', (R) 5'-ACG GCT AGG CTA GAG GTG GC-3', (P) FAM-CCA TCA CCC TCT ACA TCA CCG CCC-X-TAMRA-3' and for **MMP1** (= **nuclear DNA copy numbers**): (F) 5'-GCC AGG GTA CTG CAC TAG CAT G-3', (R) 5'-GAG GCC CTA ACA TTC

TCT GCA CT-3', (P) FAM-TGT GCT ACA CGG ATA CCC CAA GGA CAT C-X-TAMRA-3'. The PCR for each sample was run in triplicate on an ABI PRISM 7700 sequence detection system (Applied Biosystems) with a hotstart Taq polymerase (Platinum Taq). A 10 min denaturation step at 94°C was followed by 45 cycles of denaturation at 94°C for 30 s and annealing/extension at 67°C for 60 s. The TaqMan readings were analyzed using the "Sequence Detector" v1.6.3 software (Applied Biosystems). On each 96-well plate we amplified in parallel a standard dilution series ($10^0 - 10^7$ copies/μl) for every gene, which subsequently enabled us to determine absolute copy numbers while taking into account the different PCR efficiencies [13]. If the standard deviation between the reads of a triplicate sample was above 10% the measurement had to be repeated.

Western blot

Protein was extracted from tissue samples of the patient and the controls after homogenization in RIPA buffer with a proteinase inhibitor cocktail (Complete®, Roche-Diagnostics, Basel, Switzerland), 50 μg protein were separated through denaturing SDS-PAGE with the Laemmli system and blotted on nitrocellulose membranes by the semidry method (Biometra, Göttingen, Germany). The blots were first probed with antibodies against

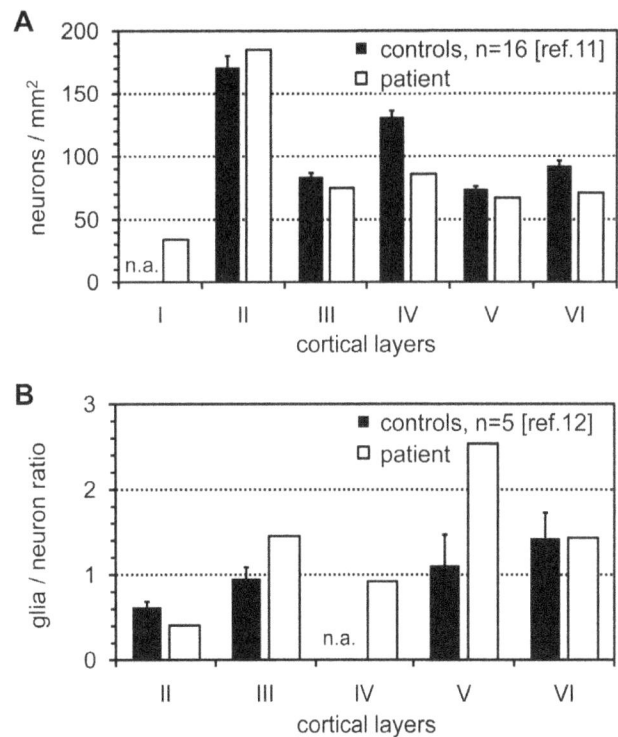

Figure 2. Morphometric analysis of neuronal cell density in the insular cortex of the index patient. (**A**) Density of cortical neurons using Abercrombie correction. The open bar from the patient represents the neuronal density from 130,000 μm^2 of cross-sectional plane per cortical layer. (**B**) Ratio between the numbers of glial *versus* neuronal cells. Black bars, control individuals from the literature (reference provided); open bars, MERRF patient; the whiskers depict the SEM; n.a., data not available.

Porin (VDAC1), TFAM, NRF1, COX IV, COX II, β-Tubulin, and GAPDH and subsequently with corresponding peroxidase-labeled secondary antibodies. Bands were visualized by chemiluminescence. All antibodies used in this study are described in Table S2. β-Tubulin and GAPDH bands were used as loading controls for brain and muscle respectively.

Results

Case history

The girl was the second child of healthy non-consanguineous German parents. Her older sister is healthy. Pregnancy, birth and postnatal development were normal. Myoclonic-astatic seizures started at 4 years of age. Henceforward symptoms progressed to severe pharmaco-resistant myoclonic epilepsy with series of bitemporal spike-waves on EEG and several seizures daily, progressive ataxia, deafness (hearing threshold of 65 dB SPL), and mental retardation (HAWIK IQ = 76 at the age of 9 years). Serum lactate (4.1 mmol/l, N<2.0) and alanine (0.60 mmol/l, N<0.48) concentrations were increased and a diagnostic muscle biopsy at the age of 9 years revealed the presence of ragged-red and COX-negative fibers (Figure 1B–F). At 14 years of age echocardiography and ECG were normal and cranial MRI revealed *ex vacuo* dilatation of the lateral ventricles and hippocampal sclerosis. Two years later she was found lifeless in bed and could not be resuscitated. Autopsy at 48 h *post mortem*, during which we were allowed to take small specimens (Table S1), did not discover any cardiac or pulmonary abnormalities, excluded asphyxia or aspiration, and finally *status epilepticus* during sleep was suspected as the cause of her death. As controls we used specimens of the same tissues from four previously healthy women (16 to 32 years), who had suffered fatal motor vehicle accidents. Additionally, we analyzed the segregation of the mutation and its mutation load in blood samples of different family members (Figure 1A).

Reduced neuronal density at the insular cerebral cortex

In our MERRF patient we found a reduction of neuronal density in the cortical layers IV, V, and VI of more than three times the SEM if compared to normal controls from the literature [11,12]. The ratio between glial and neural cells (Figure 2B) was increased in the layers III and V (no reference data were available for cortical layer IV) suggesting a replacement of neurons by glial cells. However, the reduction in the number of cortical neurons was not as obvious as described in a review by Sparaco et al. (1993), which may be due to the much younger age of our patient in whom degenerative changes might just have begun [14].

Little variation between mutation loads of different tissues

The m.8344A→G mutation loads in the blood of family members and in the tissue biopsy specimens were determined by a highly accurate Pyrosequencing® assay. This real-time sequencing technology allows quantification of two mitochondrial alleles that differ at one nucleotide position with down to 1% heteroplasmy [15,16]. In the blood of the patient we measured a mutation load of 96%. As the mutation loads in blood cells from the clinically unaffected relatives ranged from 0–93% (Figure 1A), we assume a critical threshold level for clinical manifestation in this family between 93–96% for the m.8344A→G mutation. This result confirms other studies that found mutation loads >90% in blood or muscles of MERRF patients with clinical or histochemical muscle abnormalities [17–19]. In a severely affected nephew of our patient (individual 4_1, Figure 1A), who had died also from

status epilepticus at the age of 2 years, we even detected a mutation load of 100% (= homoplasmy) in blood cells. Such a high mutation load had not been reported before and had originally been considered incompatible with life because COX-activities were extremely low in cultured myotubes with homoplasmy for the mutation [8]. Next, we determined the mutation loads in the 43 tissue samples of the index patient with the same Pyrosequencing® assay. The mutation loads were more or less evenly distributed between 89–100% (Table S1), without preference for a specific tissue type. Only liver and pancreas had lower mutation loads of 67 and 73%, respectively. Similar uniform distributions were described before [4–6], failing to explain the regionalized pathology of MERRF-syndrome.

mtDNA copy numbers are preferably increased in the most affected tissues

As cells from different tissues vary considerably in their mtDNA content, we next investigated whether the remaining wildtype mtDNA molecules per cell might correlate with the regionalized symptoms. In order to calculate this figure we determined the mtDNA copies per cell for all tissues by quantitative real-time PCR (TaqMan®) of the mitochondrial encoded *MTND1* gene (NADH:ubiquinone oxidoreductase, subunit ND1) *versus* the single copy nuclear *MMP1* gene (Matrix metalloproteinase 1). MtDNA copy numbers were increased between 3–7 fold in those tissues of the patient that were predominantly affected by the MERRF-mutation (hippocampus, cortex, striatum and skeletal muscle), but not in other tissues such as heart, lung, liver or intestinal organs (Figure 3A). Using the mtDNA copy numbers and the mutation load for each tissue we calculated the number of residual wildtype mtDNA copies per cell. There, the highly affected tissues still had the highest remaining absolute numbers of wildtype mtDNA copies per cell (Figures S1 and S2).

Effect of the storage conditions on the ratio between mtDNA and DNA

As the ratio between mtDNA and nDNA copy numbers could strongly be influenced by unequal degradation of mitochondrial *versus* nuclear DNA during storage of the body in the morgue at 4°C [20], we investigated mice carcasses which had been kept under various storage conditions. We measured the mtDNA/nDNA ratios in 7 representative mouse tissues (brain, cerebellum, heart, kidney, liver, muscle and pancreas) under two storage conditions. The qPCR experiment was performed in triplicate as previously described [21]. After atlanto-axial dislocation the animals were kept at room temperature for 6 h and then organs were removed and stored for 60 h at 4°C *versus* immediately at −20°C. With the exception of pancreas (p<0.001) we did not find significant differences in mtDNA/nDNA ratios (Figure 3B). Only the nuclear DNA of the pancreas seemed to be more prone to degradation at 4°C as compared to −20°C. These results confirmed the constancy of the mtDNA/nDNA ratio over the selected time period, especially in brain and muscle. Hence we have reason to assume that the mtDNA/nDNA ratios measured with the TaqMan®assay truly reflect those at the time of death, with the exception of the pancreas.

Determination of the mitochondrial mass

Further, we investigated whether the elevated mtDNA/nDNA ratios were solely due to enhanced mtDNA-replication or caused by a real increase of the number of mitochondrial organelles per cell (= mitochondrial mass). We thus extracted total protein from brain specimens and pectoralis muscle of patient and controls and

A

absolute mtDNA copy numbers

B

DNA degradation in different mouse tissues

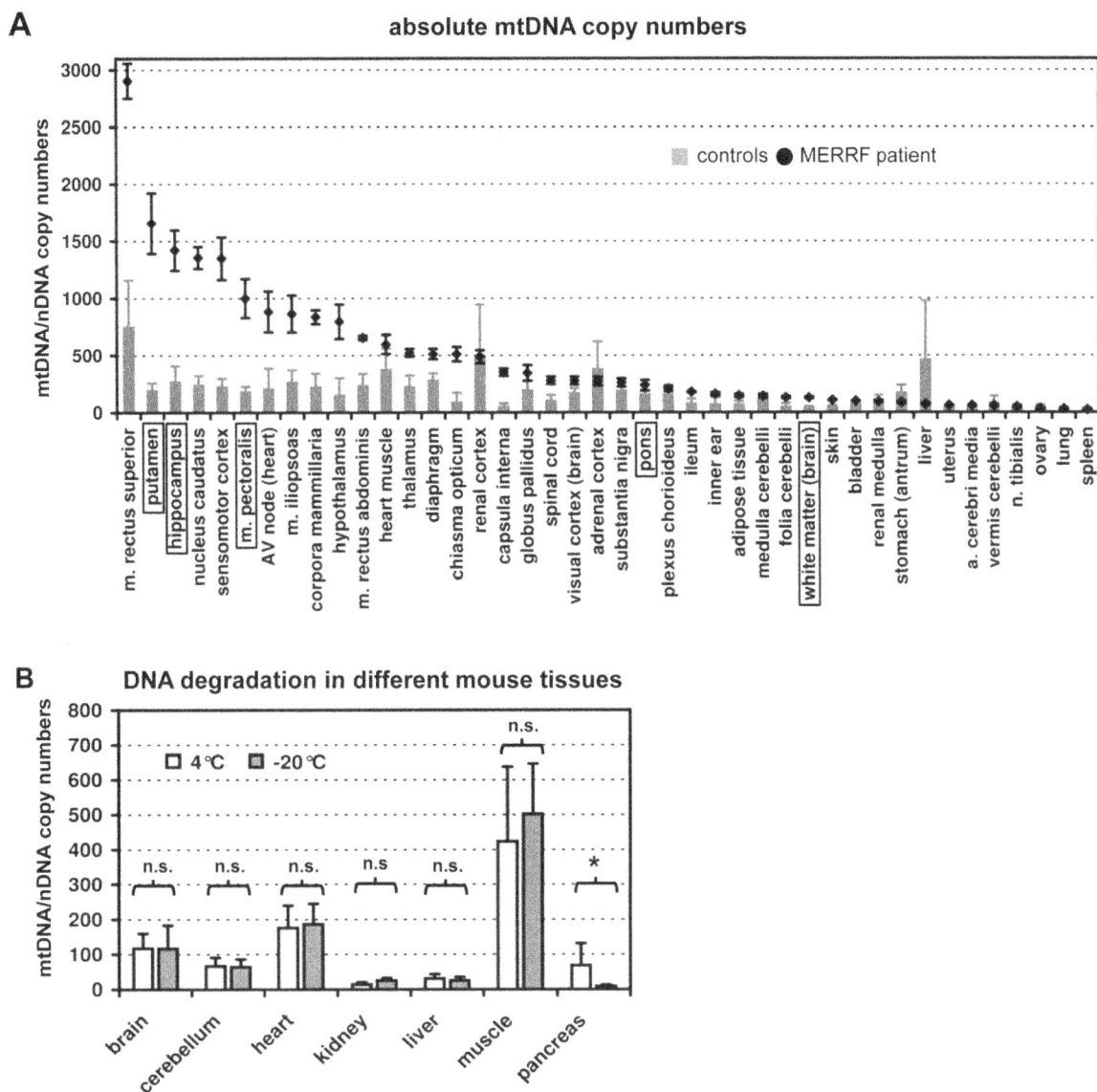

Figure 3. Determination of the absolute mtDNA copy numbers per cell in different tissues by quantitative real-time PCR (TaqMan®). (**A**) The ratio between mtDNA and nDNA copy numbers. The grey bars indicate mean values of the four controls (each sample analyzed in quadruplicate) and the black diamonds indicate mean values of the measurements from the patient's tissues. The whiskers represent the standard deviation; the tissues encircled by boxes were further investigated on the protein level. (**B**) Influence of the storage conditions on the mtDNA/nDNA ratios. With the exception of the pancreas, no significant differences on the 1% confidence level were found between the two storage conditions with regard to the mtDNA/nDNA ratios. n.s. not significant; * p<0.001. In pancreas the nuclear DNA degraded faster than the mtDNA at 4°C.

performed a semi-quantitative Western blot analysis using antibodies against Porin (VDAC1). This protein being highly expressed at the outer mitochondrial membrane [22] serves as a marker for mitochondrial mass [23]. Due to the small volumes of many biopsy specimens, we were limited in the number of tissues to be analyzed by this method but we were able to investigate hippocampus, putamen, and pectoralis muscle, representing tissues that are affected in MERRF-syndrome, and the occipital white matter and the pons, representing tissues that remain mostly unaffected. The mitochondrial mass of the patient's hippocampus and putamen was within the range of controls (Figure 4B). In contrast, a more than two-fold increase was found in pons, white matter, and skeletal muscle. Thus, we did not find a general correlation between increased mtDNA abundance and increased

mitochondrial mass. On the contrary, in the investigated brain regions we **either** found an increase in mtDNA copy numbers **or** in mitochondrial mass. Only in skeletal muscle we found a parallel increase of both parameters.

Next we examined, whether high mtDNA copy numbers might be secondary to a stimulation of mtDNA transcription *via* up-regulation of mitochondrial transcription factors. Semi-quantitative Western blot analysis of the transcription factors NRF1 (nuclear respiratory factor 1) acting on nuclear genes that encode respiratory chain subunits, and TFAM (mitochondrial transcription factor A) stimulating mtDNA transcription, revealed no correlation of their amounts with the mtDNA copy number of the analyzed brain regions (Figure 4C,D). The TFAM levels in the organ with one of the largest increase in mtDNA copy numbers

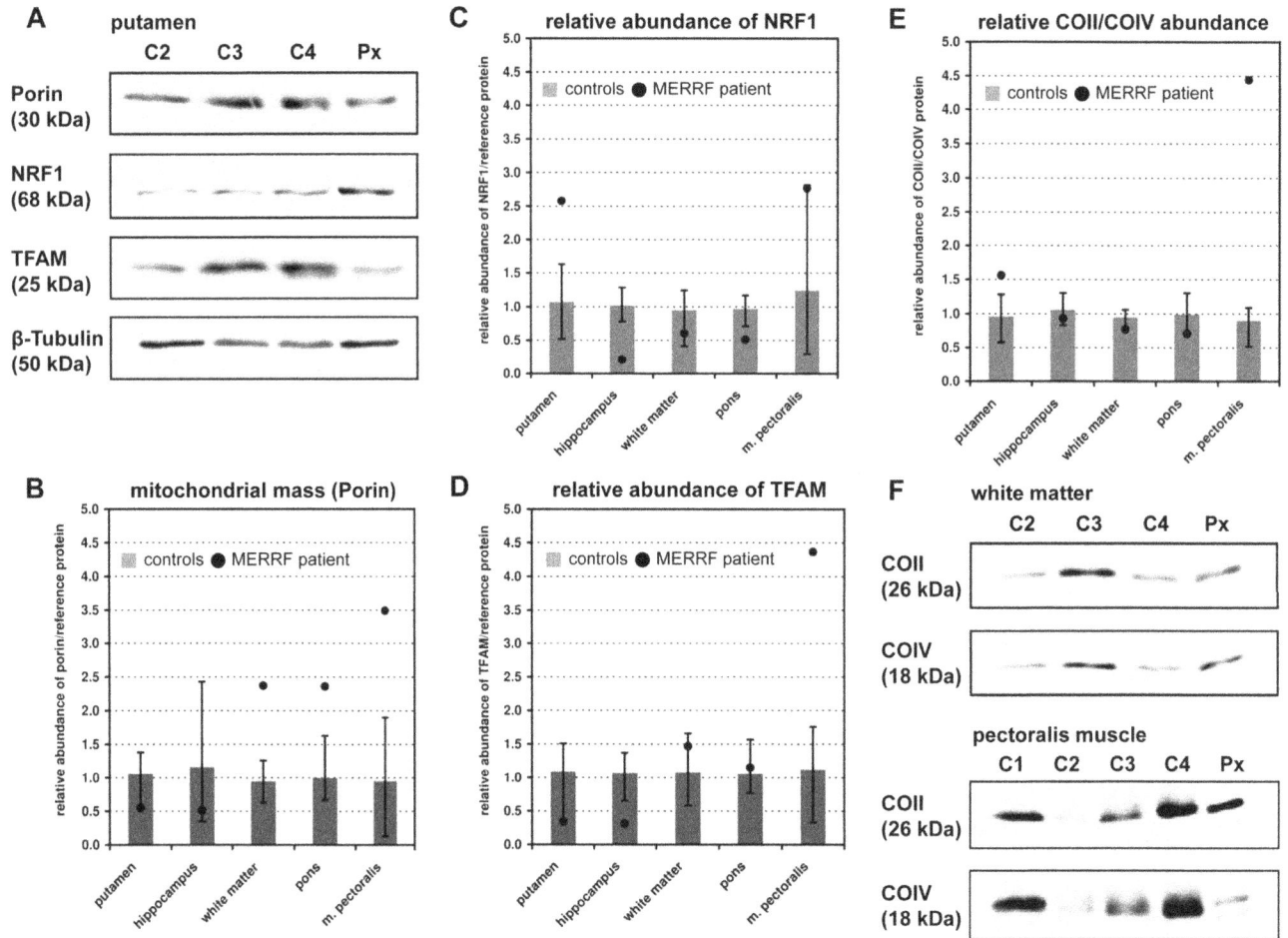

Figure 4. Determination of protein abundance for structural mitochondrial proteins and for transcription factors. (**A**) Western blot of tissue samples from the putamen of three controls (C2-4) and the patient (individual 3_2 on Figure 1A). Protein abundance was determined semi-quantitatively through densitometry. β-Tubulin was used as loading control. (**B**) Results of the semi-quantitative analysis of the mitochondrial mass as represented by anti-Porin (VDAC1) immune reactivity. The whiskers represent the absolute (100%) range of all three control measurements. The result of the patient is represented as a black dot. Figures (**C**) and (**D**) represent the quantification of the transcription factors NRF1 and TFAM. (**E**) Relative abundance of the nuclear encoded subunit of cytochrome C oxidase (COIV) *versus* an mtDNA-encoded subunit (COII) of the same complex. The immune staining with both antibodies was done on the identical blot which secured the comparability. (**F**) Only in muscle the mtDNA-encoded COII subunit was much higher expressed (4.5×) than its nDNA encoded counterpart. *Note:* Due to the lack of sufficient autopsy material the loading of each lane could not be adjusted. However, these Western blots are only intended to illustrate an equal abundance of proteins encoded by the nuclear (COIV) *versus* the mtDNA (COII) and the absence of this balance in the muscle of the MERRF patient.

(putamen) were even the lowest. The situation looked different in the patient's pectoralis muscle where a fourfold up-regulation of TFAM was paralleled by a similar increase of mitochondrial mass.

Finally we investigated the balance of abundance between proteins encoded by the mitochondrial *versus* the nuclear genome. For that we determined the integrated band densities on Western blots that had been co-stained with antibodies against COX subunit II (26 kDa, mtDNA encoded) and COX subunit IV (18 kDa, nDNA encoded). Here again, the protein expression was balanced in all investigated brain regions irrespective of their mtDNA copy number and mitochondrial mass (Figure 1E). Only in muscle we found this relation considerably and unexpectedly skewed more than fourfold towards the mtDNA encoded subunit Cox II (Figure 4E,F). As mitochondrial mass was increased in a similar range in muscle (3.5 fold) we hypothesize that synthesis and import of nuclear encoded mitochondrial proteins might not have been increased strictly in parallel. The subsequent deposition of overproduced subunits might have led to the appearance of paracrystalline inclusions in many of the muscle mitochondria as

seen on Figure 1C. As alternative explanation, the intense Cox II band might not represent intact subunits but misfolded or partially miscomposed polypeptide chains caused by a lack of tRNA^Lys which recognizes 4 of 227 codons in Cox II mRNA.

Discussion

It is generally agreed that ATP deficiency and increased production of reactive oxygen species (ROS) are crucial factors in the pathophysiology of mitochondrial disorders due to mtDNA mutations and deletions [1,24]. ROS are generated through electron leaks in a dysfunctional respiratory chain, however, their harmful effects on the mtDNA may be mitigated, at least partially, by compensatory up-regulation of mtDNA copy numbers and mitochondrial mass. H_2O_2 in the low μM range increases mtDNA copy numbers and mitochondrial mass in cultures of yeast as well as human cells and cybrids harboring the 4,977 bp deletion [25,26]. Moreno-Loshuertos *et al.* (2006) even went as far as to propose that respiration deficient phenotypes caused by certain

relation between mtDNA copy numbers and mitochondrial mass

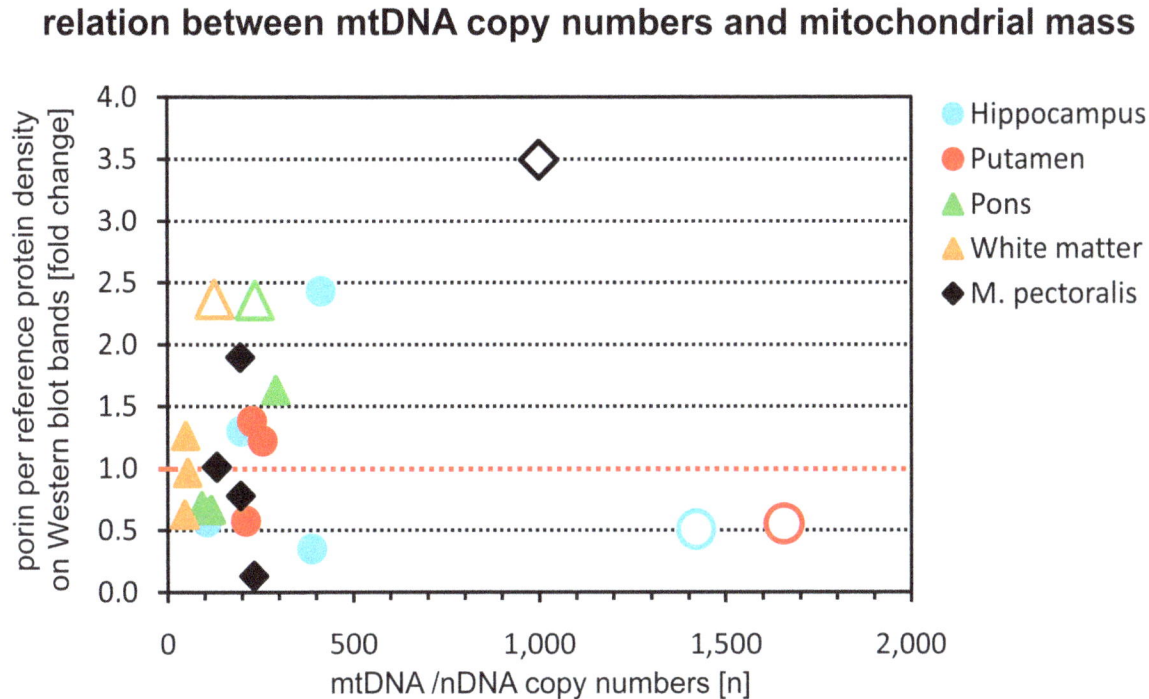

Figure 5. Relation between mtDNA copy numbers and mitochondrial mass. The figure depicts an X-Y plot of mtDNA copy numbers *versus* mitochondrial mass in five representative tissues. Mitochondrial mass is represented by the reference-corrected density of Western blot bands from the outer mitochondrial membrane protein porin. The red line depicts the average of the mitochondrial mass, which was calculated as the geometric means from all control individuals. Circles represent clinically affected tissues and triangles unaffected tissues. Closed symbols represent the control individuals and open symbols the patient. Muscle, which was clinically only mildly affected, is represented by the diamond shaped symbol.

mouse mtDNA haplotypes on a uniform cybrid background be compensated *via* ROS-mediated increase of mtDNA copy numbers [27], a view that did not remain unchallenged [28]. Hori et al. (2009) proposed an attractive link between increased ROS production and enhanced mtDNA replication *via* increased nicking by Ntg1 of oxidized single-stranded mtDNA at the origin of replication and thus initiating rolling cycle replication of yeast mtDNA [29]. Whether a homologous mechanism applies for mammalian mtDNA is currently unknown.

Here we demonstrate for the first time that the augmentation of mtDNA copy numbers in a MERRF patient is a tissue-specific phenomenon, which might help to explain the preponderance of certain organs for disease-specific symptoms. However, the question remains whether the up-regulation of mtDNA copy numbers is a compensatory, albeit insufficient step caused by increased ROS production in metabolically "demanding" tissues or whether such an up-regulation, especially if not followed by a subsequent increase in mitochondrial mass, may be harmful *per se* as it may exhaust the resources of the mitochondria. As TFAM is known to have an influence mtDNA copy numbers [24], we investigated its expression in predominantly affected and unaffected tissues. In brain we found an especially low expression for putamen and hippocampus which did not up-regulate their mitochondrial mass despite high mtDNA copy numbers (Figure 5). This stood in contrast to white matter and pons that augmented their mitochondrial mass. In the muscle of the patient, elevated mitochondrial mass and TFAM abundance went strictly parallel demonstrating that the mechanism(s) to increase mitochondrial mass are at least partially independent of TFAM. This has already been shown in muscle specific *Tfam*-knockout mice that were able to up-regulate mitochondrial mass in the absence of Tfam [30].

Unfortunately, lack of sufficient autopsy material prohibited the investigation of other tissues. We are aware that the data being obtained from a single individual have to be confirmed by further investigations of MERRF patients and preferably also in individuals with other mtDNA mutations, especially the MELAS (m.3243A→G) mutation, to explore whether a tissue-specific increase in mtDNA copy numbers is a MERRF-specific phenomenon or whether it may be generalized for other mitochondrial disorders as well.

Supporting Information

Figure S1 Increase [in %] of the mtDNA copy numbers in the patient in relation to the mean of the four controls. The tissues mainly affected by the MERRF-syndrome cluster on the left side of the chart.

Figure S2 Absolute numbers of residual wildtype mtDNA molecules per cell in the patient tissues (magenta dots). The blue bars depict the mean and the whiskers the standard deviation of the mtDNA copy numbers in the four controls.

Figure S3 Calibration curve for the Pyrosequencing assay. Measurements from the assay were plotted against the expected degrees of heteroplasmy from known mixtures between plasmid preparations containing the wildtype and mutant DNA sequence. All measurements were performed in triplicate and the standard deviation is indicated by whiskers. Due to the high precision of the method with small standard deviations, not all the whiskers can be seen. The regression line forms a smooth curve with the above mentioned equation and a very good approximation of the measurements. All raw measurements of the samples were normalized to the regression curve.

Table S1 Mutation loads (= degrees of heteroplasmy in [%]) of all the organs as measured by the Pyrosequencing assay. The numbers indicate the average of three measurements ± standard deviation.

Table S2 Primary antibodies and their dilutions used for Western blot and immunohistochemistry.

References

1. DiMauro S, Davidzon G (2005) Mitochondrial DNA and disease. Ann Med 37: 222–232.
2. Fukuhara N, Tokiguchi S, Shirakawa K, Tsubaki T (1980) Myoclonus epilepsy associated with ragged-red fibres (mitochondrial abnormalities): disease entity or a syndrome? Light-and electron-microscopic studies of two cases and review of literature. J Neurol Sci 47: 117–133.
3. Shoffner JM, Lott MT, Lezza AM, Seibel P, Ballinger SW, et al. (1990) Myoclonic epilepsy and ragged-red fiber disease (MERRF) is associated with a mitochondrial DNA tRNA(Lys) mutation. Cell 61: 931–937.
4. Oldfors A, Holme E, Tulinius M, Larsson NG (1995) Tissue distribution and disease manifestations of the tRNA(Lys) A-->G(8344) mitochondrial DNA mutation in a case of myoclonus epilepsy and ragged red fibres. Acta Neuropathol 90: 328–333.
5. Lertrit P, Noer AS, Byrne E, Marzuki S (1992) Tissue segregation of a heteroplasmic mtDNA in MERRF (myoclonic epilepsy with ragged red fibers) encephalomyopathy. Hum Genet 90: 251–254.
6. Tanno Y, Yoneda M, Tanaka K, Kondo R, Hozumi I, et al. (1993) Uniform tissue distribution of tRNA(Lys) mutation in mitochondrial DNA in MERRF patients. Neurology 43: 1198–1200.
7. Matthews PM, Hopkin J, Brown RM, Stephenson JB, Hilton-Jones D, et al. (1994) Comparison of the relative levels of the 3243 (A-->G) mtDNA mutation in heteroplasmic adult and fetal tissues. J Med Genet 31: 41–44.
8. Boulet L, Karpati G, Shoubridge EA (1992) Distribution and threshold expression of the tRNA(Lys) mutation in skeletal muscle of patients with myoclonic epilepsy and ragged-red fibers (MERRF). Am J Hum Genet 51: 1187–1200.
9. Lombes A, Diaz C, Romero NB, Ziegler F, Fardeau M (1992) Analysis of the tissue distribution and inheritance of heteroplasmic mitochondrial DNA point mutation by denaturing gradient gel electrophoresis in MERRF syndrome. Neuromuscul Disord 2: 323–330.
10. Abercrombie M (1946) Estimation of nuclear population from microtome sections. Anat Rec 94: 239–247.
11. Gittins R, Harrison PJ (2004) Neuronal density, size and shape in the human anterior cingulate cortex: a comparison of Nissl and NeuN staining. Brain Res Bull 63: 155–160.
12. Gittins R, Harrison PJ (2004) A quantitative morphometric study of the human anterior cingulate cortex. Brain Res 1013: 212–222.
13. Pfaffl MW (2001) A new mathematical model for relative quantification in real-time RT-PCR. Nucleic Acids Res 29: e45.
14. Sparaco M, Bonilla E, DiMauro S, Powers JM (1993) Neuropathology of mitochondrial encephalomyopathies due to mitochondrial DNA defects. J Neuropathol Exp Neurol 52: 1–10.
15. White HE, Durston VJ, Seller A, Fratter C, Harvey JF, et al. (2005) Accurate detection and quantitation of heteroplasmic mitochondrial point mutations by pyrosequencing. Genet Test 9: 190–199.
16. Brinckmann A, Ruther K, Williamson K, Lorenz B, Lucke B, et al. (2007) De novo double mutation in PAX6 and mtDNA tRNA(Lys) associated with atypical aniridia and mitochondrial disease. J Mol Med 85: 163–168.
17. Larsson NG, Tulinius MH, Holme E, Oldfors A, Andersen O, et al. (1992) Segregation and manifestations of the mtDNA tRNA(Lys) A-->G(8344) mutation of myoclonus epilepsy and ragged-red fibers (MERRF) syndrome. Am J Hum Genet 51: 1201–1212.
18. Hammans SR, Sweeney MG, Brockington M, Lennox GG, Lawton NF, et al. (1993) The mitochondrial DNA transfer RNA(Lys)A>G(8344) mutation and the syndrome of myoclonic epilepsy with ragged red fibres (MERRF). Relationship of clinical phenotype to proportion of mutant mitochondrial DNA. Brain 116: 617–632.
19. Huang CC, Kuo HC, Chu CC, Liou CW, Ma YS, et al. (2002) Clinical phenotype, prognosis and mitochondrial DNA mutation load in mitochondrial encephalomyopathies. J Biomed Sci 9: 527–533.
20. Foran DR (2006) Relative degradation of nuclear and mitochondrial DNA: an experimental approach. J Forensic Sci 51: 766–770.
21. Amthor H, Macharia R, Navarrete R, Schuelke M, Brown SC, et al. (2007) Lack of myostatin results in excessive muscle growth but impaired force generation. Proc Natl Acad Sci U S A 104: 1835–1840.
22. Crompton M (1999) The mitochondrial permeability transition pore and its role in cell death. Biochem J 341(Pt 2): 233–249.
23. Acquaviva F, De Biase I, Nezi L, Ruggiero G, Tatangelo F, et al. (2005) Extra-mitochondrial localisation of frataxin and its association with IscU1 during enterocyte-like differentiation of the human colon adenocarcinoma cell line Caco-2. J Cell Sci 118: 3917–3924.
24. Ekstrand MI, Falkenberg M, Rantanen A, Park CB, Gaspari M, et al. (2004) Mitochondrial transcription factor A regulates mtDNA copy number in mammals. Hum Mol Genet 13: 935–944.
25. Lee HC, Yin PH, Lu CY, Chi CW, Wei YH (2000) Increase of mitochondria and mitochondrial DNA in response to oxidative stress in human cells. Biochem J 348: 425–432.
26. Wei YH, Lee CF, Lee HC, Ma YS, Wang CW, et al. (2001) Increases of mitochondrial mass and mitochondrial genome in association with enhanced oxidative stress in human cells harboring 4,977 BP-deleted mitochondrial DNA. Ann N Y Acad Sci 928: 97–112.
27. Moreno-Loshuertos R, Acin-Perez R, Fernandez-Silva P, Movilla N, Perez-Martos A, et al. (2006) Differences in reactive oxygen species production explain the phenotypes associated with common mouse mitochondrial DNA variants. Nat Genet 38: 1261–1268.
28. Battersby BJ, Shoubridge EA (2007) Reactive oxygen species and the segregation of mtDNA sequence variants. Nat Genet 39: 571–572.
29. Hori A, Yoshida M, Shibata T, Ling F (2009) Reactive oxygen species regulate DNA copy number in isolated yeast mitochondria by triggering recombination-mediated replication. Nucleic Acids Res 37: 749–761.
30. Wredenberg A, Wibom R, Wilhelmsson H, Graff C, Wiener HH, et al. (2002) Increased mitochondrial mass in mitochondrial myopathy mice. Proc Natl Acad Sci U S A 99: 15066–15071.

Acknowledgments

The authors thank the patients and their families for participation in this study, late Professor Dr. Helmut Maxeiner (Department of Forensic Medicine, Charité, Berlin) for his help, Professor Nils-Göran Larsson, PhD (Max Planck Institute for Biology of Ageing, Cologne) for the gift of his anti-TFAM antibody, and Priv.-Doz. Dr. Werner Stenzel and Petra Matilewsky for their help with the anti-NeuN/DAPI staining of the paraffin sections of the patient.

Author Contributions

Conceived and designed the experiments: AvM MS. Performed the experiments: AB CW FW AZ MS. Analyzed the data: AB CW FW GSD MS. Contributed reagents/materials/analysis tools: AvM GSD EW MS. Wrote the paper: AB MS.

4

NQO1-Dependent Redox Cycling of Idebenone: Effects on Cellular Redox Potential and Energy Levels

Roman H. Haefeli[1,2,9], **Michael Erb**[1,9], **Anja C. Gemperli**[3], **Dimitri Robay**[1], **Isabelle Courdier Fruh**[4], **Corinne Anklin**[1], **Robert Dallmann**[5], **Nuri Gueven**[1]*

1 Santhera Pharmaceuticals, Liestal, Switzerland, 2 Biozentrum, University of Basel, Basel, Switzerland, 3 Institut Straumann AG, Basel, Switzerland, 4 Novartis Pharma AG, Basel, Switzerland, 5 Institute of Pharmacology and Toxicology, University of Zürich, Zürich, Switzerland

Abstract

Short-chain quinones are described as potent antioxidants and in the case of idebenone have already been under clinical investigation for the treatment of neuromuscular disorders. Due to their analogy to coenzyme Q_{10} (CoQ$_{10}$), a long-chain quinone, they are widely regarded as a substitute for CoQ$_{10}$. However, apart from their antioxidant function, this provides no clear rationale for their use in disorders with normal CoQ$_{10}$ levels. Using recombinant NAD(P)H:quinone oxidoreductase (NQO) enzymes, we observed that contrary to CoQ$_{10}$ short-chain quinones such as idebenone are good substrates for both NQO1 and NQO2. Furthermore, the reduction of short-chain quinones by NQOs enabled an antimycin A-sensitive transfer of electrons from cytosolic NAD(P)H to the mitochondrial respiratory chain in both human hepatoma cells (HepG2) and freshly isolated mouse hepatocytes. Consistent with the substrate selectivity of NQOs, both idebenone and CoQ$_1$, but not CoQ$_{10}$, partially restored cellular ATP levels under conditions of impaired complex I function. The observed cytosolic-mitochondrial shuttling of idebenone and CoQ$_1$ was also associated with reduced lactate production by cybrid cells from *mitochondrial encephalomyopathy, lactic acidosis and stroke-like episodes* (MELAS) patients. Thus, the observed activities separate the effectiveness of short-chain quinones from the related long-chain CoQ$_{10}$ and provide the rationale for the use of short-chain quinones such as idebenone for the treatment of mitochondrial disorders.

Editor: Annalisa Pastore, National Institute for Medical Research, Medical Research Council, United Kingdom

Funding: Santhera Pharmaceuticals (Switzerland) Ltd. (www.santhera.com) funded and approved the publication of this work.

Competing Interests: The authors have read the journal's policy and have the following conflicts: During the preparation of this manuscript, all authors were paid employees of Santhera Pharmaceuticals (Switzerland). Santhera is marketing Catena® (idebenone) for the treatment of Friedreich's Ataxia in Canada and is currently evaluating the compound in other indications in phase II and III trials.

* E-mail: nuri.gueven@santhera.com

9 These authors contributed equally to this work.

Introduction

Quinones, such as vitamin K or coenzyme Q_{10} (CoQ$_{10}$), are a chemical class containing a quinoid ring system [reviewed by 1,2] as pharmacophore. Despite significant differences between quinones, the quinoid system is the dominant feature that causes all of them to be electrophiles, oxidants and colored. However, already minor variances in their chemical and physicochemical properties lead to extensive differences in their biological and pharmacological effects. Enzymes involved in cellular quinone metabolism catalyze mainly two different redox reactions. For example, NADPH:cytochrome P450 reductase can generate semiquinones by incomplete, one-electron reduction [1,2]. Since semiquinones can react with molecular oxygen to generate reactive oxygen species (ROS), this process can lead to oxidative damage of cellular macromolecules, toxicity and mutagenicity [1,2]. In contrast, NAD(P)H:quinone oxidoreductases (NQOs) are cytosolic flavoproteins that compete with P450 reductase and catalyze the reduction of highly reactive quinones and their derivates by complete, two-electron reduction [2]. This results in the formation of relatively stable hydroquinones, often also referred to as quinols, and therefore avoids the formation of ROS. Thus, NQOs are considered key detoxifying enzymes which

are induced by stressors such as xenobiotics or oxidants [3]. Currently, NQO1 and NQO2, with substantial differences in substrate specificity and expression patterns, are described. While NQO1 uses nicotinamide adenine dinucleotide (phosphate) (NADH or NADPH) as electron donor, NQO2 shows a high preference for dihydronicotinamide riboside (NRH) [3].

NQOs have been shown to reduce numerous pharmacologically active compounds such as quinone epoxides, aromatic nitro and nitroso compounds, azo dyes and Cr(VI) compounds [4]. Notably, NQO1 has its highest affinity towards quinones; for example, β-lapachone and mitomycin C exhibit their biological activity not until their NQO1-dependent bioreduction [5,6]. Both NQO1 and NQO2 are able to reduce CoQ$_0$ [7] and CoQ$_1$ [8,9]. These quinones are short-chain analogs of CoQ$_{10}$, which is best known for its pivotal role in mitochondrial oxidative phosphorylation, although the functional significance of NQO-dependent reduction of CoQ$_0$ and CoQ$_1$ is still unclear.

Idebenone, a benzoquinone carrying exactly the same quinone moiety as CoQ$_0$, CoQ$_1$ and CoQ$_{10}$, shows multiple activities *in vitro* and *in vivo*. Most prominently associated with idebenone is its potent antioxidant capacity as substantiated by the ability to prevent lipid peroxidation and ROS in multiple systems [10–14]. Consistent with this role, idebenone proved cytoprotective after cellular exposure to various toxic insults [10,12,13,15]. Consequently, it is under investigation as a possible treatment for disorders characterized by excessive oxidative damage due to mitochondrial defects. Idebenone is quickly absorbed and is well tolerated and safe given as single or repeated daily doses [16]. Successful treatment of a patient with Leigh syndrome using idebenone, where high-dose CoQ_{10} had no effect on respiratory function, is indicative of significant levels of idebenone in the brain [17]. Thus, idebenone has been suggested for treating patients with *mitochondrial encephalopathy, lactic acidosis and stroke-like episodes* (MELAS) [18,19]. Idebenone has been most intensely studied for the treatment of Friedreich's Ataxia (FRDA) [20,21], which is a mitochondrial disorder characterized by increased sensitivity to free radicals [22]. FRDA patients also show deficient activity of mitochondrial respiratory complexes I, II and III and aconitase.

In addition to its antioxidant function, multiple activities have been reported for idebenone such as blocking of Ca^{2+}-channels [23], increased synthesis of NGF [24], stimulation of mitochondrial glycerol-phosphate shuttle [25], modulation of arachidonic acid metabolism [26] and increased mitochondrial function under low oxygen [27]. Due to its structural analogy to CoQ_{10}, idebenone was anticipated to participate in electron transport through the respiratory chain [11]. Indeed, idebenone interacts with mitochondrial complexes I, II and III [28,29]. But whereas it is a good substrate for the latter two, it inhibits both the proton pumping and redox activity of mitochondrial complex I [11,25,29–31]. To what extent this activity is responsible for the beneficial effects of idebenone is still under investigation.

Here, we describe that idebenone is a substrate for reduction by NQO1 and NQO2. The NQO1-reduced idebenone is able to donate electrons into the mitochondrial respiratory chain and it can partially restore cellular adenosine triphosphate (ATP) levels under conditions of impaired complex I function. Consistent with this cytoplasmic-mitochondrial redox cycling hypothesis, idebenone also reduces lactate production in a cell culture model of MELAS. We also show that this effect is specific to some short-chain quinones such as idebenone and is not shared with the structurally related long chain quinones such as CoQ_{10}.

Results

Reduction of short-chain quinones by NQO enzymes *in vitro*

Since NQO1 is thought to be the main cellular enzyme responsible for quinone metabolism, we were interested if this also applied to idebenone (Ide) and related quinones such as CoQ_1 and CoQ_{10}, since they share the identical substitution pattern of the quinone moiety (Figure 1). We also analyzed QS-10 (6-(9-carboxynonyl)-2,3-dimethoxy-5-methyl-1,4-benzoquinone), one of the first idebenone metabolites during oxidative side chain shortening [32]. Experiments with recombinant enzymes clearly demonstrate that these four quinones are differentially reduced by NQO1 (Table 1, Figure S1A+B). Generally, NQO1 demonstrated a slight preference of NADPH over NADH as electron donor with either idebenone, CoQ_1 or QS-10 as acceptor substrate (Table 1). Whereas maximal reduction velocity (v_{max}) for NQO1 presented in the following order: CoQ_1 > idebenone > QS-10, we could not

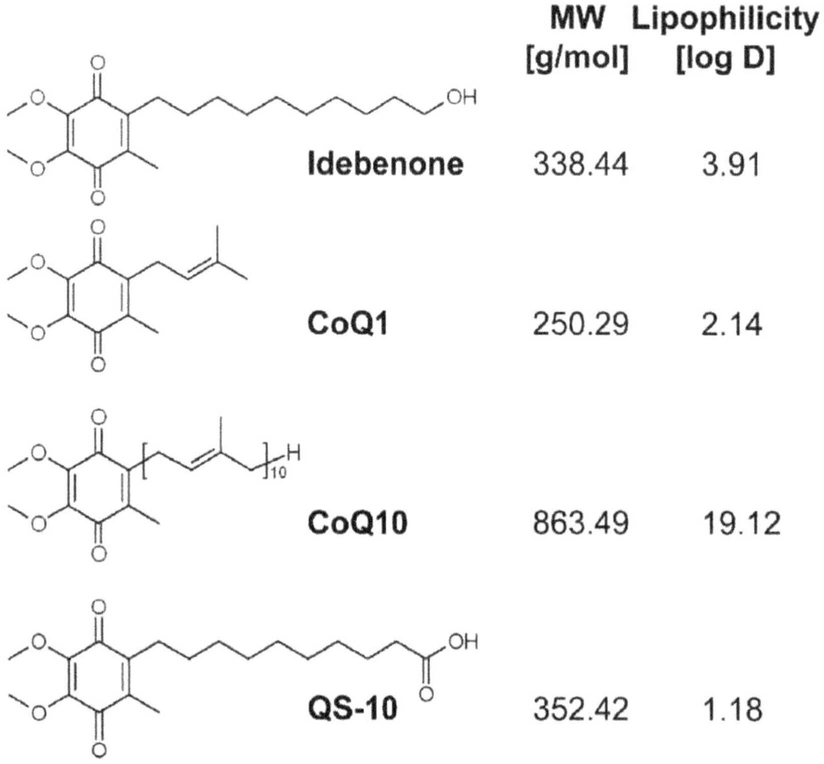

	MW [g/mol]	Lipophilicity [log D]
Idebenone	338.44	3.91
CoQ1	250.29	2.14
CoQ10	863.49	19.12
QS-10	352.42	1.18

Figure 1. Chemical structures of the quinones tested. Idebenone, CoQ_1, CoQ_{10} and QS-10 share the same substitution pattern of the quinone moiety but differ in the alkyl tail attached to the C6-carbon atom of their quinone ring. Whereas idebenone and QS-10 possess an alkyl chain with a terminal polar group (hydroxyl or carboxylic acid group), CoQ_1 and CoQ_{10} contain one or ten isoprenoid repeats, respectively. Molecular weight and calculated log D value (Advanced Chemistry Development Software Package, Version 12, ACD Labs, Toronto, Canada) for each molecule are shown. Log D values are a measure for lipophilicity incorporating ionization of the compound in which small values indicate affinity for the aqueous phase.

Table 1. Steady-state kinetic constants of NQO1 and NQO2 with different quinones.

Enzyme	NQO1				NQO2	
Substrate	NADH		NADPH		NRH-derivate[*]	
	K_m [µM]	v_{max} [µmol/mg/min]	K_m [µM]	v_{max} [µmol/mg/min]	K_m [µM]	v_{max} [µmol/mg/min]
Idebenone	27	41.9	30	53.4	38	97.4
CoQ$_1$	31	115.5	36	172.2	47	128.0
CoQ$_{10}$	-[†]	-[†]	-[†]	-[†]	-[†]	-[†]
QS-10	8	20.5	13	23.3	5	29.6

[*]For NQO2 enzymatic assays 1-(3-sulfonatopropyl)-3-carbamoyl-1,4-dihydropyrimidine (NRH-derivative) was used as electron donor as described [36];
[†]No enzymatic activity above background could be detected for CoQ$_{10}$, thus, steady-state kinetics could not be calculated.

find any evidence for a NQO1-mediated reduction of CoQ$_{10}$ (Table 1). Due to poor solubility of CoQ$_{10}$ in aqueous solutions, we repeated the assay with different formulations of CoQ$_{10}$ in accordance to its lipophilic requirements. Nevertheless, when complexed with fetal bovine serum (FBS) or incorporated into phosphatidylcholine-based liposomes [33,34], we were unable to detect any NQO1-dependent reduction of CoQ$_{10}$ (Figure S1C). In contrast, idebenone was clearly reduced by NQO1 under all conditions tested.

NQO2, although much less studied, is reported to possess similar oxidoreductase activity with some differences in substrate specificities [35]. Despite similar cDNA and amino acid sequences of NQO1 and NQO2, NQO2 has different co-factor requirements (3). We were unable to demonstrate NQO2-dependent reduction of quinones using either NADH or NADPH as electron donor (data not shown), and used 1-(3-sulfonatopropyl)-3-carbamoyl-1,4-dihydropyrimidine, a synthetic analog of NRH [36], as electron donor instead. For all four quinones, we found similar results with regards to the K_m and v_{max} for NQO2-dependent reduction compared to the data generated with NQO1 (Table 1, Figure S1D).

Cellular reduction of short-chain quinones by NQO1

To confirm the *in vitro* reduction of short-chain quinones by NQO enzymes in cells, we employed an assay that measures the reduction-associated change in absorption of WST-1 to quantify NQO1-dependent reduction of quinones. A recent publication associated the quinone-dependent reduction of the tetrazolium dye WST-1 with NQO1 activity [37]. The authors demonstrated that WST-1 is converted only in the presence of functional NQO1, since inhibition of enzymatic activity by dicoumarol (Dic) abolished WST-1 reduction. Furthermore, the dye was potently reduced in cells expressing NQO1 but failed to change absorption in NQO1 deficient cells such as CHO cells. Indeed, using this assay, idebenone, CoQ$_1$ and QS-10 were readily reduced by NQO1 in a dose-dependent manner in HepG2 cells; whereas for CoQ$_{10}$ consistently no activity was detected (Figure 2A). Prior to differentiating between NQO1- and NQO2-dependent activities, it was essential to confirm the usefulness of the NQO1 inhibitor dicoumarol, with a reported IC$_{50}$ for NQO1 of approximately 10 nM [38]. Consistent with previous reports [3,35], our results showed that dicoumarol (20 µM) potently inhibited recombinant NQO1 activity (4% residual activity), while at the same time NQO2 activity was only inhibited by 14% (86% residual activity) (Figure S2). Therefore, co-incubation of HepG2 cells with quinones and dicoumarol for 120 minutes efficiently abolished the WST-1 signal (0% and 5% for idebenone and CoQ$_1$, respectively) (Figure 2B). To rule out a cell line specific metabolism in HepG2 cells, comparable effects were also detected in primary fibroblasts and rat L6

myoblasts (Figures S3, S4). Reduction of substrates such as quinones by NQO1 uses NAD(P)H as electron donor. In agreement with previous reports using CoQ$_1$ and β-lapachone [9,39], idebenone

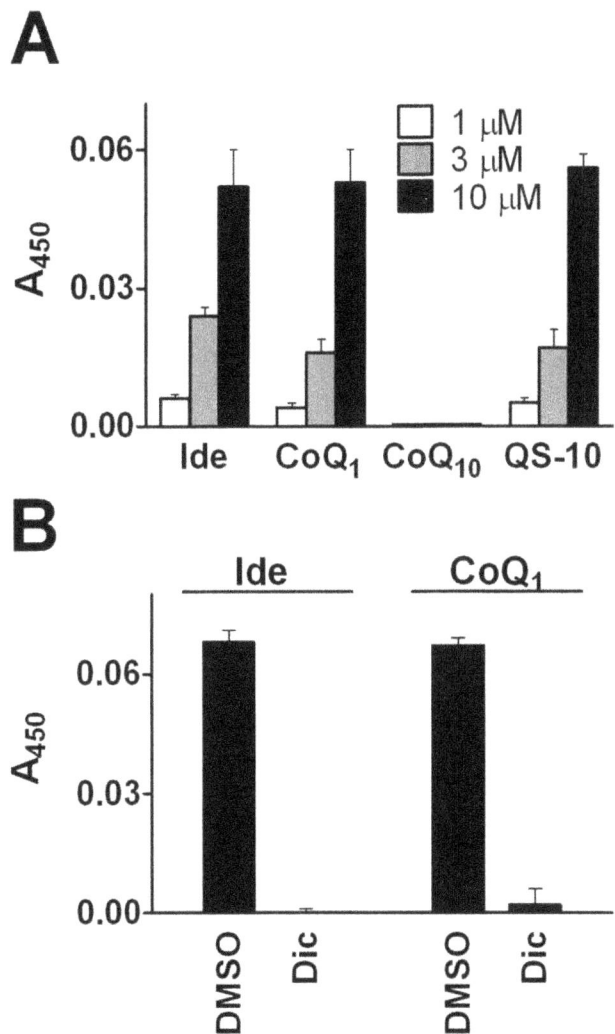

Figure 2. NQO1-dependent cellular reduction of quinones. (A) Dose-dependent cellular quinone reduction was measured as described by Tan *et al.* [37] in HepG2 cells. (B) Dicoumarol (Dic)-treatment (20 µM) efficiently blocked cellular quinone reduction in HepG2 cells. Bars represent mean +stdev of triplicates from one typical out of three independent experiments.

reduced NADH levels in human lymphoblastoid cells in a dose-dependent manner. Using the NADH-dependent conversion of resazurin into the fluorescent resofurin product, idebenone reduced the fluorescence signal by 9% and 11% at (0.1 μM), 11% and 17% (1 μM) and 27% and 40% (10 μM) after 1- or 6-hours incubation, respectively (Figure S5A). Similarly, idebenone, CoQ$_1$ and QS-10 decreased NADH levels after 3-hours incubation at a concentration of 10 μM quinone (69±4%, 62±0%, and 80±4% residual levels, respectively) (Figure S5B). In presence of dicoumarol (20 μM), the reduction of NADH was less prominent (80±5% with CoQ$_1$) or was even prevented (105±15% and 92±6% by idebenone and QS-10, respectively). CoQ$_{10}$ had no influence on NADH levels independent of a co-treatment with dicoumarol (100±1% without and 118±4% with dicoumarol).

Effect of reduced quinones on rescue of rotenone-induced loss of ATP

It has been suggested that hydroquinones such as reduced CoQ$_1$, despite their reduction in the cytosol, can donate electrons

into the mitochondrial electron transport chain [8,40,41]. As a consequence, it was described that proton flux, membrane potential and ATP synthesis increased under conditions of impaired mitochondrial complex I function. We therefore determined the individual effectiveness of the related quinones for this cytosolic-mitochondrial electron transfer (Figure 3). In HepG2 cells, acute treatment of cells with the complex I inhibitor rotenone dramatically reduced ATP levels to 2% residual ATP while all four quinones left ATP levels unaffected (idebenone: 91±12%, CoQ$_1$: 120±15%, CoQ$_{10}$: 99±10%, and QS-10: 104±9% of control) (Figure 3A). However, under conditions of rotenone-induced ATP depletion (2±1% residual ATP), idebenone and CoQ$_1$ partially restored ATP levels (71±6% or 64±6% of control levels, respectively) while CoQ$_{10}$ and QS-10 were completely unable to restore ATP levels (2±1% for both quinones).

In the light of the results obtained in the cell-free system, we investigated to what extent the observed quinone-mediated rescue of ATP levels of complex I-inhibited cells was dependent on

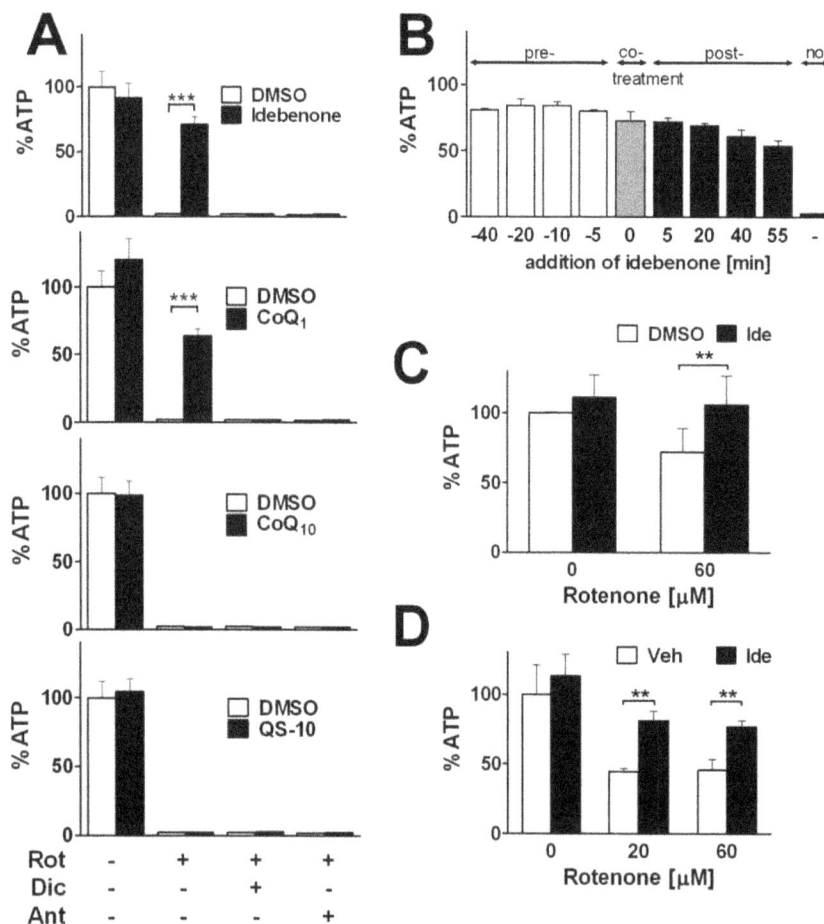

Figure 3. Idebenone and CoQ$_1$ rescue ATP levels in complex I-repressed hepatocytes. (A) HepG2 cells were incubated with rotenone (Rot; 60 μM), dicoumarol (Dic; 20 μM) or antimycin A (Ant, 6 μM) in absence (empty bars) or presence (filled bars) of different quinones (5 μM idebenone, CoQ$_1$, CoQ$_{10}$ or QS-10) for 1 hour. ATP levels were normalized to protein and expressed as percentage of DMSO-treated cells in absence of rotenone. (B) HepG2 cells were incubated with 6 μM rotenone for 60 minutes, while 10 μM idebenone was pre-, co- or post-incubated regarding the time point of rotenone addition. ATP levels are expressed as percentage of untreated cells. Bars represent mean +stdev of triplicates of one typical out of two independent experiments. (C) Rescue of ATP levels of rotenone-treated (60 μM) primary mouse hepatocytes by acute idebenone treatment (5 μM) for 1 hour. Bars represent mean +stdev of six independent experiments. (D) Idebenone (400 mg/kg/day; p.o.) was administered to mice over 4 weeks and protection of ATP levels was maintained in rotenone-treated (20 and 60 μM for 1 hour) primary hepatocytes *ex vivo* without acute addition of idebenone. Bars represent mean +stdev of duplicates from each one idebenone- and sham-treated mouse. ATP levels were normalized to cell number and expressed as percentage of sham-treated hepatocytes in absence of rotenone. $p^{**}<0.01$, $p^{***}<0.001$.

NQO1. In presence of rotenone, dicoumarol completely abolished the rescue of ATP levels normally induced by idebenone and CoQ$_1$ (Figure 3A). Specifically, addition of 20 μM dicoumarol reduced ATP levels in presence of 60 μM rotenone from 71±6% and 64±6% residual ATP for idebenone and CoQ$_1$, respectively, to 2% for both quinones (Figure 3A). Likewise, to address the question whether the quinone-dependent rescue of ATP levels is dependent on mitochondrial function we used the mitochondrial complex III inhibitor antimycin A (Ant). Analogous to the results obtained with dicoumarol, antimycin A prevented quinone dependent rescue of ATP levels (2% and 2±1% residual ATP with idebenone and CoQ$_1$, respectively).

Recently, some evidence emerged that longer incubation periods of up to one week are required to detect some protective effects by CoQ$_{10}$ [42]. Therefore, we investigated whether rescue of ATP levels, as demonstrated for acute exposure to idebenone and CoQ$_1$, would be detectable after a 1-week treatment with CoQ$_{10}$ (Figure S6). Rescue of ATP levels could not be detected for any quinone when administered only once at the beginning of a 1-week treatment. However, further addition of quinone simultaneously to the rotenone challenge after the 1-week treatment restored ATP levels in the case of idebenone and CoQ$_1$, whereas under these conditions, CoQ$_{10}$ again failed to protect ATP levels (Figure S6).

To test a possible time-dependency of the idebenone-mediated rescue of ATP levels, HepG2 cells were incubated with 6 μM rotenone for 60 minutes (Figure 3B). In addition, these cells were also treated with 10 μM idebenone for various incubation periods, either before or after the addition of rotenone (Figure 3B). Compared to rotenone-only treated cells (3±0% residual ATP), idebenone showed consistent protection of ATP levels in cells either pre-treated 40 minutes before the rotenone challenge (81±1% residual ATP) or cells simultaneous treated with rotenone and idebenone (73±7%) (Figure 3B). Interestingly, protection of ATP levels by idebenone was also evident, when it was added after the rotenone challenge. A 5-minute idebenone treatment still showed significant efficacy (54±4% residual ATP) in cells, which were already exposed to rotenone for 55 minutes (Figure 3B).

Similar results were observed in freshly isolated mouse hepatocytes. After isolation, hepatocytes were immediately treated with 60 μM rotenone in presence or absence of 5 μM idebenone. Again, idebenone protected cells from rotenone-induced ATP depletion (Figure 3C). Although, acute incubation of primary hepatocytes with rotenone did not lead to the same striking reduction of ATP levels compared to HepG2 cells (72±18% of control), idebenone fully restored ATP levels (106±21%) in this system. At the same time, in the absence of rotenone, idebenone did not alter ATP levels in these cells (111±16%).

This *ex vivo* activity of idebenone on ATP levels after rotenone-mediated impairment of complex I raised the question, whether this protective action could also be observed *in vivo*. Therefore, idebenone (400 mg/kg/day; p.o.) was administered to mice over a period of four weeks before hepatocytes were isolated and immediately treated with 20 μM or 60 μM rotenone for one hour as in previous experiments. In this experiment, however, idebenone was not freshly added to hepatocytes during this stress phase. Freshly isolated hepatocytes of idebenone-treated and sham- treated mice had similar basal ATP levels (113±16% and 100±21% respectively) (Figure 3D). Consistent with our *in vitro* and *ex vivo* data, rotenone led to a drop in ATP levels in hepatocytes of sham-treated animals (45±2% residual ATP levels at 20 μM rotenone, 46±8% at 60 μM rotenone). However, hepatocytes of idebenone-fed mice were significantly more

resistant to rotenone challenge (81±7% residual ATP at 20 μM rotenone and 77±4% at 60 μM rotenone).

ATP rescue is dependent on NQO1

Even though dicoumarol is reported to be a specific inhibitor of NQO1 [38], we wanted to rule out that other activities of dicoumarol, independent of NQO1, are responsible for the observed abolition of ATP rescue. Therefore, we investigated the ability of idebenone to rescue ATP levels after rotenone-challenge in cell lines and primary cells with different NQO1 expression levels (Figure 4). To compare the different cell lines, NQO1 mRNA levels, determined by qPCR, were normalized to HepG2 cells which showed the highest expression levels (mRNA levels: 100±2.7%; ATP rescue: 54.7±83%). In comparison, human embryonic kidney cells (HEK293) with very low NQO1 mRNA levels (0.4±1.2%) consistently failed to rescue ATP levels (−0.4±0.1%). Similarly, human neuroblastoma cells (SH-SY5Y) showed low NQO1 expression (3.7±0.3%) as well as ATP rescue capacity (−0.8±0.3%). In cells expressing higher NQO1 mRNA levels, such as human keratinocyte cell line (HaCaT) (18.9±0.0%), human myoblasts (42.8±1.2%) or human fibroblasts (52.0±0.5%), ATP rescue was more prominent (3.8±0.4%, 10.7±0.8% or 29.0±7.9%, respectively). Furthermore, downregulation of NQO1 expression in HepG2 cells by shRNA reduced mRNA levels (from 100±2.7% to 66.2±7.6%) as well as the ability to rescue ATP levels in presence of rotenone (from 54.7±8.3% to 39.0±4.4%). The data for all human cell lines tested clearly showed a positive correlation ($R^2 = 0.9458$) of ATP rescue and NQO1 expression (Figure 4).

Effect of quinones on lactate production by MELAS cybrids

Cells from *mitochondrial encephalomyopathy, lactic acidosis and stroke-like episodes* (MELAS) patients are characterized by impaired mitochondrial respiratory function. Mutations in mtDNA in these cells are generally associated with impaired function of mitochondrial complex I. As a consequence, low

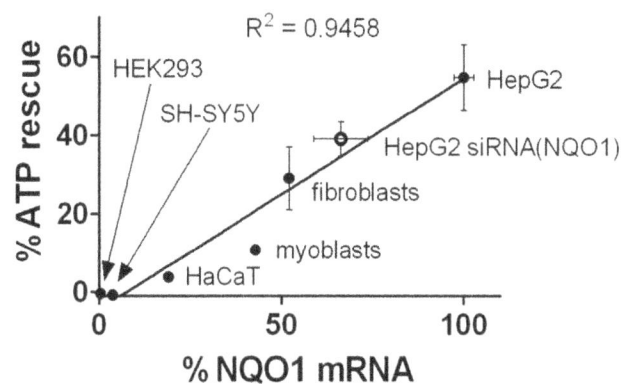

Figure 4. Rescue of ATP levels is dependent on NQO1. Correlation of ATP rescue and NQO1 mRNA expression in different human cell lines and primary cells. Percentage of ATP rescue by 10 μM idebenone in presence of 6 μM rotenone was defined as percentage of ATP levels in presence of rotenone and idebenone relative to the difference between ATP levels of DMSO- and rotenone-treated cells. mRNA levels were determined using qPCR and are relative to NQO1 expression in HepG2 cells. Results from HepG2 cells transduced with lentivirus encoding NQO1-specific shRNA are also included (open circle). Error bars represent standard deviation for both mRNA levels and ATP rescue ($R^2 = 0.9458$).

levels of ATP synthesis and excess production of lactate are described [43]. The observed excess lactate is largely a result of increased glycolysis to maintain sufficient energy levels under conditions of defective oxidative phosphorylation. The reason for producing lactate is to regenerate NAD^+ levels which were utilized in the initial steps of glycolysis. Without sufficient NAD^+, glycolysis cannot proceed. Since we showed quinone-dependent rescue of ATP levels under conditions of impaired mitochondrial complex I function (Figure 3) and NQO1-dependent metabolism is described to increase $NAD^+/NADH$ ratio [9], we investigated the role of quinones on cellular metabolism in cybrids harboring either wild type (WT) mitochondria or mitochondria from MELAS patients. If the effects of idebenone and CoQ_1 in MELAS cybrids were comparable to those observed in healthy cells, it should strengthen mitochondrial respiration and, as a result, increase mitochondrial membrane potential ($\Delta\psi_m$). Although neither quinone changed $\Delta\psi_m$ in WT cybrids after a 2-day treatment, in MELAS cells, which have a slightly lower $\Delta\psi_m$ (85.0±16.9%) compared to DMSO-treated WT, $\Delta\psi_m$ was substantially increased after treatment with idebenone (145.8±26.2%) and CoQ_1 (120.0±19.9%) (Figure 5A). Under these conditions, CoQ_{10} and QS-10 did not influence $\Delta\psi_m$ (80.3±15.2% and 78.8±23.9%). Unlike the situation where acute short-term incubation with quinones increased ATP levels after rotenone challenge (Figures 3,4), MELAS cells did not show increased ATP levels after 48-hour treatment (Figure S7). However, upon treatment with quinones for 48 hours, only idebenone and CoQ_1 significantly reduced lactate levels by 24% and 57%, respectively (Figure 5B), which was partially reversed by addition of the NQO1-inhibitor dicoumarol (Figure 5C).

Toxicological assessment of quinones

Previous studies reported that idebenone and CoQ_1 inhibit mitochondrial complex I function [11,25,29–31]. Based on results with other complex I inhibitors such as rotenone, it was suggested that some short-chain quinones could possess cytotoxic potential. Since a pro-oxidative function for some short-chain quinones was discussed [29,31], we investigated the effects of the quinones tested in this study on cellular DNA damage in different cell lines. After 24-hour incubation with 10 μM quinones in normal medium, only CoQ_1 showed a marked increase in γH2AX-positive cells (Figure 6A). This effect was most prominent in HEK293 cells (34% positive cells compared to 4% in sham-treated cells), but also in SH-SY5Y (10% compared to 2%), and amounted to only a slight increase in γH2AX-positive nuclei in HepG2 cells (33% compared to 25%). We extended this study also to primary cells. After 72-hour incubation of primary human fibroblasts with quinones (10 μM), only cells treated with CoQ_1 were positive for the nuclear DNA damage marker γH2AX, while for all other quinones, including idebenone, no increase above basal levels could be detected (Figure 6B).

Discussion

Quinones that are analogous to CoQ_{10} in the substitution pattern of their quinone moiety have often been proposed to share its biological activity. Just recently, Villalba et al. [44] suggested idebenone to be a good substitute for CoQ_{10} in different diseases. However, such predictions are questionable, since structural variances entail different chemical and physicochemical properties. Here, we have described that short-chain quinones are excellent substrates for reduction by NQO1 and NQO2, which is generally in agreement with previous reports [8,40]. For instance,

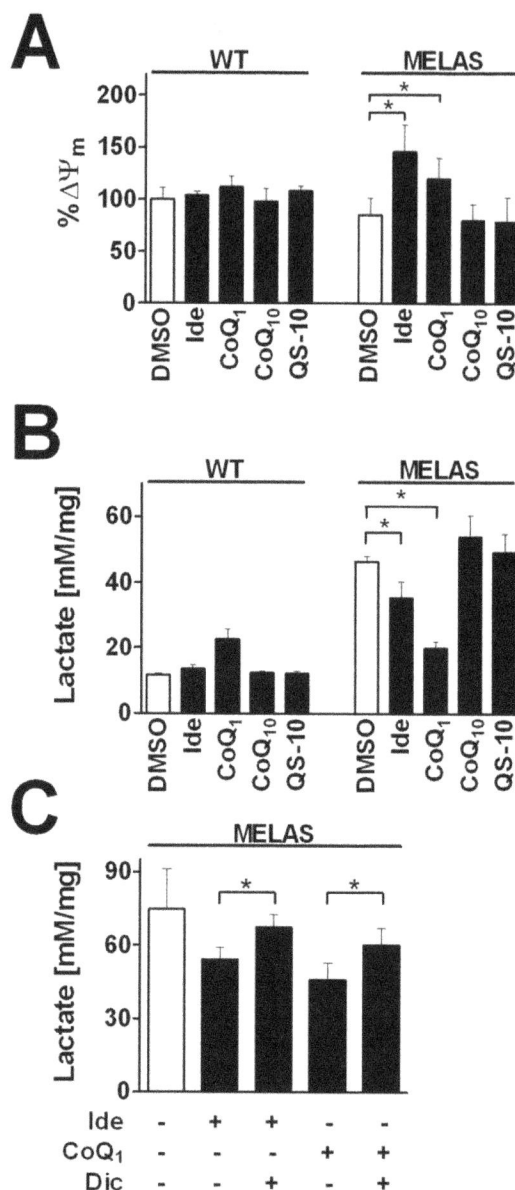

Figure 5. Effect of quinones on mitochondrial membrane potential and lactate production in MELAS cybrids. Cells were cultivated in galactose-containing media for 2 days in the presence or absence of quinones (10 μM). (A) Mitochondrial membrane potential ($\Delta\psi_m$) in wild-type (WT) and MELAS cybrids was measured using TMRM. Bars represent mean +stdev of 4 separate wells of a typical experiment as relative percentage compared to TMRM/protein in DMSO-treated WT cybrids (B) Lactate was measured in the supernatant and standardized to protein content. Data depict one typical experiment out of three and each data point represents mean + standard deviation of three individual wells. (C) Co-incubation with dicoumarol (10 μM) partially reverses the drop of lactate levels induced by idebenone or CoQ_1. Extracellular lactate levels were standardized to protein content. Bars represent mean +stdev of 4 separate dishes within a typical experiment. p^*<0.05, Student t-test.

the obtained v_{max} for CoQ_1 reduction by NQO1 is within the same range as reported by Beyer et al. [41]. In accordance to CoQ_1, we have demonstrated here that idebenone and QS-10, an early metabolite of idebenone [32], are good substrates for NQO1. Strikingly, we did not detect any NQO1 or NQO2 activities above background when the lipophilic CoQ_{10} was used as electron

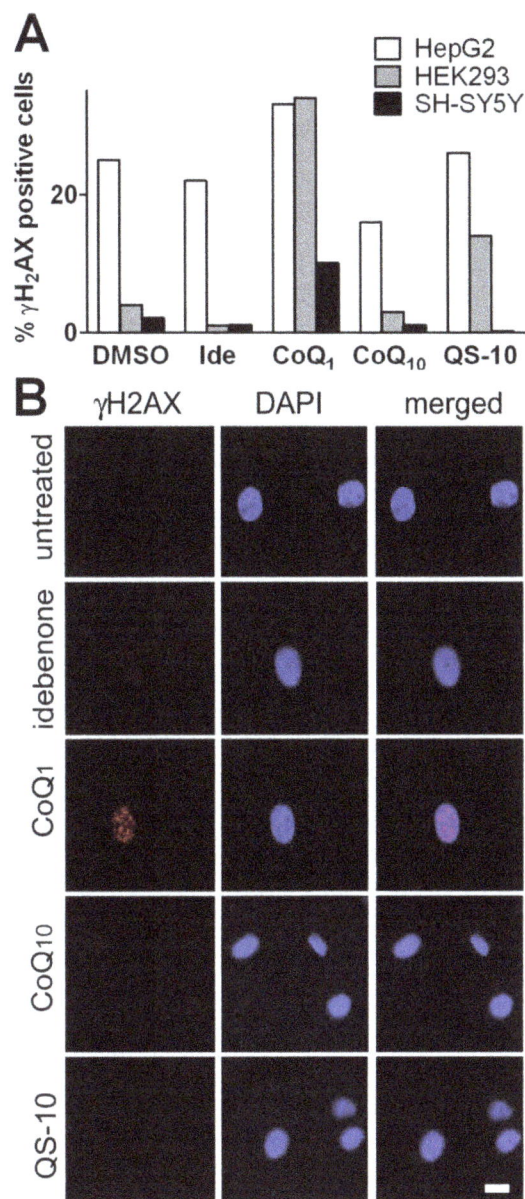

Figure 6. Genotoxic assessment of quinones. Induction of DNA damage by CoQ_1. (A) HepG2, HEK293 and SH-SY5Y cells were cultured under culture conditions in presence of quinones (10 μM) for 24 hours before cells were fixed and stained against the DNA damage marker γH2AX. More than thousand cells per condition were counted manually for each condition and γH2AX-positive cells were expressed as percentage of the total number of cells counted. (B) Human primary fibroblasts were incubated for 72 hours with quinones (10 μM) under ambient conditions before cells were fixed and stained against the DNA damage marker γH2AX (red). DAPI dye was used as nuclear counterstain (blue). Scale bar: 10 μm.

selective reduction of different quinones by NQO1, which was observed by us and others in different cellular systems, supports the idea of a general mechanism that is not cell type-dependent.

The relevance of NQO1-mediated reduction of short-chain quinones such as idebenone and CoQ_1 lies in the fact that some hydroquinones can shuttle into the mitochondria and participate in mitochondrial electron transport. We were therefore interested if this phenomenon could restore energy levels under conditions of complex I deficiency. In this study, we observed a beneficial effect of idebenone and CoQ_1 on cellular energy levels under conditions of acute inhibition of mitochondrial complex I by rotenone. Our results for CoQ_1 are consistent with previously published data [8]. In this study, we demonstrate that idebenone also rescues ATP levels after acute complex I inhibition and that this action is dependent on both NQO1 and mitochondrial complex III. The dependency of NQO1 is not only shown by dicoumarol-mediated inhibition of enzymatic activity, but NQO1 expression in different cell lines and primary cells correlates well with the capacity to rescue ATP levels after rotenone challenge. In addition, partial silencing of NQO1 by RNAi reduces the idebenone mediated ATP rescue.

Both cytosolic and mitochondrial events are required for the quinone-dependent circumvention of complex I blockage of mitochondrial electron transport. Under normal conditions, mitochondrial complex I transfers two electrons from mitochondrial NADH to CoQ_{10} in the mitochondrial membrane which then passes the electrons on to cytochrome c in complex III. In contrast, the mechanism possibly used by idebenone and CoQ_1 starts with the reduction of the quinone by NQO1 in the cytosol (Figure 7). Thereby, cytosolic NAD(P)H acts as the electron donor and substitutes for mitochondrial NADH as carrier of energy. The hydroquinone then enters the mitochondria to donate its electrons to complex III. Experiments by Degli Esposti et al. [29] revealed that reduced idebenone is a good substrate for complex III and can potently lead to reduction of cytochrome c. Since the hydroquinone is oxidized back into its quinone form by this reaction, a new cycle can be triggered resulting in a quinone-driven electron shuttle from cytosolic NAD(P)H to mitochondrial cytochrome c. Not only is this the first time that this mode of action has been described for the clinically used short-chain quinone idebenone, we have also provided evidence by treating animals with idebenone that this mechanism can operate in vivo.

Interestingly, when complex I was inhibited by rotenone for about one hour, a short, additional 5-minute incubation period with idebenone was still able to protect ATP levels. This suggests that idebenone is quickly absorbed and reduced by cellular systems and that restoration of decreased ATP levels can occur extremely fast. These findings provide a rationale why idebenone can be protective in disorders associated with impaired complex I function but normal levels of CoQ_{10}. The reason for the extremely poor reduction of CoQ_{10} by NQO enzymes most likely originates from compartmentalization of enzyme and substrate. While NQO1 and NQO2 are strictly cytosolic enzymes [1,3], CoQ_{10} is extremely hydrophobic and under physiological conditions only found integrated into biological membranes [47]. Therefore, CoQ_{10} cannot participate in this cytosolic-mitochondrial shuttling of electrons. Consistently, even prolonged cellular exposure to CoQ_{10} for up to one week failed to trigger an ATP rescue when complex I was dysfunctional. On the other hand, the surprising lack of detectable activity of QS-10, one of the first metabolites of idebenone [32], on restoring ATP levels, despite being reduced efficiently in cells and in cell-free conditions, could lie in its polarity. QS-10 is significantly more hydrophilic than idebenone and CoQ_1, as manifested in a smaller log D value (Figure 1). It is

acceptor, despite testing different formulations of CoQ_{10} such as liposomes. These results mirror a report by Siegel et al. [45], who described CoQ_{10} reduction by NQO1 with a v_{max} 3 orders of magnitude lower than the v_{max} we observed for CoQ_1. Further publications reporting reduction of CoQ_{10} by NQO1 [reviewed in 46] display similar low velocities, which fall below the detection level of our system. These differences between the long-chain CoQ_{10} and its short-chain analogs were also observed in cells. The

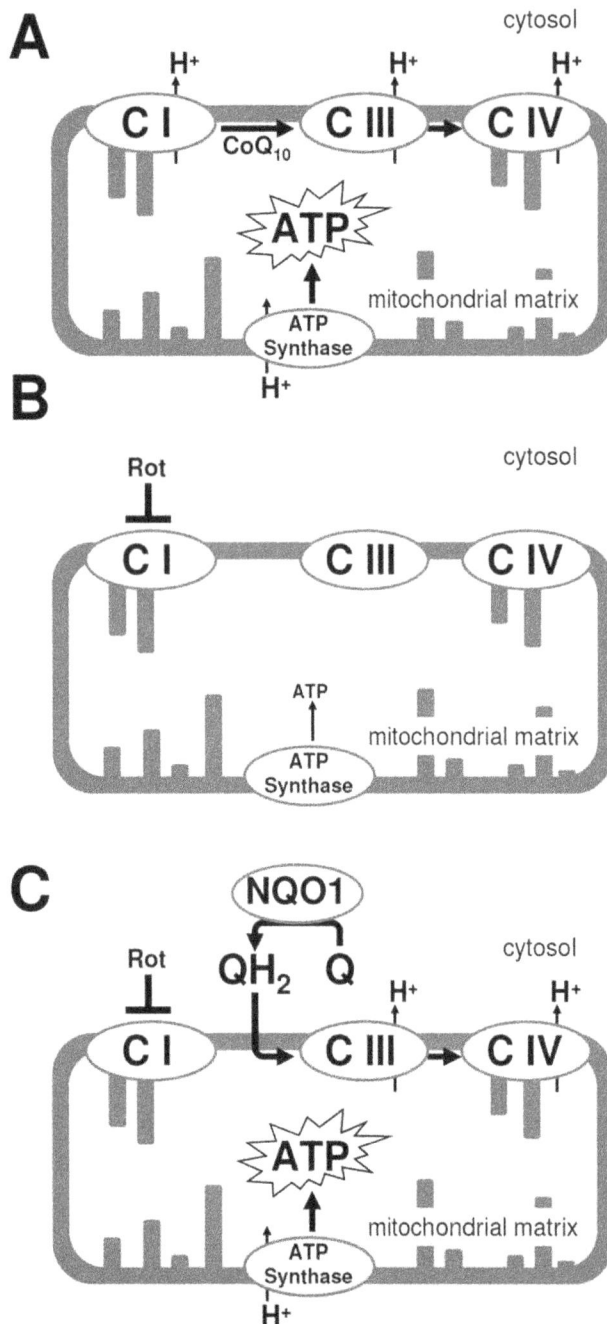

Figure 7. Schematic representation of NQO1-dependent cytosolic-mitochondrial electron shuttling. (A) During oxidative phosphorylation under normal conditions, CoQ_{10} transports electrons from complex I (CI) to complex III (CIII) and cytochrome c, reduced by complex III, transfers them to complex IV. As a consequence of this electron propagation, all three complexes translocate protons (H^+) across the mitochondrial membrane, thus generating a proton gradient. ATP synthase utilizes the energy stored in this electro-chemical gradient to generate ATP. (B) Upon rotenone-induced (Rot) inhibition of complex I, ATP levels decrease dramatically (see also results of Fig. 3). (C) Some short-chain quinones (Q) such as idebenone or CoQ_1 can bypass complex I inhibition via a cytosolic-mitochondrial shuttling of electrons. Upon reduction by cytosolic NQO1 (QH_2), these quinones can feed electrons into the mitochondrial respiratory chain in a complex III-dependent manner, thereby restoring ATP production.

therefore less likely that reduced QS-10 can pass through the lipophilic mitochondrial membrane to donate the electrons to complex III. Thus, our findings imply several requirements for this form of cytosolic-mitochondrial respiration. Not only is it necessary for quinones to enter the cytoplasm and show efficient reduction by NQO1, these compounds must also be able to enter the mitochondria. Then, within the mitochondria, they must be able to interact with complex III of the respiratory chain and release electrons that contribute to the mitochondrial proton gradient which is necessary for ATP synthesis.

Cybrid cells harboring the A3243G MELAS mutation possess a dysfunctional complex I. Thus, in order to generate sufficient ATP, they have to depend on anaerobic glycolysis. The price for increased glycolysis is the excessive production of lactate. Consistent with previous work [43], our data demonstrate that MELAS cybrids show more than 4-fold increased levels of extracellular lactate. It is interesting to note in this context that the main function of lactate production from pyruvate is entirely focused on regenerating NAD^+ that is needed as co-factor for the initial steps of glycolysis. Here we show that quinone-mediated electron transfer from cytosolic NADH to mitochondrial complex III, as we described it for idebenone and CoQ_1, is associated with increased mitochondrial membrane potential and an NQO1-dependent reduced lactate production of MELAS cybrids. The observation that at the same time both quinones were unable to increase ATP levels in cybrid cells suggests that MELAS cells are switching their metabolism from anaerobic glycolysis to mitochondrial respiration in order to generate the same levels of ATP. Since excess lactate production is considered to be one of the main pathological events in MELAS, this switch could be sufficient to alleviate some of the problems associated with the disease. Although we can not rule out a contribution of NQO1-quinone-dependent NAD^+ production in the reduction of lactate levels observed in MELAS cells, we hypothesize that the mode of action lies predominantly in a quinone-dependent increase in mitochondrial activity.

Idebenone and CoQ_1 have both been described to inhibit complex I [11,25,29–31]. As consequence of complex I inhibition, both quinones were suggested to also act as pro-oxidants under certain conditions [29,31]. However, our results demonstrate that only CoQ_1 but not idebenone triggered substantial DNA damage in different cell types. This clearly indicates that, despite sharing the protective activity against acute rotenone toxicity, idebenone does not cause DNA damage compared to CoQ_1 after long-term administration. Because of these serious cytotoxic effects of CoQ_1, we strongly caution against the use of CoQ_1 in a clinical indication. Of the four quinones tested in this study, only idebenone met all requirements for cytosolic-mitochondrial redox cycling without evoking adverse effects (Table 2). Our findings also highlight the influence of modifications to the alkylic tail of short-chain quinones on their biological activity.

In summary, our data show that short-chain quinones possess entirely different activities compared to the lipophilic CoQ_{10} which suggests that they cannot substitute for each other. Some short-chain quinones such as idebenone, upon reduction by NQO1, generate a cytosolic-mitochondrial electron shuttle that can increase cellular energy levels, which can be utilized under conditions of impaired mitochondrial function. This mode of action appears promising for disorders characterized by complex I deficiencies such as MELAS, Leber's hereditary optic neuropathy (LHON) and Leigh's syndrome. However, without further testing for additional features of short-chain quinones, such as possible toxic liabilities, as shown here for CoQ_1, extreme caution has to be exerted with regards to their therapeutic usefulness.

Table 2. Summary of the quinone characteristics.

	NQO substrate	Complex III substrate (reported)	Increased $\Delta\psi_m$	ATP rescue (in presence of rotenone)	Decrease of lactate (in MELAS)	Absence of toxicity
Idebenone	+	+*	+	+	+	+
CoQ$_1$	+	+*	+	+	+	-
CoQ$_{10}$	-	+†	-	-	-	+
QS-10	+	-	-	-	-	+

The abilities of the individual quinones to meet the requirements of cytosolic-mitochondrial shuttling and consequences thereof, as well as caveats for clinical administration, are listed.
*Idebenone and CoQ$_1$ [29], as well as †CoQ$_{10}$ [47], have been reported to be complex III substrates.

Materials and Methods

Ethical Statement

All animal experiments were approved by the governmental authorities (Kantonales Verterinäramt Basel-Land, Switzerland; permit number BL404) and were in accordance with international guidelines.

Reagents and Chemicals

All chemical reagents, if not otherwise stated, were purchased from Sigma (Sigma-Aldrich, Buchs, Switzerland). All cell culture media and solutions, if not otherwise stated, were purchased from Omnilab (Zurich, Switzerland). Idebenone and QS-10 were synthesized in-house and were solid with purity ≥95% as determined by NMR and LCMS. For all assays described, compounds were dissolved at 10 mM (stock solution) in 100% DMSO (Acros Organics, Belgium).

Cell culture and animal husbandry

Primary human fibroblasts (GM08402, Coriell, Camden NJ, USA), human neuroblastoma cell line SH-SY5Y (330154, Cell Line Services, Eppelheim, Germany), spontaneously transformed human keratinocyte cell line HaCaT (330493, CLS, Eppelheim, Germany), human embryonic kidney cell line HEK293 (CRL-1573, ATCC, Molsheim, France), rat L6 myoblasts (CRL-1458, ATCC, Molsheim, France), and human hepatic cell line HepG2 (330198, CLS, Eppelheim, Germany) cells were cultured under ambient conditions (37°C, 5% CO$_2$, 90% humidity) in DMEM, 10% fetal bovine serum (FBS), Penicillin-Streptomycin-Glutamine. Lymphoblastoid cells (GM15851, Coriell) were cultured in RPMI 1640 under conditions as described above. Primary human myoblasts (from biopsy of healthy, 14-year old male, AFM, Evry, France) were cultured in MEM EBS supplemented with 25% M-199 EBS, 10% Hyclone FCS, 10 µg/ml insulin, 100 ng/ml EGF, 100 ng/ml FGF and Penicillin-Streptomycin-Glutamine under conditions described above. Wild-type (RN236, WT, homoplastic) and MELAS (RN164, A3243G homoplastic) cybrid cells [43] were cultured in DMEM, 7% FBS, Penicillin-Streptomycin-Glutamine and 50 µg/ml uridine. If not otherwise stated all animals were held under standard laboratory conditions (12 hours light per day, 22±2°C, 40–60% humidity) with food and water available ad libitum.

NQO1 and NQO2 Activity

Recombinant NQO1 and NQO2 (Sigma, Buchs, Switzerland) activity in presence of different quinones was measured essentially according to a modified protocol by Ernster [48]. Reactions were performed in 1-ml disposable cuvettes at room temperature in reaction buffer (25 mM Tris-HCl pH 7.4, 0.7 mg/ml bovine serum albumin (BSA), 1 µg/ml enzyme, 10 µM quinone). The reaction was started by addition of NAD(P)H (for NQO1) or 1-(3-sulfonatopropyl)-3-carbamoyl-1,4-dihydropyrimidine (a NRH-derivate, for NQO2) [36]. Enzyme activity was measured as decrease of A$_{340}$ for NAD(P)H and A$_{355}$ for the NRH-derivate, respectively, during 30 seconds in a spectrophotometer (Ultrospec® 3000, Amersham Pharmaceutical Biotech, Little Chalfont, UK). All assays were performed in triplicate. Electron donor concentrations at start of linear phase of the decrease of absorbance were calculated using the absorbance coefficient ($\varepsilon_{NADH} = 6300$ M^{-1} cm^{-1}; $\varepsilon_{NADPH} = 6200$ M^{-1} cm^{-1}; $\varepsilon_{NRH\text{-}derivate} = 4480$ M^{-1} cm^{-1}). Reduction rates per mg enzyme were calculated during the linear phase of the reduction. Since NQO1 possesses a single quinone-binding site [49], steady-state kinetic constants were calculated using the Michaelis-Menten equation combined with Hanes-Woolf plot because of its independence towards variability at high substrate levels. To determine the dicoumarol sensitivity of enzymes, reactions were performed in triplicate in the presence or absence of 20 µM dicoumarol in reaction buffer (25 mM Tris-HCl pH 7.4, 0.7 mg/ml BSA, and 1 µg/ml enzyme) containing 50 µM CoQ$_1$ and started with 100 µM NADH or 1-(3-sulfonatopropyl)-3-carbamoyl-1,4-dihydropyrimidine, respectively. Electron donor consumption rate was calculated as described above and expressed as percentage of the rate in the absence of dicoumarol. For complexing quinones with serum, powdered quinones were dissolved in heat-inactivated FBS by vortexing for one minute. Alternatively, quinones were formulated in liposomes as described [33,34]. Briefly, L-α-phosphatidylcholine and quinone were dissolved in PBS at a final concentration of 25 mg/ml lipid in a molar drug/lipid fraction of 0.05 (final quinone concentration: 1.6 mM). The mixture was then subjected to five repetitive freeze-thaw cycles.

WST-1 assay for measuring NQO1-dependent quinone reduction in cells

WST-1 absorbance was determined as described previously [37]. Briefly, 96-well plates (Greiner, Frickenhausen, Germany) were seeded with 10^4 HepG2 cells per well in DMEM with 2% FBS and 0.3 g/l glucose on the day before the WST-1 experiment. Inhibitors were preincubated for one hour using the following concentrations: dicoumarol 20 µM; rotenone 6 µM; antimycin 6 µM. After the preincubation time, the medium was replaced by Hank's balanced salt solution (HBSS; Omnilab, Zurich, Switzerland) containing 450 µM WST-1 (Dojindo Laboratories, Kumamoto, Japan) with or without inhibitors. The reaction was started by the addition of the quinone. WST-1 reduction (A$_{450}$) was followed over a period of 120 minutes.

Isolation of hepatocytes

Hepatocytes were isolated from 6-week old female NMRI mice (Janvier, France) as described [8]. Briefly, animals were sacrificed by CO_2 and immediately perfused with 50 ml perfusion buffer (10 mM HEPES pH 7.4, 140 mM NaCl, 5 mM KCl, 2.5 mM Na_2HPO_4, 6 mM glucose and 0.2 mM EGTA; 37°C). The liver was removed and minced in pre-warmed collagenase buffer (10 mM HEPES pH 7.4, 140 mM NaCl, 5 mM KCl, 2.5 mM Na_2HPO_4, 6 mM glucose, 0.2 mM $CaCl_2$, 1.3 mM $MgSO_4$ and 0.05% collagenase D (Roche Diagnostics AG, Switzerland)). After incubation for 30 minutes at 37°C, hepatocytes were dissociated using a 5-ml syringe. The homogenous solution was filtered through gauze and the viability of cells was assessed using trypan blue staining. Typical viability of isolated hepatocytes was about 90%. For *ex vivo* studies with long-term treated mice, five-week-old male C57BL/6J mice were purchased from Janvier (France). After one week acclimatization period in the facility, the animals were single-housed and received a daily dose of 400 mg/kg idebenone in the food. For this, idebenone was dissolved in 0.5% carboxymethyl-cellulose by overnight stirring at 4°C. A 1:1 (w/w) mixture thereof with a normal chow/sugar (9:1 w/w ratio) mash was prepared. Portions which amounted of approximately 75% of the daily calorie intake were stored at −20°C and administered just before start of the dark period. The portions for control animals were prepared identically with the exception of omitted idebenone. Additionally, mice had access to ad libitum food. Hepatocytes were isolated and treated as described before.

Quinone-dependent rescue of ATP levels

HepG2 cells were seeded at a density of 10^5 cells per well in a 96-well plate and incubated for 24 hours in DMEM without glucose, 2% FBS and Penicillin-Streptomycin-Glutamine. Cells were treated with 10 μM quinones in presence or absence of rotenone (60 μM), dicoumarol (20 μM) and antimycin A (6 μM) for 60 minutes in DMEM without glucose. Subsequently, cells were lysed and ATP levels were determined. Immediately after isolation, 10^6 hepatocytes were diluted in 1 ml Krebs-Hensleit buffer (12.5 mM HEPES pH 7.4, 120 mM NaCl, 5 mM KCl, 1 mM KH_2PO_4, 1.2 mM $MgSO_4$, 3 mM $CaCl_2$, 24 mM $NaHCO_3$,) and treated with different concentrations of quinones and inhibitors for 60 minutes at 37°C before ATP levels were determined.

Quantification of ATP

Cellular ATP levels were quantified using luminescence from the ATP-dependent enzymatic oxidation of luciferin by luciferase. Briefly, isolated and treated cells were lysed in a volume of 200 μl (4 mM EDTA, 0.2% Triton X-100) for five minutes. In 96-well plates, 100 μl of ATP measurement buffer (25 mM HEPES pH 7.25, 300 μM D-luciferin, 5 μg/ml firefly luciferase, 75 μM DTT, 6.25 mM $MgCl_2$, 625 μM EDTA and 1 mg/ml BSA) was combined with 10 μl lysate to start the reaction. Luminescence was quantified immediately using a multimode plate reader (Tecan M1000, Tecan iControl 1.6 software; Tecan Austria GmbH, Grödig, Austria). ATP levels were standardized to cell number for isolated hepatocytes or protein levels using BCA assay (ThermoScientific, Rockford, IL, USA) for cultured cells. Changes were calculated as percentage relative to levels of DMSO-treated control cells. ATP rescue is defined as the percentage of quinone-induced increase in ATP levels in presence of rotenone relative to the ATP reduction by rotenone alone.

Lentiviral knock-down of NQO1

To knock down NQO1 expression, HepG2 cells were seeded in 12-well plates at 30000 cells per well in normal growth medium for

24 hours. Medium was replaced by 180 μl growth medium and 20 μl stock solution containing 10^5 infectious units (IFU) of lentivirus encoding shRNA against NQO1 (sc-37139-V, Santa Cruz, Santa Cruz CA, USA) for a 24-hour incubation. Cells were then immediately used for quantifying NQO1 gene expression using qPCR and for ATP rescue experiments.

mRNA levels

RNA was extracted from cultured cells using the High Pure RNA Isolation kit (Roche, Switzerland) according to the manufacturer's recommendations. Synthesis of first-strand cDNA was conducted using High Fidelity Transcriptor cDNA Synthesis kit (Roche, Switzerland) and random hexamer primers in a total volume of 20 μl containing 5 μg RNA. Real-time PCR was performed with Sybrgreen Real-Time PCR Master Mix (Roche, Switzerland) in a LightCycler 480 mastercycler and results were analyzed with the corresponding software (version 1.5.0.39). Protocol parameters used: 5 minutes at 95°C followed by 40 cycles of 10 seconds at 95°C for denaturing, 10 seconds at 56°C for annealing, and 10 seconds at 72°C for extension. GAPDH was used as internal control. Target gene sequences were amplified with the following primer pairs: NQO1 (forward: 5′-CACACTCCAGCAGACGCCCG-3′, reverse: 5′-TGCCCAAGTGATGGCCCACAG-3′) and GAPDH (forward: 5′-GAAGGTGAAGGTCGGAGTC-3′, reverse: 5′-GAAGATGGTGATGGGATTTC-3′).

Measurement of mitochondrial membrane potential

MELAS and WT cybrid cells were seeded in black 96-well plates at 7500 cells per well in normal growth medium (DMEM, 4.5 mg/ml glucose, 10% FBS, 50 μg/ml uridine, Penicillin-Streptomycin). After 24 hours, the medium was changed to challenge medium (DMEM, 2 mg/ml glucose, 10% FBS, 50 μg/ml uridine, 2.5 mg/ml galactose, 0.11 mg/ml pyruvate, Penicillin-Streptomycin) containing DMSO or 10 μM quinones. After 48 hours, 50 μl of DMEM without glucose containing 3 μM tetramethylrhodamine methyl ester perchlorate (TMRM; Sigma-Aldrich, Buchs, Switzerland) was added on top. After 15 min incubation, cells were washed with warm PBS and 50 μl PBS was used for measurement of TMRM fluorescence using a multimode plate reader (Ex.: 545 nm; Em.: 580 nm; Tecan M1000). Fluorescence, corresponding to mitochondrial membrane potential $(\Delta\psi_m)$, was standardized to protein content of lysates.

Determination of extracellular lactate

MELAS and WT cybrid cells were seeded at a density of $1.5*10^5$ cells per 3.5-cm diameter cell culture dish in normal growth medium. After 24 hours, the medium was changed to challenge medium containing either DMSO or compounds. After 48 hours, the medium was removed for lactate measurement and the cells were lysed in 500 μl lysis solution (4 mM EDTA, 0.2% NP-40, 0.2% Tween-20) for 10 minutes. In a 96-well plate, 90 μl of reaction buffer (10 mM KH_2PO_4 pH 7.8, 2 mM EDTA, 1 mg/ml BSA, 0.6 mM DCPIP, 0.5 mM PMS, 0.8 mM NAD^+, 1.5 mM gluta-mate, 5 U/ml glutamate-pyruvate-transaminase, 12.5 U/ml lactate dehydrogenase) was mixed with 10 μl medium. After incubation at 30°C for 30 minutes, absorption at 600 nm was quantified using a multimode plate reader (Tecan M1000). A lactate standard curve was run in parallel. Finally, the lactate concentration in the medium was standardized to protein content of the lysate using BCA assay.

Genotoxic assessment of quinones

HepG2 cells, HEK293 cells, SH-SY5Y neuroblastoma cells and human primary fibroblasts were seeded in 8-chamber slides (Ibidi,

Martinsried, Germany) under ambient conditions and treated for 24-hours with 10 µM quinones (72 hours for human primary fibroblasts). Cells were fixed using 4% PFA/PBS and stained against the DNA damage marker γH2AX (ab2893, Abcam, Cambridge, UK; 1:1000 in TBST, 5% horse serum). DAPI dye was used as nuclear counter stain.

Supporting Information

Figure S1 Different quinones as substrates for NQO1 and NQO2. Hanes-Woolf plots depict oxidation of (A) NADH or (B) NADPH by NQO1 in presence of different quinones as electron acceptors. Each data point represents the average of three independent measurements. (C) Effect of different quinone formulation in DMSO, liposomes (Lip) and fetal bovine serum (FBS) on metabolism by NQO1. Graph depicts electron donor oxidation rate expressed as percentage of control; mean +stdev of three independent measurements; $p^{***} < 0.001$, $p^{**} < 0.01$, two-tailed t-test. (D) Hanes-Woolf plot of NRH-derivate oxidation by NQO2 in presence of different quinone analogs. Each data point represents the average of three independent measurements.

Figure S2 Specific inhibition of NQO1 by dicoumarol. Dicoumarol (20 µM) selectively inhibited recombinant NQO1 activity (96% inhibition, filled bars) *in vitro*, whereas it reduced NQO2 activity by only 14% (empty bars). Graph depicts electron donor oxidation rate (%$V_{substrate\ oxidation}$) expressed as percentage of control; mean +stdev of three independent measurements; $p^{***} < 0.001$, $p^{**} < 0.01$, two-tailed t-test.

Figure S3 NQO1-dependent reduction of quinones in primary fibroblasts. Dose-dependent cellular quinone reduction was measured as described [32] in human fibroblast cells. Bars represent mean +stdev of triplicates from one representative out of three independent experiments.

Figure S4 NQO1-dependent reduction of quinones in rat L6 muscle cell line. Dicoumarol (Dic)-treatment (20 µM) also efficiently blocked cellular quinone reduction in rat L6 cells. Bars represent mean +stdev of triplicates from one representative out of three independent experiments.

Figure S5 NADH turnover in presence of quinones in human lymphoblastoid cells. (A) Idebenone reduces NADH levels in a dose-dependent manner. (B) NADH levels are differently affected by treatment with idebenone, CoQ$_1$, CoQ$_{10}$ and QS-10 (10 µM) in absence (empty bars) or presence (filled bars) of dicoumarol (Dic; 20 µM). NADH content was measured using the NADH-dependent conversion of non-fluorescent resazurin into the fluorescent product resofurin. For cell culture experiments, 96-well black plates (Greiner, Frickhausen, Germany) were seeded with 10^5 wild-type lymphoblastoid cells per well in 110 µl medium and compounds were added ranging from 0 to 10 µM. After one-day incubation at 37°C, cells were washed with PBS and resuspended in 110 µl phenol red-free RPMI. A volume of 10 µl cells was removed for protein determination. Resazurin was added to a final concentration of 4 µM and the cells were incubated at 37°C. Fluorescence change (Ex.: 544 nm, Em.: 590 nm) was measured at (A) 1 and 6 or (B) 3 hours. Wells containing medium and resazurin but no cells served to determine background fluorescence. Fluorescence signal was normalized to protein levels.

Figure S6 ATP rescue after 1-week treatment. HepG2 cells were seeded in to 96-well plates and treated for 1 week with 10 µM quinones under normal culture conditions. Medium was replaced by DMEM without glucose and cells were incubated for one hour in presence or absence of 6 µM rotenone. In addition, some of the wells were treated with fresh quinone (1 week + acute). After one hour, ATP levels were determined as described. Bars represent mean +stdev of one typical experiment.

Figure S7 Effect of quinones on ATP levels in cybrid cells. Cells were cultivated in galactose-containing challenge media for 2 days in the presence or absence of quinones (10 µM) and dicoumarol (10 µM). ATP levels were determined as described. Data depict one typical experiment out of three and each data point represents the mean +stdev of four individual dishes. $p^* < 0.05$, Student t-test.

Acknowledgments

We would like to thank M. Hirano and M. Davidson for the generous gift of the MELAS cybrid cells and the Association Française contre les Myopathies (AFM) for the donation of muscle biopsies.

Author Contributions

Conceived and designed the experiments: RHH ME ACG NG. Performed the experiments: RHH ME ACG DR CA NG. Analyzed the data: RHH ME ACG DR NG. Contributed reagents/materials/analysis tools: ICF CA. Wrote the paper: RHH NG. RHH ME RD NG.

References

1. O'Brien PJ (1991) Molecular mechanisms of quinone cytotoxicity. Chem Biol Interactions 80: 1–41.
2. Monks TJ, Hanzlik RP, Cohen GM, Ross D, Graham DG (1992) Contemporary issues in toxicology. Toxicol Appl Pharmacol 112: 2–16.
3. Long II DJ, Jaiswal AK (2000) NRH:quinone oxidoreductase2 (NQO2). Chem Biol Interact 129: 99–112.
4. Colucci MA, Moody CJ, Gouch GD (2008) Natural and synthetic quinones and their reduction by the quinone reductase enzyme NQO1: from synthetic organic chemistry to compounds with anticancer potential. Org Biomol Chem 6(4): 637–56.
5. Pink JJ, Planchon SM, Tagliarino C, Varnes ME, Siegel D, et al. (2000) NAD(P)H:Quinone oxidoreductase activity is the principal determinant of β-lapachone cytotoxicity. J Biol Chem 275: 5416–5424.
6. Adikesavan AK, Barrios R, Jaiswal AK (2007) In vivo role of NAD(P)H:Quinone oxidoreductase 1 in metabolic activation of mitomycin C and bone marrow cytotoxicity. Cancer Res 67: 7966–7971.

7. Boutin JA, Chatelain-Egger F, Vella F, Delagrangea P, Ferry G (2005) Quinone reductase 2 substrate specificity and inhibition pharmacology. Chem Biol Interact 151: 213–228.
8. Chan TS, Teng S, Wilson JX, Galati G, Khan S, et al. (2002) Coenzyme Q cytoprotective mechanisms for mitochondrial complex I cytopathies involves NAD(P)H: quinone oxidoreductase 1 (NQO1). Free Radic Res 36: 421–7.
9. Dragan M, Dixon SJ, Jaworski E, Chan TS, O'Brien PJ, et al. (2006) Coenzyme Q(1) depletes NAD(P)H and impairs recycling of ascorbate in astrocytes. Brain Res 1078: 9–18.
10. Suno M, Akinobu N (1984) Inhibition of lipid peroxidation by a novel compound (CV-2619) in brain mitochondria and mode of action of the inhibition. Biochem Biophys Res Comm 125: 1046–1052.
11. Sugiyama Y, Fujita T, Matsumoto M, Okamoto K, Imada I (1985) Effects of idebenone (CV-2619) and its metabolites on respiratory activity and lipid peroxidation in brain mitochondria from rats and dogs. J Pharmacobio-Dyn 8: 1006–1017.

12. Suno M, Akinobu N (1989) Inhibition of lipid peroxidation by idebenone in brain mitochondria in the presence of succinate. Arch Gerontol Geriatr 8: 291–297.

13. Rauchovà H, Vrbacky M, Bergamini C, Fato R, Lenaz G, et al. (2006) Inhibition of glycerophosphate-dependent H_2O_2 generation in brown fat mitochondria by idebenone. Biochem Biophys Res Comm 339: 362–366.

14. Ranganathan S, Harmison GG, Meyertholen K, Pennuto M, Burnett BG, et al. (2009) Mitochondrial abnormalities in spinal and bulbar muscular atrophy. Hum Molr Genet 18: 27–42.

15. Jauslin ML, Wirth T, Meier T, Schoumacher F (2002) A cellular model for Friedreich Ataxia reveals small-molecule glutathione peroxidase mimetics as novel treatment strategy. Human Mol. Genet 11: 3055.

16. Kutz K, Drewe J, Vankan P (2009) Pharmacokinetic properties and metabolism of idebenone. J Neurol 256: 31–3.

17. Haginoya K, Miyabayashi S, Kikuchi M, Kojima A, Yamamoto K, et al. (2009) Efficacy of idebenone for respiratory failure in a patient with Leigh syndrome: a long-term follow-up study. J Neurol Sci 278: 112–4.

18. Ikejiri Y, Mori E, Ishii K, Nishimoto K, Yasuda M, et al. (1996) Idebenone improves cerebral mitochondrial oxidative metabolism in a patient with MELAS. Neurology 47: 583–5.

19. Napolitano A, Salvetti S, Vista M, et al. (2000) Long-term treatment with idebenone and riboflavin in a patient with MELAS. Neurol Sci 21: 981–2.

20. Tonon C, Lodi R (2008) Idebenone in Friedreich's Ataxia. Expert Opin Pharmacother 9: 2327–2337.

21. Myers L, Farmer JM, Wilson RB, Friedman L, Tsou A, et al. (2008) Antioxidant use in Friedreich ataxia. J Neurol Sci 267: 174–6.

22. Rötig A, de Lonlay P, Chretien D (1997) Aconitase and mitochondrial iron-sulphur protein deficiency in Friedreich ataxia. Nat Genet 7: 215–17.

23. Houchi H, Azuma M, Oka M, Morita K (1991) Idebenone inhibits catecholamine secretion through its blocking action on Ca^{2+} channels in cultured adrenal chromaffin cells. Jpn J Pharmacol 57: 553–8.

24. Takuma K, Yoshida T, Lee E, Mori K, Kishi T, et al. (2000) CV-2619 protects cultured astrocytes against reperfusion injury via nerve growth factor production. Eur J Pharmacol 406: 333–9.

25. Rauchová H, Drahota Z, Bergamini Z, Fato R, Lenaz G (2008) Modification of respiratory-chain enzyme activities in brown adipose tissue mitochondria by idebenone (hydroxydecyl-ubiquinone). J Bioenerg Biomembr 40: 85–93.

26. Civenni G, Bezzi P, Trotti D, Volterra A, Racagni G (2009) Inhibitory effect of the neuroprotective agent idebenone on arachidonic acid metabolism in astrocytes. Eur J Pharmacol 370: 161–7.

27. Chapela SP, Burgos HI, Salazar AI, Nievas I, Kriguer N, et al. (2008) Biochemical study of idebenone effect on mitochondrial metabolism of yeast. Cell Biol Int 32: 146–50.

28. James AM, Cochemé HM, Smith RA, Murphy MP (2005) Interactions of mitochondria-targeted and untargeted ubiquinones with the mitochondrial respiratory chain and reactive oxygen species. Implications for the use of exogenous ubiquinones as therapies and experimental tools. J Biol Chem 280: 21295–312.

29. Degli Esposti M, Ngo A, Ghelli A, Benelli B, Carelli B, et al. (1996) The interaction of Q analogs, particularly hydroxydecyl-benzoquinone (idebenone), with the respiratory complexes of heart mitochondria. Arch Biochem Biophys 330: 395–400.

30. Brière JJ, Schlemmer D, Chretien D, Rustin P (2004) Quinone analogues regulate mitochondrial substrate competitive oxidation. Biochem Biophys Res Comm 316: 1138–1142.

31. Fato R, Bergamini C, Bortolus M, Maniero AL, Leoni S, et al. (2008) Differential effects of mitochondrial Complex I inhibitors on production of reactive oxygen species. Biochim Biophys Acta 1787: 384–92.

32. Okamoto K, Watanabe M, Morimoto H, Imada I (1998) Synthesis, metabolism, and in vitro biological activities of 6-(10-hydroxydecyl)-2,3-dimethoxy-5-methyl-1,4-benzoquinone (CV-2619)-related compounds. Chem Pharm Bull (Tokyo) 36: 178–89.

33. Mayer LD, Hope MJ, Cullis PR, Janoff AS (1985) Solute distributions and trapping efficiencies observed in freeze-thawed multilamellar vesicles. Biochim Biophys Acta 817: 193–196.

34. Paolino D, Iannone M, Cardile V, Renis M, Puglisi G, et al. (2004) Tolerability and improved protective action of idebenone-loaded pegylated liposomes on ethanol-induced injury in primary cortical Astrocytes. J Pharmaceut Sci 93: 1815–1827.

35. Wu K, Knox R, Sun XZ, Joseph P, Jaiswal AK, et al. (1997) Catalytic properties of NAD(P)H:quinone oxidoreductase-2 (NQO2), a dihydronicotinamide riboside dependent oxidoreductase. Arch Biochem Biophys 347: 221–228.

36. Knox RJ, Jenkins TC, Hobbs SM, Chen S, Melton RG, et al. (2000) Bioactivation of 5-(aziridin-1-yl)-2,4-dinitrobenzamide (CB 1954) by human NAD(P)H quinone oxidoreductase 2: A novel co-substrate-mediated antitumor prodrug therapy. Canc Res 60: 4179–4186.

37. Tan AS, Berridge MV (2010) Evidence for NAD(P)H:quinone oxidoreductase 1 (NQO1)-mediated quinone-dependent redox cycling via plasma membrane electron transport: A sensitive cellular assay for NQO1. Free Radic Biol Med 48: 421–429.

38. Ernster L, Danielson L, Ljunggren M (1962) DT Diaphorase. 1. Purification from the soluble fraction of rat-liver cytoplasm, and properties. Biochim Biophys Acta 58: 171–188.

39. Hwang JH, Kim DW, Jo EJ, Kim YK, Jo YS, et al. (2009) Pharmacological stimulation of NADH oxidation ameliorates obesity and related phenotypes in mice. Diabetes 58: 965–974.

40. Audi SH, Zhao H, Bongard RD, Hogg N, Kettenhofen NJ, et al. (2003) Pulmonary arterial endothelial cells affect the redox status of coenzyme Q_0. Free Radic Biol Med 34: 892–907.

41. Beyer RE, Segura-Aguilar J, Di Bernardo S, Cavazzoni M, Fato R, et al. (1996) The role of DT-diaphorase in the maintenance of the reduced antioxidant form of coenzyme Q in membrane systems. Proc Natl Acad Sci U S A 93: 2528–32, 1996.

42. Lopéz LC, Quinzii CM, Area E, Naini A, Rahman S, et al. (2010) PLoS One 5(7): e11897.

43. Pallotti F, Baracca A, Hernandez-Rosa E, Walker WF, Solaini G, et al. (2004) Biochemical analysis of respiratory function in cybrid cell lines harbouring mitochondrial DNA mutations. Biochem J 384: 287–93.

44. Villalba JM, Parrado C, Santos-Gonzalez M, Alcain FJ (2010) Therapeutic use of coenzyme Q_{10} and coenzyme Q_{10}-related compounds and formulations. Expert Opin Investig Drugs 19: 535–54.

45. Siegel D, Bolton EM, Burr JA, Liebler DC, Ross D (1997) The reduction of alpha-tocopherolquinone by human NAD(P)H: quinone oxidoreductase: the role of alpha-tocopherolhydroquinone as a cellular antioxidant. Mol Pharmacol 52: 300–5.

46. Dinkova-Kostova AT, Talalay P (2010) NAD(P)H:quinone acceptor oxidoreductase 1 (NQO1), a multifunctional antioxidant enzyme and exceptionally versatile cytoprotector. Arch Biochem Biophys 501: 116–123.

47. Lenaz G (2001) A critical appraisal of the mitochondrial coenzyme Q pool. FEBS Lett 509: 151–155.

48. Ernster, L (1967) DT-diaphorase. Methods Enzymol 10: 309–317.

49. Gasdaska PY, Fisher H, Powis G (1995) An alternatively spliced form of NQO1 (DT-Diaphorase) messenger RNAi the putative quinone substrate binding site is present in human normal and tumor tissues. Canc Res 55: 2542–2547.

5

Habitual Physical Activity in Mitochondrial Disease

Shehnaz Apabhai[1,9], **Grainne S. Gorman**[1,2,3,9], **Laura Sutton**[3], **Joanna L. Elson**[1], **Thomas Plötz**[4], **Douglass M. Turnbull**[1,2,3], **Michael I. Trenell**[1,2,3]*

1 Mitochondrial Research Group, Newcastle University, Newcastle upon Tyne, United Kingdom,, **2** NIHR Biomedical Research Centre for Ageing and Age-related Disease, Newcastle University, Newcastle upon Tyne, United Kingdom, **3** Newcastle Centre for Brain Ageing and Vitality, Newcastle University, Newcastle upon Tyne, United Kingdom, **4** School of Computing, Newcastle University, Newcastle upon Tyne, United Kingdom

Abstract

Purpose: Mitochondrial disease is the most common neuromuscular disease and has a profound impact upon daily life, disease and longevity. Exercise therapy has been shown to improve mitochondrial function in patients with mitochondrial disease. However, no information exists about the level of habitual physical activity of people with mitochondrial disease and its relationship with clinical phenotype.

Methods: Habitual physical activity, genotype and clinical presentations were assessed in 100 patients with mitochondrial disease. Comparisons were made with a control group individually matched by age, gender and BMI.

Results: Patients with mitochondrial disease had significantly lower levels of physical activity in comparison to matched people without mitochondrial disease (steps/day; 6883 ± 3944 vs. 9924 ± 4088, p = 0.001). 78% of the mitochondrial disease cohort did not achieve 10,000 steps per day and 48% were classified as overweight or obese. Mitochondrial disease was associated with less breaks in sedentary activity (Sedentary to Active Transitions, % per day; 13 ± 0.03 vs. 14 ± 0.03, p = 0.001) and an increase in sedentary bout duration (bout lengths / fraction of total sedentary time; 0.206 ± 0.044 vs. 0.187 ± 0.026, p = 0.001). After adjusting for covariates, higher physical activity was moderately associated with lower clinical disease burden (steps / day; $r_s = -0.49$; 95% CI -0.33, -0.63, P<0.01). There were no systematic differences in physical activity between different genotypes mitochondrial disease.

Conclusions: These results demonstrate for the first time that low levels of physical activity are prominent in mitochondrial disease. Combined with a high prevalence of obesity, physical activity may constitute a significant and potentially modifiable risk factor in mitochondrial disease.

Editor: Markus Schuelke, Charité Universitätsmedizin Berlin, NeuroCure Clinical Research Center, Germany

Funding: Dr. Gorman is funded by the UK NIHR Biomedical Research Centre for Ageing and Age-related Disease. Dr. Elson is supported by a Research Council UK Academic fellowship. Professor Turnbull acknowledges funding from the UK NIHR Biomedical Research Centre for Ageing and Age-related Disease, the Medical Research Council, Muscular Dystrophy Campaign, Newcastle University Centre for Brain Ageing and Vitality and the Wellcome Trust. Dr. Trenell acknowledges the Medical Research Council and is supported by a fellowship from Diabetes UK. The funders had no role in study design, data collection and analysis, decision to publish, or preparation of the manuscript.

Competing Interests: The authors have declared that no competing interests exist.

* E-mail: michael.trenell@ncl.ac.uk

❾ These authors contributed equally to this work.

Introduction

Mitochondria are ubiquitous intracellular organelles found in all nucleated cells and are responsible for energy production and cellular respiration. They are involved in various different cellular processes including calcium signalling [1], cellular metabolism [2], and cytochrome c mediated apoptosis [3]. Mitochondrial enzymes are integral in intermediary metabolism [4]; but, it is usually defects in the respiratory chain, the common final pathway of energy metabolism that result in what are termed mitochondrial cytopathies [5]. Mitochondrial disorders typically affect organs that are heavily dependent on oxidative metabolism such as the brain, eye and skeletal muscle and consequently are commonly characterised by multi-system involvement and variable phenotypic expression, disease severity and rate of progression [6,7,8]. Mitochondrial disease is the most common neuromuscular disease [9] and there are currently no validated therapies.

Exercise intolerance is a characteristic hallmark of patients with mitochondrial disease, with muscle weakness and fatigue reported after low levels of exertion [10]. It is not known whether the reduced exercise tolerance associated with mitochondrial disease is associated with reduced daily physical activity. As an important mediator of mortality, life expectancy, physical function and the onset of disability in normal aging [11,12,13], physical activity may represent an environmental influence that acts independently of the genetic predisposition.

Several studies have now shown that the reversal of a sedentary lifestyle in mitochondrial disease with exercise therapy confers benefits to mitochondrial function and have confirmed safety [14,15,16,17]. Before critically evaluating exercise as a potential therapy in mitochondrial disease it is important to understand the additional risks that patients with mitochondrial disease may be exposed to as a result of low levels of habitual physical activity. Consequently, the aims of this study were to characterise habitual physical activity in patients with known mitochondrial disease and evaluate its relationship with genotype and phenotype.

Methods

Subjects

One hundred patients with a diagnosis of mitochondrial disease were enrolled in the study. Forty-seven participants had a diagnosed point mutation (29 patients with m.3243A>G MELAS mutation; 8 patients with m.8344A>G MERRF mutation: 9 patients with other mitochondrial tRNA (mt-tRNA) mutations). Twenty-eight participants were diagnosed with multiple mtDNA deletions (15 patients unspecified nuclear genetic defect, three patients OPA1 (optic atrophy type 1), five patients POLG1 (polymerase gamma) and five patients PEO1 (Twinkle)). Twenty-one participants were diagnosed with heteroplasmic single-large scale mtDNA deletion. The remaining four patients had uncharacterised genetic defects, but presence of ragged red fibres and Cox negative staining from their biopsy (1–3%). From the patient group 1 participant was wheelchair bound and 1 used a wheel chair for mobilization outside the home. None of the patients were taking part in any exercise based interventions during the duration of the trial. Two of the patients had clinically identified mild cardiomyopathy but without exercise limitation, none had undergone formal evaluation of liver function. All patients had cognitive function sufficient for provision of informed consent (Mini-Mental State Examination >26). The control group consisted of 100 participants, individually matched by age, gender and body mass index (BMI). Participants were over 18 years of age and gave written informed consent. All participants provided informed consent and the study was approved by the Newcastle regional medical research ethics committee.

Physical Activity

Habitual physical activity was measured objectively using a validated multi-sensor array [18] (SenseWear Pro₃, Bodymedia Inc, PA, USA) worn over 3 days. Physical activity data are presented as average METs / day, where 1 MET = resting metabolic rate, or in steps / day. Patterns of sedentary behaviour were assessed by power law analyses of the lengths of sedentary bouts fitted from raw sedentary data, as described in more detail previously [19]. Briefly; the density $p(x)$ of sedentary bouts in a time bin width $d(x)$ was plotted against the bout length x on a logarithmic scale to derive power distribution (equation 1) from the shape of the histogram with respect to there length $_\alpha$:

$$p(x) = CX^{-\alpha} \qquad (1)$$

The type of sedentary distribution characterised by the exponent α (equation 2), can quantify different sedentary behaviour strategies, with a lower α indicating that subjects accumulate sedentary time with a larger proportion of long sedentary bouts:

$$\alpha = 1 + \left[\sum_{i=1}^{n} \ln \frac{x_i}{x_{min}} \right]^{-1} \qquad (2)$$

From these power distributions, Lorentz curves were calculated where the fraction Wx of the total sedentary time that is accumulated in bouts longer than any sedentary period of length x:

$$W_x = \frac{\int_x^\infty x \cdot p(x \cdot) dx \cdot}{\int_{x_{min}}^\infty x \cdot p(x \cdot) dx \cdot} \qquad (3)$$

The curves are then plotted as $Wx / p(x)$ pairs for each patient and control. Activity patterns were also assessed by assessing transitions from being inactive to active and normalized by the length of the recording, termed "Sedentary to Active Transitions". These data are presented as a percentage of the activity data per day. Subjective reports of habitual physical activity were assessed using the International Physical Activity Questionnaire (IPAQ) long form [20].

Clinical Presentations

Disease severity was assessed using the Newcastle Mitochondrial Disability Adult Scale (NMDAS) [21]. The NMDAS is a validated clinical rating scale consists of four domains: current function; system specific involvement; current clinical assessment; and quality of life. Each item within these domains is allocated one question with a six-point response scale scored between 0 (unaffected) and 5(severely affected). A low NMDAS score is advantageous and a high NMDAS score is disadvantageous for the patient. This tool semi-quantifies disease severity and longitudinally, can evaluate the long-term natural progression of mitochondrial myopathies.

Statistical Analysis

Assessment of normality was performed using a Shapiro Wilks Test and skewed data were transformed using natural logarithms or analysed using rank tests. Differences between patient and control group values were calculated and analysed using paired t-tests. The relationships between physical activity and clinical presentations in the patient group were determined using hierarchical regression, controlling for age, gender and BMI. Relationships between physical activity and BMI in patient and control groups were also determined using regression models, adjusted for age, gender and, where appropriate, disease severity. Variables included in the NMDAS were assessed using correlation and regression techniques to determine their relative contribution to the relationship between physical activity and disease severity. Assumption and diagnostic checks were performed on all data. All statistical analyses were performed using SPSS for Windows, version 16 (SPSS Inc., Illinois, USA). All values are expressed as mean ± SD unless otherwise stated.

Results

Baseline characteristics

General group descriptions stratified by genotype can be found in Table 1. Habitual physical activity was low, with 78% of the patient cohort taking less than 10,000 steps per day. Twenty-eight per cent of the mitochondrial disease group were overweight (BMI 25–29.9 kg/m²) and 20% were obese (BMI ≥30 kg/m²); only 4% were underweight (BMI<18.5 kg/m²). Patient characteristics (gender, age, BMI, number of steps walked per day, average METS and NMDAS score) were similar across genotype categories.

Age, gender, disease burden and physical activity

Mitochondrial disease patients performed significantly less physical activity than the control group (Table 1), with mean differences between groups of 3041 steps per day (95% CI 1966, 4117) and 0.09 average METs per day (95% CI 0.02, 0.16). A higher disease burden assessed by the NMDAS was associated

Table 1. Clinical, physical, and descriptors of habitual physical activity for all study participants and for subgroups by genetic mutation.

Genotype	N	Age	BMI	Clinical Rating (NMDAS)	Average Daily METS	Number of Steps Walked Per Day	Subjective recall of Physical activity (met.min.wk)
Point Mutations	47	47±12	25±6	21±14	1.4±0.3	6967±3760	2344±5253
Multiple Deletions	28	56±11	27±5	28±16	1.4±0.3	7162±4187	3414±1466
Single deletion	21	49±13	25±5	23±15	1.3±0.2	6360±3745	2125±2347
Complex deficiency	4	51±14	23±4	20±24	1.4±0.4	6715±7055	5494±5385
All patients	100	50±12	26±7	23±15	1.4±0.3*	6883±3944*	3356±5531
Control group	100	50±13	25±4	-	1.5±0.2	9924±4088	-

Data are expressed as Mean ± SD. * = significantly different from control group.

with a lower level of physical activity (Figure 1, steps / day; $r_s = -0.49$; 95% CI -0.33, -0.63, P<0.01; avMETs / day; $r_s = -0.30$; 95% CI -0.11, -0.47, p<0.01). After partitioning the variance accounted for by age, gender and BMI, the variance in physical activity (METs and steps, respectively) explained by disease severity was 4 – 15%.

The NMDAS subscales showing significant correlations with physical activity variables were entered into exploratory regression models; the only variable to be retained in all models following stepwise iterations was the exercise subscale, with R^2 values of 25% when steps per day was the response variable and 19% for METs. Physical activity as measured by METs was negatively associated with BMI in both patient and control groups, with a stronger relationship evident in the control group. In the patient group, METs was a significant predictor ($\beta = -0.32$, p = 0.002) of BMI and accounted for 10.3% of the variance after partialling out the effects of age, gender and disease severity. After adjusting for age and gender, METs was a significant predictor ($\beta = -0.67$, p<0.001) of, and accounted for 34.8% of the variance in, BMI in the control group. Physical activity as measured by steps per day was not a significant predictor of BMI in either patient or control groups.

Low levels of physical activity were common in the patient group, with half of the group having an average daily energy expenditure of less than 1.4 times their resting metabolic rate. Objective measures of physical activity were seen to be moderately associated with subjective reports of physical activity at work, leisure time, active transport (steps variable only) and with the amount of time (min) spent sitting per day ($0.25 < r_s < 0.35$; lowest 95% confidence limit 0.05, highest 0.51). Objective measures of physical activity were not associated with subjective reports during domestic & gardening activities.

Sedentary Activity

Power law analyses of the lengths of sedentary bouts demonstrate that patients with mitochondrial disease have a longer duration of sedentary bout (Figure 2A, Mean difference 0.02; 95% CI 0.01, 0.03, $t_{74} = 3.32$, p = 0.001). The number of transitions from being sedentary to activity were significantly lower in patients with mitochondrial disease compared with controls (Figure 2B, Mean difference -0.01; 95% CI -0.02, -0.00, $t_{75} = -2.78$, p = 0.007).

Discussion

This is the first study to report daily physical activity levels of people with mitochondrial disease. The major findings of this study

are: 1) a sedentary lifestyle is prominent in people with mitochondrial disease, 2) across all genotypes there is a significant inverse relationship between clinical rating and measures of physical activity, with patients with greater phenotypic disease burden undertaking less daily physical activity; and 3) 48% of the patient group were either overweight or obese; only 4% were underweight.

The first key observation was the low level of physical activity in the patient cohort; with 78% of the patients not achieving internationally advised levels of physical activity (10,000 steps per day [22]). The failure to achieve advised levels of physical activity is acknowledged to have an adverse influence upon healthy living, compounding metabolic diseases and reducing life expectancy [12,23,24]. Recent studies have suggested that sedentary behaviour, in contrast to active energy expenditure, is possibly a more important predictor of metabolic risk though its significant impact on metabolic regulation [24,25]. In this light, analysis of the raw physical activity data reveals that the average duration of sedentary periods is longer in patients with mitochondrial disease than controls. Breaks in sedentary time are also fewer than controls. Combined, these data suggest that patients with mitochondrial disease are at an increased risk of metabolic disease due to their low levels of physical activity and prominent sedentary behaviour, independent of their genetic predisposition.

Clinical rating was inversely related to habitual physical activity, with those undertaking less physical activity having greater physical impairment. The relationship between clinical rating and habitual physical activity is intuitive and follows similar relationships demonstrated in other metabolic disorders [24]. The large variation in physical activity data for people with similar disease burden also provides an insight into the ability of people with mitochondrial disease to maintain a physically active lifestyle. There are individuals with low clinical ratings (<4) who have no clinical reason to have low levels of physical activity, yet have very low levels of habitual physical activity (<2000 steps per day / <1.3 METS/day [Figure 1]). Conversely, there are those with high clinical ratings who do have significant physical impairment, yet achieve high levels of physical activity. As such, although clinical phenotype is broadly related to physical activity it is clear that clinical phenotype alone *does not* dictate the level of physical activity. This observation is of particular interest as several studies have now shown that the reversal of a sedentary lifestyle with exercise therapy confers benefits to mitochondrial function and have confirmed safety [14,15,16,17].

Additional information can be gleaned by analysis of the sub-scales of the NMDAS and the subjective reports of physical activity. Clinical sub-scales associated with physical function, such

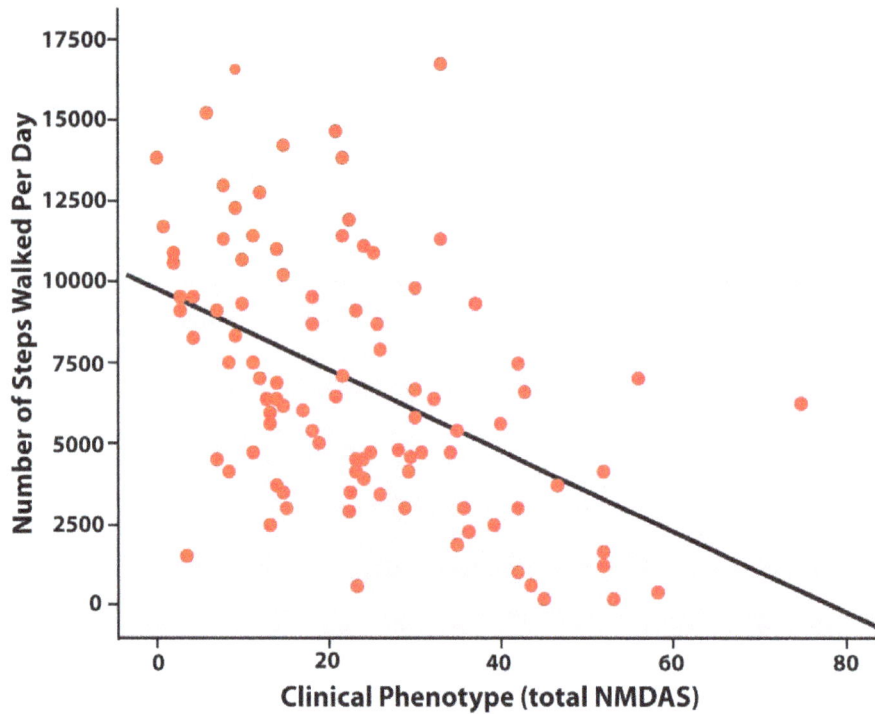

Figure 1. Scatter plot of the relationship between disease burden (total NMDAS score) and habitual physical activity (steps walked per day) (unadjusted regression line, R-Sq = 0.22, p<0.001). The red zone represents under and green zone over 10,000steps per day; the advised level of physical activity by the World Health Organisation [22] for health.

as cerebellar dysfunction and exercise intolerance were associated with low levels of physical activity. Again, there is significant breadth in the clinical presentations within these scales – with some phenotypically healthy individuals demonstrating low levels of physical activity and vice versa. There was no association between habitual physical activity and the subscales of myopathy

or neuropathy as may have been expected. This may in part be due to the mild nature of both parameters in this cohort. These observations suggest that disease burden is a strong predictor of habitual physical activity but is not the only determinant.

Subjective reports of physical activity provide information about where in everyday life people are physically active and where

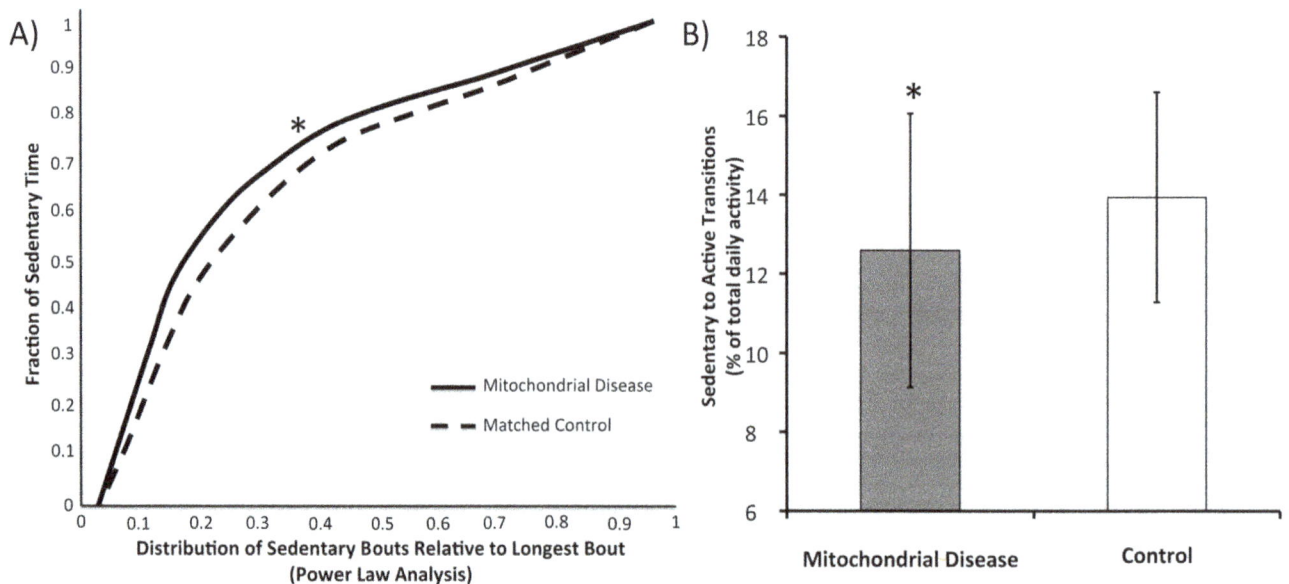

Figure 2. Power law analyses of the lengths of sedentary bouts of patients with mitochondrial disease [line] and controls [dashed] (Panel A). Sedentary to Active Transitions, indicating transition from inactive to active periods, in patients with mitochondrial disease [grey] and controls [open] (Panel B). Data are Mean ± SD. * = significantly different from control p = 0.007.

physical activity is reduced. These data reveal that work and leisure time physical activities were a key determinant of overall physical activity. Not surprisingly, low levels of daily physical activity are associated with high levels of sitting. These observations suggest that some of the key clinical presentations are associated with physical activity and that physical activity, in turn, is reduced in parts of the day where the patients'ave choice of movement, that is, work, leisure an d sitting. The high level of sitting time associated with mitochondrial disease is particularly of concern as high levels of sitting time are associated with a 2.5 times greater risk of heart disease and the development of metabolic syndrome [12,24]. The next challenge is to better understand how these areas of life can be targeted to increase physical activity, with a view to improving clinical features and reducing metabolic disease risk.

Almost half of the patients were overweight and one in five classified as obese [22]. This is contrary to historical descriptions of svelte body habitus of mitochondrial disease, particularly in relation to the 3243 A>G genotype [26]. This would suggest that people with mitochondrial disease are at added risk of high morbidity and mortality as posed by obesity and low physical activity in addition to the inherent predispositions that accompany mitochondrial disease.

These results show that the majority of people with mitochondrial disease lead an essentially sedentary lifestyle and that low levels of physical activity are related to clinical correlates of function and obesity. Combined, these observations suggest that low levels of physical activity, alongside a high prevalence of obesity, constitute significant disease risk factors in addition to the inherent predispositions that accompany mitochondrial disease and may represent a significant therapeutic target.

Author Contributions

Conceived and designed the experiments: SA GSG DMT MIT. Performed the experiments: SA GSG MIT. Analyzed the data: JLE LS TP MIT. Contributed reagents/materials/analysis tools: LS TP.

References

1. Hajnóczky G, Csordás G, Das S, Garcia-Perez C, Saotome M, et al. (2006) Mitochondrial calcium signalling and cell death: Approaches for assessing the role of mitochondrial Ca2+ uptake in apoptosis. Cell Calcium 40: 553–560.
2. Bride HM, Neuspiel M, Wasiak S (2006) Mitochondria: More Than Just a Powerhouse. Current Biology 16: R551–R560.
3. Green DR (1998) Apoptotic Pathways: The Roads to Ruin. Cell 94: 695–698.
4. Armstrong JS, Whiteman M, Yang H, Jones DP (2004) The redox regulation of intermediary metabolism by a superoxide-aconitase rheostat. BioEssays 26: 894–900.
5. Byrne E, Trounce I, Marzuki S, Dennett X, Berkovic SF, et al. (1991) Functional respiratory chain studies in mitochondrial cytopathies. Support for mitochondrial DNA heteroplasmy in myoclonus epilepsy and ragged red fibers (MERRF) syndrome. Acta Neuropathol 81: 318–323.
6. Chinnery PF, Howell N, Lightowlers RN, Turnbull DM (1997) Molecular pathology of MELAS and MERRF. The relationship between mutation load and clinical phenotypes. Brain 120: 1713–1721.
7. DiMauro S, Schon EA (2003) Mitochondrial Respiratory-Chain Diseases. N Engl J Med 348: 2656–2668.
8. Schaefer AM, Taylor RW, Turnbull DM (2001) The mitochondrial genome and mitochondrial muscle disorders. Current Opinion in Pharmacology 1: 288–293.
9. Chinnery PF, Johnson MA, Wardell TM, Singh-Kler R, Hayes C, et al. (2000) The epidemiology of pathogenic mitochondrial DNA mutations. Annals of Neurology 48: 188–193.
10. Taivassalo T, Jensen TD, Kennaway N, DiMauro S, Vissing J, et al. (2003) The spectrum of exercise tolerance in mitochondrial myopathies: a study of 40 patients. Brain 126: 413–423.
11. Gill TM, Robison JT, Tinetti ME (1997) Predictors of recovery in activities of daily living among disabled older persons living in the community. J Gen Intern Med 12: 757–762.
12. Morris JN, Heady J, Raffle P, Roberts C, Parks J (1953) Coronary heart-disease and physical activity of work. Lancet 28: 1111–1120.
13. Weller I, Corey P (1998) The Impact of Excluding Non-Leisure Energy Expenditure on the Relation between Physical Activity and Mortality in Women. Epidemiology 9: 632–635.
14. Trenell MI, Sue CM, Sachinwalla T, Kemp GJ, Thompson CH (2006) Aerobic exercise and muscle metabolism in patients with mitochondrial myopathy. Muscle Nerve 33: 524–531.
15. Murphy JL, Blakely EL, Schaefer AM, He L, Wyrick P, et al. (2008) Resistance training in patients with single, large-scale deletions of mitochondrial DNA. Brain 131: 2832–2840.
16. Jeppesen TD, Schwartz M, Olsen DB, Wibrand F, Krag T, et al. (2006) Aerobic training is safe and improves exercise capacity in patients with mitochondrial myopathy. Brain 129: 3402–3412.
17. Taivassalo T, Haller RG (2005) Exercise and Training in Mitochondrial Myopathies. Med Sci Sports Exerc 37: 2094–2101.
18. St-Onge M, Mignault D, Allison DB, Rabasa-Lhoret R (2007) Evaluation of a portable device to measure daily energy expenditure in free-living adults. Am J Clin Nutr 85: 742–749.
19. Chastin SFM, Granat MH (2009) Methods for objective measure, quantification and analysis of sedentary behaviour and inactivity. Gait & Posture 31: 82–86.
20. Hagströmer M, Oja P, Sjöström M (2006) The International Physical Activity Questionnaire (IPAQ): a study of concurrent and construct validity. Public Health Nutr 9: 755–762.
21. Schaefer AM, Phoenix C, Elson JL, McFarland R, Chinnery PF, et al. (2006) Mitochondrial disease in adults: A scale to monitor progression and treatment. Neurology 66: 1932–1934.
22. WHO (1995) Physical status: the use and interpretation of anthropometry. Geneva: World Health Organization.
23. Jonker JT, De Laet C, Franco OH, Peeters A, Mackenbach J, et al. (2006) Physical Activity and Life Expectancy With and Without Diabetes: Life table analysis of the Framingham Heart Study. Diabetes Care 29: 38–43.
24. Healy G, Wijndaele K, Dunstan D, Shaw J, Salmon J, et al. (2008) Objectively Measured Sedentary Time, Physical Activity, and Metabolic Risk: The Australian Diabetes, Obesity and Lifestyle Study (AusDiab). Diab Care 31: 369–371.
25. Hamilton MT, Hamilton DG, Zderic TW (2007) Role of Low Energy Expenditure and Sitting in Obesity, Metabolic Syndrome, Type 2 Diabetes, and Cardiovascular Disease. Diabetes 56: 2655–2667.
26. Di Mauro S, Bonilla E (1997) Mitochondrial encephalomyopathies. In: Rosenberg RN, Prusiner SB, Di Mauro S, Barch RL, eds. The molecular and genetic basis of neurological disease Boston: Butterworth-Heinemann. pp 201–235.

6

A Randomized, Controlled, Trial of Short Cycle Intermittent Compared to Continuous Antiretroviral Therapy for the Treatment of HIV Infection in Uganda

Steven J. Reynolds[1,2]*, Cissy Kityo[3], Claire W. Hallahan[1], Geoffrey Kabuye[3], Diana Atwiine[3], Frank Mbamanya[3], Francis Ssali[3], Robin Dewar[4], Marybeth Daucher[1], Richard T. Davey, Jr.[1], Peter Mugyenyi[3], Anthony S. Fauci[1], Thomas C. Quinn[1,2], Mark R. Dybul[5,6]

1 National Institute of Allergy and Infectious Diseases, National Institutes of Health, Bethesda, Maryland, United States of America, 2 Johns Hopkins University School of Medicine, Baltimore, Maryland, United States of America, 3 Joint Clinical Research Center, Kampala, Uganda, 4 SAIC-Frederick, Inc., National Cancer Institute, National Institutes of Health, Bethesda, Maryland, United States of America, 5 O'Neill Institute for National and Global Health Law, Georgetown University Law Center, Washington, D. C., United States of America, 6 George W. Bush Institute, Dallas, Texas, United States of America

Abstract

Background: Short cycle treatment interruption could reduce toxicity and drug costs and contribute to further expansion of antiretroviral therapy (ART) programs.

Methods: A 72 week, non-inferiority trial enrolled one hundred forty six HIV positive persons receiving ART (CD4+ cell count ≥ 125 cells/mm^3 and HIV RNA plasma levels <50 copies/ml) in one of three arms: continuous, 7 days on/7 days off and 5 days on/2 days off treatment. Primary endpoint was ART treatment failure determined by plasma HIV RNA level, CD4+ cell count decrease, death attributed to study participation, or opportunistic infection.

Results: Following enrollment of 32 participants, the 7 days on/7 days off arm was closed because of a failure rate of 31%. Six of 52 (11.5%) participants in the 5 days on/2 days off arm failed. Five had virologic failure and one participant had immunologic failure. Eleven of 51 (21.6%) participants in the continuous treatment arm failed. Nine had virologic failure with 1 death (lactic acidosis) and 1 clinical failure (extra-pulmonary TB). The upper 97.5% confidence boundary for the difference between the percent of non-failures in the 5 days on/2 days off arm (88.5% non-failure) compared to continuous treatment (78.4% non failure) was 4.8% which is well within the preset non-inferiority margin of 15%. No significant difference was found in time to failure in the 2 study arms (p = 0.39).

Conclusions: Short cycle 5 days on/2 days off intermittent ART was at least as effective as continuous therapy.

Editor: Sean Emery, University of New South Wales, Australia

Funding: The study was funded through the Laboratory of Immunoregulation, Division of Intramural Research, National Institute of Allergy and Infectious Diseases, National Institutes of Health. SJR, CWH, MD, RTD, ASF, TCQ & MAD were employees of the NIH during the study design and implementation period and were involved in study design, conduct and publication.

Competing Interests: The authors have declared that no competing interests exist.

* E-mail: sjr@jhmi.edu

Introduction

Combination antiretroviral therapy (ART) has significantly decreased morbidity and mortality for HIV-infected persons who have access to such therapy.[1–3] However, it is now clear that currently available medications will not eradicate or "cure" HIV disease making lifelong therapy a necessity. Although there have been advances in treatment options that have reduced pill burden and frequency of dosing, the need for daily dosing poses challenges for long term adherence. While newer formulations of antiretroviral drugs (ARVs) have reduced certain toxicities, other significant complications remain and continued exposure has revealed new toxicities.[4,5] Long term toxicities can affect adherence as well as the effectiveness of treatment.[6] Several significant international and

domestic initiatives have greatly expanded ART in resource limited settings. Further reductions in the cost of ARVs could increase the reach of such programs. Recently, guidance has shifted to earlier initiation of ART and ART has been suggested as a prevention strategy.[7,8] ART approaches that reduce cost and toxicity while potentially increasing adherence could significantly enhance the feasibility of the implementation of such strategies on a large scale.

Researchers have previously evaluated several approaches of structured treatment interruptions to enhance adherence and reduce toxicity and cost.[9–11] It is now clear that long cycle interruptions of ART that allow a rebound of plasma HIV RNA are not clinically beneficial. The SMART and TRIVICAN trials showed significant increases in death and opportunistic infections with long cycles of treatment interruptions, consistent with previous trials showing virologic and immunologic failure with such strategies.[12–14] In sharp contrast, short cycle interruptions are designed specifically to maintain suppression of plasma HIV RNA below the limit of assay detection. In pilot studies conducted in the United States of short cycle interruptions designed to maintain suppression of plasma HIV RNA below the limit of detection, we observed that 7 days on and 7 days off ARV maintained suppression of plasma HIV RNA below the limit of detection and reduced certain laboratory markers of toxicity with certain regimens.[10,15] However, strict adherence to the 7 day cycles was essential for the success of such an approach. Because of the potential difficulty for certain individuals to maintain strict adherence to such cycles, we reasoned that more "user-friendly" short cycle ARV interruption approaches could have greater implementation feasibility and clinical relevance. Based on these findings, we initiated a randomized, controlled, non-inferiority trial of two short cycle intermittent ART regimens (7 days on and 7 days off and 5 days on and 2 days off) compared to continuous ART. Because of the potential applicability of those strategies to resource limited settings, the study was conducted in Uganda. The 5 days on 2 days off regimen was based on the known kinetics of the rebound of plasma HIV RNA following a discontinuation of ART and the potential clinical applicability of a regimen that allowed treatment interruptions on weekends which could allow for novel approaches such as directly observed therapy (DOT) in certain settings such as schools and the workplace and could be useful in expanding the use of ART earlier in the course of disease.[16]

We here report an evaluation of a randomized, controlled, non-inferiority trial of two regimens of short cycle intermittent compared to continuous ART on virologic, immunologic, toxicity and adherence parameters.

Methods

The protocol for this trial and supporting CONSORT checklist are available as supporting information; see Checklist S1 and Protocol S1.

Participants

Ethics Statement: The study protocol was reviewed and approved by the Uganda National Council for Science and Technology (UNCST), and by the Institutional Review Boards (IRBs) of the National AIDS Research Committee of the UNCST, Uganda and the National Institute of Allergy and Infectious Diseases, National Institutes of Health (NIAID/NIH).

HIV-infected persons receiving ART at the Joint Clinical Research Center (JCRC) in Kampala, Uganda, with a CD4+ cell count equal to or greater than 125 cells/mm^3 of whole blood and plasma HIV RNA below 50 copies per milliliter of plasma were eligible following signed informed consent. A confirmatory HIV test was required prior to enrollment. Participants were required to be receiving at least 3 ARVs including a protease inhibitor or the non-nucleoside reverse transcriptase inhibitor, efavirenz. Patients receiving a nevirapine-based regime were required to switch to a protease inhibitor or efavirenz if they were randomized to the interrupted arm. Nine patients in the 5 days on/2 days off arm and 7 participants in the 7 days on/7 days off arm were on nevirapine and switched to efavirenz for study enrollment. Stavudine was dosed by weight, participants weighing >60 kg received 40 mg, those weighing <60 kg received 30 mg. All participants paid for their ARVs, consistent with standard practice at the JCRC. It should be noted that at the time the study was initiated, large international programs to support the cost of ART had not begun.

Such programming was not available until a large number of patients had already been enrolled. It was the decision of the investigators and the review boards that changing the payment practices mid-study could bias the results. Trial oversight was provided by and independent Data Safety and Monitoring Board (DSMB). Clinicaltrials.gov registry number NCT00339456.

Study design

The study was designed to test non-inferiority of two short cycle intermittent ART regimens (7 days on/7 days off and 5 days on/2 days off) compared to continuous ART with 57 patients (52 plus 5 allowed for attrition) randomized in a 1-1-1 manner to each arm and followed for 72 weeks (73 weeks for the interrupted arms because all lab tests were done during on-treatment periods). The primary endpoint was ART treatment failure determined by a plasma HIV RNA level equal to or greater than 10,000 copies on any one evaluation, a plasma HIV RNA level equal to or greater than 1,000 copies on two consecutive measurements, a plasma HIV RNA level greater than 400 copies/ml at the end of the study, a CD4+ cell count decrease of greater than 30 percent from baseline on 2 consecutive measurements, death attributed to study participation or occurrence of an opportunistic infection. The primary endpoint was changed during the study by the protocol team from <50 copies/ml to <400 copies/ml (end of study) to eliminate the inclusion of low-level viral blips. Patients who experienced treatment failure received standard clinical care in Uganda including switching of ARV regimen, where appropriate. They were followed until 30 days after their plasma viremia and/or CD4+ cell count returned to baseline if they changed therapy or for 30 days from the time of treatment failure if they decided not to change therapy. Laboratory safety monitoring and HIV viral load measurements (Amplicor HIV-1 Monitor v1.5 – Roche, Switzerland) were performed on site at the JCRC. HIV genotyping (Trugene HIV-1 Genotyping Kit, Visible Genetics – Siemens Healthcare Diagnostics, Inc., Tarrytown, NY) was performed off-site at SAIC-Frederick, Inc., Frederick, Maryland.

Data collection and follow-up

Participants were evaluated for standard clinical, virologic, immunologic, and adherence parameters at weeks 2 and 4 following enrollment (interrupted arms only, not included in outcome analysis) and every 6 weeks thereafter including toxicity monitoring (renal toxicity, ALT and AST were evaluated every 12 weeks and lipid profiles were done every 6 months). Lipodystropy, peripheral neuropathy and lactic acidosis were determined by the treating physician's assessment, clinical symptoms and laboratory confirmation (serum lactate). All laboratory evaluations were provided to the participants free of charge. Intervening visits were scheduled based on clinical standard of care or relevant failure parameters. All evaluations except the end of study evaluation were performed at the end of the off drug period in the intermittent arm. Adherence to ART was measured using patient maintained study calendars which were recorded at all study visits, adherence rates based on self-reported diaries were then calculated based on the percentage of drugs taken.

Interim monitoring of safety and efficacy

An independent data and safety monitoring board (DSMB) reviewed all safety data and treatment failures on a bi-annual basis and at least yearly after 50% of participants were enrolled in each treatment arm.

Statistical analysis

A sample size of 57 individuals in each treatment group (52 plus 5 allowed for attrition) was determined for a 95% non-failure rate in each study group with a non-inferiority margin of 15%, an alpha (type I error) of 0.025 and 81% power using the Farrington and Manning method.[17] The non-inferiority of the 5 days on/2 days off ART arm to continuous ART arm was assessed by constructing the upper limit of a 97.5% confidence interval for the difference in proportions, continuous ART minus 5 days on/2 days off, of those successfully completing the study.[18]

Paired differences and the median correlations, determined by the Spearman rank method, were tested for significance by the Wilcoxon sign rank test. The Wilcoxon two-sample test was used to compare independent groups, and Fisher's exact test was used to compare frequencies of categorical variables. Comparison of Kaplan-Meier survival curves was done by the log-rank test. The significance of the ratios of rates of occurrences of adverse events was determined by the exact rate ratio test based on the Poisson distribution. Exact methods were used so that p values and confidence intervals are properly defined even when the counts are very small or zero.[19] The calculations were done using the 'rateratio test' R package. [20] Adjustment of p values for multiple testing was performed by the Bonferroni method.

Role of the funding source

The study was funded through the Division of Intramural Research, NIAID/NIH. SJR, CWH, MD, RTD, ASF, TCQ & MAD were employees of the NIAID/NIH during the study design and implementation period.

Results

Study Population

A total of 146 HIV-positive participants were enrolled in the trial between 2002 and 2005: 32 in the 7 days on/7 days off arm, 57 in the 5 days on/2 days off arm and 57 in the continuous arm. Five individuals in the 5 days on 2 days off group left the study (2 lost-to-follow-up, 1 relocated, 1 reverted to continuous ART and 1 with renal failure died). Five in the continuous arm were lost-to-follow-up resulting in 52 with data in the interrupted and 51 in the continuous arm at week 72/73 (Figure 1). Fifty-six participants in the continuous arm (one withdrew without participating and was excluded from analysis) and 57 participants in the 5 days on/2 days off ART are included in the intent-to-treat analysis. Table 1 summarizes the key baseline characteristics of the participants. The groups were similar in all characteristics upon study entry.

Primary endpoint

Following the enrollment of 32 participants in the 7 days on and 7 days off arm, the DSMB agreed with the principal investigator to terminate that arm because of a failure rate of 31% found during the interim analysis in the fall of 2004 (3 participants had withdrawn and 9/29 remaining participants had failed).

Six of 52 (11.5%) participants who completed the 5 days on/2 days off arm failed. Five of these participants had virologic failure all with a viral load greater than 10,000 copies/ml (median VL = 50,130 copies/ml; interquartile range (IQR) 14,398 to 50,551 and one participant had immunologic failure. In comparison, eleven of 51 (21.6%) participants who completed the continuous treatment arm failed. Nine of these participants had virologic failure. Six failed with a viral load greater than 10,000 copies/ml, one with a viral load greater than 1,000 and 2 with a viral load greater than 400 at week 72(median VL = 24,410 copies/ml; IQR: 4,394 to 86,316 copies/ml) The

remaining 2 failures included 1 death (lactic acidosis) and 1 clinical failure (extra-pulmonary TB). The upper 97.5% confidence boundary for the difference between the percent of non-failures in the 5 days on/2 days off (88.5% non-failure) arm compared to continuous treatment (78.4% non failure) was 4.8% which is well within the preset non-inferiority margin of 15%. In the modified intent-to-treat analysis which designated the 5 in each group who discontinued treatment as failures, the upper 97.5% confidence boundary for the difference between the percent of non-failures in the 5 days on/2 days off, 80.7% (46 of 57), and that in the continuously treated, 71.4% (40 of 56) was 6.6% which is within the preset non-inferiority margin of 15%. In the intent-to-treat analysis with 57 in each group, the upper 97.5% confidence boundary for the difference between the 80.7% (46 of 57) non-failures in the 5 days on/2 days off, and the 70.2% (40 of 57) non-failures in the continuously treated arm was 5.4% which is again well within the preset non-inferiority margin of 15%. No significant difference was found in time to failure in the 2 study arms, p = 0.39 (Figure 2).

Immunologic responses to treatment

As mentioned above, only 1 participant in the 5 days on/2 days off arm failed by protocol defined immunologic criteria (CD4 decrease of >30% on 2 consecutive measurements) at week 12 of follow-up. This participant remained virologically suppressed (<50 copies/ml) through week 73 suggesting that this was not a true failure but merely a fluctuation in CD4+ T cell count. CD4+ T cell counts were correlated with weeks on treatment in the continuous treatment arm (median r = 0.54, p<0.001) and in the 5 days on, 2 days off arm (r = 0.57, p<0.001). The correlations in the two groups were not statistically different (p = 0.33). For the 46 individuals in the 5 days on/2 off arm and the 40 in the continuously treated arm who successfully completed the study the median CD4+ T cell counts at baseline were similar in the two arms (255 and 271/mm^3, respectively, p = 0.85), at week 24 (347 and 293/mm^3, respectively, p = 0.30), at week 48 (399 and 318/mm^3, respectively, p = 0.55) and marginally different at week 72/73 (p = 0.08)(Figure 3A). The median paired changes in CD4+ T cells from baseline were not statistically different at week 24 (48 and 15/mm^3, respectively, p = 0.21) nor at week 48 (90 and 69/mm^3, respectively, p = 0.90). The median paired difference in CD4+ T cells was statistically greater in the 5 days on/2 days off arm at week 72/73 (p = 0.01)(Figure 3B) None of the virologic failures experienced a corresponding immunologic failure during follow-up.

Toxicity

The rates of lactic acidosis, lipodystrophy and peripheral neuropathy were compared among participants receiving stavudine within the continuous versus 5 days on/2 days off ART groups. The data were normalized for comparison between groups by reporting data as events per 100 person years. Among the 40 participants receiving continuous stavudine, 5 cases of lactic acidosis as determined by clinical findings and arterial blood levels of lactate occurred (resulting in one death), with an incidence of 11.4/100 person years, whereas no occurrences of lactic acidosis occurred among 44 participants receiving intermittent ART that included stavudine (p = 0.04). A reduction in lipodystrophy was also observed with 5 cases in the continuous treatment arm (incidence 11.4/100 person-years) compared with 1 case in the intermittent treatment arm (incidence 1.8/100 person-years) (p = 0.13). The rate of lipodystrophy in the continuous arm was 6.2 times the rate in the 5 days on and 2 days off arm (95% confidence interval {CI}: 0.7, 293). The rates of peripheral neuropathy were similar in both arms (Table 2) with the occurrence in the continuous arm 1.5 times (95%

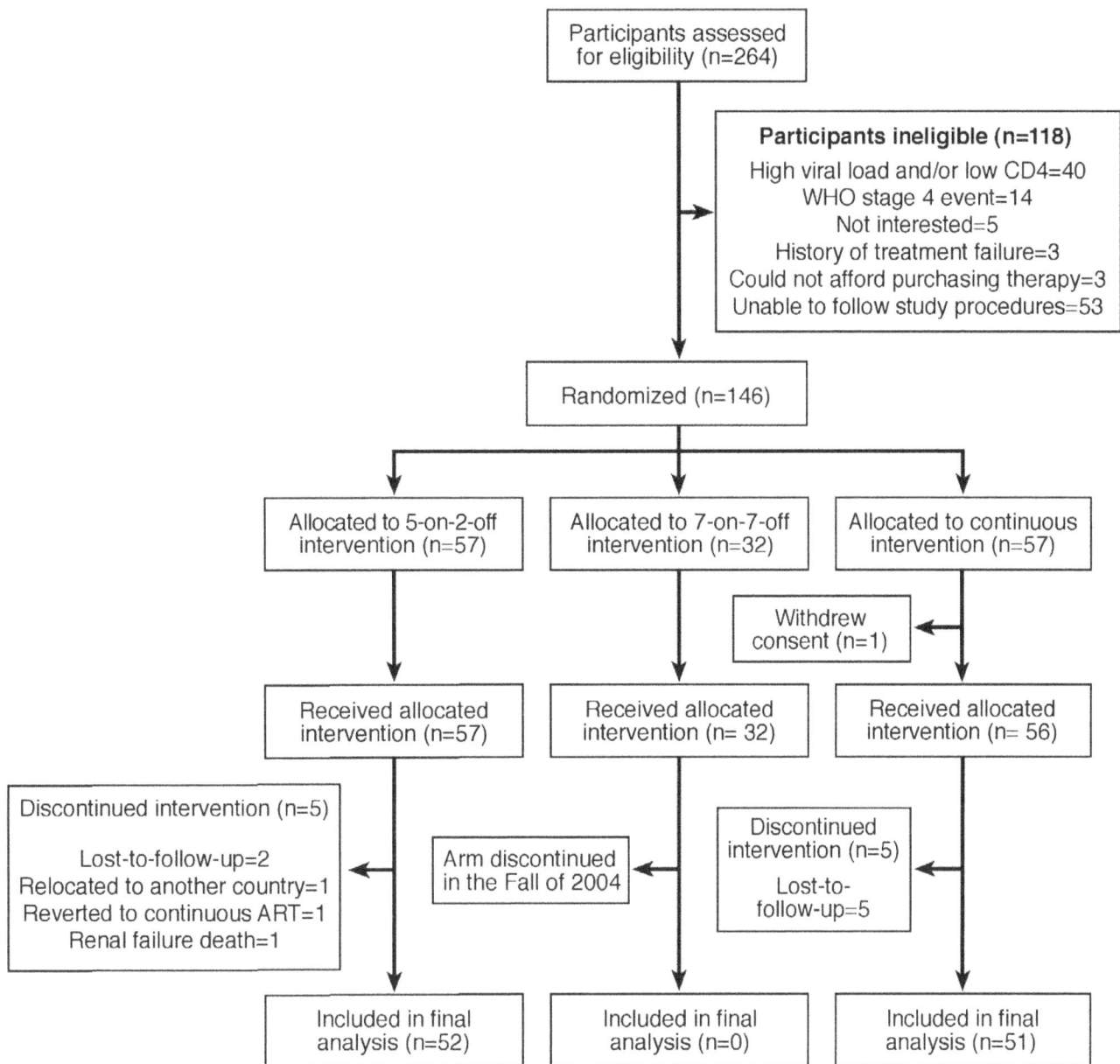

Figure 1. Flow diagram for study eligibility and follow-up.

CI: 0.4, 6.2) that in the intermittent treatment arm. Because there were no cases of lactic acidosis in the 5 days on 2 days off arm, the ratio comparing the continuous and intermittent rates was infinite with a 95% CI lower limit of 1.13, i.e. greater than 1. Participants who developed lipodystrophy, peripheral neuropathy or lactic acidosis were switched from stavudine to zidovudine as standard of care at the time.

One patient receiving 5 days on and 2 days off ART died from chronic renal failure that predated enrollment; the event was determined to be unrelated to the study by investigators in Uganda. The patient had a plasma HIV RNA level of less than 50 copies per milliliter of plasma at death and a CD4+ T cell count at baseline and death of 171 and 349, respectively. No other significant hepatotoxicity, renal toxicity or anemia were observed during follow up with similar AST, ALT and creatinine measurements between study arms at 73 weeks (Table 2). Median

LDL cholesterol levels were slightly lower at 73 weeks comparing continuous versus intermittent treatment arms (96 versus 123, $p = 0.08$).

Adherence

Overall adherence to ARVs for the study was greater than 95% in both study arms based on participant diaries. Pharmacy records were consistent with the high level of reported adherence measured during the study (data not shown).

Antiretroviral resistance

Clinical monitoring of mutations associated with antiretroviral drugs resistance was not available in Uganda during the study period. Consistent with standard clinical care at the JCRC and per protocol, and with review and monitoring by the DSMB and the IRB, patients were evaluated for failure by laboratory and clinical

Table 1. Baseline Characteristics.

Baseline Characteristic	Continuous n = 56	5 Days On/2 Days Off n = 57	7 Days On/7 Days Off** n = 32
Age (year)	38 (33,44)*	38 (34, 46)	38 (32, 43)
Females	36 (64%)	35 (61%)	21 (66%)
Males	20 (36%)	22 (39%)	11 (34%)
BMI#	25 (22,29)	25 (23, 29)	25 (22, 29)
CD4 T cells (cells/mm)	262 (192,389)	264 (219, 405)	268 (213, 375)
HIV RNA (copies/ml)	<50 (<50, <50)	<50 (<50, <50)	<50 (<50, <50)
PI based regimen	1 (1.8%)	1 (1.8%)	2 (6.2%)
NNRTI based regimen	55 (98%)	56 (98%)	30 (94%)
Stavudine backbone	40 (71%)	44 (77%)	21 (66%)
Zidovudine backbone	16 (29%)	13 (23%)	11 (34%)
Pre-study ART exposure time (weeks)(IQR)	49 (29–83)	48 (30–69)	46 (33,76)

#n = 55 in Continuous arm.
*Median (IQR).
**The 7 days on and 7 days off arm was closed following enrollment of 32 participants because of a 31% failure rate in this group found during interim analysis.

evaluations and treated according to standard clinical practice including switching of ARV regimen where appropriate. Genotypic evaluation of mutations associated with ARV resistance was performed by SAIC-Frederick, Inc., Frederick, Maryland and the results were made available to clinicians in Uganda.

Genotyping was performed on 4 out of 5 of the participants in the 5 days on 2 days off arm at the first viral load measured >1000 copies/ml. Each participant was receiving an efavirenz-based regimen that included lamivudine and each had mutations consistent with resistance to efavirenz and lamivudine (Table 3). No participant developed thymidine analogue mutations (TAMS) or evidence of nucleoside analogue resistance apart from one individual who developed an A62V insertion as previously reported.[21] Genotyping was also performed on 5 of the 7 participants in the continuous treatment arm who developed virologic failure during follow-up (first VL>1000 copies/ml). Two participants had wild type virus, 3 had mutations consistent with resistance to efavirenz and one had a mutation consistent with resistance to lamivudine. None of the participants in the

continuous arm had TAMS or nucleoside analogue resistance, as previously reported.[21]

Discussion

The present study demonstrates that short cycle intermittent ART defined as 5 days on/2 days off is at least as effective as continuous ART over a 72/73 week follow-up period. The data are consistent with the results of a pilot study that was begun in the United States after this randomized, controlled trial was underway and with a recent report of significantly increased risk of failure with interruptions beyond 2 days.[22,23] Our findings are also consistent with those of the FOTO study which found that participants on a 5 day on/2 day off interruption strategy receiving tenofovir, emtricitabine and efavirenz maintained virologic suppression at 24 weeks.[24] The primary endpoint, ART treatment failure, was reached by a lower percentage of participants in the intermittent arm than the continuous treatment arm by 73 weeks of study follow-up. The early termination of the 7 days on/7 days off arm due to a high failure rate was consistent with another trial reported after the present study was begun.[25] It is important to point out that failures that have been reported in treatment interruption studies have invariably been associated with a rebound in plasma viremia during the period of intermittent discontinuation of ARVs.[12,13] Such rebounds are generally associated with the emergence of drug resistance and the depletion of CD4+ T cells.[12,26] We chose the 5 days on/2 days off regimen of treatment interruption to study because previous experience with the kinetics of plasma rebound following interruption of ART strongly indicates that plasma viremia that had been suppressed below the level of detection (<50 copies per ml) by ART does not generally rebound during the 2 day drug-interruption period.

Although the trial was not powered to show superiority, it was interesting that there were nearly twice as many failures in the continuous arm compared to the 5 days on/2 days off arm (11 and 6, respectively). The adherence data collected indicated high levels of adherence in each arm. However, 2 of 5 participants with virologic failure in the continuous arm evaluated for drug resistance had wild-type virus, suggesting poor adherence. Those results are compatible with the possibility that scheduled

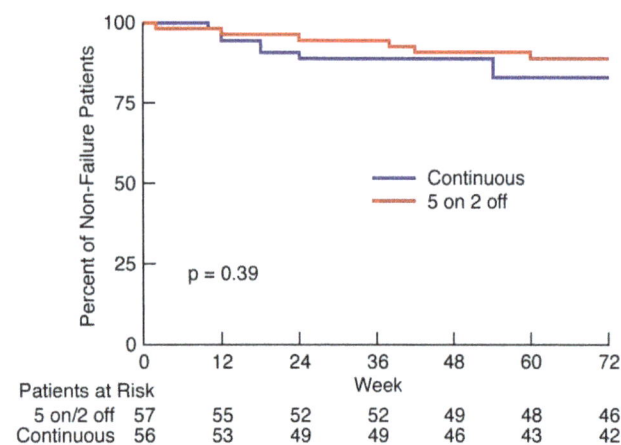

Figure 2. Kaplan-Meier Survival Curve with Time to Failure. No difference was found in the time to failure in the 2 groups during the 72/73 week study.

A **B**

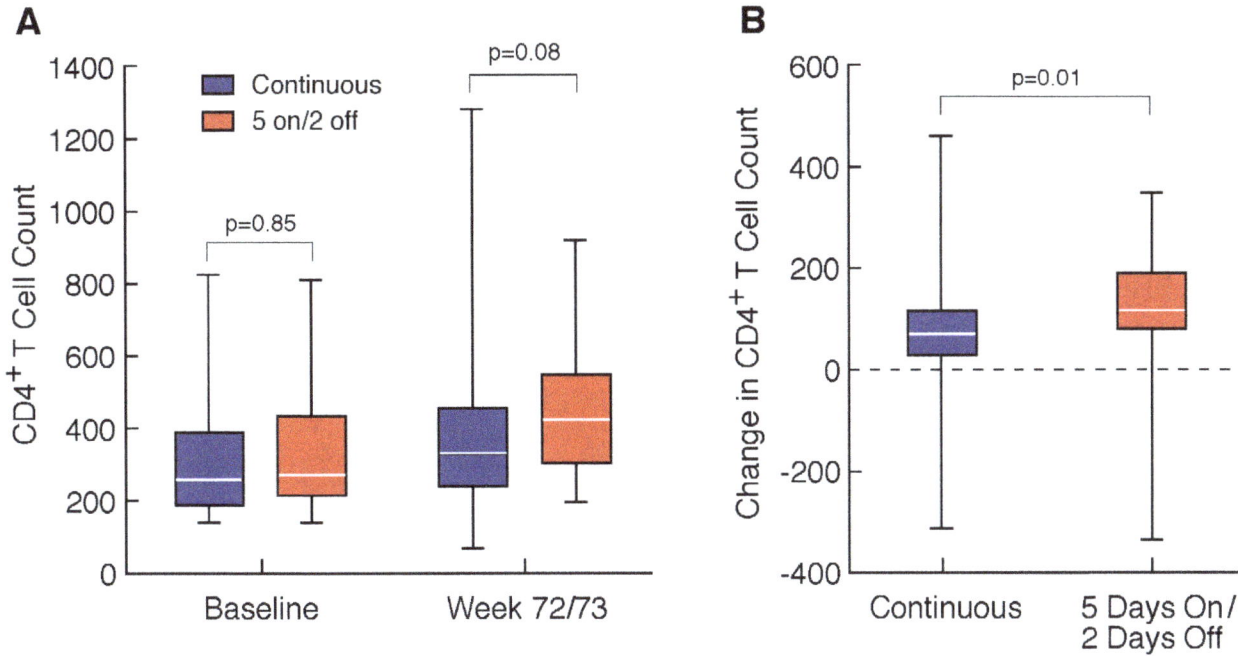

Figure 3. A. Change in CD4+ T cells for participants successfully completing 72/73 weeks. The CD4+ T cell counts in the continuously treated (N = 40) and in the 5 days on/2 days off (N = 46) arms were similar at baseline (255 and 271/mm^3, respectively, p = 0.85) and marginally different at week 72/73 (330 and 429/mm^3, respectively, p = 0.08). B. The median paired difference in CD4+ T cells between baseline and week 72/73 was greater in the 5 days on/2 days off group (114/mm^3) than in the continuously treated group (68/mm^3). (p = 0.01). The lines across the box indicates the median values; the boxes contain the 25–75% interquartile range; and the whiskers extend to the highest and lowest values.

interruptions promote adherence during the on-drug period. All participants in the 5 days on/2 days off arm developed genetic mutations consistent with resistance to both lamivudine and efavirenz while 3 of 5 participants in the continuous arm developed mutations consistent with resistance to efavirenz and only 1 developed resistance to lamivudine with a second participant developing lamivudine resistance at a later follow-up

visit. Our study was not powered to specifically look at differences in genotypic resistance patterns and also used self-reported adherence, known to be an imperfect measure, limiting our ability to draw any firm conclusions from these findings.[27]

There was evidence of reduced toxicities associated with intermittent ART. This was particularly striking among the subset of participants receiving stavudine containing ART which is

Table 2. Toxicity.

Event (cases/100py)*	Continuous	5 Days On/2 Days Off	p-value
Lactic Acidosis	11.4	0	0.04
Lipodystrophy	11.4	1.8	0.13
Peripheral neuropathy	13.7	9.2	0.72
Cholesterol/LFTs			
Creatinine**			
at week 72/73			
Median (IQR) [N]			
Total Cholesterol (mg/dL)	176 (141-194) [38]	192 (174-220) [43]	0.15
LDL Cholesterol (mg/dL)	96 (76-127) [36]	123 (106-139) [43]	0.08
HDL Cholesterol (mg/dL)	42 (35-50) [37]	45 (34-58) [43]	0.99
Triglycerides (mg/dL)	149 (88-212) [36]	144 (98-212) [42]	0.99
AST (IU/L)	21 (16-31) [27]	22 (17-24) [35]	0.99
ALT (IU/L)	20 (14-32) [27]	18 (13-25) [35]	0.99
Creatinine (mg/dL)	0.74 (0.62-0.83) [35]	0.76 (0.68-090) [43]	0.54

*stavudine patient years, subanalysis of participants receiving stavudine containing regimens.
**Cholesterol, liver function tests and creatinine for patients followed 72/73 weeks (all HAART regimens).

Table 3. Reverse Transcriptase Genotypic Resistance Among Participants with Virologic Failure.

Participant	Study Arm	Failure Week	HIV RNA Level (copies/ml)	Major RT Mutations
6	5 on/2 off	38	50 130	K103N, M184V
31	5 on/2 off	42	60 899	K103N, M184V
248	5 on/2 off	12	14 398	K101P, K103N
				M184V
258	5 on/2 off	60	50 551	K103N, V1081
				M184V, P225H
9	Continuous	18	24 400	K103N
21	Continuous	54	205 517	None
81	Continuous	72	4 394	Genotype failed
98	Continuous	24	56 800	K103N, M1841
245	Continuous	18	18 933	None
256	Continuous	54	128 231	K103N

commonly used in resource limited settings despite efforts to replace it with other nucleoside reverse transcriptase inhibitors. We observed a marked reduction in the rate of lactic acidosis among participants receiving intermittent stavudine with no cases detected in this group compared to 5 cases in the continuous treatment arm. A similar although not statistically significant reduction in lipodystrophy was also observed among participants receiving intermittent stavudine in our study. This finding is consistent with reports that mitochondrial toxicity associated with stavudine appears to be at least partially dose dependent.[28] Of note, lipodystrophy was physician defined which could result in measurement bias. If larger clinical trials validate reductions in debilitating and fatal adverse reactions observed in this trial, short cycle structured treatment interruptions could have particular relevance for earlier initiation of ART and ART as a viable prevention strategy.

Immunologic responses to ART were robust in both intermittent and continuous treatment arms. Although there was a significantly greater increase in CD4+ T cell counts between arms for patients followed more than 52 weeks, the clinical relevance of this finding is unclear. Larger trials would be needed to validate those results and to determine their clinical significance. Consistent with recent publications from other resource limited settings, immunologic failure was not observed despite several episodes of virologic failure.[29–31] Of note, none of the participants in this study who had developed virologic failure and genetic mutations associated with ARV resistance would have been detected by the current WHO guidelines for determining ARV failure and changing to second line regimens based on immunologic criteria alone, highlighting the role of virologic evaluations to determine treatment failure.[32]

The present study has several limitations. It was not powered to evaluate superiority or long term outcomes including death. The protocol included only subjects on efavirenz in the intermittent arms due to the concern of nevirapine resistance. Because nevirapine is extensively used in low and middle income countries this might limit the applicability of our findings. The continuous treatment arm had a higher than expected failure rate than used in the original statistical design which could impact on the overall conclusion of non-inferiority. The methodology used to measure adherence relied on participant diaries which may not reflect the true adherence levels of the different treatment arms in the study.

Finally, the patient population at the JCRC tended to be of higher socioeconomic status during the time of the study and thus, most were able to pay for their ART. A larger trial will be needed to more fully address short cycle intermittent therapy among patients representing a wide range of demographics.

Since 5 days on/2 days off intermittent therapy has been shown to be as least as effective as continuous therapy, this strategy could have particular importance for programs of directly observed therapy (DOT) for difficult to treat populations including children and adolescents attending school 5 days a week. It could also be relevant for workplace programs. The possibility of decreased toxicity could be relevant as treatment guidelines shift to initiating ART earlier in the course of disease. Drug treatment costs could also be 29 percent lower with a 5 days on/2 days off treatment regimen. Finally, as guidance shifts to earlier initiation of ART, a less expensive, "user-friendly" approach with reduced toxicity could be significant for scale-up of those strategies, particularly in the developing world.

Acknowledgments

The authors would like to thank the staff at the Joint Clinical Research Center in Kampala, Uganda and the study participants for their participation in this study and John Weddle for assistance with the figures included in the manuscript. Presented at the combined ICAAC/IDSA meeting in Washington, DC, October 25–28, 2009, abstract number H–1250.

Author Contributions

Conceived and designed the experiments: CK FS RTDJ PM ASF MRD. Performed the experiments: SJR CK GK DA FM FS RD RTDJ PM TCQ MRD. Analyzed the data: SJR CWH TCQ MRD. Contributed reagents/materials/analysis tools: RD MD ASF. Wrote the paper: SJR CK CWH GK DA FM FS MD RTDJ PM ASF TCQ MRD.

References

1. Bussmann H, Wester CW, Ndwapi N, Grundmann N, Gaolathe T, et al. (2008) Five-year outcomes of initial patients treated in Botswana's National Antiretroviral Treatment Program. AIDS 22: 2303–2311.
2. Jahn A, Floyd S, Crampin AC, Mwaungulu F, Mvula H, et al. (2008) Population-level effect of HIV on adult mortality and early evidence of reversal after introduction of antiretroviral therapy in Malawi. Lancet 371: 1603–1611.

3. Lowrance DW, Makombe S, Harries AD, Shiraishi RW, Hochgesang M, et al. (2008) A public health approach to rapid scale-up of antiretroviral treatment in Malawi during 2004–2006. J Acquir Immune Defic Syndr 49: 287–293.

4. McComsey GA, Libutti DE, O'Riordan M, Shelton JM, Storer N, et al. (2008) Mitochondrial RNA and DNA alterations in HIV lipoatrophy are linked to antiretroviral therapy and not to HIV infection. Antivir Ther 13: 715–722.

5. Nelson M, Azwa A, Sokwala A, Harania RS, Stebbing J (2008) Fanconi syndrome and lactic acidosis associated with stavudine and lamivudine therapy. AIDS 22: 1374–1376.

6. Parruti G, Manzoli L, Toro PM, D'Amico G, Rotolo S, et al. (2006) Long-term adherence to first-line highly active antiretroviral therapy in a hospital-based cohort: predictors and impact on virologic response and relapse. AIDS Patient Care STDS 20: 48–56.

7. Panel on Antiretroviral Guidelines for Adults and Adolescents. Guidelines for the Use of antiretroviral agents in HIV-1 infected adults and adolescents. Department of Health and Human Services. December 1, 2009; 1–161. Available at http://www.aidsinfo.nih.gov/ContentFiles/AdultandAdolescentGL.pdf.

8. Granich RM, Gilks CF, Dye C, De Cock KM, Williams BG (2009) Universal voluntary HIV testing with immediate antiretroviral therapy as a strategy for elimination of HIV transmission: a mathematical model. Lancet 373: 48–57.

9. Ananworanich J, Gayet-Ageron A, Le BM, Prasithsirikul W, Chetchotisakd P, et al. (2006) CD4-guided scheduled treatment interruptions compared with continuous therapy for patients infected with HIV-1: results of the Staccato randomised trial. Lancet 368: 459–465.

10. Dybul M, Nies-Kraske E, Daucher M, Hertogs K, Hallahan CW, et al. (2003) Long-cycle structured intermittent versus continuous highly active antiretroviral therapy for the treatment of chronic infection with human immunodeficiency virus: effects on drug toxicity and on immunologic and virologic parameters. J Infect Dis 188: 388–396.

11. Papasavvas E, Kostman JR, Mounzer K, Grant RM, Gross R, et al. (2004) Randomized, controlled trial of therapy interruption in chronic HIV-1 infection. PLoS Med 1: e64.

12. El-Sadr WM, Lundgren JD, Neaton JD, Gordin F, Abrams D, et al. (2006) CD4+ count-guided interruption of antiretroviral treatment. N Engl J Med 355: 2283–2296.

13. El-Sadr WM, Grund B, Neuhaus J, Babiker A, Cohen CJ, et al. (2008) Risk for opportunistic disease and death after reinitiating continuous antiretroviral therapy in patients with HIV previously receiving episodic therapy: a randomized trial. Ann Intern Med 149: 289–299.

14. Danel C, Moh R, Minga A, Anzian A, Ba-Gomis O, et al. (2006) CD4-guided structured antiretroviral treatment interruption strategy in HIV-infected adults in west Africa (Trivacan ANRS 1269 trial): a randomised trial. Lancet 367: 1981–1989.

15. Dybul M, Nies-Kraske E, Dewar R, Maldarelli F, Hallahan CW, et al. (2004) A proof-of-concept study of short-cycle intermittent antiretroviral therapy with a once-daily regimen of didanosine, lamivudine, and efavirenz for the treatment of chronic HIV infection. J Infect Dis 189: 1974–1982.

16. Frost SD, Martinez-Picado J, Ruiz L, Clotet B, Brown AJ (2002) Viral dynamics during structured treatment interruptions of chronic human immunodeficiency virus type 1 infection. J Virol 76: 968–979.

17. Farrington CP, Manning G (1990) Test statistics and sample size formulae for comparative binomial trials with null hypothesis of non-zero risk difference or non-unity relative risk. Stat Med 9: 1447–1454.

18. [Anonymous] (2007) StatXact 8 Statistical Software for Exact Nonparametric Inference. 433–435.

19. Agresti A, Min Y (2001) On small-sample confidence intervals for parameters in discrete distributions. Biometrics 57: 963 971.

20. Fay MP (2007) R: A language and environment for statistical computing; rateratio.test: Exact rate ratio test. R package version 1.0.

21. Reynolds SJ, Kityo C, Mbamanya F, Dewar R, Ssali F, et al. (2009) Evolution of drug resistance after virological failure of a first-line highly active antiretroviral therapy regimen in Uganda. Antivir Ther 14: 293–297.

22. Cohen CJ, Colson AE, Sheble-Hall AG, McLaughlin KA, Morse GD (2007) Pilot study of a novel short-cycle antiretroviral treatment interruption strategy: 48-week results of the five-days-on, two-days-off (FOTO) study. HIV Clin Trials 8: 19–23.

23. Parienti JJ, Das-Douglas M, Massari V, Guzman D, Deeks SG, et al. (2008) Not all missed doses are the same: sustained NNRTI treatment interruptions predict HIV rebound at low-to-moderate adherence levels. PLoS ONE 3: e2783.

24. Cohen C, Colson A, Pierone G, DeJesus E, Kinder F, et al. (2008) The FOTO study: 24-week results support the safety of a 2-day break on efavirenz-based antiretroviral therapy. Journal of the International AIDS Society 11 (Suppl 1).

25. Ananworanich J, Nuesch R, Le BM, Chetchotisakd P, Vibhagool A, et al. (2003) Failures of 1 week on, 1 week off antiretroviral therapies in a randomized trial. AIDS 17: F33–F37.

26. Fox Z, Phillips A, Cohen C, Neuhaus J, Baxter J, et al. (2008) Viral resuppression and detection of drug resistance following interruption of a suppressive non-nucleoside reverse transcriptase inhibitor-based regimen. AIDS 22: 2279–2289.

27. Levine AJ, Hinkin CH, Marion S, Keuning A, Castellon SA, et al. (2006) Adherence to antiretroviral medications in HIV: differences in data collected via self-report and electronic monitoring. Health Psychol 25: 329–335.

28. McComsey GA, Lo RV, III, O'Riordan M, Walker UA, Lebrecht D, et al. (2008) Effect of reducing the dose of stavudine on body composition, bone density, and markers of mitochondrial toxicity in HIV-infected subjects: a randomized, controlled study. Clin Infect Dis 46: 1290–1296.

29. Mee P, Fielding KL, Charalambous S, Churchyard GJ, Grant AD (2008) Evaluation of the WHO criteria for antiretroviral treatment failure among adults in South Africa. AIDS 22: 1971–1977.

30. Moore DM, Mermin J, Awor A, Yip B, Hogg RS, et al. (2006) Performance of immunologic responses in predicting viral load suppression: implications for monitoring patients in resource-limited settings. J Acquir Immune Defic Syndr 43: 436–439.

31. Reynolds SJ, Nakigozi G, Newell K, Ndyanabo A, Galiwongo R, et al. (2009) Failure of immunologic criteria to appropriately identify antiretroviral treatment failure in Uganda. AIDS.

32. World Health Organization (2006) ANTIRETROVIRAL THERAPY FOR HIV INFECTION IN ADULTS AND ADOLESCENTS IN RESOURCE-LIMITED SETTINGS: TOWARDS UNIVERSAL ACCESS Recommendations for a public health approach.

7

Modes of Metabolic Compensation during Mitochondrial Disease using the Drosophila Model of ATP6 Dysfunction

Alicia M. Celotto[1,2]*, Wai Kan Chiu[1,2], Wayne Van Voorhies[3], Michael J. Palladino[1,2]

1 Department of Pharmacology and Chemical Biology, University of Pittsburgh School of Medicine, Pittsburgh, Pennsylvania, United States of America, 2 Pittsburgh Institute for Neurodegenerative Diseases, University of Pittsburgh School of Medicine, Pennsylvania, United States of America, 3 Molecular Biology Program, New Mexico State University, Las Cruces, New Mexico, United States of America

Abstract

Numerous mitochondrial DNA mutations cause mitochondrial encephalomyopathy: a collection of related diseases for which there exists no effective treatment. Mitochondrial encephalomyopathies are complex multisystem diseases that exhibit a relentless progression of severity, making them both difficult to treat and study. The pathogenic and compensatory metabolic changes that are associated with chronic mitochondrial dysfunction are not well understood. The *Drosophila ATP6[1]* mutant models human mitochondrial encephalomyopathy and allows the study of metabolic changes and compensation that occur throughout the lifetime of an affected animal. *ATP6[1]* animals have a nearly complete loss of ATP synthase activity and an *acute* bioenergetic deficit when they are asymptomatic, but surprisingly we discovered no *chronic* bioenergetic deficit in these animals during their symptomatic period. Our data demonstrate dynamic metabolic compensatory mechanisms that sustain normal energy availability and activity despite chronic mitochondrial complex V dysfunction resulting from an endogenous mutation in the mitochondrial DNA. *ATP6[1]* animals compensate for their loss of oxidative phosphorylation through increases in glycolytic flux, ketogenesis and Kreb's cycle activity early during pathogenesis. However, succinate dehydrogenase activity is reduced and mitochondrial supercomplex formation is severely disrupted contributing to the pathogenesis seen in *ATP6[1]* animals. These studies demonstrate the dynamic nature of metabolic compensatory mechanisms and emphasize the need for time course studies in tractable animal systems to elucidate disease pathogenesis and novel therapeutic avenues.

Editor: Michael N. Nitabach, Yale School of Medicine, United States of America

Funding: This work was supported by National Institutes of Health (NIH) R01 AG025046 and AG027453 to Dr. Palladino and U.S. National Cancer Institute (NCI U56 CA96286) to Dr. Van Voorhies. The funders had no role in study design, data collection and analysis, decision to publish, or preparation of the manuscript.

Competing Interests: The authors have declared that no competing interests exist.

* E-mail: amc41@pitt.edu

Introduction

Normal metabolic pathways in animals have been elucidated and extensively studied for decades; however, the response of each pathway to the loss or disturbance of another is poorly understood. The eukaryotic cell and its mitochondria have evolved different methods of energy production from the catabolism of most food products. However, there are many human diseases that disrupt, typically via genetic hypomorphic mutations, one of these pathways. Such heritable diseases known collectively as inborn errors of metabolism do not immediately cause death; they do, however, lead to poorly understood diseases including enzymo-pathies and mitochondrial encephalomyopathies. Metabolic pathways are complex networks, therefore a single perturbation resulting from a single gene mutation can lead to dramatic changes in an animal's ability to maintain its normal physiological functions as well as homeostatic impairment that affects its ability to cope with environmental stresses [1].

Our current understanding of mitochondrial disease has been facilitated by the study of cellular cybrids bearing human disease mutations. However, such systems have not yielded a clear picture of the bioenergetics and compensatory mechanisms that exist within the tissues of an intact animal with mitochondrial disease. Thus, no comprehensible understanding of the associated pathogenesis has

resulted, demonstrating the inherent difficulty in using cellular models to study multisystem diseases [2,3]. Additionally, these diseases typically exhibit an asymptomatic period varying from days to decades, onset, and a stereotyped progression of the disease making them difficult to model in cellular systems. Little is known about disease pathogenesis in an intact animal with functional neurons and muscle fibers that can be examined over the life of the animal. Thus, it is essential to study the progressive nature and tissue-specific attributes of these diseases with the goal of identifying endogenous compensatory mechanisms that might be exploited as therapeutic avenues.

Here we utilize a novel, well-characterized, endogenous mitochondrial mutation in the *ATP6* gene (NC_001709.1) of *Drosophila melanogaster* with a nearly complete loss of ATP synthase activity [4]. These *Drosophila* mutants have a missense mutation in *ATP6* (G to A transition resulting in a glycine to glutamate change at position 116 in the protein), the mitochondrial gene encoding subunit 6 of the F_1F_o-ATP synthase (complex V of the respiratory chain) [4,5,6,7,8]. ATP6 allows for the hydrogen ion translocation required for the rotation of the F_o motor and the production of ATP from ADP [9]. *Drosophila ATP6[1]* mutants model human mitochondrial encephalomyopathy and demonstrate phenotypes associated with degenerative disease, including: reduced longevity, mitochondrial pathology, progressive neural dysfunction, tissue degeneration and locomotor impairment [4]. In humans, 8 missense and two frame shift mutations lead to ATP6 impairment and are known to cause the related mitochondrial disorders: maternally inherited Leigh's syndrome (MILS), neuropathy, ataxia, and retinitis pigmentosa (NARP), and familial bilateral striatal necrosis (FBSN) [10,11,12,13,14,15,16,17,18]. These diseases are characterized by reduced longevity, progressive neuromuscular impairment, seizures, myodegeneration and a range of devastating complications resulting from renal, cardiac, endocrine and hepatic system dysfunction [19,20,21,22,23,24,25,26,27,28]. The diversity of symptoms and phenotypes associated with ATP6 dysfunction in humans and flies likely reflects this protein's important and highly conserved role in cellular bioenergetics. The pathological basis of diseases associated with ATP6 impairment in humans is not understood but it has been hypothesized that there may be uncoupling of complex V resulting in bioenergetic impairment and oxidative stress owing to respiratory chain dysfunction [29,30].

Our results demonstrate that there are dynamic adjustments made within many of the metabolic pathways over the lifetime of animals with ATP6 dysfunction, which allow them to maintain a normal level of energy, despite the severe reduction in ATP production through oxidative phosphorylation (OXPHOS). Glycolysis and ketogenesis compensate for the OXPHOS defect earlier in life. We also demonstrate that a loss in mitochondrial supercomplex formation and complex II activity are associated with pathogenesis. These data demonstrate that mitochondrial encephalomyopathies results in dynamic metabolic compensation and that disease pathogenesis does not result from a loss of energy and involves a cascade of events broadly affecting metabolic and mitochondrial function.

Results

$ATP6^1$ survival and behavioral changes

$ATP6^1$ Drosophila mutants exhibit a stereotyped phenotypic progression that is analogous to the symptomatic progression reported for many human mitochondrial disease patients [5,14]. $ATP6^1$ mutant flies demonstrate stress sensitivity, shortened lifespan, muscle degeneration and abnormal mitochondrial morphology [4]. $ATP6^1$ animals eclose looking and acting completely normal and are morphologically and behaviorally indistinguishable from wildtype animals. $ATP6^1$ animals exhibit a stereotypical progression of disease following onset (~day 8) when the animals begin to have reduced locomotor activity (Figure 1A and 1B). By day 13, $ATP6^1$ animals are sensitive to mechanical stress resulting in paralysis, suggesting neuromuscular impairment. At ~day 20, $ATP6^1$ animals can be observed having sporadic and unprovoked seizure-like activity. Late in pathogenesis $ATP6^1$ phenotypes continue to worsen until their premature death (Figure 1B).

We discovered that $ATP6^1$ animals have a similar developmental survival rate as wildtype animals whether they are raised at 22°C or 29°C (Figure 1C). Interestingly, $ATP6^1$ animals show a modest but significant shortening in the time of development during the larval and pupal stages at 22°C and during the larval stage at 29°C (Figure 1D). Additionally, $ATP6^1$ females lay significantly more eggs than wildtype animals during their first week of life (Figure 1E). These data demonstrate that the altered physiology of $ATP6^1$ animals results in an accelerated development and increase in female fecundity. Such effects could cause increase utilization of energy early in life to ensure survival despite the dramatically altered physiology.

To examine the seizure behavior we asked whether sensory hyperstimulation, such as a strobe light, could elicit seizure behavior in $ATP6^1$ flies. Video analysis of locomotor function prior to, during, and following 1450 fpm (flashes per minute) strobe lighting (20 seconds) was used to examine the ability to induce seizure behavior by sensory hyperstimulation alone. Although strobe lighting did not affect the locomotion of wildtype flies (Video S1, Video S2, Video S3), $ATP6^1$ animals exhibited convulsive behavior with a high penetrance both during and after the strobe light (Video S4, Video S5, Video S6). Surprisingly, the convulsive behavior was followed by full paralysis that continued well after resumption of normal lighting (Figure 1F, Video S6). This phenotype was also progressive, as young animals did not exhibit convulsions or paralysis (Figure 1F).

Energy buffering capacity and energy levels over time in $ATP6^1$ animals

We examined the effect altered $ATP6^1$ physiology had on animal bioenergetics. We examined phosphoarginine (P-Arg), arginine (Arg) as well as the adenylate pool using distinct HPLC protocols (Figure 2). P-Arg is the invertebrate equivalent to phosphocreatine, which buffers ATP levels and provides a reliable measure of bioenergetics [31]. Since we observe progressive pathogenesis in $ATP6^1$ animals, we analyzed the bioenergetic state over a relevant time course from asymptomatic to late-stage pathogenesis. Wildtype animals exhibit a reduction in P-Arg:Arg ratios over the first two weeks of their adult life that appear to plateau around 0.18 (Figure 2A). Surprisingly, $ATP6^1$ animals also plateau at ~0.18 when aged, however, in the first week of their adult life P-Arg:Arg ratios are significantly reduced from that of age-matched wildtype control animals (Figure 2A).

We also examined the adenylate pool (ATP, ADP and AMP) from mutant and control animals using the same time course and the identical trend was observed (Figure 2B). A surprising decrease in the ATP:ADP ratio can be seen at days 3 and 6 (when mutants are largely aphenotypic) but no change was noted at later time points when the phenotypes are marked in severity. These data are in agreement with the data from the P-Arg:Arg assays. We also noted an age dependent decrease in AMP unique to $ATP6^1$ animals (day 20; Figure 2C). However, no change in overall total adenylate pool was noted (data not shown). These data surprisingly demonstrate that bioenergetic impairment is not likely to cause pathogenesis and suggests the importance of compensatory metabolic pathways in delaying disease pathogenesis.

Metabolic compensation: glycolysis

Substrate level phosphorylation occurs in glycolysis when phosphoenol pyruvate is converted to pyruvate and in the Kreb's cycle when succinyl-CoA is converted to succinate. It is thus predicted that without a functional ATP synthase (Complex V), 2 net ATP per glucose are produced through glycolysis and 1 GTP per acetyl-CoA can be produced through the Kreb's cycle. Additionally, it has been demonstrated in cell cybrid models that defects in respiratory chain complexes leads to an upregulation of glycolysis [32]. Using steady state lactic acid as a measure of glycolytic flux, a dramatic increase can be seen in young $ATP6^1$ animals (day 5) compared to age matched controls (Figure 3). Later in life (days 10 and 20) these levels have dropped to wildtype levels. These data demonstrate that increased glycolysis is an important early compensatory mechanism that is ineffective at fully abating the reduced bioenergetics observed prior to pathogenesis. These data also imply that lactic acidosis is not likely to account for the severe pathogenesis observed late in life (~days 15–25).

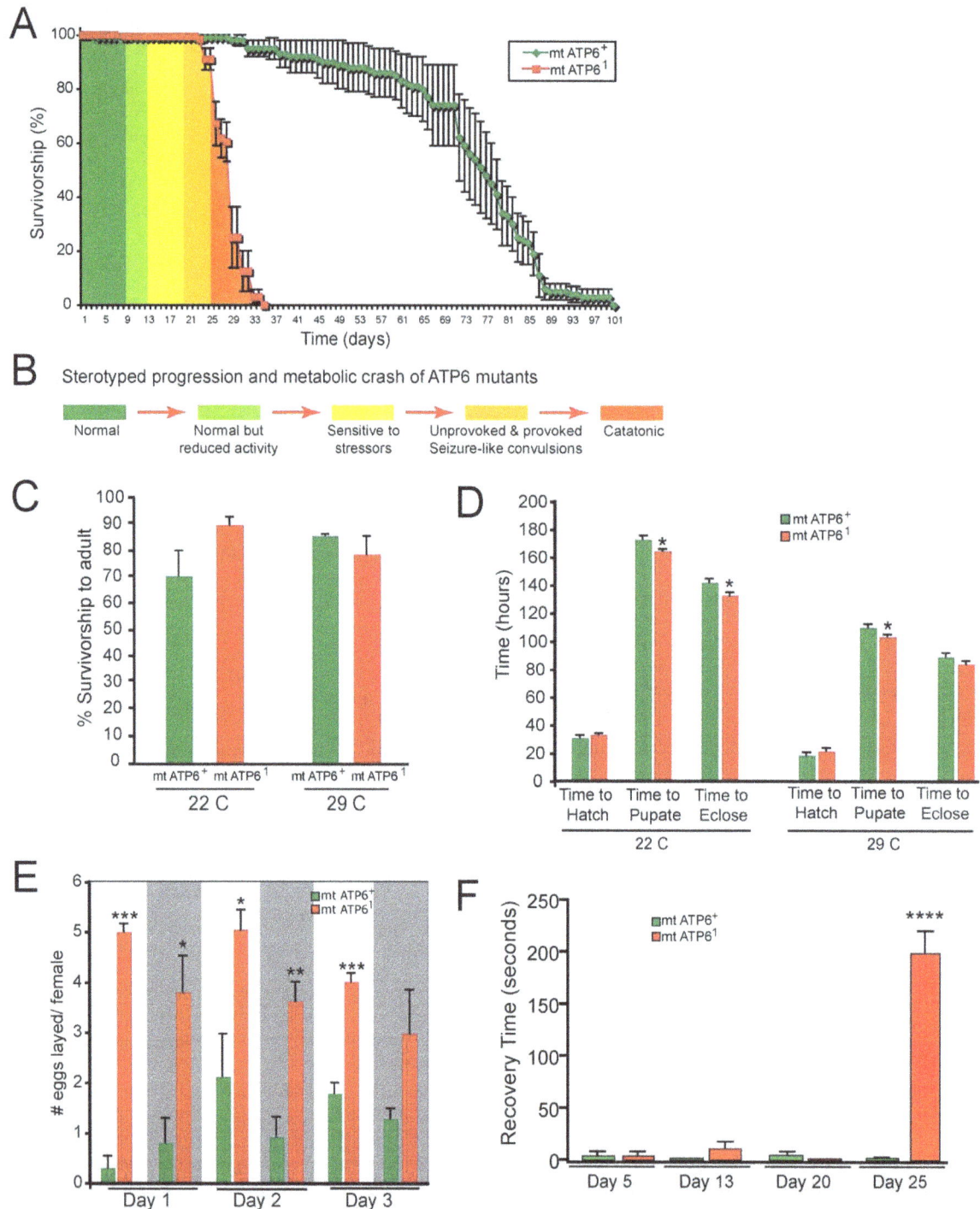

Figure 1. Phenotypic progression of _ATP6[1]_ animals. A) Longevity curve showing wildtype (green) and _ATP6[1]_ (red) demonstrating an ~40% reduction in lifespan. Green, yellow and orange shading describes the change in animal behavior over _ATP6[1]_ lifespan. Life spans are based upon 80 total animals per genotype. Error is S.E.M. Statistical analysis is log-rank. B) Summary of phenotypic progression of _ATP6[1]_ animals. C) Graph showing normal developmental survival rate for _ATP6[1]_ compared to wildtype at 22°C and 29°C. N = 510 _ATP6[1]_ at 22°C, N = 173 wildtype at 22°C, N = 696 _ATP6[1]_ at 29°C, N = 586 wildtype at 29°C. Error is S.E.M. Statistical analysis is student's t-test. D) _ATP6[1]_ mutants develop significantly faster than controls at 22°C (to eclosion) and at 29°C (to pupation). N = 30 both genotypes both temperatures. Error is S.E.M. Statistical analysis is student's t-test. E) _ATP6[1]_ animals exhibit a higher fecundity early in adulthood. Gray represents dark intervals of a 12:12 light dark regime. N = 462 _ATP6[1]_, N = 139 wildtype. Error is S.E.M. Statistical analysis is student's t-test. F) Strobe lighting induces seizure-like convulsions followed by paralysis only in aged _ATP6[1]_ animals. Young mutants and controls did not exhibit convulsions or paralysis. _ATP6[1]_ day 5 N = 17; day 13 N = 19; day 20 N = 13; day 25 N = 23. Wildtype day 5 N = 14; day 13 N = 23; day 20 N = 13; day 25 N = 25. Error is S.E.M. Statistical analysis at day 25 is a two-tailed Mann-Whitney U test. Also see S1A–C and S2A–C.

A

B

C

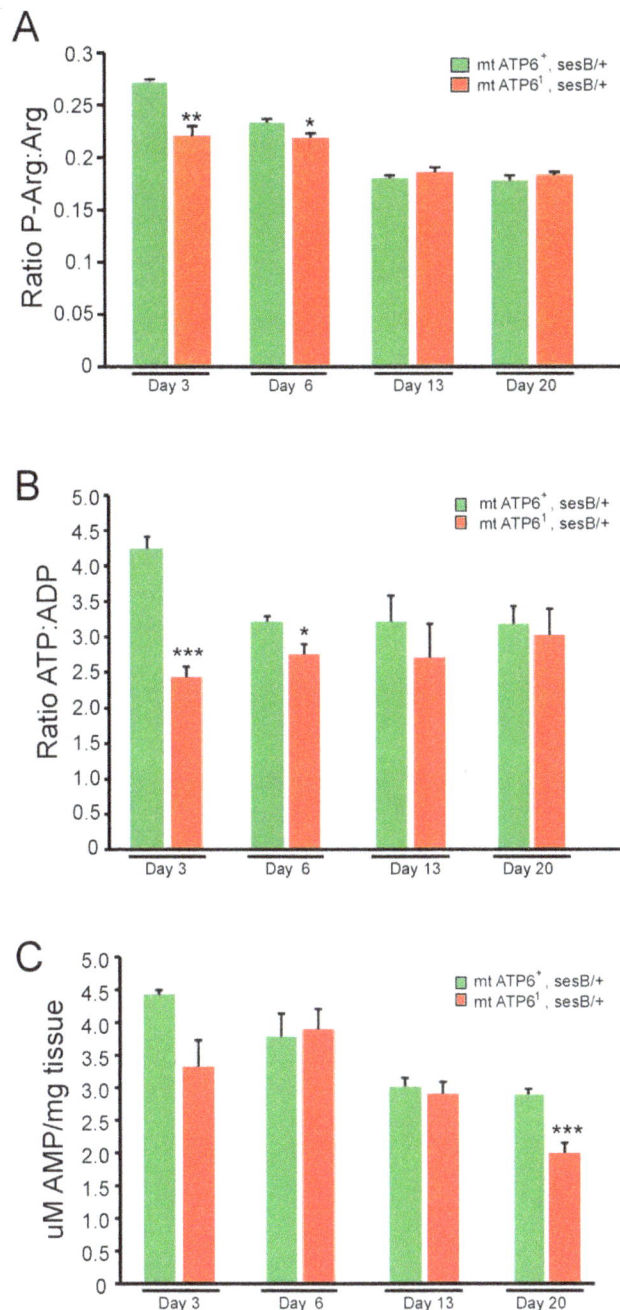

Figure 2. Bioenergetics of wildtype and *ATP6[1]* animals. A) P-Arg:Arg ratios exhibit impaired bioenergtics in *ATP6[1]* animals only at adult day 3 and 6 compared to age-matched wildtype. All mutant genotypes are mt *ATP6[1]*, *sesB[1]*/+ and wildtype controls are *mt ATP6[+]*, *sesB/+*. *sesB[1]* (recessive stress sensitive B mutation) is the fly homologue to ANT (adenine nucleotide translocase) and *ATP6[1]* is maintained in this mutant background and the heteroplasmy is verified by RFLP analysis prior to experimentation (Data not shown). F1 female progeny heterozygous for *sesB[1]* are of high mutant heteroplasmy and were analyzed compared to *sesB[1]* heterozygote controls. N = 9 wildtype at each time point, N = 6 *ATP6[1]* day 3 and 13, N = 9 *ATP6[1]* day 6 and 20. Error is S.E.M. Statistical analysis is student's t-test. B) The ATP:ADP ratio analyses show a similar reduction in bioenergetics only in young mutants. N = 9 wildtype at each time point, N = 6 *ATP6[1]* day 3 and 13, N = 9 *ATP6[1]* day 6 and 20. Error is S.E.M. Statistical analysis is student's t-test. C) Comparison of uM AMP per mg of tissue between wildtype and *ATP6[1]* animals show a modest decrease in AMP in aged mutants at day 20. No significant changes are seen in total adenylate pool in *ATP6[1]* animals. N = 9 wildtype at each time point, N = 6 *ATP6[1]* day 3 and 13, N = 9 *ATP6[1]* day 6 and 20. Error is S.E.M. Statistical analysis is student's t-test.

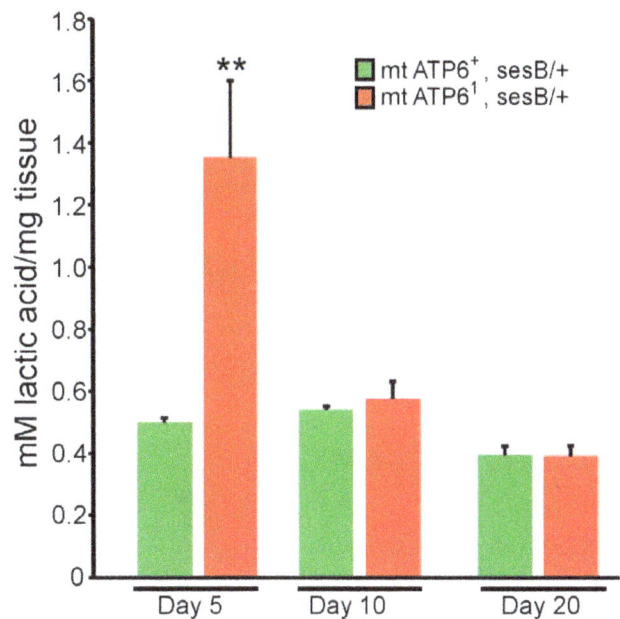

Figure 3. Glycolytic compensation in young *ATP6[1]* animals. A significant increase in lactic acid levels is seen in *ATP6[1]* animals on day 5 compared to wildtype animals. Steady state lactic acid is unchanged between wildtype and mutants at day 10 and 20. N = 9 wildtype at each time point, N = 9 *ATP6[1]* day 5 and 10, N = 6 *ATP6[1]* day 20. Error is S.E.M. Statistical analysis is student's t-test.

Metabolic compensation

Ketogenesis. When animals are metabolically stressed, such as during starvation, they transition to utilizing fatty acids through beta-oxidation and ketogenesis. We investigated the hypothesis that *ATP6[1]* animals are utilizing ketogenesis to compensate for OXPHOS impairment. Ketogenesis is a multi-step pathway that converts acetyl-CoA to ketone bodies (acetoacetate, acetone and beta-hydroxybutyrate) that can be utilized by numerous tissues in the body, including the brain, to produce energy (Figure 4A). The expressions of two key enzymes, involved in ketogenesis, were measured over the life of *ATP6[1]* animals to determine the likelihood that this pathway is up-regulated. Both thiolase and 3-hydroxy-3-methylglutaryl-CoA synthase (HMGS) are up-regulated in *ATP6[1]* animals compared to wildtype animals beginning at day 13 (Figure 4B and 4C, respectively). Additionally, elevated beta-hydroxybutyrate was observed in *ATP6[1]* animals versus control animals early in adult life (Figure 4D). However, the ~6-fold increase in steady state beta-hydroxybutyrate levels seen in young mutants are not maintained as *ATP6[1]* animals age and there is a reduction compared to wildtype by day 20, a time coincident with a marked worsening of *ATP6[1]* phenotypes (Figure 4D).

To understand whether this decrease in beta-hydroxybutyrate was due to the inability to maintain elevated ketone bodies or an increase in catabolism, 3-oxoacid-CoA transferase was measured. This enzyme is involved in ketone body catabolism converts of succinyl-CoA and acteoacetate (a ketone body) to succinate and acetoacetyl-CoA (Figure 4E). The expression level of this enzyme, in *ATP6[1]* animals, shows an ~2.5-fold increase in expression compared to wildtype at days 13 and 20 (Figure 4F). These data suggest that both synthesis and catabolism are increased and that catabolism must be increased relative to synthesis to produce lower steady state beta-hydroxybutyrate levels.

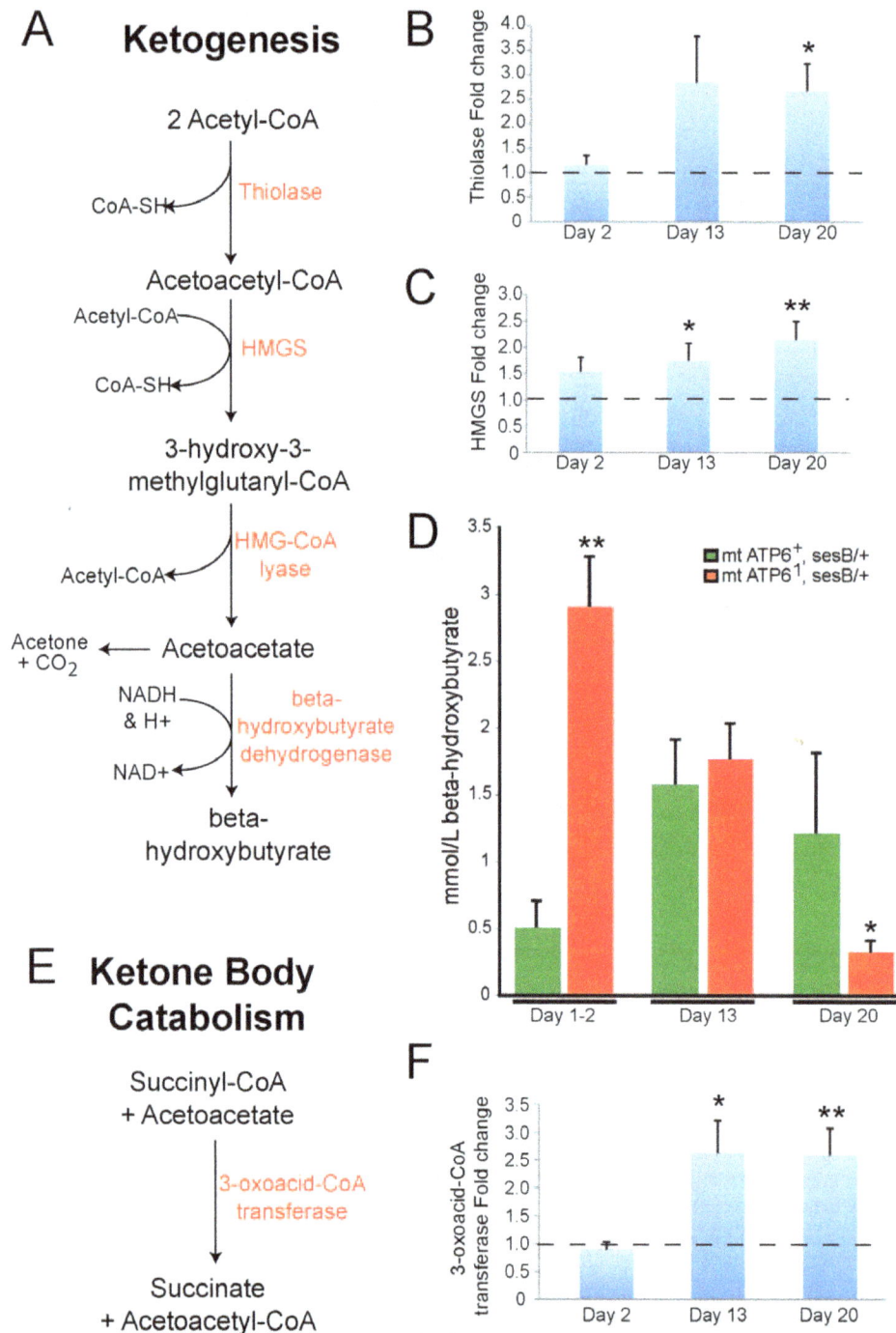

Figure 4. Ketogenic compensation in *ATP6[1]* animals. A) The ketogenic metabolic pathway is used to produce ketone bodies (acetoacetate, acetone and beta-hydroxybutyrate). Enzymes shown in red. B & C) Real-time quantitative RT-PCR of the enzyme thiolase and 3-hydroxy-3-methyl-glutaryl-CoA synthase (HMGS) reveal an increasing trend in *ATP6[1]* animals with age compared to wildtype. N = 12 wildtype each time point. N = 12 *ATP6[1]* each time point. Error is S.E.M. Statistical analysis is student's t-test. D) Quantitation of beta-hydroxybutyrate shows a marked increase in young animals with a decreasing trend with age compared with wildype. N = 9 wildtype day1–2, N = 5 wildtype days 13 and 20. N = 6 *ATP6[1]* day 1–2, N = 5 *ATP6[1]* days 13 and 20. Error is S.E.M. Statistical analysis is student's t-test. E) The enzyme 3-oxoacid-CoA transferase is involved in ketone body catabolism. F) Real-time quantitative RT-PCR of 3-oxoacid-CoA transferase reveals an increasing trend with age in *ATP6[1]* animals versus controls. N = 12 wildtype each time point. N = 12 *ATP6[1]* each time point. Error is S.E.M. Statistical analysis is student's t-test.

Respiration rate changes in *ATP6[1]* and wildtype animals over lifespan

During OXPHOS, oxygen is the final acceptor of electrons that are passed across the inner mitochondrial membrane at complex IV and is ultimately reduced to water. CO2 is produced during the transition from glycolysis to the Kreb's cycle where pyruvate dehydrogenase converts pyruvate to acetyl-CoA and within the Kreb's cycle at the conversion of isocitrate to alpha-ketoglutarate and the conversion of alpha-ketoglutarate to succinyl-CoA. Respiration is typically intimately coupled to mitochondrial energy production and *ATP6^1* are severely deficient in OXPHOS, suggesting respiration would be a key parameter to understand bioenergetics and pathogenesis resulting from ATP6 impairment. To determine whether there is an age-specific change in metabolic rate, we assayed rates of CO_2 production in wildtype and *ATP6^1* flies.

Respiration rate was measured in individual animals at days 5, 10, 15 and 20 as the emergence of CO_2 (Figure 5A and 5B). A natural trend emerged in wildtype animals, where the respiration rate increased over time plateauing between days 15–20. These data demonstrate a normal change in respiration and metabolic physiology associated with aging in our wildtype strain. Interestingly, *ATP6^1* animals also exhibit a similar trend, however, the increase observed through day 15 dramatically reverses by day 20 (Figure 5A). By examining the single animal data the trend of increasing at day 15 and the dramatic reduction observed by day 20 for most animals can be clearly seen with only a few outliers (Figure 5B). These data demonstrate that *ATP6^1* animals exhibit modestly elevated respiration during the aphenotypic period, and that onset of pathogenesis is associated with a striking increase in respiration followed by a dramatic drop in respiration corresponding to severe phenotypic impairment.

The dynamic changes observed in metabolic physiology and respiration over time could also be mediated through changes in mitochondrial metabolic substrate utilization. An estimate of substrate use can be obtained by comparing the ratio of CO_2 produced during respiration to the amount of O_2 consumed. This ratio termed the respiratory quotient (RQ) varies from approximately 0.7 for pure lipid metabolism to 1.0 for mitochondrial carbohydrate metabolism [33]. We determined the RQ for 5, 10 and 20 day old animals (Figure 5C). The RQ values for wildtype and *ATP6^1* animals were between 0.8 and 1.0 indicative of a largely carbohydrate based metabolism. However, young *ATP6^1* animals' exhibit a lower RQ value consistent with an increased usage of fatty acids. Overall, these respiration and RQ data suggest that *ATP6^1* animals may be increasing their utilization of the Kreb's cycle and thus producing modestly more CO_2.

Kreb's Cycle compensation in *ATP6^1* animals

To test the hypothesis that the Kreb's cycle activity has increased in *ATP6^1* animals, aconitase and succinate dehydrogenase (complex II) were measured. Aconitase converts citrate to isocitrate and succinate dehydrogenase converts succinate to fumarate after GTP production in the Kreb's cycle (Figure 6A). Aconitase activity is significantly increased in *ATP6^1* mutant mitochondria compared to wildtype (Figure 6B). However, succinate dehydrogenase activity is decreased in *ATP6^1* mitochondria compared to wildtype (Figure 6C). These data suggest that *ATP6^1* animals may be attempting to increase their utilization of the Kreb's cycle to maintain elevated energy levels as is seen with an increase in the aconitase step; however, later steps (succinate dehydrogenase) are unable to keep up a wildtype level of activity.

Complex V instability and loss of Supercomplex formation in *ATP6^1* mitochondria

TEM tomography of *ATP6^1* mitochondria demonstrated a vesicular inner mitochondrial membrane appearance lacking the normal flattened cristae morphology seen in wildtype mitochondria [4]. Using blue-native gel electrophoresis and western blot analysis, we found impairment in complex V dimerization in *ATP6^1* animals (Figure 7A and 7C). These data imply that mutant

ATP6 protein is being expressed, yet only a small fraction of the complex V is able to dimerize. Amazingly, this mutation also leads to the disruption of complex I containing supercomplexes (Figure 7B and 7C). The changes observed in complex I supercomplexes suggest a functional connection between complex I and V, that has not previously been appreciated and may also explain the observed decrease in complex II activity in *ATP6^1* animals.

Discussion

Mitochondrial encephalomyopathies are devastating diseases that are difficult to diagnose and treat. Mitochondrial dysfunction results directly from mutations in the proteins involved in mitochondrial function, such as components required for OXPHOS, as is the case for archetypal mitochondrial diseases. Numerous other common disorders such as Alzheimer's disease, diabetes, cardiovascular disease, obesity and premature aging have also been associated with mitochondrial dysfunction [34,35,36,37,38,39,40,41]. Understanding metabolic compensatory mechanisms that occur during chronic mitochondrial dysfunction will be needed to fully understand pathogenesis and develop effective treatments for these disorders. Utilizing an amenable intact animal model of mitochondrial encephalomyopathy has allowed for the study of disease progression and a more complete understanding of the associated pathogenesis.

The *ATP6^1* pathogenic phenotypes are not due to bioenergetic crisis. P-Arg:Arg ratios, as well as ATP:ADP ratios, show a significant decrease compared to wildtype animals during *ATP6^1* animals' first week of life. However, these lower levels are during a time when *ATP6^1* animals do not exhibit signs of mitochondrial pathogenesis. When *ATP6^1* animals begin to exhibit locomotor phenotypes as well as later in pathogenesis, energy levels are maintained at normal levels. These data demonstrate that bioenergetic crisis does not underlie pathogenesis.

The phenotypic progression in *ATP6^1* animals includes: reduced locomotor function, sensitivity to mechanical stress, unprovoked seizure behavior, and light-induced convulsions that result in paralysis. Seizure behavior and induced convulsions demonstrates, in this invertebrate model, a neurological link between mitochondrial dysfunction and seizure activity that is also commonly seen in mitochondrial disease patients [42,43,44]. Conditional paralysis associated with bang- or stress-sensitivity was originally reported many decades ago and this phenotype has remained mysterious and controversial [45]. Our data demonstrate that sensory hyperstimulation alone is sufficient to cause paralysis in this bang-sensitive mutant and that this stimulation causes convulsive seizure behavior that leads to the observed paralysis.

ATP6^1 animals compensate for their reduced ability to produce ATP through OXPHOS by increasing their usage of other metabolic pathways (Figure 8). The pathogenesis seen in *ATP6^1* animals does not appear when the activity of the ketogenic and glycolytic pathways remain elevated, suggesting their ability to effectively compensate for the OXPHOS dysfunction. It is likely that pathogenesis results from an inability to maintain these compensatory mechanisms chronically or that chronic compensation is toxic. Further studies will be needed to distinguish between these possibilities.

Respiration has previously been measured over the lifespan of several wildtype organisms resulting in conflicting reports on metabolic rate changes with age [46,47,48,49,50]. We have found wildtype animals demonstrate an increase in respiration early in life that plateaus as they age. *ATP6^1* animals exhibit an early increase in CO_2 production during the first 2 weeks of their

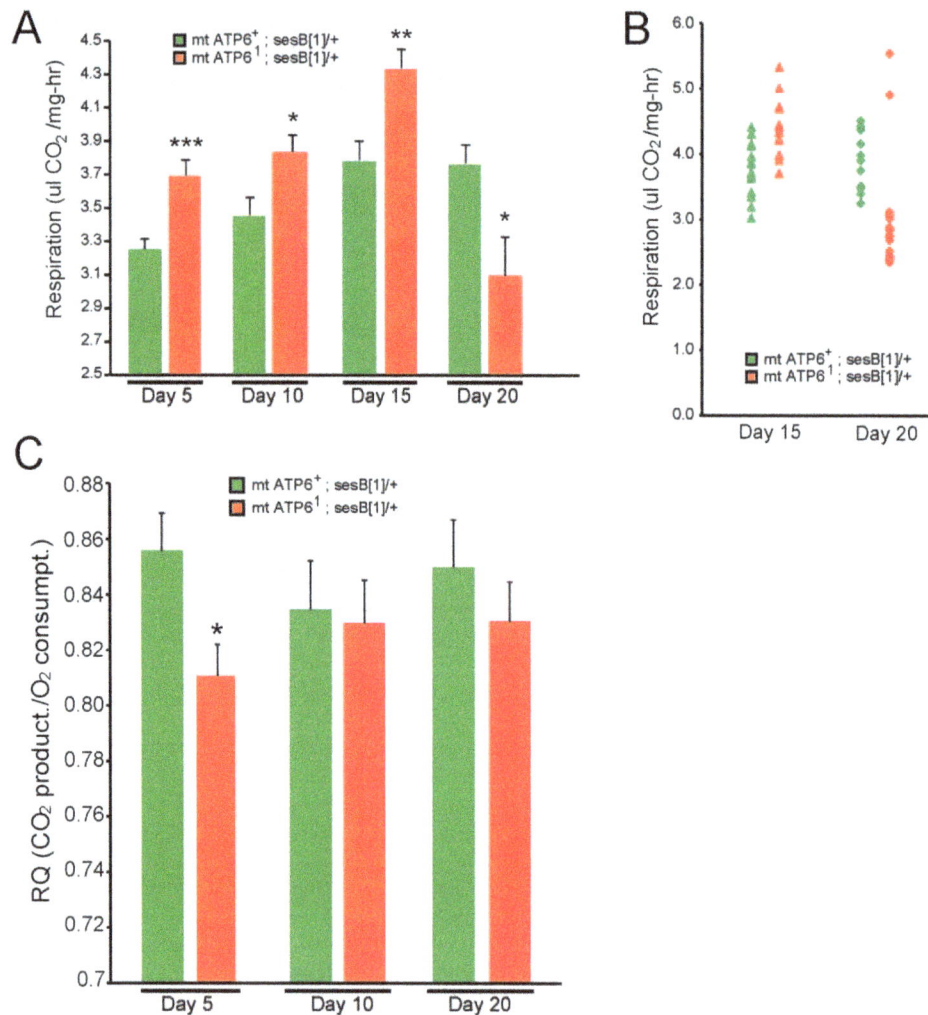

Figure 5. Respiration and respiratory quotient (RQ) changes over lifespan. A) Average respiration rate (ul C02/mg-hr) in wildtype (green) and *ATP6¹* (red) animals over time. On days 5, 10 and 15 *ATP6¹* animals have a modest but significantly higher respiration rate than wildtype animals; however, by day 20 *ATP6¹* mutants show a significant decrease in respiration rate. N = 21 − 24 animals per time point per genotype. Error is S.E.M. Statistical analysis is student's t-test. B) Individual animal respiration rates at days 15 and 20. C) Respiratory quotient (RQ) of wildtype and *ATP6¹* animals. There is a modest but significant, decrease of the RQ of *ATP6¹* animals at day 5 compared to wildtype. N = 6 − 9 chambers per time point per genotype. Error is S.E.M. Statistical analysis is student's t-test.

life that is elevated relative to wildtype, however, this is followed by a drastic reduction by day 20. This suggests that these animals are trying to increase their utilization of the Kreb's cycle early in their life; however they may be unable to maintain this level of activity later in life. Additionally, *ATP6¹* animals have a lower RQ value at day 5 and a similar value to wildtype throughout the rest of their life. This decrease in RQ value at day 5 is consistent with the observed increase in utilization of ketogenesis, a lipid-utilizing pathway.

The aberrant mitochondrial morphology seen in these *ATP6¹* animals can be attributed to the lack of complex V dimerization. Recent work demonstrates that complex V dimer formation is necessary for the bending of the inner mitochondrial membrane giving cristae their characteristic elongated appearance and placing complex V in the proper position to utilize the highest concentration of hydrogen ions for catalysis [2,51,52,53,54,55,56]. The loss of efficient ATP synthase activity is either due to the inability of complex V to dimerize or due to the malformed cristae, which need to be elongated to concentrate the hydrogen ions for

proper ATP synthesis. Additionally, we show that this single missense mutation disrupts the formation of supercomplexes containing complex I. This loss of supercomplex formation may have a causal relationship to the decrease in succinate dehydrogenase (complex II) activity observed, thus preventing the Kreb's cycle from functioning at an increased level.

In conclusion, we have studied the metabolic pathways within *ATP6¹* animals and discovered a dynamic interplay between compensatory mechanisms that results when efficient production of ATP through OXPHOS is not possible. These compensatory responses allow the animal to maintain largely normal levels of ATP, demonstrating that bioenergetic crisis does not underlie pathogenesis. This normal level of ATP may be at the expense of the animals' normal activity level during the second half of their lives and thus may contribute to the observed locomotor phenotypes. Importantly, nearly every parameter examined was dynamic over the lifespan of *ATP6¹* animals, underscoring the importance of studying such diseases as a time course in an intact animal model.

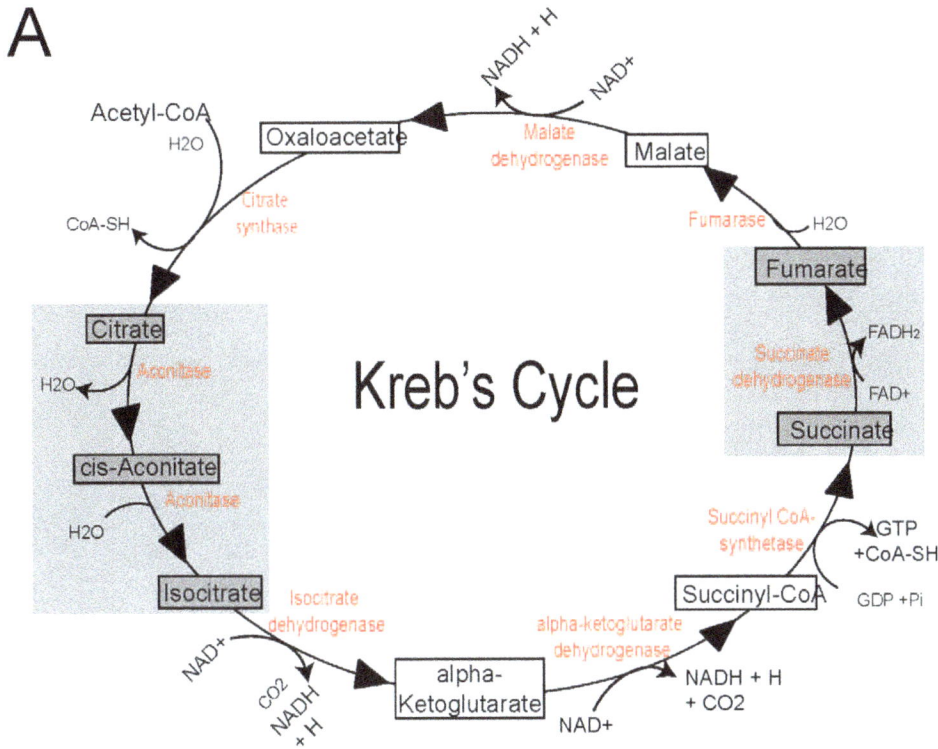

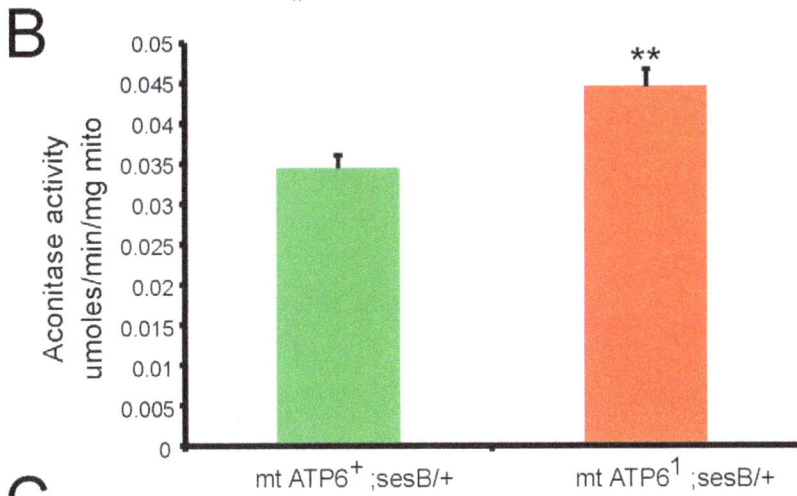

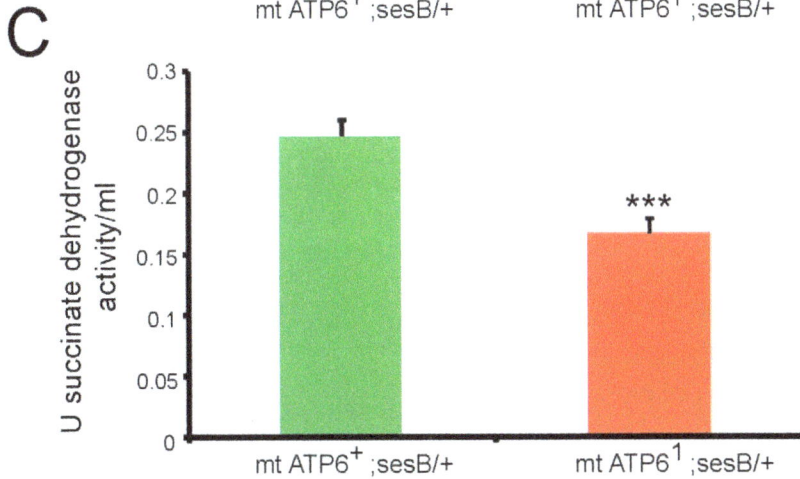

Figure 6. Succinate dehydrogenase and aconitase enzyme activity measurements. A) Kreb's cycle pathway; intermediates shown in boxes, enzymes shown in red. Gray boxes represent steps where enzyme activity level was measured in isolated mitochondria. B) Aconitase activity measured in wildtype (green) and $ATP6^1$ (red) mitochondria. $ATP6^1$ mitochondria have increased aconitase activity compared to wildtype. N = 15 per

genotype (0–100 ug mitochondria). Error is S.E.M. Statistical analysis is student's t-test. C) Succinate dehydrogenase activity measured in wildtype (green) and *ATP6^1* (red) mitochondria. *ATP6^1* mitochondria have reduced succinate dehydrogenase activity compared to wildtype. N = 9 per genotype. Error is S.E.M. Statistical analysis is student's t-test.

Materials and Methods

Fly Strains, longevity, survival, egg laying and development

All mutant genotypes were mt *ATP6^1*, *sesB^1*/+, wildtype controls were *mt ATP6$^+$*, *sesB*/+. *sesB^1* (recessive stress sensitive B mutation) is the fly homologue to ANT (adenine nucleotide translocase) and *ATP6^1* is maintained in this mutant background and the

heteroplasmy is verified by RFLP analysis prior to experimentation (Data not shown). F1 female progeny heterozygous for *sesB^1* are of high mutant heteroplasmy and were analyzed compared to *sesB^1* heterozygote controls, unless otherwise noted. Longevity was examined as previously published [57,58,59,60,61,62,63]. *Survival:* females were allowed to lay eggs in a new vial for 4 consecutive days, each day the eggs were counted and the females were moved to a new vial (adjustment made for unfertilized eggs). *Egg laying:*

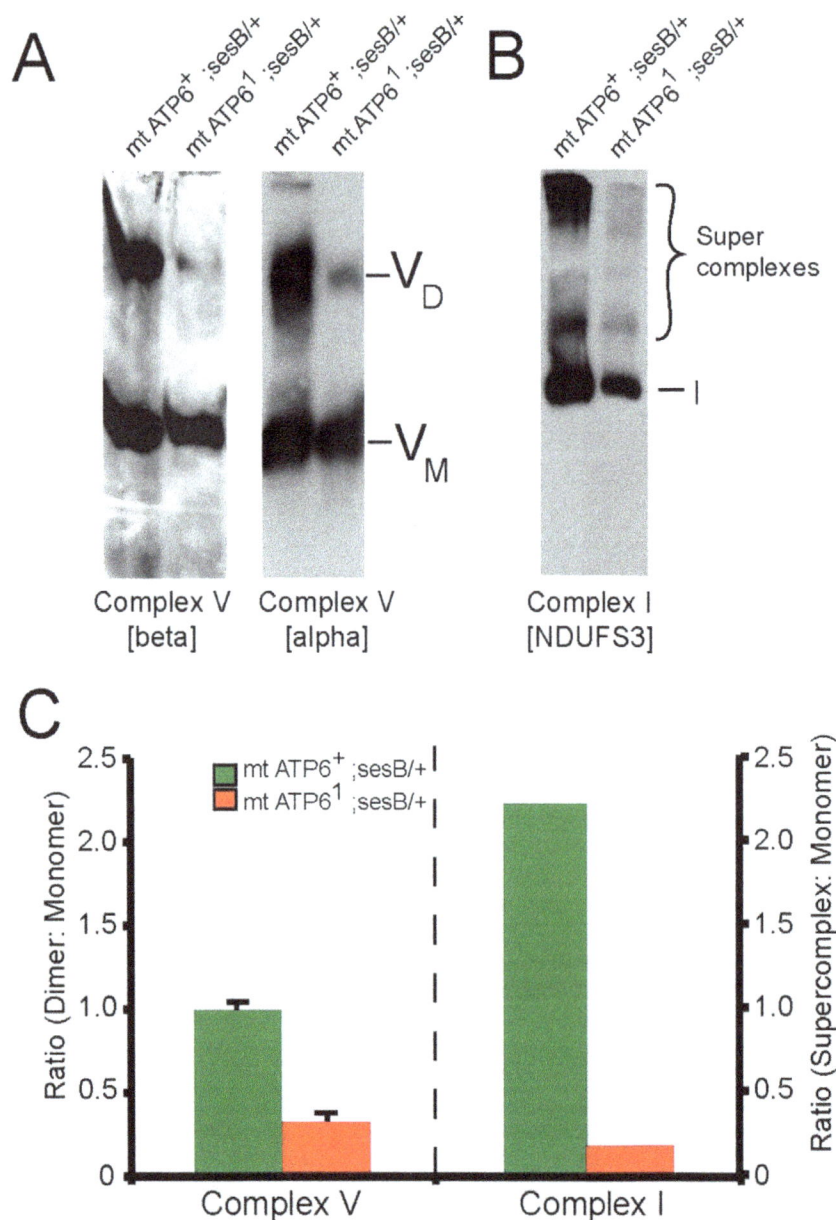

Figure 7. Impaired complex V dimerization and complex I supercomplex formation. A) BN-western analysis with beta and alpha subunit antibodies reveals a marked reduction in complex V dimer (VD) relative to monomer (VM) in *ATP6^1* mitochondrial isolates compared to wild type controls. B) BN-western analysis using an antibody to complex I (NDUFS3) reveals a loss in normal supercomplexes in *ATP6^1* mitochondria. C) Quantitation of the westerns shown in panels A and B comparing WT (green) to *ATP6^1* (red): dimer to monomer ratio of complex V and supercomplex to monomer ratio of complex I.

A Normal Metabolic Activity

B Compensatory metabolic response in ATP6¹ mutants

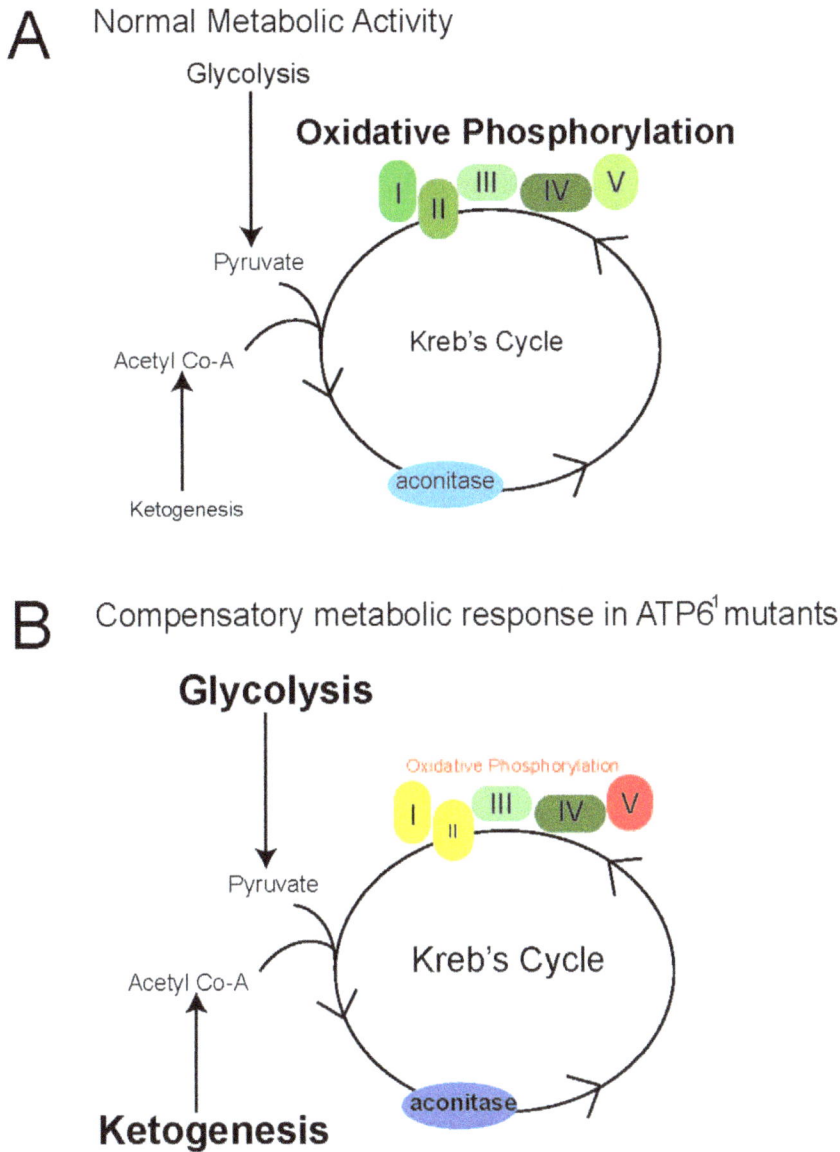

Figure 8. Model summarizing the dynamic metabolic changes resulting from ATP6 impairment compared with normal metabolism. A) During normal metabolic activity, oxidative phosphorylation is the major producer of ATP in the cell. Glycolysis, ketogenesis and the Kreb's cycle contribute as needed. B) During chronic ATP6 dysfunction these less utilized pathways (glycolysis and ketogenesis) are upregulated to compensate for the loss of oxidative phoshorylation. Complex V is unable to form a dimer and lacks ATP synthase capacity. Complex I supercomplexes are missing and complex II activity is down, however, there is a measurable increase in aconitase activity (an additional component of the Kreb's cycle).

number of embryos laid per female was determined in 12-hour intervals over a 3-day period. *Development:* times to transition to the next stage was monitored every 12 hours at each temperature.

Extract preparation for HPLC assays

Animals were rapidly frozen using liquid nitrogen, weighed then homogenized with an electric homogenizer in 200 µl 0.6 M perchloric acid and were then neutralized by the addition of 25 µl of 2 M potassium carbonate. Samples were centrifuged at 12,000xg for 10 minutes at 4°C. The supernatant was then filtered through a PVDF 0.45 µm spin column at 12,000xg for 5 minutes at 4°C.

Phosphoarginine

Arginine ratios. HPLC protocol to measure phospho-arginine and arginine ratios was adapted from an established

method [64]. Ten µl of extract was injected. HPLC conditions: Phenomenex Luna 5 µm NH2 250×4.6 mm column and 4.6×3 mm 3 µm NH2 Guard column. Flow rate of 0.6 ml/min and detection wavelength of 205 nm. A linear mobile phase consisting of 95:5 20 mM KH2PO4 pH 2.6: Acetonitrile. Arginine standard was used in the linear range of 0.1–5 mM. Phosphoarginine standard was synthesized using arginine kinase from Homarus vulgaris longitudinal muscle similar to a published method [65]. Retention times were 3.7 and 5.3 minutes for arginine and phosphoarginine, respectively.

Adenylate Pool. HPLC protocol to measure ATP, ADP and AMP levels was adapted from an established method [66]. Twenty µl of extract was injected. HPLC conditions: Waters XBridge Shield RP18 150×4.6 mm 5 µm column and guard column. Flow rate of 0.8 ml/min, detection wavelength of 257 nm and column temperature of 30°C. A gradient mobile phase was used: time 0–6.5 minutes 0% B, 6.5–12.5 minutes 100% B, 12.5–25 minutes 0%B. Buffer A was 50 mM NH4H2PO4 pH 5.7, Buffer B was 60:40 Acetonitrile: H2O. ATP, ADP and AMP standards were linear through the range of 100–250 µM. Approximate retention times were 4.2 minutes for ATP, 4.7 minutes for ADP and 6.2 minutes for AMP.

Lactic acid levels

HPLC protocol to measure lactic acid levels was adapted from an established method [67]. Twenty five µl of extract was injected. HPLC conditions: Waters Atlantis dC18 150×4.6 mm 3 µm column and 4.6×20 mm 3 µm Guard column. Flow rate of 0.5 ml/min, detection wavelength of 190 nm and column temperature of 30°C. A linear mobile phase consisting of 10 mM NaH2PO4 pH 2.5. Lactic acid standard was used in the linear range of 2–10 mM with an approximate retention time of 7.6 mintues.

Beta-hydroxybutyrate assay

Animals were cold slowed on ice before being homogenized in 10 µl PBS using a plastic pestle in a centrifuge tube. Extract was immediately read using an Optium Xceed Meter (Abbott) containing an Optium Plus β–ketone test strip. Readout was given in mmol/L.

Quantitative RT-PCR. RNA was prepped using Qiagen RNAeasy kit. Quantitative RT-PCR was performed as previously published [60].

Respiration rate

Resting metabolic rates were measured on individual wildtype and *ATP6¹* flies at 4 ages (5, 10, 15 and 20 days post-emergence, n = 21−24 animals per time point per genotype) using methods similar to those we have previously described [68,69].

RQ measurements. To determine the relationship between CO2 production and O2 consumption, both variables were measured in wildtype and *ATP6¹* flies at 4 ages (5, 10 and 20 days post-emergence). Groups of 5–6 flies (n = 6–9 chambers per time point per genotype) were measured using a previously described protocol [69].

Mitochondria isolation

A continuous percoll gradient was used to isolate mitochondria from 1.5–2 g of wildtype or *ATP6¹* adults. Protocol was adapted from an established method [70]. Between 1.5 g and 2 g of adult flies between the ages of 1–7 days were placed in 10 ml of cold buffer A (250 mM sucrose, 1 mM EDTA, 50 mM Tris-HCl pH 7.4 with protease inhibitors added before use) homogenized and centrifuged. The supernatant was centrifuged at 10,000xg for 15 minutes and was washed. The pellet was then resuspended in 1 ml buffer B (250 mM sucrose, 1 mM EGTA, 10 mM Tris-HCl pH 7.4), placed on top of a continuous percoll gradient (2.2 ml 2.5 M sucrose, 6.65 ml 100% percoll, 12.25 ml 10 mM Tris-HCl pH 7.4, 84 µl 0.25 EDTA) and centrifuged at 47,000xg for 45 minutes. The mitochondria layer was removed with a syringe and washed.

Aconitase activity. Mitosciences kit MS745 was used. Aconitase activity is measured by following the conversion of isocitrate to cis-aconitate through the increase of absorbance at 240 nm.

Succinate dehydrogenase activity

Protocol was adapted from an established method [71]. Activity of sucinate dehydrogenase (U/min) was calculated as the change of absorbance over time and multiplied by 5.18 (due to the molar absorbance of INT-formazan).

Blue native gel electrophoresis and western analysis

Blue Native protocol was adapted from an established method [72]. 150 µg of mitochondrial protein was loaded per well. A gradient gel was poured with 5% acrylamide:bis-acrylamide for the light component and 12% for the heavy component (plus glycerol at 11.4%), a final concentration of 50 mM bis-tris and 0.5 M 6-aminohexanoic acid (APS and temed for polymerization). Gels were run at 4°C, 50 V for 20 hours. Western analysis used the following antibodies: complex V beta subunit (Invitrogen A21351), complex V alpha subunit (Mitosciences MS507), complex I NDUFS3 (Mitosciences MS112).

Seizure-like activity movie analysis

Flies were recorded using PAX-it version 6 software (Midwest Information Systems, Inc., Villa Park, IL) through a PAXCAM (camera) mounted on a ZEISS microscope (W.E.L. Instrument Co). Fly movements were recorded for 5 minutes then were treated with a strobe light (SHIMPO, Itasca, IL) at a frequency of 1450 flashes per minute for 20 seconds. After the strobe light treatment, videotaping of the fly movements continued for an additional 5 minutes. Video analysis was performed using iMovie (Apple, Cupertino, CA). The recovery time was measured as the time between the end of strobe light treatment and the first normal fly movement (i.e. walking forward or grooming). A two-tailed Mann-Whitney U test was used for statistical analysis at day 25 (****p<0.0001).

Statistical analysis

In all experiments standard error is represented as standard error of the mean (S.E.M.). All analyses are student's T-test where the stars represent: **** p<0.0001, ***p<0.001, **p<0.01, *p<0.05.

Supporting Information

Video S1 Video analysis of wildtype before strobe light, demonstrating normal behavior.

Video S2 Video analysis of wildtype during 20 second strobe light, demonstrating that wildtype animals do not change their behavior during this sensory stressor.

Video S3 Video analysis of wildtype after strobe light, again demonstrating that wildtype animals were unaffected by the strobe light.

Video S4 Video analysis of *ATP6¹* before strobe light, demonstrating that *ATP6¹* animals have reduced but normal activity.

Video S5 Video analysis of *ATP6¹* during 20 second strobe light, demonstrating the convulsive seizure behavior induced by the strobe light.

Video S6 Video analysis of *ATP6¹* after strobe light, some *ATP6¹* animals continue convulsive seizure behavior while others exhibit paralysis.

Acknowledgments

The authors would like to thank Ravi Patel for help in purifying phospharginine, Dr. Bennett Van Houten for many thought provoking discussions and helpful advice, Dr. Teresa Hastings and Dr. Victor Van Larr for the use of their lyophilizer and help with running blue-native electrophoresis. Dr. Daniel Keubler for advice with the strobe light sensitivity, and Dr. Billy Day for help with the chemistry needed to verify phosphoarginine.

Author Contributions

Conceived and designed the experiments: AMC MJP. Performed the experiments: AMC WKC WVV. Analyzed the data: AMC WKC MJP. Contributed reagents/materials/analysis tools: AMC WVV MJP. Wrote the paper: AMC MJP.

References

1. Vockley J (2008) Metabolism as a complex genetic trait, a systems biology approach: implications for inborn errors of metabolism and clinical diseases. J Inherit Metab Dis 31: 619–629.

2. Kucharczyk R, Zick M, Bietenhader M, Rak M, Couplan E, et al. (2009) Mitochondrial ATP synthase disorders: molecular mechanisms and the quest for curative therapeutic approaches. Biochim Biophys Acta 1793: 186–199.

3. Wallace DC (2010) Mitochondrial DNA mutations in disease and aging. Environ Mol Mutagen 51: 440–450.

4. Celotto AM, Frank AC, McGrath SW, Fergestad T, Van Voorhies WA, et al. (2006) Mitochondrial encephalomyopathy in Drosophila. J Neurosci 26: 810–820.

5. Palladino MJ (2010) Modeling mitochondrial encephalomyopathy in Drosophila. Neurobiol Dis 40: 40–45.

6. Valiyaveetil FI, Fillingame RH (1998) Transmembrane topography of subunit a in the Escherichia coli F1F0 ATP synthase. J Biol Chem 273: 16241–16247.

7. Vik SB, Ishmukhametov RR (2005) Structure and function of subunit a of the ATP synthase of Escherichia coli. J Bioenerg Biomembr 37: 445–449.

8. Rastogi VK, Girvin ME (1999) Structural changes linked to proton translocation by subunit c of the ATP synthase. Nature 402: 263–268.

9. Fernandez-Vizarra E, Tiranti V, Zeviani M (2009) Assembly of the oxidative phosphorylation system in humans: what we have learned by studying its defects. Biochim Biophys Acta 1793: 200–211.

10. Schon EA, Santra S, Pallotti F, Girvin ME (2001) Pathogenesis of primary defects in mitochondrial ATP synthesis. Semin Cell Dev Biol 12: 441–448.

11. Jung J, Mauguiere F, Clerc-Renaud P, Ollagnon E, Mousson de Camaret B, et al. (2007) NARP mitochondriopathy: an unusual cause of progressive myoclonic epilepsy. Neurology 68: 1429–1430.

12. Castagna AE, Addis J, McInnes RR, Clarke JT, Ashby P, et al. (2007) Late onset Leigh syndrome and ataxia due to a T to C mutation at bp 9,185 of mitochondrial DNA. Am J Med Genet A 143A: 808–816.

13. Carelli V, Baracca A, Barogi S, Pallotti F, Valentino ML, et al. (2002) Biochemical-clinical correlation in patients with different loads of the mitochondrial DNA T8993G mutation. Arch Neurol 59: 264–270.

14. Debray FG, Lambert M, Lortie A, Vanasse M, Mitchell GA (2007) Long-term outcome of Leigh syndrome caused by the NARP-T8993C mtDNA mutation. Am J Med Genet A 143A: 2046–2051.

15. D'Aurelio M, Vives-Bauza C, Davidson MM, Manfredi G (2009) Mitochondrial DNA background modifies the bioenergetics of NARP/MILS ATP6 mutant cells. Hum Mol Genet 19: 374–386.

16. Tatuch Y, Christodoulou J, Feigenbaum A, Clarke JT, Wherret J, et al. (1992) Heteroplasmic mtDNA mutation (T—G) at 8993 can cause Leigh disease when the percentage of abnormal mtDNA is high. Am J Hum Genet 50: 852–858.

17. Santorelli FM, Shanske S, Macaya A, DeVivo DC, DiMauro S (1993) The mutation at nt 8993 of mitochondrial DNA is a common cause of Leigh's syndrome. Ann Neurol 34: 827–834.

18. Enns GM, Bai RK, Beck AE, Wong LJ (2006) Molecular-clinical correlations in a family with variable tissue mitochondrial DNA T8993G mutant load. Mol Genet Metab 88: 364–371.

19. Beal MF (1996) Mitochondria, free radicals, and neurodegeneration. Curr Opin Neurobiol 6: 661–666.

20. Di Donato S (2000) Disorders related to mitochondrial membranes: pathology of the respiratory chain and neurodegeneration. J Inherit Metab Dis 23: 247–263.

21. Di Donato S (2009) Multisystem manifestations of mitochondrial disorders. J Neurol 256: 693–710.

22. Schon EA, Manfredi G (2003) Neuronal degeneration and mitochondrial dysfunction. J Clin Invest 111: 303–312.

23. DiMauro S, Schon EA (2003) Mitochondrial respiratory-chain diseases. N Engl J Med 348: 2656–2668.

24. Schapira AH (1999) Mitochondrial disorders. Biochim Biophys Acta 1410: 99–102.

25. Vilarinho L, Barbot C, Carrozo R, Calado E, Tessa A, et al. (2001) Clinical and molecular findings in four new patients harbouring the mtDNA 8993T>C mutation. J Inherit Metab Dis 24: 883–884.

26. Lopez-Gallardo E, Solano A, Herrero-Martin MD, Martinez-Romero I, Castano-Perez MD, et al. (2009) NARP syndrome in a patient harbouring an insertion in the MT-ATP6 gene that results in a truncated protein. J Med Genet 46: 64–67.

27. Chakrapani A, Heptinstall L, Walter J (1998) A family with Leigh syndrome caused by the rarer T8993C mutation. J Inherit Metab Dis 21: 685–686.

28. Rantamaki MT, Soini HK, Finnila SM, Majamaa K, Udd B (2005) Adult-onset ataxia and polyneuropathy caused by mitochondrial 8993T-->C mutation. Ann Neurol 58: 337–340.

29. Hartzog PE, Cain BD (1993) Mutagenic analysis of the a subunit of the F1F0 ATP synthase in Escherichia coli: Gln-252 through Tyr-263. J Bacteriol 175: 1337–1343.

30. Hartzog PE, Cain BD (1993) The aleu207-->arg mutation in F1F0-ATP synthase from Escherichia coli. A model for human mitochondrial disease. J Biol Chem 268: 12250–12252.

31. Nation JL (2008) Insect Physiology and Biochemistry. Boca RatonFL: CRC Press and Taylor & Francis Group. pp 509.

32. Pallotti F, Baracca A, Hernandez-Rosa E, Walker WF, Solaini G, et al. (2004) Biochemical analysis of respiratory function in cybrid cell lines harbouring mitochondrial DNA mutations. Biochem J 384: 287–293.

33. Schmidt-Nielsen K (1997) Animal Physiology. Cambridge: Cambridge University Press.

34. Yoon Y, Galloway CA, Jhun BS, Yu T (2011) Mitochondrial dynamics in diabetes. Antioxid Redox Signal 14: 439–457.

35. Ren J, Pulakat L, Whaley-Connell A, Sowers JR (2010) Mitochondrial biogenesis in the metabolic syndrome and cardiovascular disease. J Mol Med 88: 993–1001.

36. Gonzalez CD, Lee MS, Marchetti P, Pietropaolo M, Towns R, et al. (2011) The emerging role of autophagy in the pathophysiology of diabetes mellitus. Autophagy 7: 2–11.

37. de Moura MB, dos Santos LS, Van Houten B (2010) Mitochondrial dysfunction in neurodegenerative diseases and cancer. Environ Mol Mutagen 51: 391–405.

38. Tillement L, Lecanu L, Papadopoulos V (2011) Alzheimer's disease: effects of beta-amyloid on mitochondria. Mitochondrion 11: 13–21.

39. Seo AY, Joseph AM, Dutta D, Hwang JC, Aris JP, et al. (2010) New insights into the role of mitochondria in aging: mitochondrial dynamics and more. J Cell Sci 123: 2533–2542.

40. Ferreira IL, Resende R, Ferreiro E, Rego AC, Pereira CF (2010) Multiple defects in energy metabolism in Alzheimer's disease. Curr Drug Targets 11: 1193–1206.

41. Forester BP, Berlow YA, Harper DG, Jensen JE, Lange N, et al. (2010) Age-related changes in brain energetics and phospholipid metabolism. NMR Biomed 23: 242–250.

42. Thorburn DR, Rahman S (1993) Mitochondrial DNA-Associated Leigh Syndrome and NARP; Pagon RA, Bird, T.D., Dolan, C.R. et al., editor. Seattle: University of Washington.

43. Tucker EJ, Compton AG, Thorburn DR (2010) Recent advances in the genetics of mitochondrial encephalopathies. Curr Neurol Neurosci Rep 10: 277–285.

44. Zsurka G, Kunz WS (2010) Mitochondrial dysfunction in neurological disorders with epileptic phenotypes. J Bioenerg Biomembr 42: 443–448.

45. Ganetzky B, Wu CF (1982) Indirect Suppression Involving Behavioral Mutants with Altered Nerve Excitability in DROSOPHILA MELANOGASTER. Genetics 100: 597–614.

46. Lints FA, Lints CV (1968) Respiration in Drosophila. II. Respiration in relation to age by wild, inbred and hybrid Drosophila melanogaster imagos. Exp Gerontol 3: 341–349.

47. Hulbert AJ, Else PL (2004) Basal metabolic rate: history, composition, regulation, and usefulness. Physiol Biochem Zool 77: 869–876.

48. Van Voorhies WA, Ward S (1999) Genetic and environmental conditions that increase longevity in Caenorhabditis elegans decrease metabolic rate. Proc Natl Acad Sci U S A 96: 11399–11403.

49. Van Voorhies WA (2003) The metabolic rate of Caenorhabditis elegans dauer larvae: comments on a recent paper by Houthoofd et al. Exp Gerontol 38: 343–344.

50. Van Voorhies WA (2002) Metabolism and aging in the nematode Caenorhabditis elegans. Free Radic Biol Med 33: 587–596.

51. Goyon V, Fronzes R, Salin B, di-Rago JP, Velours J, et al. (2008) Yeast cells depleted in Atp14p fail to assemble Atp6p within the ATP synthase and exhibit altered mitochondrial cristae morphology. J Biol Chem 283: 9749–9758.

52. Paumard P, Vaillier J, Coulary B, Schaeffer J, Soubannier V, et al. (2002) The ATP synthase is involved in generating mitochondrial cristae morphology. EMBO J 21: 221–230.

53. Rak M, Tetaud E, Godard F, Sagot I, Salin B, et al. (2007) Yeast cells lacking the mitochondrial gene encoding the ATP synthase subunit 6 exhibit a selective loss of complex IV and unusual mitochondrial morphology. J Biol Chem 282: 10853–10864.

54. Strauss M, Hofhaus G, Schroder RR, Kuhlbrandt W (2008) Dimer ribbons of ATP synthase shape the inner mitochondrial membrane. EMBO J 27: 1154–1160.

55. Wittig I, Schagger H (2008) Structural organization of mitochondrial ATP synthase. Biochim Biophys Acta 1777: 592–598.

56. Wittig I, Velours J, Stuart R, Schagger H (2008) Characterization of domain interfaces in monomeric and dimeric ATP synthase. Mol Cell Proteomics 7: 995–1004.

57. Ashmore LJ, Hrizo SL, Paul SM, Van Voorhies WA, Beitel GJ, et al. (2009) Novel mutations affecting the Na, K ATPase alpha model complex neurological diseases and implicate the sodium pump in increased longevity. Hum Genet 126: 431–447.

58. Seigle JL, Celotto AM, Palladino MJ (2008) Degradation of functional triose phosphate isomerase protein underlies sugarkill pathology. Genetics 179: 855–862.

59. Fergestad T, Olson L, Patel KP, Miller R, Palladino MJ, et al. (2008) Neuropathology in Drosophila mutants with increased seizure susceptibility. Genetics 178: 947–956.

60. Celotto AM, Frank AC, Seigle JL, Palladino MJ (2006) Drosophila model of human inherited triosephosphate isomerase deficiency glycolytic enzymopathy. Genetics 174: 1237–1246.

61. Fergestad T, Ganetzky B, Palladino MJ (2006) Neuropathology in Drosophila membrane excitability mutants. Genetics 172: 1031–1042.

62. Palladino MJ, Bower JE, Kreber R, Ganetzky B (2003) Neural dysfunction and neurodegeneration in Drosophila Na+/K+ ATPase alpha subunit mutants. J Neurosci 23: 1276–1286.

63. Palladino MJ, Hadley TJ, Ganetzky B (2002) Temperature-sensitive paralytic mutants are enriched for those causing neurodegeneration in Drosophila. Genetics 161: 1197–1208.

64. Viant MR, Rosenblum ES, Tjeerdema RS (2001) Optimized method for the determination of phosphoarginine in abalone tissue by high-performance liquid chromatography. J Chromatogr B Biomed Sci Appl 765: 107–111.

65. Morrison JF, Griffiths DE, Ennor AH (1957) The purification and properties of arginine phosphokinase. Biochem J 65: 143–153.

66. Xue X, Wang F, Zhou J, Chen F, Li Y, et al. (2009) Online cleanup of accelerated solvent extractions for determination of adenosine 5′-triphosphate (ATP), adenosine 5′-diphosphate (ADP), and adenosine 5′-monophosphate (AMP) in royal jelly using high-performance liquid chromatography. J Agric Food Chem 57: 4500–4505.

67. Matthews RT, Yang L, Jenkins BG, Ferrante RJ, Rosen BR, et al. (1998) Neuroprotective effects of creatine and cyclocreatine in animal models of Huntington's disease. J Neurosci 18: 156–163.

68. Van Voorhies WA, Khazaeli AA, Curtsinger JW (2004) Testing the "rate of living" model: further evidence that longevity and metabolic rate are not inversely correlated in Drosophila melanogaster. J Appl Physiol 97: 1915–1922.

69. Van Voorhies WA, Melvin RG, Ballard JW, Williams JB (2008) Validation of manometric microrespirometers for measuring oxygen consumption in small arthropods. J Insect Physiol 54: 1132–1137.

70. Gasnier F, Rousson R, Lerme F, Vaganay E, Louisot P, et al. (1993) Use of Percoll gradients for isolation of human placenta mitochondria suitable for investigating outer membrane proteins. Anal Biochem 212: 173–178.

71. Munujos P, Coll-Canti J, Gonzalez-Sastre F, Gella FJ (1993) Assay of succinate dehydrogenase activity by a colorimetric-continuous method using iodonitrotetrazolium chloride as electron acceptor. Anal Biochem 212: 506–509.

72. Brookes PS, Pinner A, Ramachandran A, Coward L, Barnes S, et al. (2002) High throughput two-dimensional blue-native electrophoresis: a tool for functional proteomics of mitochondria and signaling complexes. Proteomics 2: 969–977.

8

A Risk-Factor Guided Approach to Reducing Lactic Acidosis and Hyperlactatemia in Patients on Antiretroviral Therapy

Lynn T. Matthews[1]*, Janet Giddy[2], Musie Ghebremichael[3], Jane Hampton[2], Anthony J. Guarino[4], Aba Ewusi[5], Emma Carver[6], Karen Axten[3], Meghan C. Geary[7], Rajesh T. Gandhi[3,8], David R. Bangsberg[3,9,10]

1 Division of Infectious Disease, Beth Israel Deaconess Medical Center, Boston, Massachusetts, United States of America, 2 HIV Program, McCord Hospital, Durban, South Africa, 3 Ragon Institute of Massachusetts General Hospital, Massachusetts Institute of Technology, and Harvard University, Boston, Massachusetts, United States of America, 4 Institute of Health Professions, Massachusetts General Hospital, Boston, Massachusetts, United States of America, 5 Division of Internal Medicine, Harvard Vanguard Medical Associates, Boston, Massachusetts, United States of America, 6 Department of Emergency Medicine, University Hospital of Wales, Cardiff, Wales, 7 Albany Medical College, Albany, New York, United States of America, 8 Division of Infectious Disease, Massachusetts General Hospital, Boston, Massachusetts, United States of America, 9 Mbarara University of Science and Technology, Mbarara, Uganda, 10 Center for Global Health, Massachusetts General Hospital, Boston, Massachusetts, United States of America

Abstract

Background: Stavudine continues to be used in antiretroviral treatment (ART) regimens in many resource-limited settings. The use of zidovudine instead of stavudine in higher-risk patients to reduce the likelihood of lactic acidosis and hyperlactatemia (LAHL) has not been examined.

Methods: Antiretroviral-naïve, HIV-infected adults initiating ART between 2004 and 2007 were divided into cohorts of those initiated on stavudine- or zidovudine-containing therapy. We evaluated stavudine or zidovudine use, age, sex, body mass index (BMI), baseline CD4 cell count, creatinine, hemoglobin, alanine aminotransferase, and albumin as predictors of time to LAHL with Cox Proportional Hazards (PH) regression models.

Results: Among 2062 patients contributing 2747 patient years (PY), the combined incidence of LAHL was 3.2/100 PY in those initiating stavudine- and 0.34/100 PY in those initiating zidovudine-containing ART (RR 9.26, 95% CI: 1.28–66.93). In multivariable Cox PH analysis, stavudine exposure (HR 14.31, 95% CI: 5.79–35.30), female sex (HR 3.41, 95% CI: 1.89–6.19), higher BMI (HR 3.21, 95% CI: 2.16–4.77), higher creatinine (1.63, 95% CI: 1.12–2.36), higher albumin (HR 1.04, 95% CI: 1.01–1.07), and lower CD4 cell count (HR 0.96, 95% CI: 0.92–1.0) at baseline were associated with higher LAHL rates. Among participants who started on stavudine, switching to zidovudine was associated with lower LAHL rates (HR 0.15, 95% CI: 0.06–0.35). Subgroup analysis limited to women with higher BMI≥25 kg/m2 initiated on stavudine also showed that switch to zidovudine was protective when controlling for other risk factors (HR 0.21, 95% CI .07–0.64).

Conclusions: Stavudine exposure, female sex, and higher BMI are strong, independent predictors for developing LAHL. Patients with risk factors for lactic acidosis have less LAHL while on zidovudine- rather than stavudine-containing ART. Switching patients from stavudine to zidovudine is protective. Countries continuing to use stavudine should avoid this drug in women and patients with higher BMI.

Editor: Landon Myer, University of Cape Town, South Africa

Funding: Dr. Matthews' work was supported by the Mark and Lisa Schwartz Family Foundation and by a postdoctoral fellowship in tropical infectious diseases from the Burroughs Wellcome Fund/American Society for Tropical Medicine and Hygiene. Dr. Gandhi is supported by NIH R01 AI066992-04A1 and NIH G08LM008830-01 and by grants to the AIDS Clinical Trials Group (NIH U01 AI 694722) and the Harvard University Center for AIDS Research (NIH 2P30 AI060354-06). Dr. Bangsberg was supported by NIH grant MH K-24 87227. The authors are also grateful to Dr. Heather Ribaudo of the Harvard University Center for AIDS Research Biostatistical Core (NIH #AI060354). The funders had no role in study design, data collection and analysis, decision to publish, or preparation of the manuscript.

Competing Interests: The authors have declared that no competing interests exist.

* E-mail: ltmatthe@bidmc.harvard.edu

Introduction

Lactic acidosis is a potentially fatal side effect of nucleoside analog reverse transcriptase inhibitors (NRTIs) [1,2], which are commonly used in combination antiretroviral therapy (ART). This complication is related to NRTI-induced mitochondrial toxicity possibly due to structural similarities between mitochondrial DNA polymerase and HIV-reverse transcriptase (the target of NRTIs) [3]. The incidence of lactic acidosis among patients on ART ranges from 1–4 per 100 patient years in resource-rich settings and is as high as 10 per 100 patient years in sub-Saharan African cohorts [4,5,6,7,8,9,10,11]. The lactic acidosis case-fatality rate in resource-limited settings can be as high as 60% [12].

Of the NRTIs, the dideoxynucleosides (stavudine and didanosine) confer the highest risk of lactic acidosis [1,2,5]. While stavudine is rarely used in resource-rich settings and is no longer recommended by the World Health Organization for initial treatment of HIV-1 infection [13], it remains an important component of standard ART regimens in many resource-limited countries, largely due to cost [14,15]. In South Africa where stavudine is no longer recommended for use in first-line therapy, patients receiving stavudine-containing ART are only switched if there is evidence of toxicity, again because of financial constraints. In settings where stavudine is widely prescribed, lactic acidosis is a frequent cause of morbidity and mortality [1,2,4,5,6,7,8,9,10,16] and is associated with high losses to follow-up and treatment discontinuation [15].

Observational studies suggest that specific risk factors associated with the development of hyperlactatemia include female sex [1,4,7,11,16,17,18], elevated weight or body-mass index (BMI) [1,11,16,17,18], older age (>40 years) [1,11], and lower CD4 cell counts [1]. Where financial constraints prevent comprehensive adoption of less-toxic agents, a risk factor-guided approach to choosing an initial regimen may reduce the incidence of lactic acidosis. Studies have shown that after resolution of lactic acidosis it is safe to treat patients with zidovudine (an alternative thymidine analog NRTI which is widely used in resource-limited settings) [10,19], but none have examined whether avoiding stavudine in patients with lactic acidosis risk factors reduces incidence of lactic acidosis or hyperlactatemia.

Until April 2010, first-line therapy in South Africa included stavudine, lamivudine, and either efavirenz or nevirapine. Based on observational findings from a site-specific study that identified a high incidence of lactic acidosis in women with BMI≥28 kg/m^2, in August 2005 the HIV Clinic at McCord Hospital in Durban, South Africa substituted zidovudine for stavudine in initial ART for patients with these two risk factors [7]. The policy continued until March 2007, when the clinic was accredited as a Department of Health site and required to follow Department of Health guidelines for ART, including the use of stavudine as part of initial regimens.

To evaluate the impact of risk factor-guided selection of initial therapy, we compared the combined incidence of lactic acidosis and hyperlactatemia among treatment-naive patients initiating stavudine-containing therapy with those starting zidovudine-containing therapy. We hypothesized that risk-factor-guided ART (initiating women with BMI≥28 kg/m2 on zidovudine rather than stavudine) would be associated with decreased incidence of lactic acidosis and hyperlactatemia. We also assessed predictors of lactic acidosis and hyperlactatemia.

Methods

Ethics statement

Ethics approvals were obtained from the McCord Hospital Medical Ethics Research Committee and from the Partners Healthcare Institutional Review Board (Boston, MA). Given the nature of the study (retrospective chart review), the requirement for informed consent was waived by the ethics committees.

Study design and population

Patient data were collected from the outpatient HIV clinic at McCord Hospital in Durban, South Africa which has initiated over 8000 patients on ART. During the study period, initial ART included two NRTIs and one NNRTI: stavudine (30 mg twice daily; 40 mg twice daily if weight >60 kg) or zidovudine plus lamivudine and either efavirenz or nevirapine.

The study population included antiretroviral (ARV)-naïve, HIV-infected adults (age ≥18 years) with baseline laboratory data and at least one follow-up visit after ART initiation. Two retrospective cohorts were identified. The first cohort included patients who initiated stavudine-containing therapy between July 2004 and March 2007. The second cohort included patients who initiated zidovudine-containing ART between July 2004 and March 2007. Both cohorts included patients who initiated ART between August 2005 and March 2007 when the clinic made women with BMI≥28 kg/m2 eligible for initiation of zidovudine - containing therapy or for regimen switch from stavudine to zidovudine.

Outcomes and their measurement

The primary outcome was event-free survival defined as the time from treatment initiation to development of lactic acidosis (symptomatic or asymptomatic) or hyperlactatemia (symptomatic or asymptomatic) (Table 1). Lactic acidosis and hyperlactatemia were defined based on AIDS Clinical Trials Group criteria [20]. Lactic acidosis is defined as having a lactate level above the upper limit of normal (4.4 mmol/L) along with evidence of acidosis (bicarbonate level <20 mmol/L or pH<7.35). Hyperlactatemia is defined as a lactate level greater than the upper limit of normal without evidence of acidosis. Cases of symptomatic lactic acidosis or hyperlactatemia met the above criteria and had new, otherwise unexplained symptoms of nausea, vomiting; abdominal pain, discomfort, or distention; increased hepatic transaminases; fatigue; dyspnea; weight loss (≥5%); or muscle weakness. Because these patients were ambulatory and often did not have repeat measurements, confirmed elevation of lactate levels was not required if at least two symptoms were present.

Blood was drawn for lactate levels without use of a tourniquet and specimens were transported on ice and processed within four hours (Beckman Coulter, Synchron systems, California, USA). A handheld lactate detection device, a reliable proxy for serum samples, was introduced in 2006 (Accutrend model #3012522) [21,22] and was used for initial screening in addition to serum lactate testing.

Outcomes were classified from a review of the medical records of patients initiating ART during the study period. This review was facilitated by the requirement that clinicians record the reason for any change or discontinuation in ARV regimen from an electronic pull down menu. For patients who had a regimen change noted in the electronic record, paper charts were reviewed for the following: 1) documentation of a regimen change due to lactic acidosis; 2) documentation of a regimen change and signs or symptoms that could be consistent with lactic acidosis or hyperlactatemia (nausea, vomiting, abdominal discomfort, bloating, increased hepatic transaminases, fatigue, dyspnea, weight loss, muscle weakness); 3) documentation of a regimen change without specific reason listed; 4) death. Serum lactate test results for all study patients were reviewed. A lactate value above 3 mmol/L prompted review of the medical record for symptoms of hyperlactatemia, all available lactate values, other possible causes for symptoms or elevated lactate levels, and clinical outcome. Data were abstracted using standardized abstraction forms (LM, AE, JH). For a subset of patients (n = 20), two physicians carried out the abstractions with 100% agreement on outcome classification (JH, LM). Cases with unclear outcomes were adjudicated by a senior clinician (RG).

We also identified patients for whom clinicians had changed ART due to peripheral neuropathy, lipodystrophy, high BMI, and drug resistance, as indicated in the electronic medical record. We identified patients with regimen switch for clinical suspicion of LA

Table 1. Criteria for lactic acidosis and hyperlactatemia outcomes[1].

	Asymptomatic lactic acidosis	Symptomatic lactic acidosis	Asymptomatic hyperlactatemia	Symptomatic hyperlactatemia
Lactate (mmol/L)	≥4.4	≥4.4	≥4.4	≥4.4
Abnormal values required	≥2	≥1	≥2	≥1
Acidosis[2]	+	+	−	−
Symptoms[3]	−	+	−	+

[1]Based on AACTG criteria [19].
[2]Bicarbonate <20 mmol/L or pH<7.35.
[3]New or otherwise unexplained symptoms of nausea or vomiting, abdominal pain or discomfort, abdominal distention, increased hepatic transaminases, unexplained fatigue, dyspnea, weight loss (≥5%), or muscle weakness.

or HL but who did not meet criteria. These subjects were not censored at change in regimen but followed out to a total two years of follow-up from treatment initiation. In addition, we identified subjects who changed clinic site, stopped ART, died or were lost to follow up.

Covariates

Covariates were obtained from paper chart abstractions and included weight at treatment initiation (within 3 months) and height. Weights obtained during pregnancy were excluded. BMI was calculated (kg/m^2) for all subjects in whom height and baseline weight were available. Sex, date of birth and baseline (the last value prior to ART initiation, or within 2 weeks) CD4 count, creatinine, hemoglobin, alanine aminotransferase, and albumin were extracted from the electronic record or the paper chart. All specimens were processed using standardized methods at laboratories in Durban.

Time to event or censor

The primary outcome was 2-year event-free survival (EFS) defined as the time from treatment initiation up to development of lactic acidosis or hyperlactatemia. Patients were also censored for loss to follow-up, change in clinic site, termination of treatment, death, or at study end. All others were followed for two years or until the primary outcome. Time on stavudine and zidovudine was calculated from start and stop dates entered by clinicians in the medical record.

Analysis

We calculated crude incidence rates for the combined primary outcome (LAHL), the combined incidence of peripheral neuropathy and lipodystrophy, death, and loss-to-follow-up. Confidence intervals for event rates based on initial therapy with stavudine or zidovudine were estimated using methods for exact binomial confidence intervals and compared using Chi-square tests [23]. Kaplan-Meier curves were plotted for event-free survival based on initial treatment and rates were compared using the log-rank test statistic. Univariate and multivariate analyses using Cox proportional hazards (PH) regression models were utilized to assess the effect of treatment on time to event [24]. We evaluated time on zidovudine or stavudine as a time-varying covariate to account for variable time on drug among patients whose regimens were switched in the absence of the outcome of interest (e.g. switch for peripheral neuropathy or increased BMI). Covariates for multivariate analysis were selected based on significance (p value<0.05) in univariate analysis and significant covariates in the literature. CD4 count was modeled as a continuous variable with the effect

size reported per 10-cell increment. BMI was modeled on a natural logarithmic scale with effect size reported per 30% shift. In the full model, BMI deviated from the proportional hazards assumption and was modeled with a time-dependent association for early (within the first year) and late (after one year) failure. In subgroup analysis, BMI followed proportional hazards. All statistical analyses were carried out using SAS version 9.2 for Windows.

Results

Baseline patient and disease characteristics

Two-thousand-sixty-two patients contributing 2747 person years of follow-up were included in the study. The median age was 34.7 years (IQR 29.8, 40.6) and 60% were women. Eighty-nine percent initiated therapy with a stavudine-containing regimen. One-hundred sixty one (77%) of those who were initiated on a zidovudine-containing regimen were started because of higher BMI or other perceived lactic acidosis risk factors. The remaining patients were initiated on zidovudine because of pre-existing lipodystrophy (<1%), peripheral neuropathy (<1%), pregnancy (10%), or unknown reason (10%).

Median CD4 count at entry was 80 cells/mm3 (IQR 29–142). Median BMI for subjects with complete data (88% had documented weight at entry, 76% had documented height) was 22 kg/m2 (IQR 20, 26). Compared with those initiated on a stavudine-containing regimen, patients started on zidovudine were older, more likely to be female, had a higher BMI, higher CD4 cell count, higher albumin and higher hemoglobin. Other characteristics are described in Table 2.

Outcomes for full cohort

In intention to treat analysis, combined incidence of LAHL was 3.2/100 PY in the stavudine- and 0.34/100 PY in the zidovudine-initiated group (RR 9.26, 95% CI 1.28–66.93, p = .007). There were 36 lactic acidosis and 43 hyperlactatemia events in the stavudine group. In contrast, there was 1 lactic acidosis event in the zidovudine group: this occurred in a woman who initiated zidovudine-based therapy because of high BMI (31 kg/m2); one year later, she was switched to stavudine because of anemia; after eight months on stavudine-containing ART, she was diagnosed with lactic acidosis. Mortality due to causes other than LAHL was 8.3% and 2.8% in stavudine- and zidovudine-initiated patients, respectively (RR = 2.89, 95% CI:1.45–5.78, p = 0.001). The combined incidence of physician-reported peripheral neuropathy and lipodystrophy was 16.8/100 PY in stavudine- and 0.34/100 PY in zidovudine-initiated groups (RR = 59.84, 95% CI: 8.36–

Table 2. Patient characteristics at study entry by treatment arm.

Variable	Initial ART includes:		
	Stavudine	Zidovudine	p-value[1]
Number (patient years follow-up)	1853 (2460)	209 (287)	
Age, years Mean (SD)	35.7 (8.3)	37.8 (9.6)	<.001
Patient years of follow up Mean (SD)	1.3 (0.7)	1.4 (0.6)	<.001
Female n (%)	1078 (58.2)	188 (90)	<.001
BMI (kg/m^2) Median (IQR)	22 (19, 24)	30 (28, 33)	<.001
CD4 (cells/mm^3) Median (IQR)	75 (27, 138)	129 (61, 172)	<.001
Creatinine (mg/dL) Median (IQR)	1.0 (0.4)	0.9 (0.3)	.21
ALT (IU/L) Median (IQR)	24 (18, 35)	23 (17, 32)	.27
Albumin (g/L) Median (IQR)	31.2 (7.3)	34.9 (5.3)	<.001
Hemoglobin (g/dL) Median (IQR)	10.8 (2.1)	11.6 (1.3)	<.001

[1]Chi-square test was used for categorical variables, T-test for continuous where mean and standard deviation reported, and Wilcoxon rank sum where median and IQR reported.

428.12, p<0.001). Loss to follow-up was equivalent between the two groups (RR = 1.42, 95% CI: 0.68–2.96, p = 0.35). (Table 3)

In univariate Cox proportional hazards analysis, stavudine in the initial treatment regimen, female sex, higher BMI, and higher baseline albumin were each associated with increased risk of LAHL (Table 4). The Kaplan Meier curve for time to LAHL based on initial treatment regimen is shown in Figure 1 (p = .006).

In multivariable Cox PH regression to assess predictors of event-free survival, hemoglobin and ALT were removed but age and CD4 cell count were included because prior data and a priori knowledge suggested an association with lactic acidosis [1]. Creatinine was into the full model when it was found to be significant in subgroup analysis. The adjusted hazards of experiencing LAHL was higher for those on stavudine (HR = 14.31, 95% CI 5.79–35.30), women (HR = 3.41, 95% CI: 1.89–6.19), subjects with higher BMI in the first year (HR = 3.21, 95% CI: 2.16–4.77), higher albumin (HR = 1.04, 95% CI:1.01–1.07), higher creatinine (HR = 1.63, 95% CI 1.12–2.36), or lower baseline CD4 cell count (HR = 0.96, 95% CI: 0.92–1.00) at baseline (Table 5). Among those initiated on stavudine, the hazards of experiencing LAHL was lower for those who were switched to zidovudine during follow-up (HR 0.15, 95% CI 0.06–0.35).

Outcomes for women with higher BMI

Women with BMI greater than or equal to 25 kg/m2 comprised 326 patients with 434 years of follow-up. The 194 women initiated on stavudine were younger; with lower BMI, baseline CD4 cell count, creatinine, albumin, and hemoglobin compared with 132 women initiated on zidovudine (Table 5). Obese women initiated on stavudine had 22 LAHL events (8.0/100 woman years), compared with 1 (0.53/100 woman years) among those initiated on zidovudine (RR = 9.94, 95% CI, 1.46–67.91, p = .0002). When controlling for BMI, CD4 cell count, albumin, creatinine, and age, stavudine use was associated with a 13-fold increase in hazards of LAHL (HR 13.37, 95% CI 4.31–41.53) (Table 6). For women in this subgroup who initiated on stavudine-containing therapy, switching to zidovudine was protective (HR 0.21, 95% CI 0.07–0.64, p = 0.006).

Of the 194 women with higher BMI who initiated stavudine-inclusive therapy, 137 were switched to zidovudine for reasons other than LAHL. Baseline characteristics (age, BMI, CD4 cell count, creatinine albumin, ALT, hemoglobin) were not significantly different from women with higher BMI initiated on stavudine-treatment who did not switch treatment arms. Women were switched for high BMI (79, 56%); lipodystrophy, peripheral neuropathy, or these plus elevated BMI (47, 34%); lab values and/or symptoms suggestive of hyperlactatemia that did not meet criteria for LAHL (7, 5%); and the remainder were switched for anemia, pregnancy, rash or other reasons. These participants subsequently contributed an additional 131.7 woman-years of follow-up (mean 1.1 years ±0.5) during which there were 5 LAHL events (3.8/100 woman years). All but one event occurred within 2–8 weeks of switching off stavudine after an average of 0.6±0.4 years on stavudine, suggesting that the recent and cumulative stavudine exposure contributed to the toxicity. When controlling for other LAHL risk factors, switch to zidovudine conferred 80% lower hazards of LAHL for this subgroup (HR 0.21, 95% CI 0.07–0.64, p = .006). The remainder of women in this subgroup of obese women, initiated on stavudine and switched to zidovudine, included two who subsequently had anemia and two who died; the rest were followed until the end of the study, change in service provider, or a maximum of two years of follow-up without adverse events.

Discussion

In our study of 2062 HIV-positive patients who initiated ART, stavudine use confers a fourteen-fold increased risk of developing hyperlactatemia or lactic acidosis when controlling for other risk factors (HR 14.31, 95% CI 5.79–35.30). Other risk factors for the primary outcome of LAHL were female sex, higher baseline BMI,

Table 3. Incidence of mitochondrial toxicity, death and loss to follow-up by initial treatment.

Outcome	Initial ART includes:		Relative Risk Ratio [95% CI]	Chi-Square p-value
	Stavudine (Incidence/100 PY)	Zidovudine (Incidence/100 PY)		
Lactic acidosis or hyperlactatemia[1]	79 (3.2)	1 (0.3)	9.26 [1.28, 66.93]	.007
Mortality due to cause other than LAHL	205 (8.3)	8(2.8)	2.89 [1.45, 5.78]	.001
Peripheral neuropathy or lipodystrophy[2]	414 (16.8)	1 (0.3)	59.84 [8.36, 428.12]	<.001
Loss to follow-up	99 (4.0)	8 (2.8)	1.42 [0.68, 2.96]	.35

[1]Primary endpoint: 37 lactic acidosis, 43 hyperlactatemia.
[2]As indicated by clinician report in the medical record.

Table 4. Univariate and multivariate Cox Regression Analysis for time to lactic acidosis or hyperlactatemia.

Variable	Hazards Ratio [95% CI]	p-value	Adjusted Hazards Ratio [95% CI]	p-value
Age (years)	1.02 [0.99, 1.04]	.14	–	.22
Female sex	2.22 [1.31, 3.75]	.003	**3.42 [1.89, 6.19]**	**<.0001**
BMI in first year (30% change kg/m^2)	1.53 [1.10, 2.12]	.01	**3.21 [2.16, 4.77]**	**<.0001**
BMI after first year (30% change kg/m^2)	0.76 [0.44, 1.32]	.33	–	.55
Stavudine use	5.81 [2.52, 13.43]	<.0001	**14.31 [5.79, 35.30]**	**<.0001**
Initial CD4 count (10 cells/mm^3)	0.99 [0.96, 1.03]	.80	**0.96 [0.92, 1.00]**	**.04**
Initial Albumin (g/L)	1.04 [1.01, 1.07]	.004	**1.04 [1.01, 1.07]**	**.004**
Initial Creatinine (mg/dL)	1.00 [0.99, 1.01]	.09	**1.63 [1.12, 2.36]**	**.010**
Initial ALT (IU/L)	1.00 [0.99, 1.01]	.38	–	–
Hemoglobin (g/dL)	1.07 [0.95, 1.19]	.26	–	–

Multivariate model with 80 events, 1546 subjects with complete data for all variables.

higher baseline creatinine or albumin, and lower initial CD4 cell count. For patients who started a stavudine-containing regimen, switching to zidovudine was associated with 85% lower hazards of developing LAHL (HR 0.15, 95% CI 0.06–0.35). For the high-risk subgroup of women with BMI≥25 kg/m2 who initiated therapy on stavudine-containing ART, switch to zidovudine was also protective when controlling for other risk factors (HR 0.21, 95% CI 0.07–0.64).

Our study adds to the literature by demonstrating that female sex is a strong independent risk factor for developing LAHL [1,4,7,11,16,17,18]. Higher weight has been associated with these outcomes in prior studies, but this is the first to confirm a relationship with BMI and LAHL when controlling for other covariates [1,11,16,17,18]. For every 30% change in BMI (i.e. 18 to 23 kg/m^2 or 24 to 31 kg/m^2), we observed a three-fold increase in the LAHL rate (HR = 3.21, 95% CI: 2.16–4.77). For the full dataset, the effect was only significant in the first year of follow-up which may reflect increased risk earlier in treatment or insufficient power to detect an association after the first year. During the study, patients with weight >60 kg received 80 mg of stavudine daily, which has been linked to worse mitochondrial toxicities compared to use of 60 mg [25]. We were unable to

control for stavudine dose; thus, the high incidence of LAHL in patients with higher BMI might be related to higher stavudine dose. This possibility is supported by observations that patients on higher dose stavudine (40 mg twice daily) have a higher incidence of elevated lactate than those who receive lower doses (20 or 30 mg twice daily) [16,25]. However, given that multiple studies involving varying stavudine dose have found an association between higher weight or BMI and lactic acidosis [7,11,17] while, in some cases, controlling for dose [16,18], it is unlikely that drug dosing explains the entire effect. Furthermore, a three-fold increase in hazards of LAHL was observed in our subgroup analysis of women with BMI≥25 kg/m2 (who likely received uniform stavudine dosing).

Higher creatinine was associated with increased hazards of LAHL, about 25% per 1 mg/dL unit increase in creatinine. This risk factor has not been reported in prior univariate analyses and has not been included in studies that control for other risk factors, but is not unexpected given the kidney's role in lactate metabolism [26]. We also found that higher albumin is associated with an increased risk of LAHL and a small protective effect of higher CD4 cell count at treatment initiation (4% decrease in hazards for each 10-point increase in baseline CD4 cell count). Two other

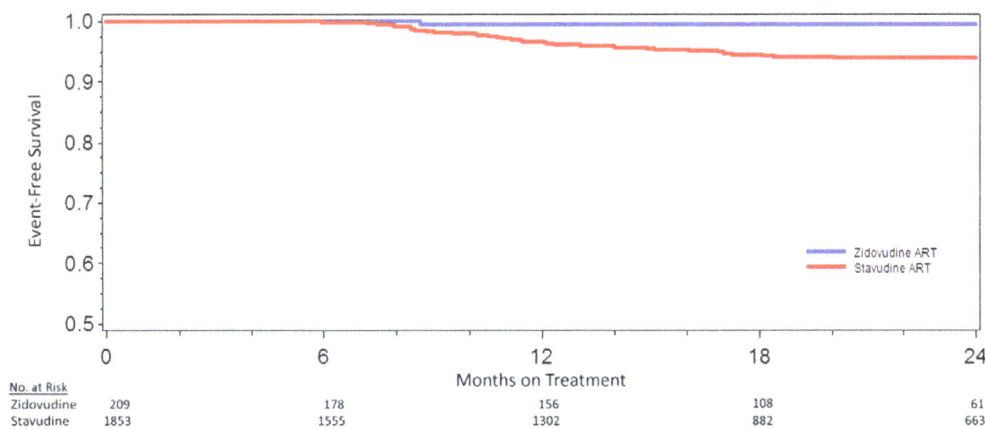

No. at Risk				
Zidovudine	209	178	156	108	61
Stavudine	1853	1555	1302	882	663

Figure 1. Kaplan Meier curves for lactic acidosis/hyperlactatemia-free survival for patients initiated on either stavudine- or zidovudine-containing antiretroviral therapy (p = .006).

Table 5. Patient characteristics at study entry by treatment arm, limited to women with BMI≥25 kg/m².

| Variable | Initial ART includes: | | p-value[1] |
	Stavudine	Zidovudine	
Number (patient years follow-up)	194 (274)	132 (190)	
Age (years) *Mean (SD)*	36 (7)	38 (9)	.03
Patient years of follow up *Mean (SD)*	1.4 (0.6)	1.4 (0.6)	.64
BMI (kg/m²) *Median (IQR)*	27 (26, 30)	30 (29, 34)	<.0001
CD4 (cells/mm³) *Median (IQR)*	99 (64)	122 (58)	.0003
Creatinine (mg/dL) *Median (IQR)*	0.85 (0.77, 0.94)	0.88 (0.80, 0.98)	.02
ALT (IU/L) *Median (IQR)*	22 (17, 32)	22 (17, 30)	.97
Albumin (g/L) *Median (IQR)*	32 (6)	36 (4)	<.0001
Hemoglobin (g/dL) *Median (IQR)*	11.1 (1.7)	11.7 (1.1)	.0001

[1]T-test for continuous where mean and standard deviation reported, and Wilcoxon rank sum where median and IQR reported.

Table 6. Multivariate Cox Regression Analysis for time to lactic acidosis or hyperlactatemia limited to women with BMI≥25 kg/m2.

Variable	Adjusted Hazards Ratio [95% CI]	p-value
BMI (30% change kg/m²)	**3.15 [1.39, 7.17]**	**.005**
Stavudine use	**13.37 [4.31, 41.53]**	**<.0001**
Initial CD4 (10 cells/mm³)	–	0.99
Initial Albumin (g/L)	1.01 [0.94, 1.08]	0.83
Initial Creatinine (mg/dL)	**1.75 [1.17, 2.62]**	**.006**

Multivariate model with 20 events, 298 subjects with complete data for all variables.

studies have also found an association between CD4 cell count and lactic acidosis [1], [27]. Each of these associations (CD4 cell count, creatinine and albumin) was small with confidence intervals close to one.

The Lactic Acidosis International Study group showed an association of older age (age >40 years) with the development of LAHL. This was not seen in our cohort nor in other studies based in Southern Africa [16,17,18]. The majority of their subjects were from Europe and the Americas with an older age distribution than in our study (mean of 42 years for cases vs. 35 years).

For the subgroup of women with higher BMI, stavudine use, when controlling for other risk factors, remained associated with a significant increase in risk of LAHL. Switching these women to zidovudine conferred an 80% reduction in hazards of LAHL. These data suggest that higher-risk individuals should be switched off stavudine-based therapy in order to reduce adverse events.

There are several limitations to this study. The two treatment groups were quite different as demonstrated in Table 1. In our model we were able to control for the variables in the model, but not for unmeasured confounders (e.g. HIV clinical stage). Clinicians may have been more likely to test for hyperlactatemia in patients on stavudine resulting in a detection bias. However, 14% of subjects initiated on stavudine and 18% of subjects initiated on zidovudine had at least one serum lactate level checked during the study period, suggesting that serum lactate testing was not biased towards subjects on stavudine. We do not think deployment of the handheld lactate machine for screening (introduced in 2006) differentially affected case finding between the two groups. Any patient with a positive handheld device test required confirmatory serological testing; as above, testing rates were not higher for subjects initiated on stavudine. Our data, in combination with prior data evaluating risk factors for lactic acidosis and hyperlactatemia, strongly suggest that women and patients with higher BMI treated with stavudine are at high risk for developing LAHL. In addition, our data demonstrate that using zidovudine rather than stavudine, even among patients at highest risk for mitochondrial toxicities, dramatically reduces the risk of developing lactic acidosis. Further, for patients initiated on stavudine-based therapy, switching to zidovudine is protective. Although a recent Cochrane Review concluded there is no difference in treatment outcomes (toxicity, death, disease progression) for stavudine- compared with zidovudine-based ART, the randomized-controlled trials on which their analyses were based included patients from North America, the Caribbean, Australia and China [28]. However, most studies observing high rates of mitochondrial toxicities include patients from sub-Saharan Africa.

As of April 2010, first-line ART in South Africa includes tenofovir, lamivudine, and either efavirenz or nevirapine [29]. However, because of drug shortages many clinics remain unable to initiate all patients on tenofovir-based therapy and are not able to routinely switch patients to tenofovir-containing regimens. Thus, in South Africa (and other countries still using stavudine) these findings will be helpful in identifying patients who are at highest risk for stavudine-induced complications. While all patients will benefit from using alternatives to stavudine, avoiding this drug in women and patients with higher BMI may offer an effective and practical strategy for reducing the incidence of lactic acidosis and hyperlactatemia until countries can completely eliminate use of this agent.

Acknowledgments

We would like to acknowledge the patients, clinicians and monitoring and evaluation staff at Sinikithemba. We would also like to acknowledge data capturers and McCord volunteers Lisa Bevilacqu, Anthony Sawyer, Winn Seay, Mary Gallo, Dr. Hannah Willoughby, and Dr. Eileen Scully. We are also grateful to Dr. Heather Ribaudo of the Harvard University Center for AIDS Research Biostatistical Core and Dr. Roger Davis for statistical support.

Author Contributions

Conceived and designed the experiments: LTM JG JH RTG DRB. Performed the experiments: LTM JH AE EC KA MCG. Analyzed the data: LTM MG AJG. Wrote the paper: LTM JG RTG DRB. Chart abstraction and data entry: LTM JH AE EC KA MCG.

References

1. Lactic Acidosis International Study Group (2007) Risk factors for lactic acidosis and severe hyperlactataemia in HIV-1-infected adults exposed to antiretroviral therapy. AIDS 21: 2455–2464.
2. Wohl DA, McComsey G, Tebas P, Brown TT, Glesby MJ, et al. (2006) Current concepts in the diagnosis and management of metabolic complications of HIV infection and its therapy. Clin Infect Dis 43: 645–653.
3. Shibuyama S, Gevorkyan A, Yoo U, Tim S, Dzhangiryan K, et al. (2006) Understanding and avoiding antiretroviral adverse events. Current Pharmaceutical Design 12: 1075–1090.
4. Bolhaar MG, Karstaedt AS (2007) A high incidence of lactic acidosis and symptomatic hyperlactataemia in women receiving highly active antiretroviral therapy in Soweto, South Africa. Clin Infect Dis 45: 254–260.
5. Boubaker KMF, Sudre P, Furrer H, Haensel A, Hirschel B, Boggian K, Chave J.-P, Bernasconi E, Egger M, Opravil M, Rickenbach M, Francioli P, Telenti A (2001) Hyperlactataemia and antiretroviral therapy: The Swiss HIV cohort study. Clin Infect Dis 33: 1931.
6. Fabian J, Venter WD, Mkhabela L, Levin JB, Baker L, et al. (2008) Symptomatic hyperlactataemia in adults on antiretroviral therapy: a single-centre experience. S Afr Med J 98: 795–800.
7. Geddes R, Knight S, Moosa MY, Reddi A, Uebel K, et al. (2006) A high incidence of nucleoside reverse transcriptase inhibitor (NRTI)-induced lactic acidosis in HIV-infected patients in a South African context. S Afr Med J 96: 722–724.
8. Kumarasamy N, Venkatesh KK, Cecelia AJ, Devaleenol B, Saghayam S, et al. (2008) Gender-based differences in treatment and outcome among HIV patients in South India. J Womens Health (Larchmt) 17: 1471–1475.
9. Moyle GJ, Datta D, Mandalia S, Morlese J, Asboe D, et al. (2002) Hyperlactataemia and lactic acidosis during antiretroviral therapy: relevance, reproducibility and possible risk factors. Aids 16: 1341–1349.
10. Stead D, Osler M, Boulle A, Rebe K, Meintjes G (2008) Severe hyperlactataemia complicating stavudine first-line antiretroviral therapy in South Africa. Antivir Ther 13: 937–943.
11. Wester CW, Okezie OA, Thomas AM, Bussmann H, Moyo S, et al. (2007) Higher-than-expected rates of lactic acidosis among highly active antiretroviral therapy-treated women in Botswana: preliminary results from a large randomized clinical trial. J Acquir Immune Defic Syndr 46: 318–322.
12. Stenzel MS, Carpenter CC (2000) The management of the clinical complications of antiretroviral therapy. Infect Dis Clin North Am 14: 851–878, vi.
13. World Health Organization (2010) Antiretroviral therapy for HIV infection in adults and adolescents: recommendations for a public health approach-2010 revision. Geneva: World Health Organization.
14. Murphy RA, Sunpath H, Kuritzkes DR, Venter F, Gandhi RT (2007) Antiretroviral therapy-associated toxicities in the resource-poor world: the challenge of a limited formulary. J Infect Dis 196 Suppl 3: S449–456.
15. Rosen S, Long L, Fox M, Sanne I (2008) Cost and cost-effectiveness of switching from stavudine to tenofovir in first-line antiretroviral regimens in South Africa. J Acquir Immune Defic Syndr 48: 334–344.
16. van Griensven J, Zachariah R, Rasschaert F, Mugabo J, Atte EF, et al. Stavudine- and nevirapine-related drug toxicity while on generic fixed-dose antiretroviral treatment: incidence, timing and risk factors in a three-year cohort in Kigali, Rwanda. Trans R Soc Trop Med Hyg 104: 148–153.
17. Boulle A, Orrel C, Kaplan R, Van Cutsem G, McNally M, et al. (2007) Substitutions due to antiretroviral toxicity or contraindication in the first 3 years of antiretroviral therapy in a large South African cohort. Antivir Ther 12: 753–760.
18. Osler M, Stead D, Rebe K, Meintjes G, Boulle A (2009) Risk factors for and clinical characteristics of severe hyperlactataemia in patients receiving antiretroviral therapy: a case-control study. HIV Med 11: 121–129.
19. Lonergan JT, Barber RE, Mathews WC (2003) Safety and efficacy of switching to alternative nucleoside analogues following symptomatic hyperlactatemia and lactic acidosis. AIDS 17: 2495–2499.
20. Adult AIDS Clinical Trial Group (2003) AACTG toxicity evaluation group, Chair Rob Murphy.
21. Ivers LC, Mukherjee JS (2006) Point of care testing for antiretroviral therapy-related lactic acidosis in resource-poor settings. AIDS 20: 779–780.
22. Kiragga AK, Ocama P, Reynolds SJ, Kambugu A, Ojiambo H, et al. (2008) Validation of a portable hand-held lactate analyzer for determination of blood lactate in patients on antiretroviral therapy in Uganda. J Acquir Immune Defic Syndr 49: 564–566.
23. Cox D, Snell E (1989) Analysis of Binary Data, 2nd Edition. London: Chapman and Hall.
24. Harrell FE, Jr. (2001) Regression modeling strategies: With applications to linear models, logistic regression, and survival analysis. New York: Springer-Verlag.
25. Hill A, Ruxrungtham K, Hanvanich M, Katlama C, Wolf E, et al. (2007) Systematic review of clinical trials evaluating low doses of stavudine as part of antiretroviral treatment. Expert Opinion in Phamacotherapy 8.
26. Bellomo R (2002) Bench-to-bedside review: lactate and the kidney. Crit Care 6: 322–326.
27. Bonnet F, Bonarek M, Morlat P, Mercie P, Dupon M, et al. (2003) Risk factors for lactic acidosis in HIV-infected patients treated with nucleoside reverse-transcriptase inhibitors: a case-control study. Clin Infect Dis 36: 1324–1328.
28. Spaulding A, Rutherford GW, Siegfried N Stavudine or zidovudine in three-drug combination therapy for initial treatment of HIV infection in antiretroviral-naive individuals. Cochrane Database Syst Rev CD008651.
29. South African National AIDS Council (2010) The South African Antiretroviral Treatment Guidelines Department of Health; Republic of South Africa. 8 p.

9

Screening for Active Small Molecules in Mitochondrial Complex I Deficient Patient's Fibroblasts, Reveals AICAR as the Most Beneficial Compound

Anna Golubitzky[1]9, Phyllis Dan[1]9, Sarah Weissman[1], Gabriela Link[1], Jakob D. Wikstrom[2], Ann Saada[1]*

1 Monique and Jacques Roboh Department of Genetic Research, Department of Genetics and Metabolic Diseases, Hadassah, Hebrew University Medical Center, Jerusalem, Israel, 2 Department of Endocrinology and Metabolism, Hadassah, Hebrew University Medical Center, Jerusalem, Israel

Abstract

Congenital deficiency of the mitochondrial respiratory chain complex I (CI) is a common defect of oxidative phosphorylation (OXPHOS). Despite major advances in the biochemical and molecular diagnostics and the deciphering of CI structure, function assembly and pathomechanism, there is currently no satisfactory cure for patients with mitochondrial complex I defects. Small molecules provide one feasible therapeutic option, however their use has not been systematically evaluated using a standardized experimental system. In order to evaluate potentially therapeutic compounds, we set up a relatively simple system measuring different parameters using only a small amount of patient's fibroblasts, in glucose free medium, where growth is highly OXPOS dependent. Ten different compounds were screened using fibroblasts derived from seven CI patients, harboring different mutations. 5-Aminoimidazole-4-carboxamide ribotide (AICAR) was found to be the most beneficial compound improving growth and ATP content while decreasing ROS production. AICAR also increased mitochondrial biogenesis without altering mitochondrial membrane potential ($\Delta\psi$). Fluorescence microscopy data supported increased mitochondrial biogenesis and activation of the AMP activated protein kinase (AMPK). Other compounds such as; bezafibrate and oltipraz were rated as favorable while polyphenolic phytochemicals (resverastrol, grape seed extract, genistein and epigallocatechin gallate) were found not significant or detrimental. Although the results have to be verified by more thorough investigation of additional OXPHOS parameters, preliminary rapid screening of potential therapeutic compounds in individual patient's fibroblasts could direct and advance personalized medical treatment.

Editor: Orian S. Shirihai, Boston University, United States of America

Funding: This work was funded by the Israeli Academy of Sciences, ISF grant, #1462/09 (AS). The funders had no role in study design, data collection and analysis, decision to publish, or preparation of the manuscript.

Competing Interests: The authors have declared that no competing interests exist.

* E-mail: annsr@hadassah.org.il

9 These authors contributed equally to this work.

Introduction

The congenital disorders of mitochondrial oxidative phosphorylation (OXPHOS) are common inborn errors of metabolism, with an incidence of 1:5000–8000 live births [1,2]. Among these, deficiency of mitochondrial respiratory chain complex I (NADH CoQ oxidoreductase, EC 1.6.5.3) is the most common and accounts for one-third of all patients referred for OXPHOS evaluation [3].

Complex I (CI), is the first complex of the mitochondrial respiratory chain. It is a large multimeric complex composed of 45 structural subunits; seven are encoded by the mitochondrial DNA (mtDNA) while 38 structural subunits and a number of CI assembly factors are all nuclear encoded [4]. Some of the subunits are post transcriptionally modified by phosphorylation, acetylation or glutathionylation [5–7].

Disease causing mutations have been identified in all mtDNA encoded subunits as well as in a number of the nuclear encoded complex I subunits and assembly factors [8,9].

The clinical phenotype of complex I deficiency is varied and includes severe neonatal lactic acidosis, Leigh disease, cardiomy-opathy-encephalopathy, hepatopathy-tubulopathy, leukodystrophy with macrocephaly optic atrophy, cerebellar ataxia, retinitis pigmentosa and growth retardation [10]. The extensive damage observed in patients with complex I deficiency is most probably due to energy depletion and to over- production of reactive oxygen species (ROS) with subsequent initiation of the apoptotic cascade [11–13].

Despite major advances in the biochemical and molecular diagnostics and the deciphering of the CI structure, function, assembly and pathomechanism, there is currently no satisfactory cure for patients with mitochondrial complex I defects. Small molecules provide one feasible therapeutic option, however their use has not been systematically evaluated using a standardized experimental system, and treatment has been based on "trial and error" [14–16]. Vitamins (vitamin K, riboflavin, B1,B2), cofactors (CoQ, carnitine, creatine), and ROS scavengers (vitamin E, CoQ_{10}), have all been administered to improve OXPHOS, by providing alternate substrates, removing lactate accumulation (by dichloroacetate) and ameliorating oxidative damage (reviewed by Dimauro and Mancuso) [15–16]. The favorable effect of Coenzyme Q_{10} supplementation for CoQ deficiency is undisputable however the efficacy of riboflavin has been demonstrated only in a few cases of complex I deficiency [11,17]. For other compounds, results have been equivocal or were reported anecdotally. In recent years, a large number of compounds with therapeutic potential have been described. These include polyphenolic phytochemicals such as resveratrol, grape seed extract, green tea extract and genistein. Resveratrol is a natural phytoalexin found in a wide variety of plant species, including grapes. Among its numerous properties, resveratrol has been reported to have anti-oxidant activities and to activate the genetic expression of key genes in energy metabolism such as peroxisome proliferator-activated receptor gamma coactivator 1 alpha (PGC1α). Resveratrol and grape seed extract (a proanthocyanidin) were demonstrated to have beneficial effects on mitochondrial function in several experimental models [18–20]. Green tea polyphenols attenuated mitochondrial dysfunction in glucose deprived glial cell cultures [21]. Genistein is a soy derived isoflavone which has been evaluated in substrate reduction therapy for mucopolysaccharidoses and was also reported to induce mitochondrial biogenesis [22–23].

In addition to polyphenols, other substances such as compounds enhancing energy metabolism, antioxidants and chemical chaperones are potentially beneficial.

Representative of this type are 5-Aminoimidazole-4-carboxamide ribotide (AICAR), oltipraz, bezafibrate and sodium phenylbutyrate.

AICAR is a pharmacological activator of AMP activated protein kinase (AMPK). This heterotrimeric protein complex plays a key role in the regulation of energy homeostasis. The kinase is activated by an elevated AMP/ATP ratio caused by cellular and environmental stress, such as heat shock, hypoxia and ischemia. AMPK regulates energy expenditure by modulating $NADH^+$ dependent-type III deacetylase SIRT1, resulting in the deacetylation of downstream targets including PGC1α forkhead box O1 and 3 transcription factors [24]. Notably, Thr172 phosphorylation on the AMPK protein is a prerequisite for its activation [25]. Oltipraz is a 1,2-dithiole-3-thione compound with antioxidant properties. Oltipraz has also been demonstrated to reduce apoptosis in cells with chemically inhibited CI by exerting its cytoprotective effect though AMPK [26–27]. Bezafibrate is an agonist of peroxisome proliferator-activated receptors (PPARs) stimulating oxidative metabolism and has a documented positive effect on mitochondria. On the other hand, fenofibrate was reported to have a negative effect on CI [16,28–29]. Sodium phenyl butyrate is a, histone deacetylase (HDAC) inhibitor, affecting protein phosphorylation and relief of endoplasmic reticulum stress. Although the mechanism of action of this compound is poorly defined, it has been found to be beneficial in a number of diseases including cancer, neurodegenerative diseases and metabolic diseases [30–33]. All of the above mentioned compounds have been documented to exert positive effects, however to our knowledge, they have not been systematically screened in OXPHOS deficient patient's cells together in the same system.

The objectives of this research were two-fold; to develop an *in vitro* system for the rapid screening of multiple compounds using a small amount of fibroblasts from individual patients and to identify compounds with a therapeutic potential for mitochondrial complex I deficiency.

Materials and Methods

Subjects

Fibroblasts previously derived (with informed consent, approved by the IRB), from six patients with mitochondrial respiratory chain complex I (CI) deficiency, were included in the study. Most of these patients have been previously described and all harbored known mutations in different nuclear encoded complex I subunits: NDUFS2[34,8]. NDUFS4 or assembly factors; C6ORF66 (NDU-FAF4)[35], C20ORF7[36], FOXRED1 [37,8] B17.2.L (NDU-FA12L)[38]. Their clinical and biochemical data are briefly summarized in Table 1.

Tissue cultures

Fibroblasts were maintained in DMEM (Biological Industries, Kibbutz Beit Haemek, Israel) medium containing 4.5 g glucose per liter and supplemented with 10% fetal calf serum, 50 µg/ml uridine, and 110 µg/ml pyruvate (GLU, permissive medium) at 37°C, 5%CO_2.

For assessment of various compounds, 3×10^3 cells/100 µl were seeded in triplicate on three identical 96 well microtiter plates. The following day, the medium was removed, the wells were washed once with phosphate buffered saline (PBS) and replaced with 100 µl GLU medium or a restrictive glucose-free DMEM medium (Biological Industries, Kibbutz Beit Haemek, Israel) supplemented with 10% dialyzed fetal calf serum and 5 mM galactose (GAL) with or without additives as follows: 0.5 mM AICAR (Tocris, Bioscience, Bristol UK); 50 µM Genistein (GENI) (Cayman Chemicals Ann Arbor MI USA; 100 µM, Bezafibrate (BEZA); 10 µM Oltipraz (OLTIP); 5uM Resveratrol (RSV); 10 uM Epigallocatechin gallate (EGCG)(Sigma-Aldrich, Steinheim, Germany) or grape seed extract (GSE) (Ttianjin Jianfeng Natural Products, China). 72h post-treatment the tissue cultures were analyzed for growth, reactive oxygen species (ROS) and ATP. (Biological Industries, Kibbutz Beit Haemek, Israel).

Assays

Cell growth was measured by a colorimetric method based on the staining of basophilic cellular compounds (mainly nucleic acids, independent on redox status) with methylene blue at A_{620}nm, as modified by Jones et al [39]. For the evaluation methylene blue assay (MB) control cells were serially diluted in GLU medium, seeded in six wells. After 48h triplicate wells were measured by MB and triplicate wells were subjected to viable count by trypan blue. For evaluation of time course, 3×10^3 control cell and cells from a patient were seeded in GLU medium. The following day the medium was replaced either with fresh GLU or GAL. The amount of cells was quantified by MB after 24 h, 48 h, 72 h and 144 h (medium was replaced with fresh after 72 h).

The intracellular ROS production was measured using 2',7'-dichlorodihydrofluorescein diacetate (DCF) (Biotium Harvard CA USA)[40]. Briefly, growth medium was removed and replaced by 100ul/well of 10 µM DCF in PBS-Ca^{2+} Mg^{2+} (PBS containing 0.9 mM calcium chloride and 0.5 mM magnesium chloride) and the plates were incubated for 20 min at 37°C, 5%CO_2. After removal of DCF, the ROS production was monitored for 20 minutes in 100ul PBS-Ca^{2+} Mg^{2+} at λ_{ex} 485 nm and λ_{em} 520 nm.

ATP content was measured by luciferin-luciferase using the ATPlite® luminescence assay system according to the manufacturer's instruction (Perkin Elmer Waltham MA, USA).

Luminescence, fluorescence and absorbance measurements were performed with a Synergy HT microplate reader (Bio-Tek instruments, Vinoosky VT, USA).

Relative fluorescence units (RFU) and relative luminescence units (RLU) were calculated by normalizing to growth as measured by MB in parallel wells for each separate experiment. The mean of all experiments was calculated and compared to that of GAL without additive (containing vehicle only). All experiments were performed in triplicate wells on at least two separate

Table 1. Patient data.

patient/ mutated gene	C20ORF7	NDUFS2	NDUFS4	C6ORF66 (NDUFAF4)	FOXRED1	B17.2L (NDUFA12L)
age of onset	1 year	6 months	3 months	birth	4 months	8 months
clinical details	Leigh's syndrome, mild lactic acidosis, died at 6years	optic atrophy, hypo dense basal ganglia, cardio-myopathy, died at 2years	lactic acidosis, seizures	encephalo-myopathy, severe lactic acidosis, died at 2 months	Micro-cephaly, encephalo-pathy, lactic- acidosis	hypotonia, motor delay, horizontal nystagmus, bilateral optic atrophy, abnormal MRI, mild lactic acidosis
residual muscle enzymatic activities	CI 54% CIV 38% CII,III within normal range	CI 17% C II-V within normal range	CI 25% C II-V within normal range	CI 14% C II-V within normal range	CI 7% C II-V within normal range	CI 24% C II-V within normal range
reference	36	34,11	unpublished	35,12	37	37,13

occasions. Statistical significance (p<0.05) was calculated by 2-tailed student's t-test. Data were also visualized using the matrix2png software [41]. http://www.bioinformatics.ubc.ca/matrix2png/.

Fluorescence microscopy

Fibroblasts, were seeded at 3.5×10^4 cells/ml in GLU medium. The following day the medium was replaced with GLU, GAL or GAL containing 0.5 mM AICAR for 72hrs. For assessment of

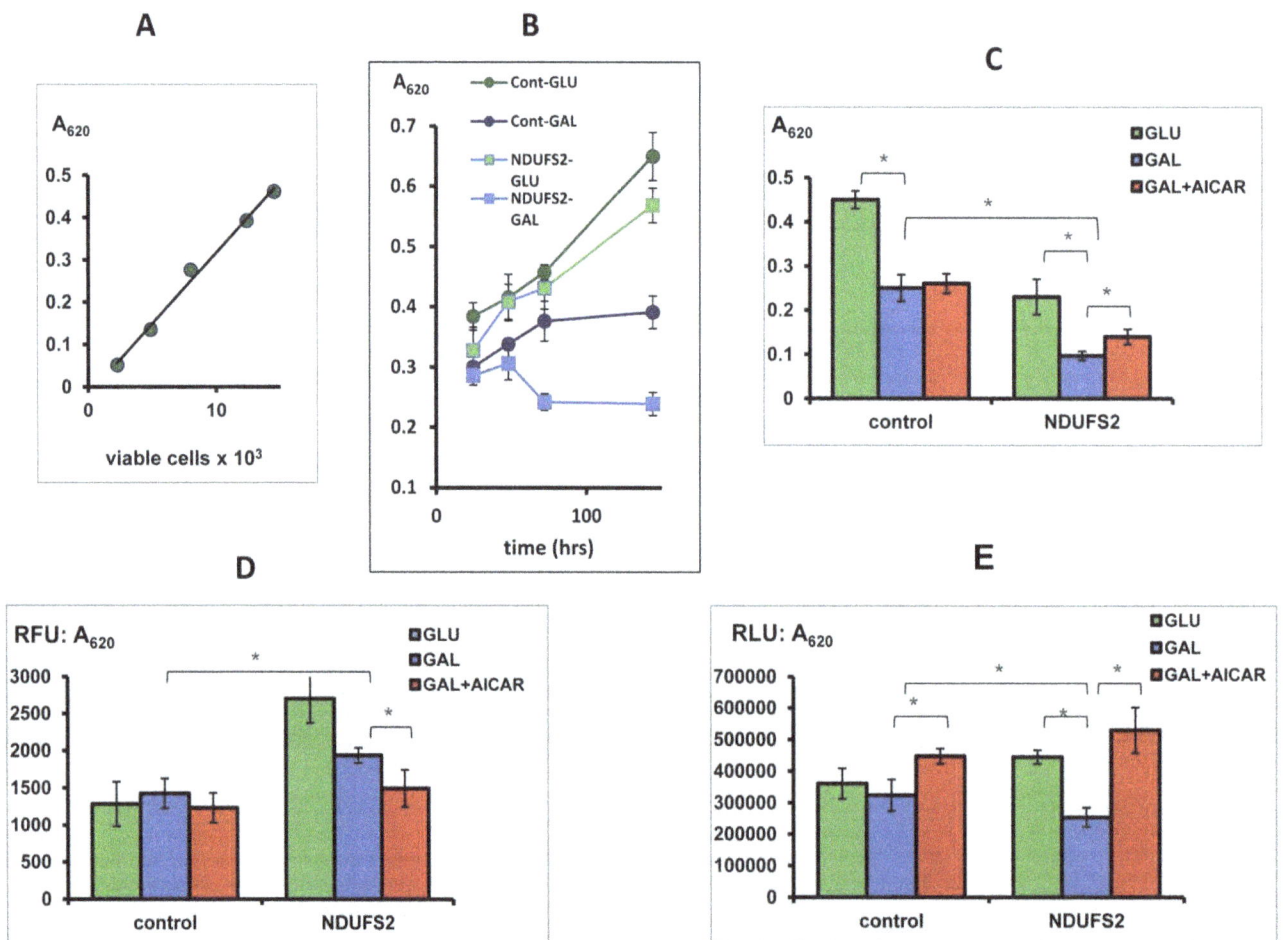

Figue 1. Measurement of growth, ROS and ATP in control and patient fibroblasts. Fibroblast from control and patient (NDUFS2) were grown in microtiter wells in GLU, GAL or GAL supplemented with AICAR. The amount of control cells, measured by methylene blue (MB) at A_{620} was compared to viable count by trypan blue at 72h (A). Growth of control and patient cells was measured at 24,48,72h and 144h by MB at A_{620} (B,C). Growth with AICAR was assessed at 72h (C). ROS measured by DCF at 72h is expressed as relative fluorescent units (RFU) divided by the amount of cells measured by MB at A_{620} (D). ATP was measured at 72h by luciferin-luciferase is expressed as relative luminescence units (RLU) divided by the amount of cells measured by MB at A_{620} (E). Values are presented as mean of triplicates +/- standard deviation. *p<0.05.

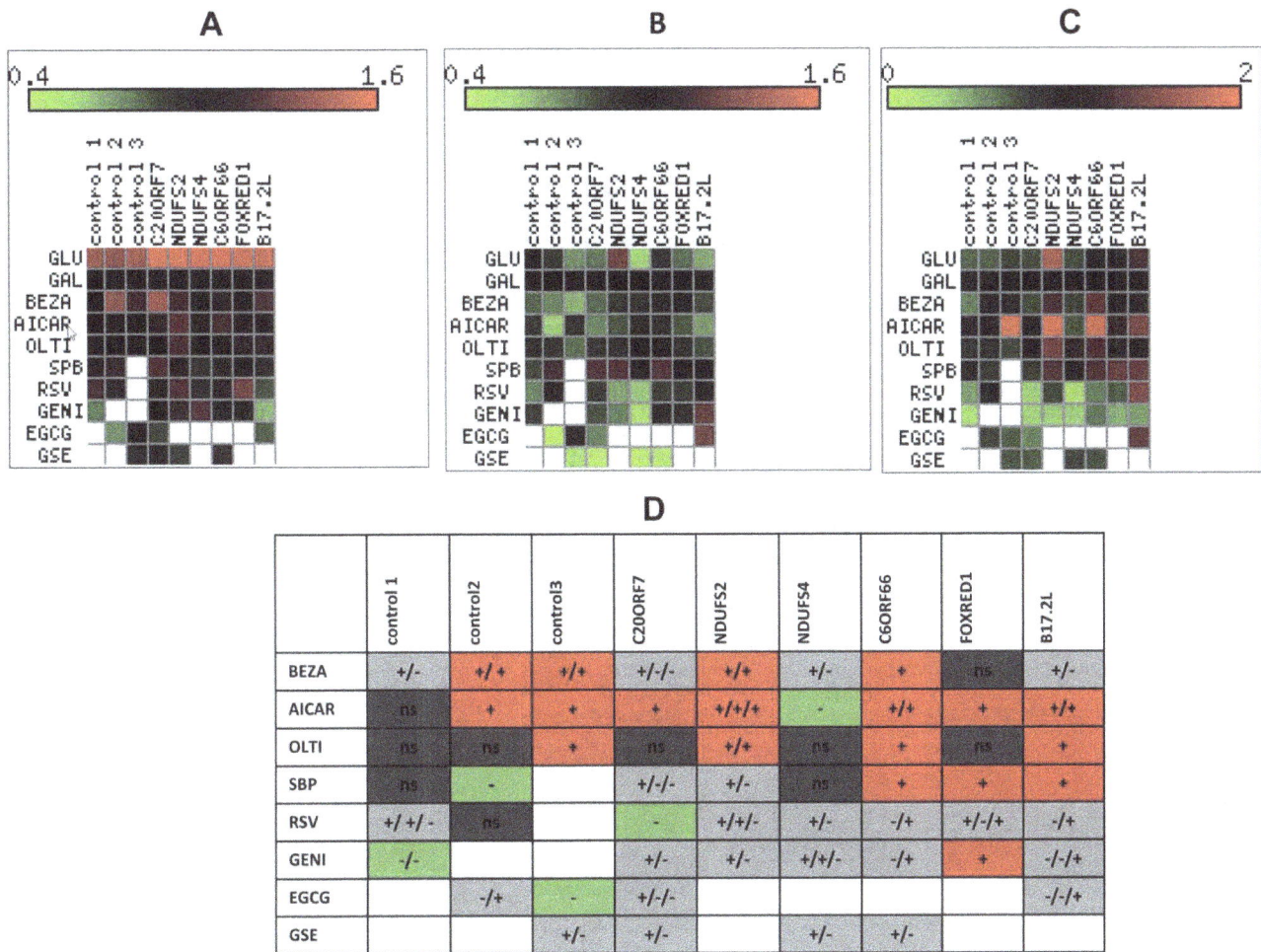

Figure 2. The effect of various compounds on growth, ROS and ATP in control and patient fibroblasts. Fibroblast from three separate controls and seven patients (C20ORF7,NDUFS2,NDUFS4,C6ORF66, FOXRED1 and B17.2L) were grown in microtiter wells in GLU or GAL medium or in GAL medium, supplemented with one of eight various compounds (BEZA,AICAR,OLTI,SBP,RZV,GENI,EGCG,GSI) in GAL for 72hrs. Growth was assessed by MB (A). ROS was measured by DCF and normalized to MB (B). ATP was measured by luciferin-luciferase and normalized to MB (C). Values (A-C) are presented as relative values graphically presented as heatmaps representing the mean of triplicates performed on at least 2 separate occasions. Growth in GAL without additives was set as the value of 1(black). Values < 1 are presented in increasingly green and values >1 in increasingly red. All parameters are summarized in (D) and evaluated as a significantly positive (+), negative (−) or nonsignificant (ns) effect. Increased values for growth and ATP were regarded as positive while negative for increased ROS. Positive only is shaded in red, negative only in green, nonsignificant in dark grey and mixed responses in gray.

mitochondrial content and $\Delta\psi$, the cells grown in 35 mm glass bottom tissue culture, plates and incubated with 200 nM Mito-Tracker Green FM (MTG) and 50 nM tetramethylrhodamine ethyl ester (TMRE) (Molecular Probes Eugene, Oregon USA), for 90 and 45 minutes respectively at 37°C, 5%CO$_2$ [42]. For phospho-AMPK (pAMPK) immunocytochemistry and Mitotracker stain, cells were grown on fibronectin coated coverslips and incubated with 1.5 μM MitoTracker Red CM-H2XRos (MTR, Molecular Probes Eugene, Oregon USA) for 45minutes at 37°C, 5%CO$_2$, chased for 30 minutes with the respective growth medium, fixed with 4% paraformaldehyde in PBS, permeabilized with 0.25% Triton X-100, stained with 1:75 Phospho-AMPKα-(Thr172) primary antibody (Cell Signalling Technology Inc.Denver MA,USA) and subsequently, with Dylight 488 conjugated anti rabbit secondary antibody (Jackson Thermo Scientific, Rockford IL,USA). Cells were visualized by fluorescent confocal microscopy (10×4). Image analysis was done with MetaMorph image analysis software. All micrographs in a series were taken under the same conditions.

Oxygen consumption

Oxygen consumption rate (OCR) was measured using an XF24 extracellular flux analyzer (Seahorse Biosciences, North Billeric,MA,USA). Fibroblast were seeded at 12- 14×10^3 cells/well in 300 μl in GLU medium on an XF 24 well plate at 37°C, 5%CO$_2$. The following day the medium was replaced with GLU, GAL or GAL containing 0.5 mM AICAR. After 72hrs the growth medium was changed to 500 μl unbuffered DMEM medium with the same constituents as above (GLU, GAL or GAL with AICAR) and incubated at 37°C for 1h for equilibration before the measurements. After 10 minutes of OCR baseline measurements, 50 μl carbonylcyanide-3-chlorophenylhydrazone (CCCP) was injected to reach a working concentration of 20 μM and the maximal OCR was measured. Background OCR was measured after injection of rotenone and antimycin to a final concentration of 5 μM each. After the experiment, cell content was estimated by MB and OCR was calculated as OCR minus background divided by MB.

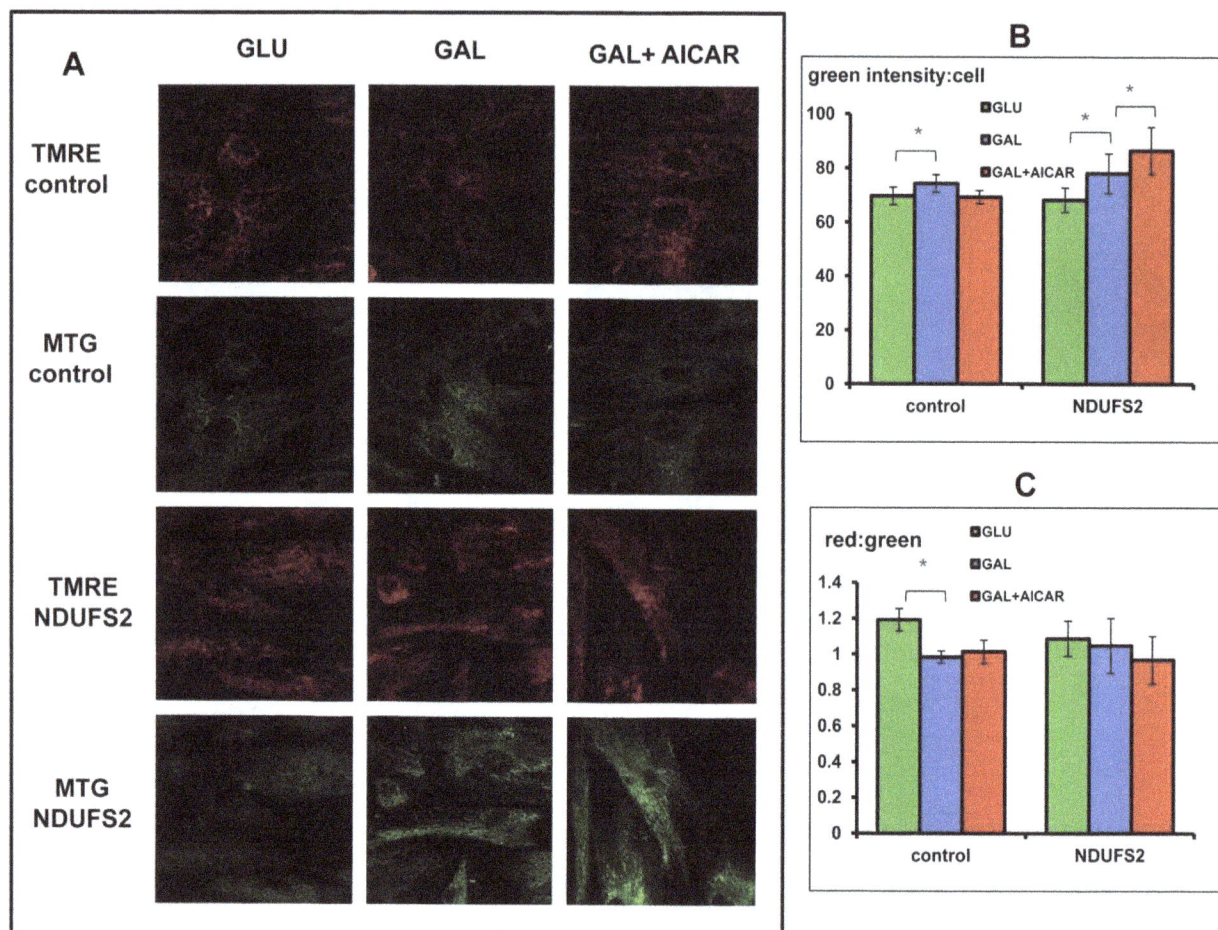

Figure 3. The effect of AICAR on mitochondrial content and Δψ. Control 1 and an NDUFS2 patient's fibroblasts were grown in GLU or GAL medium and in GAL supplemented with 0.5 mM AICAR (GAL+AICAR) for 72 hrs. Cells were then incubated with TMRE (red) and Mitrotracker green (green) and examined by confocal fluorescent microscopy. A: depicts a representative micrograph TMRE stain in red and MTG stain in green. The graphs represent green intensity per cell (B) and red:green ratio (C), +/− standard deviation (*p<0.05). All micrographs were taken under the same conditions.

Results

All patients presented in infancy, were severely affected and diagnosed with isolated CI deficiency in muscle, with the exception of patient C20ORF7 who had a combined partial deficiency of both CI and CIV. All patients were molecularly defined with mutations either in a nuclear encoded CI subunit or in a CI assembly factor (Table 1). Fibroblasts from these patients were initially assessed for growth, ROS production and ATP content. Preliminary experiments demonstrated that 3×10^3 cells/well was sufficient to obtain clear readings and reproducible results (Fig. 1A). As it was not possible to measure all parameters in the same well, 3 identical plates treated in parallel were measured in each experiment. Still it was possible to screen ten variables in triplicate wells using less than 3×10^5 cells (less than a T25 confluent flask). In order to relate values to cell content, we initially evaluated the MB assay and compared those values to values obtained by viable counts. There was a linear relationship between the number of cells and methylene blue absorption (Fig. 1A). As MB staining is much more feasible to perform than viable counting of hundreds of microtiter wells, we therefore continued to evaluate growth by the MB assay. Accordingly, all RFU and RLU values were normalized to MB in order to compare values per cell

content. To establish a suitable time frame for the experiments we compared the time course of growth in GLU and GAL. While patient's cell growth was comparable to control cells in GLU media, impaired growth of patient's cells in GAL media was evident after 72h (Fig. 1B). Therefore, 72h was chosen as the optimal time frame for examining compounds.

A typical experiment with control and patient fibroblasts is depicted in Fig. 1C–D. Since it is difficult to present and summarize a large number (1000<) of measurements, the summary of all data are depicted as a heatmaps in Fig. 2 A–C. (The values on GAL were set at 1 in the middle of the scale (black). Values less than 1 were increasingly green and higher then 1 increasingly red) The growth in GAL medium relative to GLU was slightly decreased in control fibroblasts while growth was markedly decreased in all patients cells (Fig. 2A). These results were anticipated, as GAL medium is devoid of substrates for glycolysis and therefore growth is highly dependent on the oxidation of fatty acids (derived from FCS) by intact OXPHOS for energy production [43]. Intracellular ROS production was generally increased in GAL medium. The increase was evident in one control and four of the patients (Fig. 2B). In patient NDUFS2 the ratio was reversed, presumably because of the severe growth defect in GAL (Fig. 1 B). This is also be the reason for the very low ATP

A

B

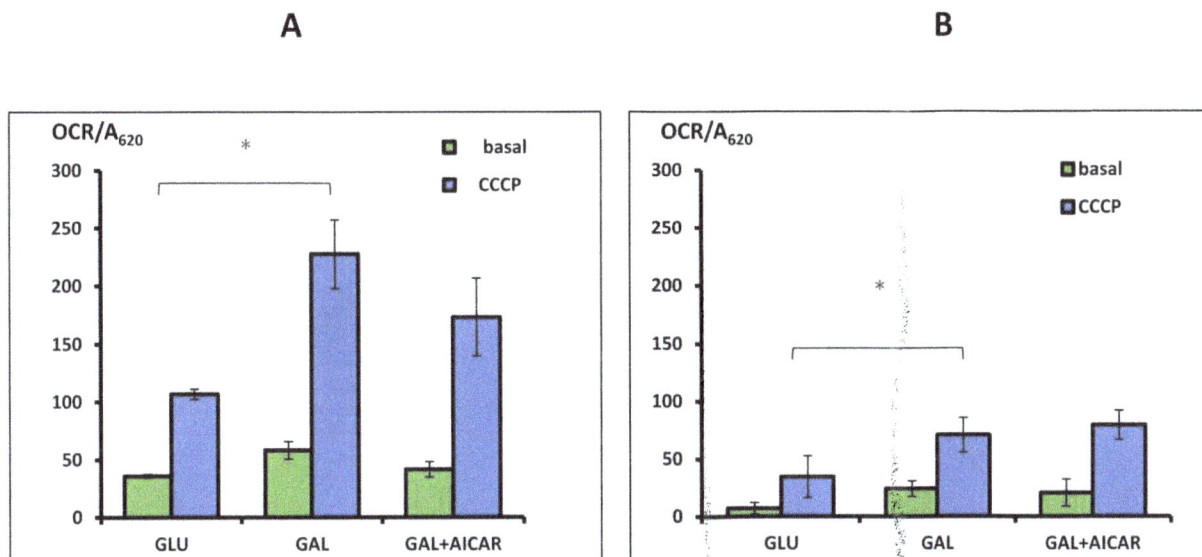

Figure 4. Oxygen consumption. Control 1 (A) and NDUFS2 patient's (B) fibroblasts were grown in GLU or GAL medium and in GAL supplemented with 0.5 mM AICAR (GAL+AICAR) for 72 hrs. Media were changed to unbuffered media and oxygen consumption rates (OCR) were measured by an XF24 instrument. Basal OCR was measured (basal) before the addition of uncoupler and maximal rate (CCCP) after. The results are presented as rates subtracted by non mitochondrial oxygen consumption (in the presence of rotenone and antimycin) and normalized to cell amount measured by methylene blue (MB)at A_{620}, +/− standard deviation. *$p<0.05$.

content in GAL medium (Fig. 1C). Notably all control cells had higher ATP content in GAL medium, reflecting the higher efficiency of ATP production by OXPHOS than by glycolysis. This was not the case for four of the six patients and reflects the CI defect. Notably cells with a high ATP content in GAL were derived from controls or patients C2ORF7 and NDUFS4 with a relatively high residual CI activity in muscle (Table 1, Fig. 2C).

Next, the effect of various compounds was examined. The compounds tested were polyphenols, and other compounds with reported effects on ROS production and mitochondrial biogenesis. Untreated cells in the presence of vehicle (DMSO), cells grown in GAL and control cells were included in each experiment. It should be noted that the examination of the effect of different compounds required a prior set of experiments initially based on data available from the literature, in order to optimize conditions with respect to medium and concentration. As these experiments required larger quantities of cells, they were performed in normal cells and in some of the patient's cells. From the preliminary data, we concluded that the effect of additives was best demonstrated under stressful conditions i.e in GAL medium compared to growth with vehicle only in the same medium (Fig. 1B). The effect of each compound on each cell on each of the above parameter is presented in Fig. 2A–C. Many compounds either lacked any effect or had a beneficial effect on growth. For example, bezafibrate increased growth in C20ORF7 approaching that in GLU medium. On the contrary, genistein, EGCG and grape seed extract had a negative effect on growth. Therefore, the investigation of these compounds was not continued in the remaining cells (Fig. 2A). Intracellular ROS production was also favorably affected by many compounds, although mostly by bezafibrate and AICAR. The only compound with an overall negative effect on ROS was sodiumphenylbutyrate (Fig. 2B). AICAR exerted a positive effect on ATP content in four of the six patient cells and one control cell line. Other cells were not affected with the exception of the negative effect on NDUFS4 (Fig. 1C, Fig. 2C).

In order to create a simplified overview, we rated a compound as beneficial when it increased growth, ATP and decreased ROS compared to the values on GAL. The evaluation was designated with a plus sign for each favorable parameter while a negative effect was designated with a minus sign. When no parameter was significantly altered by a compound it was designated non significant (ns). Mixed effects were designated plus/minus (Fig. 2D). To summarize, AICAR was the most favorable compound with positive effects on several parameters in five out of six patient cells. Bezafibrate was also beneficial to two patient' cells but to a lesser extent. Interestingly, Otipraz had a beneficial effect on half the patient's. Although sodium phenylbutyrate slightly increased ROS in some cells, the overall score was positive in fifty percent of the patients (Fig. 2D). No positive but many mixed and some negative effects were observed with resveratrol, EGCG and grapeseed extract. The effect of genistein was unclear since it had a positive effect on only FOXRED1 cells while negatively affected the control.

In order to further investigate the effect of AICAR we conducted an extended study of a representative cell (NDUFS2) to include the evaluation of mitochondrial content and mitochondrial $\Delta\psi$ by fluorescence microscopy and oxygen consumption (Figs. 3 and 4). Mitochondrial content estimated by MTG was found slightly but significantly increased in both control and patients cells in GAL medium. AICAR induced a clear increase in mitochondrial content only in the patient's cells (Fig. 3A and B). The alteration of TMRE stain relative to mitochondrial content in the presence of AICAR was minor and not significant, indicating that $\Delta\psi$ was not substantially affected (Fig. 3A and C). While uncoupled oxygen consumption was increased in GAL medium, AICAR had no significant effect (Fig. 4A and B) although the basal uncoupled OCR was somewhat, not significantly relative to basal OCR in the patient's cells (Fig. 4B).

To examine to the downstream effect of AICAR, we performed immunostaining with an antibody towards Thr172 phosphorylated AMPK (pAMPK) while co-staining with MTR (Fig. 5A–C).

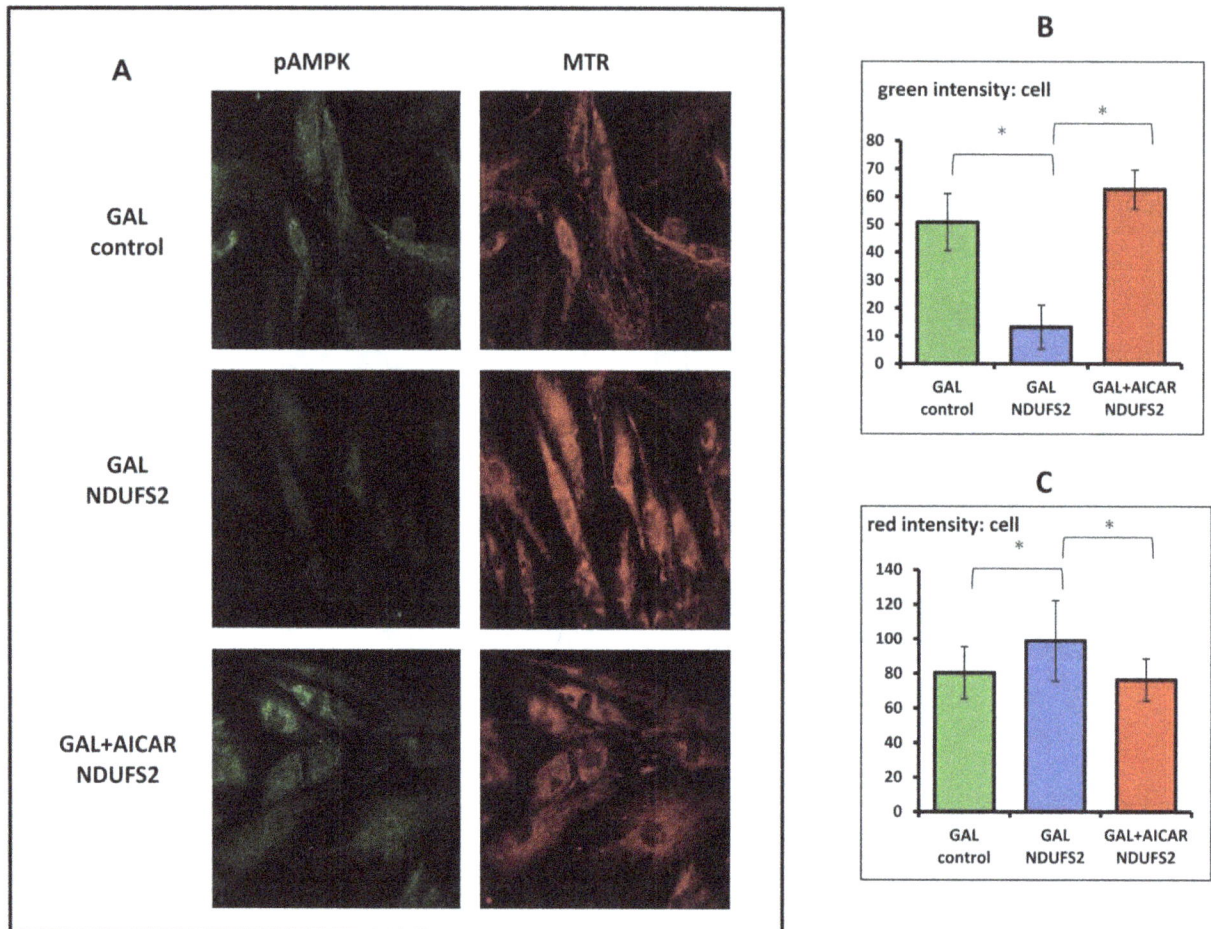

Figure 5. The effect of AICAR on pAMPK and mitotracker red stain in control and patient fibroblasts. Control and patient fibroblasts were grown on coverslips in GLU or GAL medium and in GAL supplemented with 0.5 mM AICAR (GAL+AICAR) for 72 hrs. Cells were than incubated with mitotracker red (MTR), fixed, stained with anti pAMPK antibodies and visualized by fluorescent (pAMPK) secondary antibodies. The coverslips were examined by confocal fluorescent microscopy (10×40). A: depicts a representative migrograph of pAMPK stain in green and MTR stain in red. The graphs represent green intensity per cell (B) and red intensity per cell (C) +/− standard deviation (*p<0.05). All micrographs were taken under the same conditions.

While clearly present in control cells, pAMPK stain was very weak in NDUFS2 cells grown on GLU (Fig. 5A and B). AICAR supplementation caused a marked and significant increase of pAMPK in the patients cells. Mitotracker stain was increased in patient's cells on GAL but approached control values in the presence of AICAR (Fig. 5A and C).

Discussion

The search for therapeutic agents for mitochondrial complex I deficiency and OXPHOS defects in general, is seriously hampered by the lack of a standardized model system for evaluating treatment. Many studies focused on small groups of patients simultaneously treated with several agents leading to difficulties in interpreting data and patient responses to therapy *in vivo*. Documented *in vitro* assays usually focus on a specific compound or a specific parameter using a relatively large sample size (11–13,17).

We developed an accessible and relatively simple system in 96 well plates assessing a number of different parameters by the use of one instrument. This enabled us screen multiple compounds on a small amount of fibroblasts simultaneously while measuring a

number of different parameters. The small sample size allowed the use of primary cells which is advantageous not only for practical reasons but also because immortalized cells frequently do not retain their original phenotype and thus respond differently than primary cells (personal experience).

The fibroblasts for this study were chosen to represent CI deficiency, the most common OXPHOS defect. The cells were derived from patients with different CI defects, in order to assess individual responses to different compounds. Indeed the responses differed in some instances between the patients. This is exemplified by bezafibrate which was beneficial for NDUFS2 ATP content but not for C20ORF7, emphasizing the need to evaluate compounds on an individual basis. Individual evaluation is especially important when attempting to treat disorders where the mitochondrial function is already *a priori* compromised. The necessity to measure different parameters was evident when observing the effect of the various polyphenolic cytochemicals (resveraterol, EGCG, grape seed extract and geneticin) included in the study. Generally they decreased ROS formation which is advantageous, but concomitantly decreased growth and ATP content. Although some of these results contradict studies reporting positive effects previously mentioned in the introduction, they are actually in accord with other studies reporting that some polyphenols can induce cancer cell death though mitochondrial membrane depolarization and apoptosis [44,45]. On the other hand, AICAR was found to be the most promising compound with no detected negative effect and an overall positive score in most of the patient's cells. The positive effect on mitochondrial biogenesis was also clearly visible by the MTG stain while the $\Delta\psi$ was not affected. Immunocytochemistry also supported activation of AMPK. Remarkably AICAR has been given intravenously to humans in clinical trials for the treatment of hyperinsulinemia [46]. Recently AICAR was also reported to be favorable in cytochrome c oxidase deficiency [47,48].

Apparently there is a discrepancy between the mixed effect of resveratrol and the positive effect of AICAR since they both activate the same SIRT1, PGC1α axis pathway [18,24,49]. The underlying mechanism for this inconsistency remains unclear and requires further thorough investigation. Nevertheless, we suggest that the positive effects of resveratrol on patients cells might be masked by some additional negative effects. Notably, resveratrol was reported to inhibit the mitochondrial FoF1 ATPsynthase (complex V) and oxygen consumption while depleting ATP content [50,51]. In fact, resveratrol alone is suggested to act as an anticancer compound by targeting mitochondria through the activation of pro-apoptotic pathways [52]. It is therefore conceivable that resveratrol might exert a negative effect on some parameters on some individual patient's cells with an *a priori* mitochondrial dysfunction. Apart from AICAR, oltipraz and bezafibrate disclosed a general positive effect, but to a lesser extent. Sodium phenylbutyrate increased ATP but also caused a slight increase of ROS and therefore the use of this compound in OXPHOS defects could be questionable.

We detected only a partial correlation between individual responses in fibroblasts and residual enzymatic complex I activity in muscle, genotype or clinical presentation (Table and Fig. 2). Moreover, the clinical correlation between fibroblasts responses and patients response to treatment has only been proved in a few instances and further correlation studies are warranted [11,17]. Nevertheless patient's fibroblasts provide an accessible tissue for testing individual responses to additives and drugs [48].

Taken together, we present an accessible and relative simple system using a small amount of patient's fibroblasts for screening potential treatments in OXPHOS defects. This enables the screening to be performed on an individual basis while measuring a number of different parameters which are not limited to the measurement of a specific respiratory chain complex. Consequently the system has a wide applicability, and could be used for other defined and undefined OXPHOS defects. The authors are aware that this system is suitable for preliminary screening only, and that the results will have to be verified by precise investigation of additional parameters and mechanisms by other methods measuring OXPHOS by enzymatic assays and expression analysis on the protein and mRNA levels. Nonetheless these assays are more complex and require a larger number of cells making them much less applicable for screening purposes. We propose that rapid preliminary screening of potential therapeutic compounds in individual patient's fibroblasts could direct and advance personalized medical treatment.

Acknowledgments

We thank Prof. Orly Elpeleg, Hadassah-Hebrew University Medical Center, for clinical and molecular data, and Prof. Yuval Dor, Hebrew University, for antibodies.

Author Contributions

Conceived and designed the experiments: AG GL AS JDW. Performed the experiments: AG PD SW AS. Analyzed the data: AG PD AS JDW. Contributed reagents/materials/analysis tools: AS GL. Wrote the paper: AS.

References

1. Schaefer AM, Taylor RW, Turnbull DM, Chinnery PF (2004) The epidemiology of mitochondrial disorders—past, present and future. Biochim Biophys Acta 1659: 115–120.
2. Skladal D, Halliday J, Thorburn DR (2003) Minimum birth prevalence of mitochondrial respiratory chain disorders in children. Brain 126: 1905–1912.
3. Kirby DM, Crawford M, Cleary MA, Dahl HH, Dennett X, et al. (1999) Respiratory chain complex I deficiency: an underdiagnosed energy generation disorder. Neurology 52: 1255–1264.
4. Carroll J, Fearnley IM, Skehel JM, Shannon RJ, Hirst J, et al. (2006) Bovine complex I is a complex of 45 different subunits. J Biol Chem 281: 32724–132727.
5. Chen R, Fearnley IM, Peak-Chew SY, Walker JE (2004) The phosphorylation of subunits of complex I from bovine heart mitochondria. J Biol Chem 279: 26036–26045.
6. Ahn BH, Kim HS, Song S, Lee IH, Liu J, et al. (2008) A role for the mitochondrial deacetylase Sirt3 in regulating energy homeostasis. Proc Natl Acad Sci 105: 14447–14452.
7. Hurd TR, Requejo R, Filipovska A, Brown S, Prime TA, et al. (2008) Complex I within oxidatively stressed bovine heart mitochondria is glutathionylated on Cys-531 and Cys-704 of the 75-kDa subunit: potential role of CYS residues in decreasing oxidative damage. J Biol Chem 283: 24801–24815.
8. Janssen RJ, Nijtmans LG, van den Heuvel LP, Smeitink JA (2006) Mitochondrial complex I: structure, function and pathology. J Inherit Metab Dis 29: 499–51.
9. Mckenzie M, Ryan MT (2010) Assembly factors of human mitochondrial complex I and their defects in disease. IUBMB Life 62: 497–502.
10. Pitkanen S, Feigenbaum A, Laframboise R, Robinson BH (1996) NADH-coenzyme Q reductase (complex I) deficiency: heterogeneity in phenotype and biochemical findings. J Inherit. Metab Dis 19: 675–686.
11. Bar-Meir M, Elpeleg ON, Saada A (2001) Effect of various agents on adenosine triphosphate synthesis in mitochondrial complex I deficiency. J Pediatr 139: 868–870.
12. Saada A, Bar-Meir M, Belaiche C, Miller C, Elpeleg O (2004) Evaluation of enzymatic assays and compounds affecting ATP production in mitochondrial respiratory chain complex I deficiency. Anal Biochem 335: 66–72.
13. Verkaart S, Koopman WJ, van Emst-de Vries SE, Nijtmans LG, van den Heuvel LW, et al. (2007) Superoxide production is inversely related to complex I activity in inherited complex I deficiency. Biochim Biophys Acta 1772: 373–381.
14. Briere JJ, Chretien D, Benit P, Rustin P (2004) Respiratory chain defects: what do we know for sure about their consequences in vivo? Biochim Biophys Acta 1659: 172–7.
15. DiMauro S, Mancuso M (2007) Mitochondrial diseases: therapeutic approaches. Biosci Rep 27: 125–137.
16. DiMauro S (2010) Pathogenesis and treatment of mitochondrial myopathies: recent advances. Acta Myol 29: 333–338.
17. Rötig A, Appelkvist EL, Geromel V, Chretien D, Kadhom N, et al. (2000) Quinone-responsive multiple respiratory-chain dysfunction due to widespread coenzyme Q10 deficiency. Lancet 356: 391–395.
18. Lagouge M, Argmann C, Gerhart-Hines Z, Meziane H, Lerin C, et al. (2006) Resveratrol improves mitochondrial function and protects against metabolic disease by activating SIRT1 and PGC-1alpha. Cell 127: 1109–1122.
19. Plin C, Tillement JP, Berdeaux A, Morin D (2005) Resveratrol protects against cold ischemia-warm reoxygenation-induced damages to mitochondria and cells in rat liver. Eur J Pharmacol 528: 162–168.
20. Pajuelo D, Diíaz S, Quesada H, Fernaíndez-Iglesias A, Mulero M, et al. (2011) Acute Administration of Grape Seed Proanthocyanidin Extract Modulates Energetic Metabolism in Skeletal Muscle and BAT Mitochondria. J Agric Food Chem 59: 4279–4287.
21. Panickar KS, Polansky MM, Anderson RA (2009) Green tea polyphenols attenuate glial swelling and mitochondrial dysfunction following oxygen-glucose deprivation in cultures. Nutr Neurosci 12: 105–13.
22. Kloska A, Jakóbkiewicz-Banecka J, Narajczyk M, Banecka-Majkutewicz Z, Węgrzyn G (2011) Effects of flavonoids on glycosaminoglycan synthesis: implications for substrate reduction therapy in Sanfilippo disease and other mucopolysaccharidoses. Metab Brain Dis 26: 1–8.
23. Rasbach KA, Schnellmann RG (2008) Isoflavones promote mitochondrial biogenesis. J Pharmacol Exp Ther 325: 536–543.
24. Cantó C, Gerhart-Hines Z, Feige JN, Lagouge M, Noriega L, et al. (2009) AMPK regulates energy expenditure by modulating NAD+ metabolism and SIRT1 activity. Nature 458: 1056–1060.

25. Hardie DG (2004) The AMP-activated protein kinase pathway--new players upstream and downstream. J Cell Sci 117: 5479–5487.

26. Shin SM, Kim SG (2009) Inhibition of arachidonic acid and iron-induced mitochondrial dysfunction and apoptosis by oltipraz and novel 1,2-dithiole-3-thione congeners. Mol Pharmacol 75: 242–253.

27. Kwon YN, Shin SM, Cho IJ, Kim SG (2009) Oxidized metabolites of oltipraz exert cytoprotective effects against arachidonic acid through AMP-activated protein kinase-dependent cellular antioxidant effect and mitochondrial protection. Drug Metab Dispos 37: 1187–197.

28. Wenz T, Wang X, Marini M, Moraes CT (2010) A metabolic shift induced by a PPAR panagonist markedly reduces the effects of pathogenic mitochondrial tRNA mutations. J Cell Mol Med. 2010 in press. PMID: 21129152.

29. Brunmair B, Lest A, Staniek K, Gras F, Scharf N, et al. (2004) Fenofibrate impairs rat mitochondrial function by inhibition of respiratory complex I. J Pharmacol Exp Ther 311: 109–114.

30. Burlina AB, Ogier H, Korall H, Trefz FK (2001) Long-term treatment with sodium phenylbutyrate in ornithine transcarbamylase-deficient patients. Mol Genet Metab 72: 351–355.

31. Camacho LH, Olson J, Tong WP, Young CW, Spriggs DR, et al. (2007) Phase I dose escalation clinical trial of phenylbutyrate sodium administered twice daily to patients with advanced solid tumors. Invest New Drug 25: 131–138.

32. Cudkowicz ME, Andres PL, Macdonald SA, Bedlack RS, Choudry R, et al. (2009) Phase 2 study of sodium phenylbutyrate in ALS. Amyotroph Lateral Scler 10: 99–106.

33. Xiao C, Giacca A, Lewis GF (2011) Sodium phenylbutyrate, a drug with known capacity to reduce endoplasmic reticulum stress, partially alleviates lipid-induced insulin resistance and beta-cell dysfunction in humans. Diabetes 60: 918–924.

34. Loeffen J, Elpeleg O, Smeitink J, Smeets R, Stöckler-Ipsiroglu S, et al. (2001) Mutations in the complex I NDUFS2 gene of patients with cardiomyopathy and encephalomyopathy. Ann Neurol 49: 195–201.

35. Saada A, Edvardson S, Rapoport M, Shaag A, Amry K, et al. (2008) C6ORF66 is an assembly factor of mitochondrial complex I. Am J Hum Genet 82: 32–38.

36. Saada A, Edvardson E, Shaag A, Chung WK, Segel R, et al. Combined OXPHOS complex I and IV defect, due to mutated complex I assembly factor C20ORF7. J Inherit Metab Dis, in press. DOI: 10.1007/s10545-011-9348-y.

37. Fassone E, Duncan AJ, Taanman JW, Pagnamenta AT, Sadowski MI, et al. (2010) FOXRED1, encoding an FAD-dependent oxidoreductase complex-I-specific molecular chaperone, is mutated in infantile-onset mitochondrial encephalopathy. Hum Mol Genet 2010 19: 4837–4847.

38. Barghuti F, Elian K, Gomori JM, Shaag A, Edvardson S, et al. (2008) The unique neuroradiology of complex I deficiency due to NDUFA12L defect. Mol Genet Metab 94: 78–82.

39. Jones CN, Miller C, Tenenbaum A, Spremulli LL, Saada A (2009) Antibiotic effects on mitochondrial translation and in patients with mitochondrial translational defects. Mitochondrion 9: 429–437.

40. Kukidome D, Nishikawa T, Sonoda K, Imoto K, Fujisawa K, et al. (2006) Activation of AMP-activated protein kinase reduces hyperglycemia-induced mitochondrial reactive oxygen species production and promotes mitochondrial biogenesis in human umbilical vein endothelial cells. Diabetes 55: 120–127.

41. Pavlidis P, Noble WS (2003) Matrix2png: A Utility for Visualizing Matrix Data. Bioinformatics 19: 295–296.

42. Wang T, Si Y, Shirihai OS, Si H, Schultz V, et al. (2010) Respiration in adipocytes is inhibited by reactive oxygen species. Obesity (Silver Spring) 18: 1493–502.

43. Robinson BH (1996) Use of fibroblast and lymphoblast cultures for detection of respiratory chain defects. Methods Enzymol 264: 454–464.

44. Qanungo S, Das M, Haldar S, Basu A (2005) Epigallocatechin-3-gallate induces mitochondrial membrane depolarization and caspase-dependent apoptosis in pancreatic cancer cells. Carcinogenesis 26: 958–967.

45. Sánchez Y, Amrán D, Fernández C, de Blas E, Aller P (2008) Genistein selectively potentiates arsenic trioxide-induced apoptosis in human leukemia cells via reactive oxygen species generation and activation of reactive oxygen species-inducible protein kinases (p38-MAPK, AMPK). Int J Cancer 123: 1205–14.

46. Bosselaar M, Smits P, van Loon LJ, Tack CJ (2010) Intravenous AICAR During Hyperinsulinemia Induces Systemic Hemodynamic Changes but Has No Local Metabolic Effect. J Clin Pharmacol. in press. PMID: 2114805147.

47. Viscomi C, Bottani E, Civiletto G, Cerutti R, Moggio M, et al. (2011) In vivo correction of COX deficiency by activation of the AMPK/PGC-1α Axis. Cell Metab 14: 80–90.

48. Saada A (2011) The use of individual patient's fibroblasts in the search for personalized treatment of nuclear encoded OXPHOS diseases. Mol Genet Metab. In press. doi: 10.1016/j.ymgme.2011.07.016.

49. Lagouge, M. Argmann C, Grhart-Hines Z, Mezaine H, Lerin C, et al. (2006) Resveratrol improves mitochondrial function and protects against metabolic disease by activating SIRT1 and PGC-1α. Cell 127: 1–14.

50. Zheng J, Ramirez VD (2000) Inhibition of mitochondrial proton F0F1-ATPase/ATP synthase by polyphenolic phytochemicals. Br J Pharmacol 130: 1115–23.

51. Szkudelska K, Nogowski L, Szkudelski T (2011) Resveratrol and genistein as adenosine triphosphate-depleting agents in fat cells. Metabolism 60: 720–729.

52. Wenner CE (2011) Targeting mitochondria as a therapeutic target in cancer. J Cell Physiol. In press. doi: 10.1002/jcp.22788.

53. Gogada R, Prabhu V, Amadori M, Scott R, Hashmi S, et al. (2011) Resveratrol Induces p53-Independent, XIAP-Mediated Bax Oligomerization on Mitochondria to Initiate Cytochrome c Release and Caspase Activation. J Biol Chem. PMID 21712378. In press.

10

Detection of Heteroplasmic Mitochondrial DNA in Single Mitochondria

Joseph E. Reiner[1]*, Rani B. Kishore[1], Barbara C. Levin[2], Thomas Albanetti[3], Nicholas Boire[3], Ashley Knipe[3], Kristian Helmerson[1], Koren Holland Deckman[3]

1 Physical Measurement Laboratory, National Institute of Standards and Technology, Gaithersburg, Maryland, United States of America, **2** Material Measurement Laboratory, National Institute of Standards and Technology, Gaithersburg, Maryland, United States of America, **3** Department of Chemistry, Gettysburg College, Gettysburg, Pennsylvania, United States of America

Abstract

Background: Mitochondrial DNA (mtDNA) genome mutations can lead to energy and respiratory-related disorders like myoclonic epilepsy with ragged red fiber disease (MERRF), mitochondrial myopathy, encephalopathy, lactic acidosis and stroke (MELAS) syndrome, and Leber's hereditary optic neuropathy (LHON). It is not well understood what effect the distribution of mutated mtDNA throughout the mitochondrial matrix has on the development of mitochondrial-based disorders. Insight into this complex sub-cellular heterogeneity may further our understanding of the development of mitochondria-related diseases.

Methodology: This work describes a method for isolating individual mitochondria from single cells and performing molecular analysis on that single mitochondrion's DNA. An optical tweezer extracts a single mitochondrion from a lysed human HL-60 cell. Then a micron-sized femtopipette tip captures the mitochondrion for subsequent analysis. Multiple rounds of conventional DNA amplification and standard sequencing methods enable the detection of a heteroplasmic mixture in the mtDNA from a single mitochondrion.

Significance: Molecular analysis of mtDNA from the individually extracted mitochondrion demonstrates that a heteroplasmy is present in single mitochondria at various ratios consistent with the 50/50 heteroplasmy ratio found in single cells that contain multiple mitochondria.

Editor: Tadafumi Kato, RIKEN Brain Science Institution, Japan

Funding: The authors have no support or funding to report.

Competing Interests: The authors have declared that no competing interests exist.

* E-mail: joseph.reiner@nist.gov

Introduction

Viral pathogenesis, tumor genesis and metastasis, progression of genetic disorders, and apoptosis are complex biological processes that rely on multiple biochemical signals to define the cell physiology. Gene expression levels and covalent modification of biomolecules are just two types of biochemical responses that lead to cellular heterogeneity, which may trigger variations in pathogenic steps like viral infection or variable drug responsiveness. As recently discussed by Snijder *et al.* [1], the pathway by which a disease develops is not always clear, therefore novel methods are needed to characterize subtle differences between cells. These methods could help explain disease development, which in turn could lead to new detection methods and therapies.

A growing number of diseases have been linked to mutations within the mitochondrial genome. Examples of these mitochondria-based diseases include myoclonic epilepsy with ragged red fiber disease (MERRF), mitochondrial myopathy, encephalopathy, lactic acidosis and stroke (MELAS) syndrome, and Leber's hereditary optic neuropathy (LHON) [2,3,4]. It is generally believed that the severity of a mitochondrial disorder is related to the percentage of mutant mtDNA within a given cell and tissue [5,6].

A dynamic picture of mitochondria in mammalian cells has emerged where the mitochondrial genome is impacted via direct mitochondrial mixing [7]. Little is known about the resulting distribution of mutated mtDNA throughout the mitochondrial matrix and its corresponding effect on the development of mitochondria-related diseases. Studying mtDNA from individual mitochondria could help elucidate the connection between the intracellular distribution of mtDNA and the onset of a corresponding disease.

Analyzing mtDNA from single mitochondria requires methods for both isolation and analysis of individual mitochondria [8]. Cavelier *et al.* employed fluorescence microscopy and flow cytometry to isolate individual mitochondria, from a large aggregate of cells [9]. They observed both homoplasmy and heteroplasmy (the latter being a mixture of wild-type and mutated mtDNA containing a single MERRF point mutation) within single mitochondria. Using the same flow cytometry method and a cybrid cell line (containing wild-type and a genome with a deletion of 45% of the genome) Poe *et al.* found homoplasmic distributions within smaller nucleoids of less than 13 mtDNA copies [10]. Because the technique in both studies requires mitochondrial separation from a suspension of many cells, it is impossible to study the intracellular mtDNA distribution from a single cell with their reported methodology. Several reports describe the detection and analysis of organelles extracted from single cells [11,12,13] with the work of Wang and collaborators [13] being of particular interest because an optical tweezer was used to extract single chromosomes for offline genomic analysis.

In addition to trapping chromosomes, optical tweezers have also been used to trap individual mitochondria for several purposes including the study of mitochondrion transport along microtubules *in vivo* [14], the immobilization of single mitochondria for near infrared Raman spectroscopic studies [15], the extraction of individual mitochondria from isolated cells [12,16], and the separation of individual mitochondria from a purified mitochondrial pellet extracted from *Physarum polycephalum* (slime mold) [17]. In this final example, the individual mitochondria were applied to a glass surface, dried, and the glass was cut and subjected to PCR amplification. This method required a minimum of nine mitochondria to produce a detectable amplicon [17]. References [13,16,17] imply that an optical tweezer-based extraction method may permit the use of single mitochondria separated from the same cell for further analysis over time.

In this paper we describe a method for isolating a single mitochondrion and sequencing its mtDNA. Here, we use this technique to verify that a heteroplasmy (a single nucleotide polymorphism [SNP]) exists within a single mitochondrion. This technique could be used to further study the propagation and properties of mitochondrial nucleoids and connections between the intracellular distribution of mtDNA mutations and the development of mitochondrial disorders. It could also be applied to the study of other organelles in cells from a single organism considered to have genetically identical cells to determine how cellular heterogeneity leads to changes in cell physiology and pathology.

Results

Isolation and Capture of a Single Mitochondrion Particle

To trap a single mitochondrion, we developed an optical tweezer based approach similar to that used for chromosome extraction from single rice cells [13]. We first isolate, by dilution, a human cell stained with a mitochondria indicator dye (Mitotracker Green FM), which specifically labels the membranes of respiring mitochondria. Figure 1 shows a brightfield and confocal fluorescence image of a typical dyed HL-60 cell. A schematic diagram of the experimental apparatus and extraction process are shown in Figure 2. The cell is lysed with one or several pulses from a Q-switched UV laser and a single-focus optical tweezer traps a

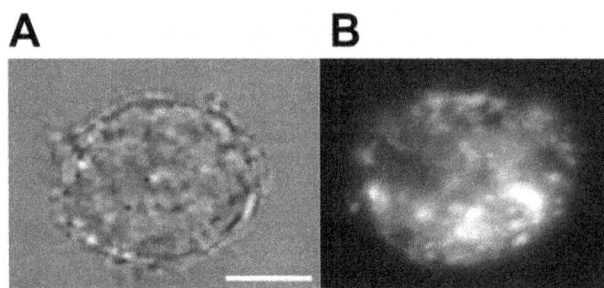

Figure 1. An isolated HL-60 cell. (A) A brightfield image of an HL-60 cell and (B) A confocal scan of the same cell showing mitochondria fluorescently labeled with Mitotracker Green FM. The scale bar corresponds to 5 microns.

freely diffusing organelle. The trapped organelle is identified as a mitochondrion with laser induced fluorescence. The trapped mitochondrion is raised above the cell to a femtopipette tip and directly inserted or suctioned, along with a small volume of buffer, into the empty tip. A time-edited video of this process is included in the supplementary material (Supplementary Video S1).

Amplification and Sequencing mtDNA from a single mitochondrion

Extracted mtDNA from an aggregate of HL-60 cells was previously shown to contain an approximate 1:1 C to T heteroplasmy at nucleotide position (np) 12071 [18]. We developed PCR and sequencing methodologies to examine the limited DNA contained in a single mitochondrion. Our study demonstrates that the heteroplasmy seen in the aggregate was also present in the mtDNA of the isolated mitochondrion, albeit at various ratios.

DNA amplification (PCR) was performed using two distinct primer sets (PS 1 and PS 43) from NIST Standard Reference Materials SRM 2392 and 2392-I [18,19]. PS 43 amplifies the region containing the heteroplasmy of interest located at np 12071. This region was then sequenced to identify the presence of the heteroplasmy at the single mitochondrion level. As a further control, PS 1 amplified the hypervariable region 2 (HV2) of the mtDNA genome [20,21]. We sequenced the HV2 region and compared this to the published sequence of HL-60 [18] to verify that the tested heteroplasmic mtDNA originated from HL-60 (Table 1).

Twenty mitochondrion particles were trapped and captured for mtDNA amplification and sequencing. A subset of the resulting PCR reactions is shown in Figure 3A. Mitochondrial DNA from five of the twenty particles (25%) was successfully amplified with PS 43 (Figure 3A). Two of these five were successfully co-amplified with PS 1 (Figure 3A), which was used to verify the identity of the mitochondrial genome as originating from HL-60 (Table 1).

To ensure the lack of PCR contamination products, a series of controls were prepared. The Control A series consisted of eleven blank femtopipette tips that were collected after being submerged for 20 minutes at a depth of 10 μm with 3 UV-lysed cells in the chamber. Control A samples were subjected to three rounds of PCR reactions. For each round of PCR reactions, one positive control (lanes 1–3, Figure 3B) and one negative control (lanes 21–23, Figure 3B) were included. In addition, two ddH$_2$O controls were amplified through three rounds of PCR (lanes 15–16, 17–18, and 19–20 for rounds 1, 2 and 3 respectively, Figure 3B). Finally, the PCR amplification results of the eleven Control A femtopipette tips are shown in lanes 4–14 in Figure 3B. No amplicons were detected in any of the blank or negative ddH$_2$O controls.

In a second series of controls (Control B), quantitative PCR (qPCR) was used to detect whether mtDNA was present in the media and drawn into the femtopipette tips during these experiments. Seven femtopipette tips were collected in a similar manner to the trapped mitochondrion samples and outlined in the experimental section. Control B tips were analyzed using TaqMan® AmpliTaq qPCR (Applied Biosystems, Inc., Foster City, CA) and primers that targeted the conserved cytochrome c oxidase subunit I (COI) region. The C_t value refers to the qPCR cycle number (C) at which fluorescence is detected above a threshold value (t). Primer artifacts are often seen past 40 qPCR cycles, as was the case in this experiment. The average C_t value for the Control B samples was above the C_t values for the ddH$_2$O and the no template media controls (Table 2). The qPCR amplification data can be found in the Supplementary Figure S1.

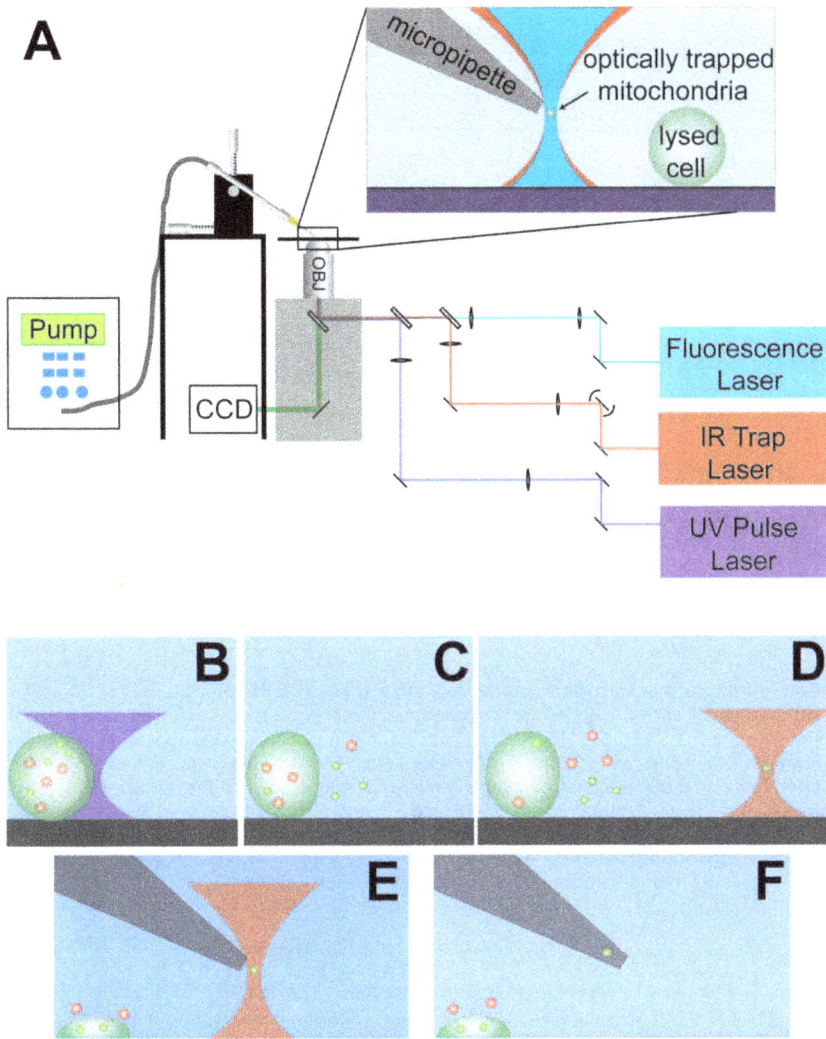

Figure 2. Schematic illustrations of the experimental setup and the extraction process. (A) Light from three different lasers is coupled into the back aperture of a microscope objective. The ultraviolet (UV) pulse, fluorescence, and infrared (IR) trap lasers are overlapped and used for cell lysing, mitochondrion identification and trapping respectively. A pump applies positive pressure to a femtopipette tip to balance against the capillary draw of fluid up inside the tip. (B) A single cell, isolated from other cells, is lysed with a UV pulse laser (violet hourglass). (C) Cell lysis occurs and organelles escape from the cell. (D) A trapped organelle is identified as a fluorescently-labeled mitochondrion with the fluorescence laser (IR trap is designated by the red hourglass; overlapping fluorescence excitation laser is not shown). (E) The trapped organelle is positioned near the end of a femtopipette tip. (F) The tip is positioned sufficiently close to directly capture the mitochondrion or backing pressure from the pump is removed and capillary action draws the mitochondrion into the femtopipette. Full details of the extraction protocol are described in the methods section. A time-edited video showing the entire process is found in the Supplementary Video (S1) available online.

Table 1. The sequence variation of the hypervariable region 2 (HV2).

NT position*	rCRS*	HL-60^	This study^	Sci #1	Sci #2	Sci #3	Sci #4	Sci #5
150	C	T	T	C	C	T	T	C
152	T	C	C	C	T	T	T	T
199	T	T	T	T	C	T	T	T
263	A	G	G	G	G	A	G	G
295	C	T	T	C	C	C	C	C
309	C	CC (insert)	CC (insert)	C	CC (insert)	CC (insert)	CC (insert)	CC (insert)
315	C	CC (insert)	CC (insert)	CC (insert)	CC (insert)	CC (insert)	CC (insert)	CC (insert)

*The HV2 region was sequenced between np 100–350 and compared to the revised Cambridge Reference Sequence (rCRS) [36,37].
^For the two samples amplified with PS 1 (single mitochondrion C and D), we found agreement with the published HL-60 sequence [18]. Sci #1 – Sci #5 refer to the five researchers that had contact with the mitochondrion or blank samples.

A   Gel electrophoresis of five single mitochondria

B   Controls

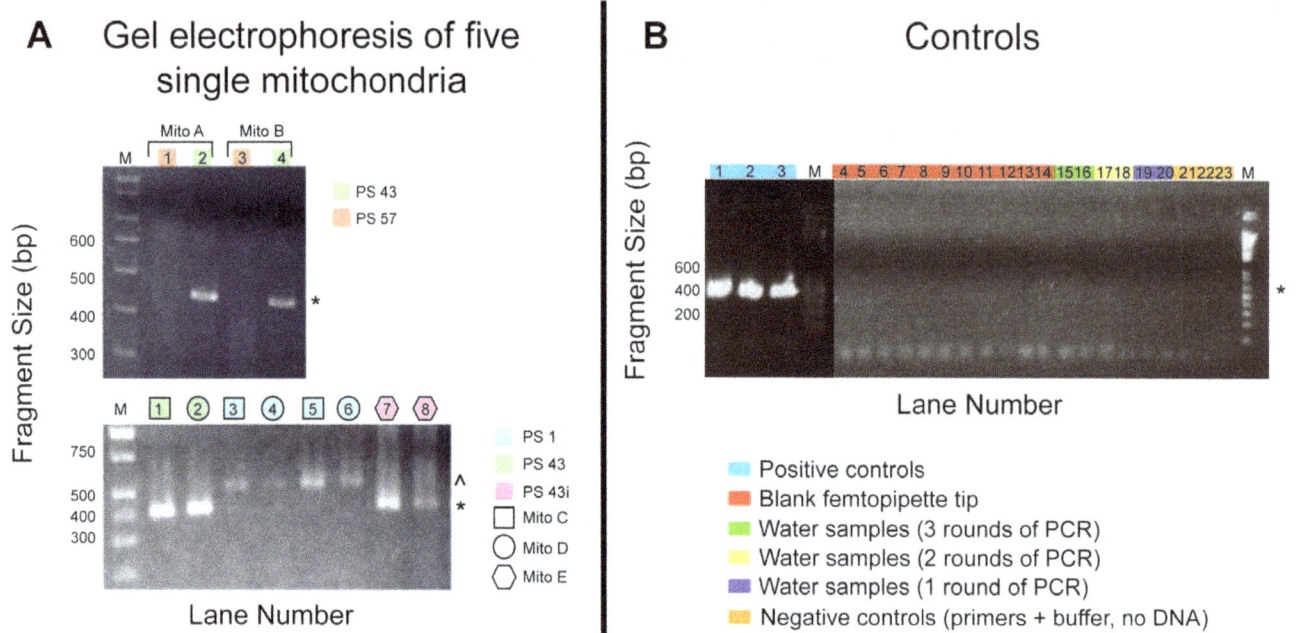

Figure 3. Agarose gel electrophoresis of amplified single mitochondrion samples A-E after three rounds of PCR. (A, top) Amplified product using PS 43 and single mitochondrion A and B (Lanes 2 and 4). Lanes 1 and 3 represent failed amplification with PS 57 and single mitochondrion samples A and B. (A, bottom) Amplified products with PS 43 (Lane 1) and PS 1 (Lanes 3 and 5) from single mitochondrion C. Amplified products with PS 43 (Lane 2) and PS 1 (Lanes 4 and 6) from single mitochondrion D. Amplified products from PS 43i for single mitochondrion E (Lanes 7 and 8). (B) Eleven Control A blank femtopipette tips inserted into the cell suspension for approximately 20 minutes after three rounds of PCR (Lanes 4–14) with PS 43. Water samples carried through 3 rounds (Lanes 15–16), 2 rounds (Lanes 17–18) and 1 round of PCR (Lanes 19–20.) Positive controls for each round of PCR (1.16 ng human DNA) with PS 43, one round PCR for each; Lanes 1, 2 and 3 for successive PCR rounds 1, 2 and 3 respectively. Negative controls for each round of PCR (no DNA) with PS 43, one round of PCR for each; Lanes 21–23 for round 1–3 respectively. *M* = molecular weight size markers. Primer set 43 and PS 43i showed PCR products of approximately 0.43 kb (*), while those amplified with PS 1 showed bands of about 0.47 kb (^).

The sequencing chromatograms, resulting from the five single mitochondrion samples successfully amplified with PS 43, are shown in Figure 4. Each chromatogram is centered around np 12071. All five samples show a heteroplasmy at np 12071, albeit at different ratios. Two samples (A and B, Figure 4) contained an abundance of T, two samples (C and E, Figure 4) contained an abundance of C, while one sample (D, Figure 4) contained

approximately equal ratios of C and T. While the absolute quantity is not calculated, reproducibility between PCR rounds of the same sample is demonstrated in Supplementary Figure S2.

Table 2. Ct values for Control B samples.

Sample	C_t*
ddH$_2$O	42.18
RPMI Media	41.77
RPMI Media	Undetected
Tip-1	47.87
Tip-2	44.10
Tip-3	46.41
Tip-4	Undetected
Tip-5	42.16
Tip-6	47.07
Tip-7	44.70

*The COI region was amplified using PS COI and TaqMan® probe COI. A series of seven dilutions were run in replicate to calculate the standard curve. Standard curve $y = -3.628x - 1.677$, $R^2 = 0.997$.

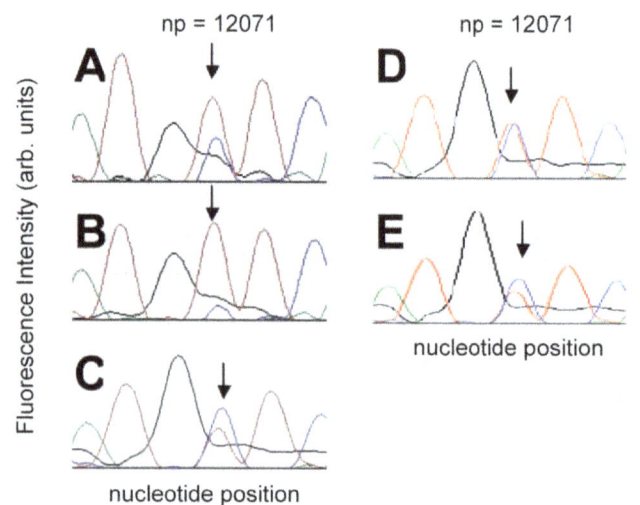

Figure 4. Sequencing chromatograms of single mitochondrion A–E. After optical tweezers capture, transfer and PCR amplification, the five samples that successfully amplified with primer set 43 or 43i were sequenced. Each sample showed the heteroplasmy (C nucleotide (blue) and T nucleotide (red)) at np 12071 highlighted with the arrow.

Discussion

Of the twenty trapped and isolated mitochondrion particles, five samples successfully amplified the SNP region of interest, and all five samples had some degree of heteroplasmy in the np 12071 position. We were able to rule out the possibility that any of the five reported samples resulted from false positives. A false positive in this case would be either the amplification of DNA from more than one mitochondria or from the wrong DNA (e.g., DNA from non-HL-60 sources or nuclear DNA). We address these concerns by noting that the primers used in these studies are mitochondrial-specific and the heteroplasmy, or simply the presence of a C homoplasmy at np 12071, is unique to the HL-60 cell line [18]. Examination of the 5,857 existing NCBI [22] whole-mtDNA sequences, MITOMAP [23] coding region variations and the mtDNA tree [24] revealed no heteroplasmy or cytosine homoplasmy at np 12071. The heteroplasmy existing at 12071 was only identified in the HL-60 cells [18]. Furthermore, the C nucleotide at 12071 was not found in any of the researchers' mtDNA (data not shown). This finding strongly implies that the three isolated mtDNA samples that amplified with PS 43 but failed with PS 1 still originated from an HL-60 cell. Our results indicate that the heteroplasmy is present at the single mitochondrial level and originated from the lysed HL-60 cell.

To establish the unlikelihood of contamination from PCR products, we amplified at least two blank control samples (ddH$_2$O only) through three rounds of PCR and purification as described in the methods section for each set of femtopipette tip samples. No amplicons were detected from these blank control samples.

We also rule out the possibility of whole cell contamination because we see no evidence of amplification at the early stages of PCR analysis. Earlier work on amplifying the mtDNA from individual HL-60 cells typically showed PCR products after one round of amplification (Kishore, Levin, Deckman, and Helmerson, unpublished observations). To minimize the possibility of mitochondria or mitochondrial DNA adhering to the outside of the femtopipette tip, we kept the end of the femtopipette tip approximately 100 microns above the settled cells (cell diameter $\approx$10 micron) during all experiments. Also sample holders containing the cells were discarded after only one to three cell lysings. Finally, the exterior surface of the femtopipette tip is hydrophobic (Eppendorf, Inc., personal communication, Westbury, NY). Thus, the polar membrane surfaces of cells and mitochondria or its DNA are unlikely to adhere to the outside of the femtopipette tip.

In addition to these experimental design controls, we characterized the likelihood of mitochondria adhering to the outside of the femtopipette tip by performing "blank-tip" controls. Eleven femtopipette tips (described above as series Control A) were submerged in solutions containing HL-60 cells at experimentally relevant cellular concentrations. Three cells were then lysed with UV laser pulses and the femtopipette tip was maintained 100 microns above the coverglass surface for a period of 20 minutes within the vicinity of the three lysed cells. If the five positive results occurred because of unwanted mitochondria adhering to the outside of the femtopipette tip, then the 25% success rate (assumes each mitochondria contains at least one mtDNA copy) implies that we should see two to three blank-tip positives (binomial distribution). We observed no amplicon production, which had a 4.2% chance of occurring given a 25% success rate from any of the eleven blank tips. This suggests, with greater than 95% confidence that our five positive samples did not result from excess mitochondria non-specifically binding to the outside of the femtopipette tip.

To minimize the possibility that a free mitochondrial DNA molecule diffused through the media to the femtopipette tip and was drawn into the tip alone or with a mitochondrial particle, the cell was lysed and a mitochondrion was collected over a maximum time frame of twenty minutes. Second, quantitative real-time PCR studies were conducted as follows: seven femtopipette tips (as described above as Control B experiments) were collected following the standard protocol with one modification. A single, optically trapped mitochondrion particle was raised to the femtopipette tip and then released by blocking the trapping beam. The mitochondrion particle was observed to float away. After which, a parcel of media blank solution ($\approx$ pL's) was drawn into the tip. The average C_t value for each sample was greater than or equal to our no template control (ddH$_2$O and media) samples (see Supplementary Figure S2).

The inability of the five successful samples to amplify with both PS 43 and PS 1 was most likely due to the very limited amount of mtDNA and stochastic effects with the amplification reaction. Cavelier et al. reported that the average mtDNA genome copy number in a single mitochondrion was around two and ranged from zero to eleven copies [9]. In addition, mtDNA was not detected in 41 to 53% of collected mitochondria (Cavelier et al., [9]). A more recent flow cytometry study, with a reported PCR efficiency of 80%, found that 35% of the mitochondria, containing mtDNA, showed no amplified PCR product [10]. Both studies suggest various technical issues that minimize the success of flow cytometry studies. Therefore, our trapping and PCR amplification success rate, albeit lower than these studies, is not unreasonable.

Our results are reasonably consistent with the reported work of Cavelier et al. [9] where approximately 50% of the isolated mitochondria contained no detectable mtDNA, approximately 13% contained heteroplasmic mixtures of wild-type and MERRF (SNP) genomes, and the remaining 37% contained homoplasmic distributions. Although we see no homoplasmic mitochondria in our five samples that amplified, they note that approximately 18% of the cells from their study were homoplasmic to begin with. This, along with the fact that mitochondria containing a low copy number of mtDNA genomes tend to bias towards homoplasmic distributions [9], partially explains the higher rate of homoplasmic detection they report.

Mitochondria in vivo have various morphologies ranging from spheres (in HL-60 cells and neutrophils [25]) to branched tubular networks (e.g. [26]; for reviews see references [27] and [28]). The fibroblast cell line employed by Cavelier et al. are elongated and networked [9]. They emphasized, though, that through mitochondrial fission, their manipulation of the cells and their sorting selection process prevented elongated or larger mitochondrial particles from being selected. We expect that our method will self select a spherical particle as well. Nevertheless, even though many organelles are not spherical in shape, this should not hinder the technique described herein because single focus optical tweezers have been shown to trap non-spherical objects including semiconducting nanowires [29,30], rod-shaped cilium [31] and chromosomes [13,32,33]. Line scan optical tweezers [34] and holographic optical trapping [35] are two examples of modifications that have also been used to trap non-spherical particles.

In this paper, we employed an optical tweezer based method [13] for extracting single mitochondria from UV lysed cells with an optical tweezer and femtopipette tip. Optical tweezers separate the mitochondria from the vicinity of the lysed cell and a single focus fluorescence laser identifies the organelle, which had been stained with Mitotracker Green FM, as a mitochondrion particle. The single mitochondrion is transferred from the femtopipette tip to a centrifuge tube followed by lysing, PCR amplification, and sequencing. This work indicates that a heteroplasmy in the mtDNA, previously shown in our laboratory to exist at the single cell level, also exists at the single mitochondrion level. By applying this technique to multiple mitochondria from the same cell, it should be possible to measure the intracellular distribution of a mtDNA mutation and learn what role, if any, this distribution plays in the development of mitochondrial-based diseases. Finally, the optical tweezer method described herein along with qPCR fluorescence analysis could be used to accurately quantify genome copy numbers and mutant to wild-type ratios of mtDNA.

Methods

Chemicals

Mitotracker Green FM and oligonucleotide primers as described in Table 3 were purchased from Invitrogen, Inc. (Carlsbad, CA). *Taq* DNA polymerase was purchased from Promega, Inc. (Madison, WI). All other chemicals were purchased from Sigma-Aldrich, Inc. (St. Louis, MO) unless otherwise noted.

Cell line

The promyelocytic leukemic cell line HL-60 consisting of peripheral blood leukocytes from a 36-year-old woman (ATCC CCL-240) was maintained in RPMI growth medium without glutamine (containing 10% fetal bovine serum, 100 µg/mL penicillin G, 100 µg/mL streptomycin sulfate and 0.25 µg/mL amphotericin B) at 37°C, 5% CO_2 and humidity. One milliliter of this culture was pelleted at 14,000 RPM centrifugation for 1 min, and the pellet was resuspended in 1 mL of growth medium (RPMI-1640 described above) containing 0.1 µmol/L Mitotracker Green FM in DMSO. The cells were incubated (37°C, 15 min), pelleted again, and washed (2x in 1 mL fresh growth media). Cells were resuspended in 1 mL of fresh growth media at an appropriate dilution, identified below, and stored at 4°C in preparation for the optical tweezer extraction.

Isolation and Capture of a Single Mitochondrion Particle

A 120 microliter well was created by mounting a #0 coverslip with vacuum silicone grease to a microscope slide containing a 1 cm diameter hole. Ten microliters of the previously prepared HL-60 culture were mixed with 110 µL of isotonic PBS buffer (137 mmol/L NaCl, 10 mmol/L potassium phosphate,

2.7 mmol/L KCl, pH 7.2), and the solution was transferred to the well. The cells in solution were allowed to settle onto the glass cover slip for 10 minutes. The cells were observed to remain intact and did not swell or lyse for the duration of the experiment. The settled cell concentration was on the order of 50 cells/mm². Three overlapped, collimated, laser beams were reflected off a dichroic mirror (505DRLP, XF2010, Omega Optical, Brattleboro, VT) and sent through the back aperture of an oil-immersion 100× microscope objective (NA = 1.3, Plan Neofluar, Carl Zeiss, Thornwood, NY) mounted on an inverted microscope (Axiovert 100, Carl Zeiss). Individual cells were lysed with a pulsed (pulse duration ≈5 ns, pulse energy ≈50 µJ) UV laser operating in triggered single pulse mode at 355 nm (ML-II, Continuum, Inc., Santa Clara, CA). A continuous wave (CW) infrared (IR) laser operating at 500 mW and 1064 nm (YLD-10-LP, IPG Photonics, Oxford, MA) was used to optically trap each mitochondrion particle. Each trapped particle was identified as a Mitotracker Green FM labeled mitochondrion by fluorescence excitation from an Ar^+ laser (CVI Melles Griot, Albuquerque, NM) operating at 488 nm and approximately 5 mW–10 mW. Emitted fluorescence from the trapped mitochondria was collected back through the 100× objective and focused onto a CCD camera (Sunstar 300, Electrophysics Inc., Fairfield, NJ) mounted onto the microscope. The presence of more than one organelle in the trap could be seen at the video rate (15 Hz) under bright field illumination. If more than one mitochondria was visualized or the trapped organelle did not fluoresce with 488 nm excitation, then the IR tweezer laser was blocked and the contents of the trap were allowed to diffuse away. A recent study reported the use of a 1064 nm optical tweezer leads to two-photon fluorescence and subsequent photobleaching of MitoTracker Green labeled mitochondria over a period of 5 seconds [16]. We do not observe this rapid degree of photobleaching in our system. Photobleaching of this magnitude would lead to a prohibitive number of false negatives (rejected mitochondria) in our protocol. The supplemental video shows a time-edited sequence of the trapping and fluorescence based identification steps and very little detectable 1064 nm induced photobleaching. The protocol was repeated until a single mitochondrion was trapped.

To acquire a mitochondrion particle for genotyping analysis, a hydrophobically treated femtopipette tip (Eppendorf, Inc. personal communication, Westbury, NY) with an attached pump (Femtojet,

Table 3. Primer sequences used for PCR, sequencing and qPCR.

Primer Set (PS)	Nucleotide Position*	Sequence^
1F	15	5′ CACCCTATTAACCACTCACG 3′
1R	484	5′ TGAGATTAGTAGTATGGGAG 3′
43F	11760	5′ ACGAACGCACTCACAGTCG 3′
43R	12189	5′ AAGCCTCTGTTGTCAGATTCAC 3′
43iF	11779	5′ CATCATAATCCTCTCTCAAGG 3′
43iR	12176	5′ AATCTGATGTTTTGGTTAAAC 3′
57F	15971	5′ TTAACTCCACCATTAGCACC 3′
57R	16451	5′ GCGAGGAGAGTAGCACTCTTG 3′
COIF	6048	5′ GGTAACGACCACATCTACAACGTT 3′
COIR	6134	5′ GCCTCCGATTATGATGGGTATTACT 3′
COI-Probe	6074	FAM-CGTCACAGCCCATGCATTTGTAATAATCTTCTTC-TAMRA

*The nucleotide position in the mtDNA genome is based on the rCRS [36,37].
^Primer sets 1, 43 and 57 are based on the SRM-2392-I by Levin *et al.* [18].

Eppendorf Inc., Westbury, NY) applying a continuous positive pressure of approximately 1 atm to prevent capillary suction of fluid, was positioned less than 1 micron from the trapped mitochondrion with a micromanipulator (MP-285, Sutter Instrument Co., Novato, CA). The positive pressure was reduced over a period of 2-3 seconds while the IR tweezer laser was blocked; this resulted in the mitochondrion being drawn into the tip. In a few cases, the suction step was unnecessary because the femtopipette tip was positioned sufficiently close to the trapped mitochondrion and the mitochondrion was directly captured by the end of the femtopipette tip (see Supplementary Video S1). The rate of success of capture was dependent upon the distance and position of the mitochondrion from the center of the tip. Approximately 75% of the trapped single mitochondria were drawn into the tip. To the best of our knowledge, each tip contained one trapped mitochondrion. The contents of the femtopipette tip were transferred into a sterile 250 µL centrifuge tube containing 10 µL sterile deionized distilled H$_2$O (ddH$_2$O, Gibco-BRL, Gaithersburg, MD) by touching the end of the tip to the bottom of the tube. A fragment of the glass femtopipette tip was intentionally broken which resulted in a capillary draw of buffer into the broken tip. Several positive pressure pulses (1 atm applied for 100 ms) flushed this excess solution back into the tube. The single mitochondrion sample was then stored in a −20°C freezer until further analysis could be performed. This process was repeated with approximately 1-3 well-separated cells before discarding the slide and repeating with a fresh sample of cells.

To demonstrate that the hydrophobic exterior surface of the femtopipette tip did not bind free mtDNA or mitochondrion particles, Control A experiments were completed. Eleven femtopipette tips were submerged in solutions containing HL-60 cells at experimentally relevant cellular concentrations. Three cells were then lysed with UV laser pulses and the femtopipette tip remained 100 microns above the coverglass surface for a period of 20 minutes within the vicinity of the three lysed cells. The contents of these eleven blank negative control tips were transferred to a sterile centrifuge tube in a manner similar to that highlighted above.

To determine whether free (intact or fragmented) mtDNA or unidentified mitochondrion particles were drawn into the tip with the trapped mitochondrion, seven buffer-only tip controls (Control B) were collected utilizing the same protocol as described in the capture section except that the IR trapping beam was blocked after the mitochondria had been identified and positioned near the end of the femtopipette tip. The trapped mitochondrion particle was allowed to diffuse away and the backing-pressure was lowered to allow only the buffer to be drawn up into the tip.

PCR Protocol

Each sample consisting of the end piece of the femtopipette tip and its single mitochondrion (or tips from Controls A or B) was sonicated (Sonifier 450, Branson, Danbury, CT) with 120 W, 2-second pulses for 2 minutes. Heat (95°C, 10 min) was then used to continue to disrupt the mitochondrion membranes. The single mitochondrion sample posed two general problems. First, a single mitochondrion sample could not be divided in order to complete the independent amplification of two regions. Second, the mtDNA genome copy number in a mitochondrion is unknown at the time of sampling and can vary from zero to 10 or more [9]. Therefore, in order to successfully amplify these samples mitochondrial DNA was subjected to three rounds of PCR using standard conditions and 2.5 units Taq DNA polymerase (Promega Corp., Madison, WI) following the manufacturer's protocol. Typical PCR parameters were: 95°C for 10 min, 35 cycles (94°C for 20 sec, 50°C for

20 sec, 72°C for 40 sec), and 72°C for 7 min. Each primer concentration was 200 nmol/L. All PCR reactions were analyzed with 2% agarose gels in TBE (100 mmol/L Tris, 90 mmol/L boric acid and 1 mmol/L EDTA, pH 8.3) and stained with 0.5 µg/mL ethidium bromide. A thermocycler (9700 or 2400, Perkin Elmer Inc., Waltham, MA) was used for all PCR amplifications. Primer sequences are highlighted in Table 3, which includes the nucleotide position for the 5′ end of the primer within the mtDNA genome [36,37].

Initially, primer set (PS) 43 and either PS 1 or PS 57 were added to the single mitochondrion sample. After each round of PCR, the amplicons were purified using QIAquick PCR columns (Qiagen, Inc., Valencia, CA) according to the manufacturer's protocol. The PCR products were eluted with 50 µL ddH$_2$O. Aliquots (1 to 10 µL) of the first and second rounds of purified amplicons were used in subsequent PCR reactions to determine the best method for PCR amplification success. Primer combinations and volume used in the series of PCR reactions are available in Table 4 and are summarized here. In Round 1, both sets of primers (PS 43 and PS 57 or PS 1) were co-amplified. Five or ten µL of Round 1 amplicon (not visible by agarose gel electrophoresis) were reamplified in Round 2. One, five or ten µL of the Round 2 PCR product (not visible by agarose gel electrophoresis) were reamplified in Round 3. Samples A and B had co-amplification of PS 43 and PS 57 in Round 2, while samples C, D and E were divided and PS 43 and PS 1 were amplified independently. Sample E utilized PS 43i, a nested primer set, for Rounds 2 and 3. PS 57 was used in earlier captured mitochondria but it failed to amplify any sample. Subsequent samples were amplified with PS 1.

The eleven blank Control A samples and ddH$_2$O blanks (no tip) were analyzed in an identical manner, including three rounds of amplification and purification of each PCR reaction between amplifications. At a minimum, two blank ddH$_2$O samples were analyzed for each series of femtopipette tip experiments.

The seven buffer blank tip samples from Control B were subjected to quantitative PCR (qPCR) analysis utilizing a TaqMan® (Applied Biosystems, Inc.) probe and primers designed to amplify a region within the highly conserved cytochrome c oxidase subunit I gene (COI). FastStart TaqMan® Probe Master Mix (Roche, Inc., Indianapolis, IN) was used following the manufacturer's procedure. The primers (400 nmol/L each) and probe (200 nmol/L) sequences are identified in Table 3. The probe was labeled with fluorescamine (5′-FAM) and the quencher 3′-TAMRA. Typical qPCR conditions were: 50°C for 2 min, 95°C for 10 minutes, and 50 cycles (95°C for 15 sec and 60°C for 1 min.)

All positive PCR amplification controls contained the appropriate primer set and 1.6 ng HL-60 total DNA (CCL 240D, ATCC, Manassas, VA). All PCR negative controls contained the appropriate primer set but lacked any amplifiable DNA. These positive and negative PCR controls reactions were prepared in separate laboratory spaces isolated from the extracted tip samples and tip controls to prevent contamination. DNA samples taken from researchers, involved in the trapping or amplification procedure, were amplified and sequenced with PS 1 and PS 43. All DNA sequences were compared to the revised Cambridge Reference Sequence (rCRS) [37,38].

Any negative water controls that contained evidence of contamination were discarded and a new set of samples was collected. These discarded samples are not included in any calculation demonstrating overall success.

DNA sequencing protocol

One to five microliters of each PCR reaction was mixed with 0.5 µmol/L of the appropriate forward or reverse primer and

Table 4. Sample manipulation for PCR amplification of mtDNA from a single mitochondrion.

Sample	PCR Round	Template	Final Reaction Volume	Primers
A	1	Single mitochondrion A in 30 μL dH$_2$O	50 μL	PS43 and PS57
	2	10 μL round 1 amplicon	50 μL	PS43 and PS57
	3	10 μL round 2 amplicon	50 μL	PS43 or PS57
B	1	Single mitochondrion B in 30 μl dH$_2$O	50 μL	PS43 and PS57
	2	10 μL round 1 amplicon	50 μL	PS43 and PS57
	3	10 μL round 2 amplicon	50 μL	PS43 or PS57
C	1	Single mitochondrion C in 10 μl dH$_2$O	25 μL	PS43 and PS1
	2	5 μL round 1 amplicon	25 μL	PS43 or PS1
	3	1 μL round 2 amplicon	25 μL	PS43 or PS1
D	1	Single mitochondrion D in 10 μl dH$_2$O	25 μL	PS43 and PS1
	2	5 μL round 1 amplicon	25 μL	PS43 or PS1
	3	5 μL round 2 amplicon	25 μL	PS43 or PS1
E	1	Single mitochondrion E in 10 μl dH$_2$O	25 μL	PS43 and PS1
	2	5 μL round 1 amplicon	25 μL	PS43i or PS1
	3	5 μL round 2 amplicon	25 μL	PS43i or PS1

8 μL BigDye Terminator v1.1 Cycle Sequencing Kit according to the manufacturer's protocol (Applied Biosystems, Inc., Foster City, CA). Sequencing reactions were utilized the following thermocycler parameters: 95°C for 2 min and 25 cycles (95°C for 15 sec, 50°C for 5 sec, and 60°C for 2 min). Products were purified using the Performa DTR gel cartridge (Edge Biosystems, Inc., Gaithersburg, MD) and dried in a vacuum microcentrifuge (SpeedVac, Thermo Fisher Scientific, Waltham, MA). Twenty μL of Template Suppression Reagent (Applied Biosystems, Inc.) or formamide was added to each sample and analyzed by capillary gel electrophoresis (Genetic Analyzer 310, Applied Biosystems, Inc.). Sequence Navigator v1.0.1 (Applied Biosystems, Inc.) was used for sequence alignment.

The successful sequencing of mtDNA from the five samples shows that the UV laser had no detectable damaging effect on the mtDNA.

Supporting Information

Supplementary Figure S1 The log of fluorescence intensity, which is proportional to the concentration of amplified DNA, is plotted against the number of PCR amplification cycle (C). The fluorescence threshold (t) for detecting mtDNA is set to 0.2 (orange solid line) as determined with a standard curve. The cycle at which fluorescence reaches the threshold value is Ct. Blank controls consisted of distilled water (purple line) and RPMI media (light blue line). Each shows a Ct above 41 cycles. Two (red and orange lines) of the seven blank tips for control B (see main text) and four other blank Control B tips (not shown) show similar results with Ct values between 42 and 48 cycles. One blank tip and one media control sample did not have detectible products (see Table 2 in main text). This suggests the buffer drawn into the femtopipette tip for the Control B samples "amplify" below the limit of detection of the qPCR analysis.

Supplementary Figure S2 Chromatograms A–D display the sequencing results of a single mitochondria (mitochondrion A from figure 4 of the main text) measured after subsequent rounds of PCR. The black arrows indicate the heteroplasmic nucleotide position 12071. Chromatograms E–F show subsequent rounds of PCR on a single cell, which also shows no discernable change of heteroplasmic ratio from multiple rounds of PCR. Note the vertical axis is the same between A–D and only a slight shift in the vertical axis exists between E and F, which has little affect on the heteroplasmic ratio.

Supplementary Video S1 Time-edited video of the mitochondrion extraction process. A UV laser pulse lyses a single HL-60 cell open. An organelle diffuses away from the lysed cell. The microscope stage is adjusted so the IR optical tweezer laser, fixed in the middle of the screen, traps the organelle. The bright field light is blocked and the 488 nm fluorescence laser, overlapped with the tweezer laser, illuminates the organelle to verify it is a mitochondrion particle. The bright field light is turned back on and the femtopipette tip is positioned to capture the mitochondrion. After capture the fluorescence laser is turned back on and the femtopipette tip is moved in a controlled fashion to verify the mitochondrion is trapped inside the femtopipette tip.

Acknowledgments

Certain commercial equipment, instruments, or materials are identified in this work to specify the experimental procedure adequately. Such identification is not intended to imply recommendation or endorsement by the National Institute of Standards and Technology, nor is it intended to imply that the materials or equipment identified are necessarily the best available for this purpose.

Author Contributions

Conceived and designed the experiments: JER RBK BCL KH KHD. Performed the experiments: JER RBK TA AK NB KHD. Analyzed the data: JER RBK TA AK NB KHD. Contributed reagents/materials/analysis tools: JER RBK BCL KH KHD. Wrote the paper: JER BCL KH KHD. Contributed to sections of the paper: RBK. Contributed to sections of the paper and editing: BCL KH.

References

1. Snijder B, Sacher R, Ramo P, Damm E-M, Liberali P, et al. (2009) Population context determines cell-to-cell variability in endocytosis and virus infection. Nature 461: 520–523.
2. Dahl HH, Thorburn DR (2001) Mitochondrial diseases: beyond the magic circle. Am J Med Genet 106: 1–3.
3. Greaves LC, Taylor RW (2006) Mitochondrial DNA mutations in human disease. IUBMB Life 58: 143–151.
4. Taylor RW, Turnbull DM (2005) Mitochondrial DNA mutations in human disease. Nat Rev Genet 6: 389–402.
5. Cree LM, Samuels DC, de Sousa Lopes SC, Rajasimha HK, Wonnapinij P, et al. (2008) A reduction of mitochondrial DNA molecules during embryogenesis explains the rapid segregation of genotypes. Nat Genet 40: 249–254.
6. DiMauro S, Schon EA (2003) Mitochondrial Respiratory-Chain Diseases. N Engl J Med 348: 2656–2668.
7. Nakada K, Inoue K, Ono T, Isobe K, Ogura A, et al. (2001) Inter-mitochondrial complementation: Mitochondria-specific system preventing mice from expression of disease phenotypes by mutant mtDNA. Nat Med 7: 934–940.
8. Fuller KM, Arriaga EA (2003) Advances in the analysis of single mitochondria. Curr Opin Biotechnol 14: 35–41.
9. Cavelier L, Johannisson A, Gyllensten U (2000) Analysis of mtDNA copy number and composition of single mitochondrial particles using flow cytometry and PCR. Exp Cell Res 259: 79–85.
10. Poe BG, Duffy CF, Greminger MA, Nelson BJ, Arriaga EA (2010) Detection of heteroplasmy in individual mitochondrial particles. Anal Bioanal Chem 397: 3397–3407.
11. Chen Y, Xiong G, Arriaga EA (2007) CE analysis of the acidic organelles of a single cell. Electrophoresis 28: 2406–2415.
12. Shelby JP, Edgar JS, Chiu DT (2005) Monitoring cell survival after extraction of a single subcellular organelle using optical trapping and pulsed-nitrogen laser ablation. Photochem Photobiol 81: 994–1001.
13. Wang H, et al. (2004) Isolation of a single rice chromosome by optical micromanipulation. J Opt A: Pure Appl Opt 6: 89.
14. Ashkin A, Schutze K, Dziedzic JM, Euteneuer U, Schliwa M (1990) Force generation of organelle transport measured in vivo by an infrared laser trap. Nature 348: 346–348.
15. Tang H, Yao H, Wang G, Wang Y, Li Y-q, et al. (2007) NIR Raman spectroscopic investigation of single mitochondria trapped by optical tweezers. Opt Express 15: 12708–12716.
16. Jeffries GD, Edgar JS, Zhao Y, Shelby JP, Fong C, et al. (2007) Using polarization-shaped optical vortex traps for single-cell nanosurgery. Nano Lett 7: 415–420.
17. Kuroiwa T, Ishibashi K, Takano H, Higashiyama T, Sasaki N, et al. (1996) Optical isolation of individual mitochondria of *Physarum polycephalum* for PCR analysis. Protoplasma 194: 275–279.
18. Levin BC, Holland KA, Hancock DK, Coble M, Parsons TJ, et al. (2003) Comparison of the complete mtDNA genome sequences of human cell lines– HL-60 and GM10742A–from individuals with pro-myelocytic leukemia and leber hereditary optic neuropathy, respectively, and the inclusion of HL-60 in the NIST human mitochondrial DNA standard reference material–SRM 2392-I. Mitochondrion 2: 387–400.
19. Levin BC, Cheng H, Reeder DJ (1999) A human mitochondrial DNA standard reference material for quality control in forensic identification, medical diagnosis, and mutation detection. Genomics 55: 135–146.
20. Butler JM, Levin BC (1998) Forensic applications of mitochondrial DNA. Trends in Biotech 16: 158–162.
21. Coble MD, Just RS, OrsquoCallaghan JE, Letmanyi IH, Peterson CT, et al. (2004) Single nucleotide polymorphisms over the entire mtDNA genome that increase the power of forensic testing in Caucasians. Int J Legal Med 118: 137–146.
22. Gertz EM (2005) BLAST Scoring Parameters http://wwwncbinlmnihgov/.
23. Ruiz-Pesini E, Lott MT, Procaccio V, Poole J, Brandon MC, et al. (2007) An enhanced MITOMAP with a global mtDNA mutational phylogeny. Nucleic Acids Res 35: D823–D828.
24. van Oven M, Manfred K (2009) Updated comprehensive phylogenetic tree of global human mitochondrial DNA variation. Hum Mutat 30: E386–E394.
25. Niu H, Kozjak-Pavlovic V, Rudel T, Rikihisa Y. Anaplasma phagocytophilum Ats-1 Is Imported into Host Cell Mitochondria and Interferes with Apoptosis Induction. PLoS Pathog 6: e1000774.
26. Legros F, Malka F, Frachon P, Lombes A, Rojo M (2004) Organization and dynamics of human mitochondrial DNA. J Cell Sci 117: 2653–2662.
27. Westermann B (2002) Merging mitochondria matters. Cellular role and molecular machinery of mitochondrial fusion. EMBO Reports 3: 527–531.
28. Chan DC (2006) Mitochondria: Dynamic Organelles in Disease, Aging, and Development. Cell 125: 1241–1252.
29. Pauzauskie PJ, Radenovic A, Trepagnier E, Shroff H, Yang P, et al. (2006) Optical trapping and integration of semiconductor nanowire assemblies in water. Nat Mater 5: 97–101.
30. Agarwal R, Ladavac K, Roichman Y, Yu G, Lieber C, et al. (2005) Manipulation and assembly of nanowires with holographic optical traps. Opt Express 13: 8906–8912.
31. Resnick A (2011) Use of optical tweezers to probe epithelial mechanosensation. J Biomed Opt 15: 015005–015008.
32. Berns MW, Wright WH, Tromberg BJ, Profeta GA, Andrews JJ, et al. (1989) Use of a laser-induced optical force trap to study chromosome movement on the mitotic spindle. Proc Nat Acad Sci U S A. 86: 4539–4543.
33. Vorobjev IA, Liang H, Wright WH, Berns MW (1993) Optical trapping for chromosome manipulation: A wavelength dependence of induced chromosome bridges. Biophys J 64: 533–538.
34. Nambiar R, Meiners J-C (2002) Fast position measurements with scanning line optical tweezers. Opt Lett 27: 836–838.
35. Dufresne ER, Spalding GC, Dearing MT, Sheets SA, Grier DG (2001) Computer-generated holographic optical tweezer arrays. Rev Sci Instrum 72: 1810–1816.
36. Anderson S, Bankier AT, Barrell BG, de Bruijn MH, Coulson AR, et al. (1981) Sequence and organization of the human mitochondrial genome. Nature 290: 457–465.
37. Andrews RM, Kubacka I, Chinnery PF, Lightowlers RN, Turnbull DM, et al. (1999) Reanalysis and revision of the Cambridge reference sequence for human mitochondrial DNA. Nat Genet 23: 147.
38. Agarwal A, Zudans I, Weber EA, Olofsson J, Orwar O, et al. (2007) Effect of cell size and shape on single-cell electroporation. Anal Chem 79: 3589–3596.

11

Anopheles Immune Genes and Amino Acid Sites Evolving Under the Effect of Positive Selection

Aristeidis Parmakelis[1,2,3]*, Marina Moustaka[1], Nikolaos Poulakakis[2,3], Christos Louis[2,4], Michel A. Slotman[5], Jonathon C. Marshall[3,6], Parfait H. Awono-Ambene[7], Christophe Antonio-Nkondjio[7], Frederic Simard[7,8], Adalgisa Caccone[3], Jeffrey R. Powell[3]

1 Department of Ecology and Taxonomy, Faculty of Biology, National and Kapodistrian University of Athens, Panepistimioupoli Zografou, Athens, Greece, 2 Department of Biology, University of Crete, Heraklion, Crete, Greece, 3 Department of Ecology and Evolutionary Biology, Yale University, New Haven, Connecticut, United States of America, 4 Institute of Molecular Biology and Biotechnology, Foundation of Research and Technology Heraklion, Vassilika Vouton, Heraklion, Crete, Greece, 5 Department of Entomology, Texas A&M University, College Station, Texas, United States of America, 6 Department of Zoology, Weber State University, Ogden, Utah, United States of America, 7 Organisation de Coordination pour la Lutte Contre les Endémies en Afrique Centrale (OCEAC), Yaoundé, Cameroon, 8 Institut de Recherche pour le Développement (IRD), Bobo Dioulasso, Burkina Faso

Abstract

Background: It has long been the goal of vector biology to generate genetic knowledge that can be used to "manipulate" natural populations of vectors to eliminate or lessen disease burden. While long in coming, progress towards reaching this goal has been made. Aiming to increase our understanding regarding the interactions between *Plasmodium* and the *Anopheles* immune genes, we investigated the patterns of genetic diversity of four anti-*Plasmodium* genes in the *Anopheles gambiae* complex of species.

Methodology/Principal Findings: Within a comparative phylogenetic and population genetics framework, the evolutionary history of four innate immunity genes within the *An. gambiae* complex (including the two most important human malaria vectors, *An. gambiae* and *An. arabiensis*) is reconstructed. The effect of natural selection in shaping the genes' diversity is examined. Introgression and retention of ancestral polymorphisms are relatively rare at all loci. Despite the potential confounding effects of these processes, we could identify sites that exhibited dN/dS ratios greater than 1.

Conclusions/Significance: In two of the studied genes, *CLIPB14* and *FBN8*, several sites indicated evolution under positive selection, with *CLIPB14* exhibiting the most consistent evidence. Considering only the sites that were consistently identified by all methods, two sites in *CLIPB14* are adaptively driven. However, the analysis inferring the lineage-specific evolution of each gene was not in favor of any of the *Anopheles* lineages evolving under the constraints imposed by positive selection. Nevertheless, the loci and the specific amino acids that were identified as evolving under strong evolutionary pressure merit further investigation for their involvement in the *Anopheles* defense against microbes in general.

Editor: Simon Joly, McGill University, Canada

Funding: This research was supported by the National Institutes of Health grant RO1 A1 046018 to J.R.P. and A.C. A.P. was supported by a Marie Curie Outgoing International Fellowship (Contract No. MOIF-CT-2006-021357) and a "Kapodistrias" Research Grant from the Research Secretariat of the University of Athens. The funders had no role in study design, data collection and analysis, decision to publish, or preparation of the manuscript.

Competing Interests: The authors have declared that no competing interests exist.

* E-mail: aparmakel@biol.uoa.gr

Introduction

It has long been a goal of vector biology to generate genetic knowledge that can be used to "manipulate" natural populations of vectors to ammeliorate the impact of diseases spread by vectors. While long in coming, progress towards reaching this goal has accelerated. Some of the explored methods for generating refractoriness involve using antibodies that kill parasites within the mosquito [1] and discovering genes that govern refractoriness in natural populations [2]. To this end, a great deal is being discovered about the immune system of mosquitoes [3,4,5], leading to the hope that the development of an effective gene construct that reduces the ability of mosquitoes to transmit malaria is not far away.

It is clear that species-specific (on both the mosquito and parasite side) interactions guide the co-evolution of *Anopheles* and *Plasmodium*. That *An. gambiae* has undergone an adaptive response to *P. falciparum* infection is suggested by several lines of evidence. Both *An. gambiae* and *An. stephensi* mosquitoes infected with *P. berghei*, for which this parasite species are not natural hosts, produce 50–80 oocysts, whereas an infection with *P. falciparum* results in far fewer oocysts. Furthermore, a specific strain of *An. gambiae* selected to be refractory to *P. cynomolgi* (monkey malaria) has very limited refractoriness to strains of *P. falciparum* isolated in Africa [6]. Genetic crosses between refractory and susceptible strains indicate that different genes are involved in the encapsulation response to different species of *Plasmodium* [7,8,9,10]. A strain of *An. stephensi* selected for refractoriness to *P. falciparum* transmission showed no detectable resistance to other *Plasmodium* species [11,12]. Furthermore, the immune response of *An. gambiae*, as detected by changes in gene regulation of immune-related genes, is different in response to *P. falciparum* and *P. berghei* infections [13]. Finally, a gene silencing assay of three immunity genes of *An. gambiae* infected with *P. falciparum*, indicated that the immune response is quite different from that manifested after infection with *P. berghei* [14]. The results of the latter study highlight one more issue, namely the importance of following up discoveries in laboratory model systems with studies on natural parasite–mosquito interactions.

Presently, few studies [15,16,17,18,19,20,21,22] have investigated the patterns of genetic diversity and the evolution of the *Anopheles* innate immunity genes involved in *Plasmodium* infection. A total number of approximately 65 innate immunity genes have been studied, representing several immunity gene families. Purifying selection was found to be the most common form of selection operating on immune genes [15,16,17,18,19,20,21,22], whereas a single case of positive selection acting on the lineage leading to *Anopheles arabiensis* was found in *LRIM1* [22]. Investigating selection patterns in a species complex of closely related species such as the *An. gambiae* complex imposes some limitations [18]. These limitations stem mainly from the phylogenetic and population genetic history of the complex [18,19]. Researchers are concerned with phylogenetic analysis within the complex, and argue that the use of an appropriate outgroup when investigating patterns of selection in *Anopheles* immunity genes is of critical importance as is the level of within species recombination [18,19]. In an effort to overcome these issues, researchers have applied modifications of well established positive selection methods to *Anopheles* immunity genes that at least partially circumvent these problems [18]. The recently approved genome sequences [23] from 13 more species of *Anopheles* mosquitoes should resolve the outgroup issue. However, until the new *Anopheles* sequences become available, phylogenetic analysis within the *An. gambiae* complex will have to use *An. melas* and *An. merus* sequences as outgroups. The divergence of these species from the *An. gambiae/ An. arabiensis* clade should be sufficient in the case of genes evolving under strong positive selection [18].

In the present work we investigated patterns of genetic diversity of four anti- *Plasmodium* genes in the *Anopheles gambiae* complex of species, using a population genetics and phylogenetic framework. The complex is composed of seven species, *An. gambiae*, *An. arabiensis*, *An. melas*, *An. merus*, *An. bwambae* and *An. quadriannulatus* A and B. *An. gambiae* and *An. arabiensis* are the two primary African human malaria vectors, whereas *An. melas*, *An. merus* and *An. bwambae* occasionally transmit human malaria locally but do not have sufficiently wide distributions to be considered primary malaria vectors. The species *An. quadriannulatus* (A and B) are zoophilic and are never or rarely exposed to the human malaria parasite *P. falciparum*.

Results

Four immunity genes were included in the study (Table 1). These genes are *MDL1*, *MDL2*, *CLIPB14* and *FBN8* and all of them have been implicated to be involved in the defense of *Anopheles* against malaria. *MDL1* is composed of 4 exons and has a transcript length of 750 bp. We amplified a fragment ranging from 618 to 739 bp from all specimens (76 sequences, Table 2). This fragment includes the complete sequence of exons one, two and three, part of exon four, and codes for 151 amino acids (Table S1). *MDL2* comprises four exons and has a total length of 3915 bp. The transcript however is only 710 bp long and only 498 bp are translated into amino acids. A total of 49 sequences were obtained from the studied species (Table 2). Sequence length varied from 540 to 868 bp, and included all 498 bp that translate into amino acids (Table S2). *CLIPB14* is composed of three exons. We obtained 49 sequences. The fragments amplified in all species was 1364 bp long, with the exception of the fragments amplified from *An. bwambae*, which were 1271 bp in length. We obtained almost the complete sequence of exon one (except 186 bp in the 5′ end of the exon), and the complete sequence of exon three (Table S3). However, we have not been able to amplify a large fragment (208 bp in *An. bwambae* and 116 in the remaining five species) of the second exon. The sequences amplified translate into a total of 318 amino acids. For the *FBN8* locus we successfully determined 50 sequences from the six species. From this gene, which is not

Table 1. Details of the loci analyzed and sequences of primers used in the study for the amplification of the immunity genes.

Locus (*Anopheles* chromosome)	Locus length (number of exons)	Length of transcript (bp)	Translation length (aa)	Sequences of primers used	
				Initial PCR	**Nested PCR**
MDL1 (3L)	992 bp (4)	750	157	*Intron_248F*: TCTGTTGGCTGCCATGTCAG	*Exon_294F*: CATCACTGTTGGCGTGAGTC
				Intron_1086R: TACACGGTCGTCCCACCAGC	*Exon_1013R*: TGGTGATGTTGATCTGCACG
MDL2 (2R)	3915 bp (4)	710	166	*Intron_073F*: CGCAGATTTTATCCCACGAT	*Exon_092F*: TTCGAGTGGCTACCGAGAGT
				Intron_944R: TCATAACCCAACAGCTCACG	*Exon_880R* GACCAGCAGCATGCTATTCA
CLIPB14 (3L)	1554 bp (3)	1225	389	*Exon1_011F (primer pair A)*: CGGATCGTTTACCACACTGTG	*Exon1_011F (primer pair A)*: CGGATCGTTTACCACACTGTG
				Exon2_1164R (primer pair A): CTGATTCGGTCGAACCCCAG	*Exon2_946R (primer pair A)*: ATTGTACTCCACGTCCGCTG
				Exon2_1073F (primer pair B): GACCGAATCAGGGAAGGAGT	*Intron3_1157F (primer pair B)*: GATTCCCTCCTCCCGAATAG
				Intron4_1664R (primer pair B): TCCTGGCATTTGTATCACCA	*Intron4_1556R (primer pair B)*: TAAACAACTTCCGACGCTCA
FBN8 (3L)	645 bp (1)	645	214	*Exon_407F*: TCGACGAAAACCCCCGTTCG	-
				Exon_959R: CCAACATATAGCTTTTGGGTCCAC	

If the initial PCR was not successful or produced very low signal a nested PCR protocol was implemented.

Table 2. Loci polymorphism (coding and non-coding sequence).

	Locus																							
	MDL1						MDL2						CLIPB14						FBN8					
	Parameters																							
	N	n	A	Hd	PiSyn	PiNonS	N	n	A	Hd	PiSyn	PiNonS	N	n	A	Hd	PiSyn	PiNonS	N	n	A	Hd	PiSyn	PiNonS
Species																								
ARA	8	15	10	0.89	0.011	0.002	6	9	7	0.92	0.014	0.015	6	11	11	1.00	0.019	0.006	5	10	8	0.95	0.064	0.015
BWA	6	12	8	0.94	0.008	0.002	7	7	2	0.29	0.012	0.000	5	6	6	1.00	0.020	0.004	4	8	4	0.78	0.021	0.007
GAM	7	12	12	1.00	0.027	0.002	6	12	12	1.00	0.023	0.002	6	8	8	1.00	0.013	0.001	5	10	10	1.00	0.068	0.014
MEL	7	10	9	0.98	0.008	0.004	6	6	2	0.60	0.000	0.000	6	7	6	0.95	0.005	0.002	5	7	6	0.95	0.062	0.018
MER	7	12	12	1.00	0.032	0.004	5	5	5	1.00	0.006	0.001	6	9	9	1.00	0.019	0.004	6	7	3	0.52	0.052	0.016
QUA/ KNP905/ SQUA	9	15	15	1.00	0.025	0.005	10	10	6	0.78	0.010	0.000	6	8	8	1.00	0.012	0.003	5	8	6	0.93	0.081	0.019
Total n	76						49						49						50					

N: number of individuals, n: number of produced sequences; A: number of unique alleles; Hd: haplotype (allelic) diversity; PiSyn: within species diversity (coding sequence) in synonymous sites; PiNonS: within species diversity (coding sequence) in non-synonymous sites. Species names are abbreviated as follows: *An. arabiensis*: ARA, *An.bwambae*: BWA, *An. gambiae*: GAM, *An. melas*: MEL, *An. merus*: MER, *An. quadriannulatus*: QUA (KNP905 and SQUA are also abbreviated as QUA for presentation purposes).

interrupted by an intron (Table 1), we amplified fragments ranging from 512 to 582 bp long. The amplified fragments translate into 194 amino acids (Table S4) out of the 214 residues that constitute the FBN8 protein.

Diversity, Polymorphism and Phylogeny Inference

Out of the 76 sequences of *MDL1*, 66 different alleles were found (Table 2), and one allele was shared between species (*An. bwambae-An. quadriannulatus*). The within species nucleotide diversity (Pi) varied from 0.008 to 0.032 and 0.002 to 0.005 in the synonymous and non-synonymous sites, respectively (Table 2). Dxy (average number of nucleotide substitutions per site between species) ranged from 1.10 to 2.83% (Table S5). The phylogenetic tree of *MDL1* was not fully resolved and multiple polytomies were present (Fig. 1). Nevertheless, *MDL1* was subjected to the maximum likelihood tests for positive selection with PAML and HyPhy.

Out of the 49 *MDL2* sequences 34 different alleles were detectd (Table 2). No alleles were shared between species. Dxy ranged from 1.10 to 3.02% (Table S5). Within species nucleotide diversity (Pi) ranged between 0.000 to 0.014 and 0.000 to 0.015 in the synonymous and non-synonymous sites, respectively (Table 2). With the exception of one allele from *An. bwambae* and three alleles from *An. gambiae*, all *MDL2* alleles were grouped according to species of origin (Fig. 2).

Out of the 49 sequences of *CLIPB14*, 48 alleles were found (Table 2); none were shared between species. Dxy ranged from 1.39 to 3.39% between species (Table S6). The within species nucleotide diversity (Pi) varied from 0.005 to 0.020 in the synonymous sites, and from 0.001 to 0.006 in the non-synonymous sites (Table 2). The alleles of each *Anopheles* species formed a strongly supported monophyletic clade (Fig. 3), with the exception of *An. bwambae*, in which two alleles were closely related to the alleles of *An. gambiae*.

In *FBN8*, 37 out of the 50 sequences were different alleles (Table 2). Five alleles were shared between species. More specifically, alleles (one in each case) were shared between *An. gambiae* and *An. quadriannulatus*, *An. gambiae* and *An. melas*, *An.*

arabiensis and *An. merus*, *An. bwambae* and *An. merus* and *An. melas* and *An. merus*. Dxy ranged from 2.82 to 5.59% between species. Nucleotide diversity within species (Pi) in the synonymous sites was higher compared to the previous genes and varied from 0.021 to 0.081, whereas in the non-synonymous sites ranged from 0.007 up to 0.019. In the *FBN8* tree (Fig. 4) many alleles appear to be more closely related to alleles of species other than their nominal ones. This is particularly the case in *An. quadriannulatus* in which 3 out of the 8 alleles are scattered across the phylogenetic tree and cluster with alleles of *An. merus* and *An. bwambae*. The situation is similar for the *An. gambiae* alleles that appear closely related to *An. quadriannulatus* alleles. Finally, some of the *An. arabiensis* alleles group with *An. gambiae* and *An. merus* alleles.

The F_{ST} values (permutation tests were significant in all cases) for all studied loci in the majority of the species pairwise comparisons were well above 0.4. In several cases the F_{ST} exceeded 0.7. However, there were two cases, one in *FBN8* (*An. gambiae-An. quadriannulatus*) and one in *MDL1* (*An. gambiae-An. quadriannulatus*) where the F_{ST} values were lower than 0.25.

Recombination Detection

The analysis using the RDP software did not detect any statistically significant recombination events in the *MDL1* and *MDL2* datasets. In total, four recombination events were detected in the *CLIPB14* and *FBN8* datasets (two events in each locus). The results from the implementation of the GARD module in detecting recombination in the datasets are presented in conjunction with the selection analysis results.

Results of Selection Analyses Using PAML and HyPhy

In *MDL1* and *MDL2* no sites evolving under positive selection could be inferred, only indications of varying selection pressure (M0 vs. M3) among codons were found (Table 3). The GARD module of HyPhy detected no recombination breakpoints in *MDL1* and *MDL2*, and no sites under positive selection were found by the consecutive analyses of HyPhy as well.

In *CLIPB14* multiple sites were indicated as having a dN/dS ratio greater than 1; they were identified both by the naive

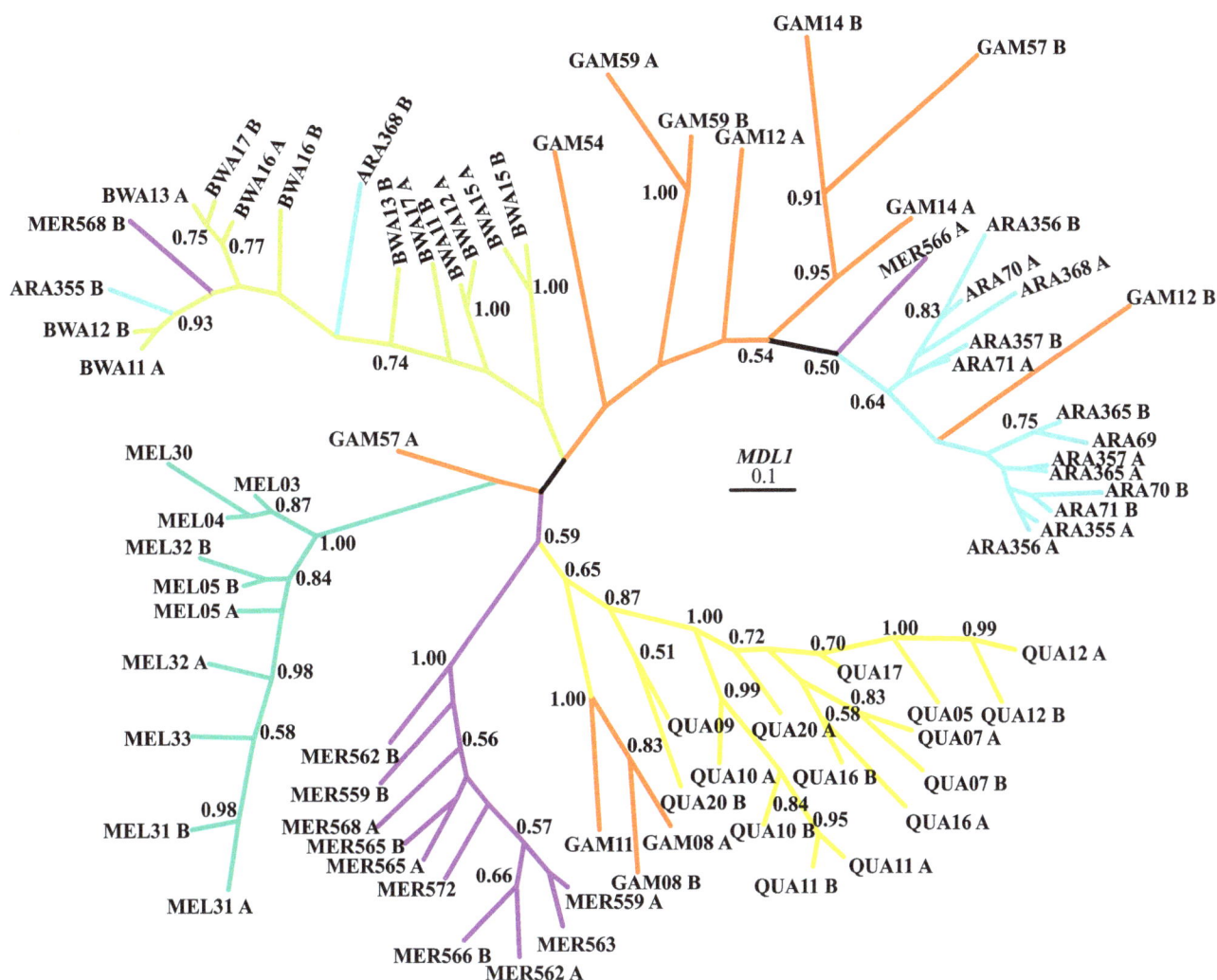

Figure 1. 50% majority-rule consensus Bayesian (unrooted) tree of *MDL1*. Numbers on branches are the posterior probabilities of clades, only values above 0.5 are presented. Species names have been abbreviated as follows: ARA: *An. arabiensis*, BWA: *An. bwambae*, GAM: *An. gambiae*, MEL: *An. melas*, MER: *An. merus*, and KNP905: *An. quadriannulatus*. The number following the species abbreviation refers to the individual specimen code, whereas the letters A and B differentiate between the two alleles of a single individual specimen.

empirical Bayes (NEB) and the Bayes empirical Bayes (BEB) analyses (see Table 3) of PAML. All the sites suggested by the BEB and the NEB analysis as having a dN/dS ratio greater than 1 (probability >0.99) are presented in Table 3. Three of them (78, 202 and 347: Table S3) were consistently identified by all pair wise tests. The dN/dS ratios in these sites were estimated to be well above 1 in all cases, even when considering the standard error of the estimates. Signs of recombination were detected in *CLIPB14* with the GARD module of HyPhy. A single breakpoint was found at position 567 by GARD. Following that, the dataset was partitioned accordingly to take the specific breakpoint into account. At least one of the selection models of the HyPhy analyses, identified sites 78 and 202 as being under positive selection. The estimated dN/dS ratios for these sites by far exceeded those detected by the PAML analysis.

In the *FBN8* gene the maximum likelihood tests of PAML indicated several sites as exhibiting values of dN/dS greater than 1. Two sites were repeatedly identified by the likelihood ratio tests. These sites were 34 and 72 (Table 3, Table S4) and their dN/dS values were greater than 1 in all cases (standard error considered).

A single recombination breakpoint was detected by the GARD module of HyPhy at position 277. After partitioning the dataset to avoid the results being affected by recombination, a single site (64) was found to be exhibiting a dN/dS (normalized) value of 3.43.

Lineage Specific Positive Selection

The branch-site 2 test (PAML) was applied for all the genes with indications of positive selection by any of the preceding tests. In both schemes applied in the branch-site 2 test, and regardless of which species was designated as the foreground branch, the likelihood ratio tests (PAML) were not in favor of positive selection acting on any of the *Anopheles* lineages in any of the genes (results not shown).

PAML Analyses and Recombination

The RDP analysis detected two sequences as the result of recombination in each one of the *CLIPB14* and *FBN8* datasets. Following that, the recombinant sequences were removed from the respective datasets and a new Bayesian tree was inferred for each locus. These trees were used as input trees in a second series of analyses with PAML. The results of these analyses were identical

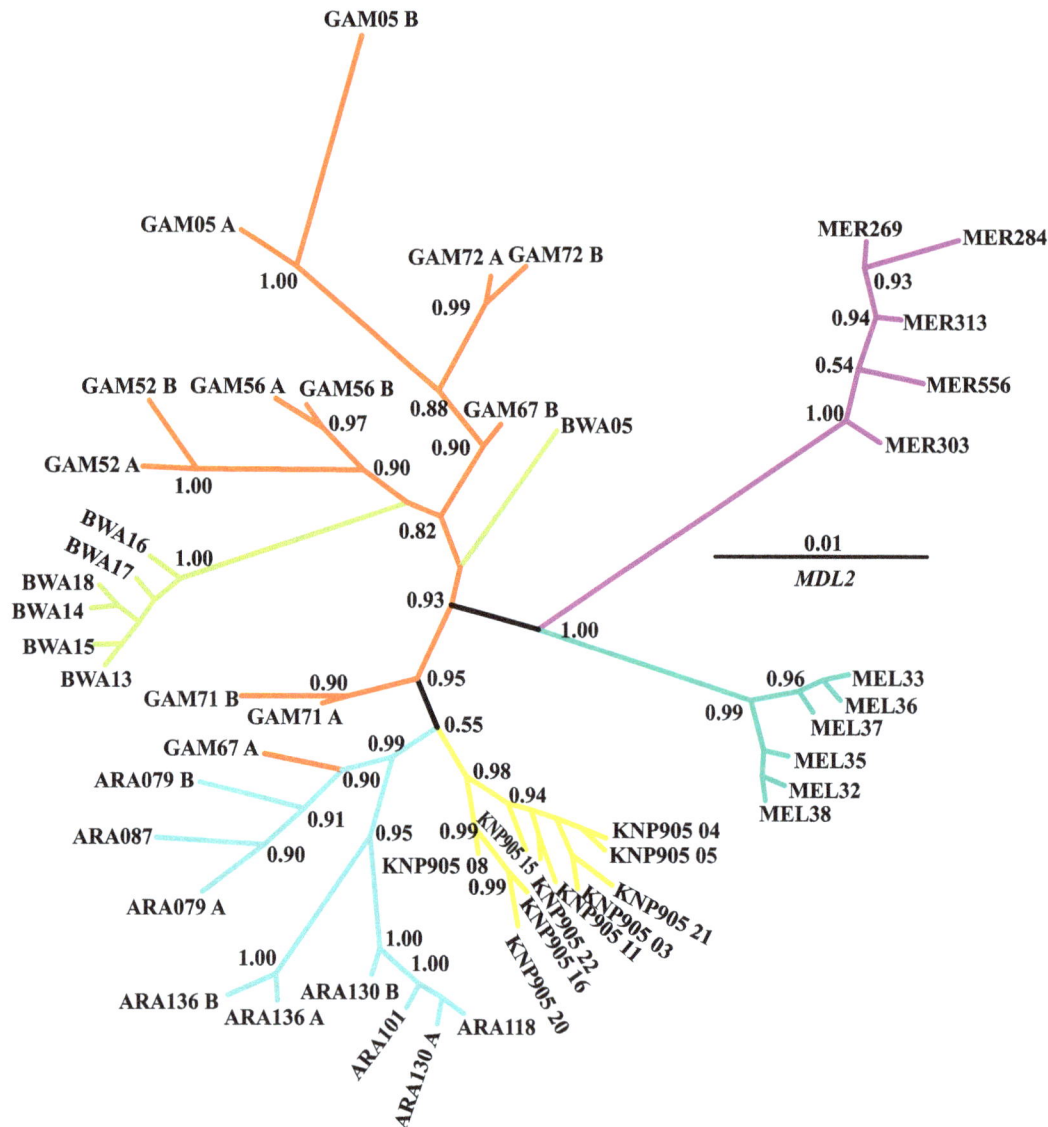

Figure 2. 50% majority-rule consensus Bayesian (unrooted) tree of *MDL2*. Numbers on branches are the posterior probabilities of clades, only values above 0.5 are presented. Species names have been abbreviated as follows: ARA: *An. arabiensis*, BWA: *An. bwambae*, GAM: *An. gambiae*, MEL: *An. melas*, MER: *An. merus*, and KNP905: *An. quadriannulatus*. The number following the species abbreviation refers to the individual specimen code, whereas the letters A and B differentiate between the two alleles of a single individual specimen.

to the initial one, thus neither the phylogenetic trees nor the PAML outputs are presented separately.

Selection Analyses Using the McDonald-Kreitman Test

Regarding the McDonald-Kreitman tests, no positive selection acting on any of the studied loci (Tables S5, S6) was detected.

Discussion

As anticipated the within species diversity is higher in the synonymous sites in all loci. The levels of within species diversity both in the synonymous (PiSyn) and the non-synonymous sites (PiNonSyn) are significantly higher in the *FBN8* locus in all six species (Fig. S1, S2). The other loci exhibit similar levels of within species diversity in the synonymous and the non-synonymous sites. An exception is the level of non-synonymous diversity within *An. arabiensis* in *MDL2*, which matches that of *FBN8* (Table 2, Fig. S1,

S2). The levels of divergence of *MDL1* and *MDL2* between the different species (Dxy) are in the same range, having a mean value of 1.96 and 2.00%, respectively (Table S5). The between species divergence is higher in *CLIPB14* compared to *MDL1* and *MDL2* with a mean value of 2.56%, whereas this value is 4.20% for *FBN8* (Table S6). The levels of divergence recorded both within and between the species for the four studied loci, are comparable to those that have been estimated for other innate immunity genes of *Anopheles* [19,20,22].

In all four loci some alleles were shared between species. This is an indication that introgression and/or retention of ancestral polymorphisms have affected the distribution of the genetic diversity of these immune genes within the *Anopheles gambiae* complex. This is also evident from the fact that in all studied loci, some alleles are more closely related to alleles other than their nominal ones. To evaluate the effect of introgression and/or retention of ancestral polymorphisms, we have estimated F_{ST}

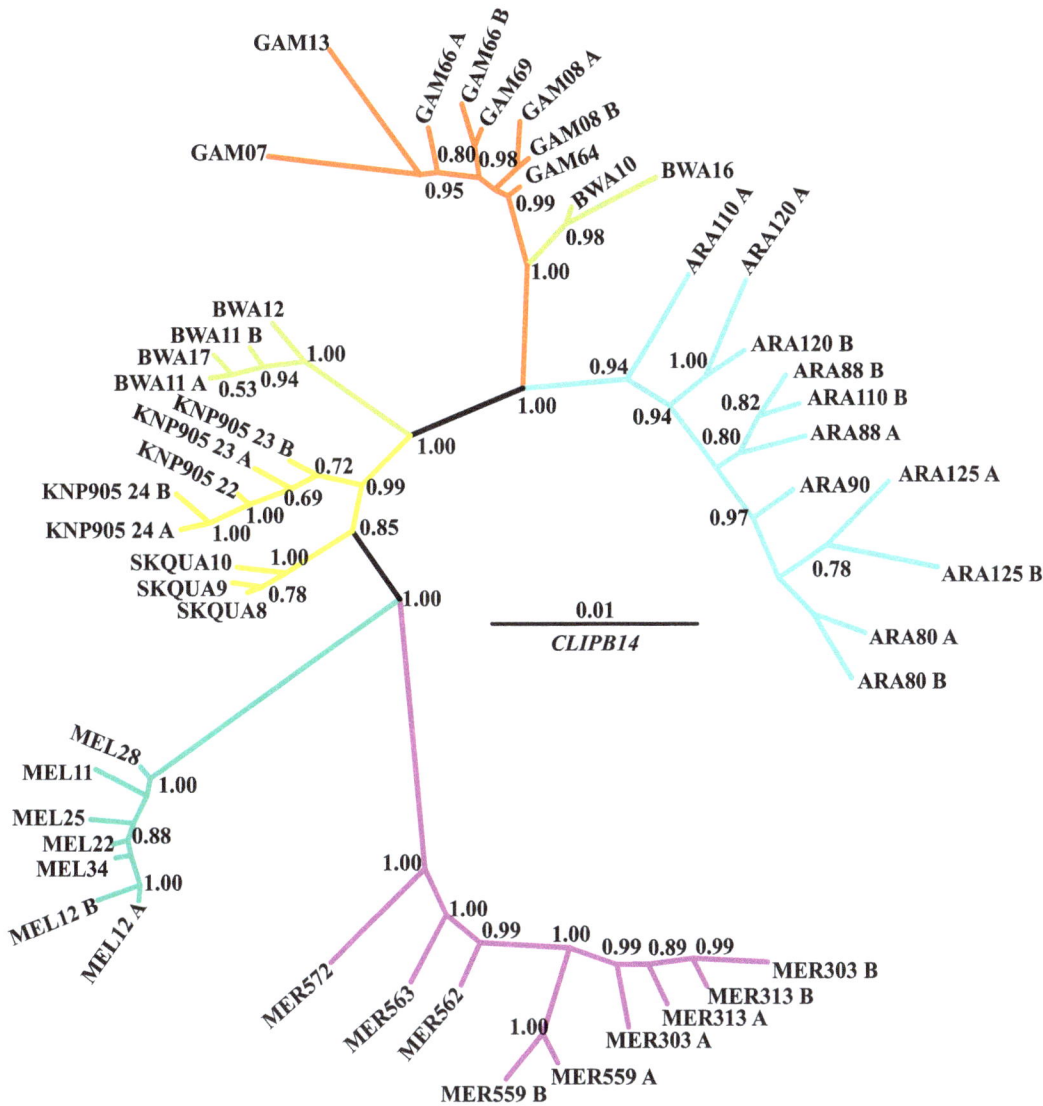

Figure 3. 50% majority-rule consensus Bayesian (unrooted) tree of *CLIPB14*. Numbers on branches are the posterior probabilities of clades, only values above 0.5 are presented. Species names have been abbreviated as follows: ARA: *An. arabiensis*, BWA: *An. bwambae*, GAM: *An. gambiae*, MEL: *An. melas*, MER: *An. merus*, and KNP905/SQUA: *An. quadriannulatus*. The number following the species abbreviation refers to the individual specimen code, whereas the letters A and B differentiate between the two alleles of a single individual specimen.

values between the species of the complex for each locus separately. The F_{ST} values reported herein are within the range reported for other *Anopheles* innate immunity genes [19] and indicative of great genetic differentiation between the species of the complex. It is very important to note at this point that allele sharing between species is restricted to a single allele in *MDL1*, and 5 alleles in *FBN8* out of a total of 185 alleles detected at all four loci. Furthermore, no shared alleles were detected between *An. gambiae s.s.* and *An. arabiensis*. It seems that allele sharing and retention of ancestral polymorphisms is present only at a very low level, at least for the four genes we studied. Therefore, all the species are significantly differentiated (Tables S5, S6) with no or very little indication of gene flow for these four loci (F_{ST} values and Tables S5, S6). This degree of differentiation and isolation minimizes the confounding effects of these processes in the investigation of selection patterns.

In all the studied loci relatively few fixed non-synonymous differences (Tables S5, S6) were found and the McDonald-

Kreitman tests did not detect positive selection acting on any of them. We concur with [18] that this is probably due to the limitations relating to our datasets in conjunction with the inherent properties of the McDonald-Kreitman test.

Regarding *MDL1*, the result of the McDonald-Kreitman test is corroborated by the maximum likelihood tests implemented in the PAML and HyPhy analysis.

Similarly to *MDL1*, *MDL2* was also found to be evolving under purifying selection. This gene has been shown to exhibit significant induction in the midgut tissue upon *P. falciparum* ookinete invasion. However, it did not show specificity to *P. falciparum* infection [3]. At the same time, the maximum likelihood tests of PAML and HyPhy did not detect any branches and/or sites evolving under positive selection.

In *CLIPB14*, both the PAML and the HyPhy analyses suggest that there may be specific sites of the CLIPB14 protein that exhibit a dN/dS ratio greater than 1. Sites 78 and 202, were identified as exhibiting a dN/dS ratio above 1 in both analyses.

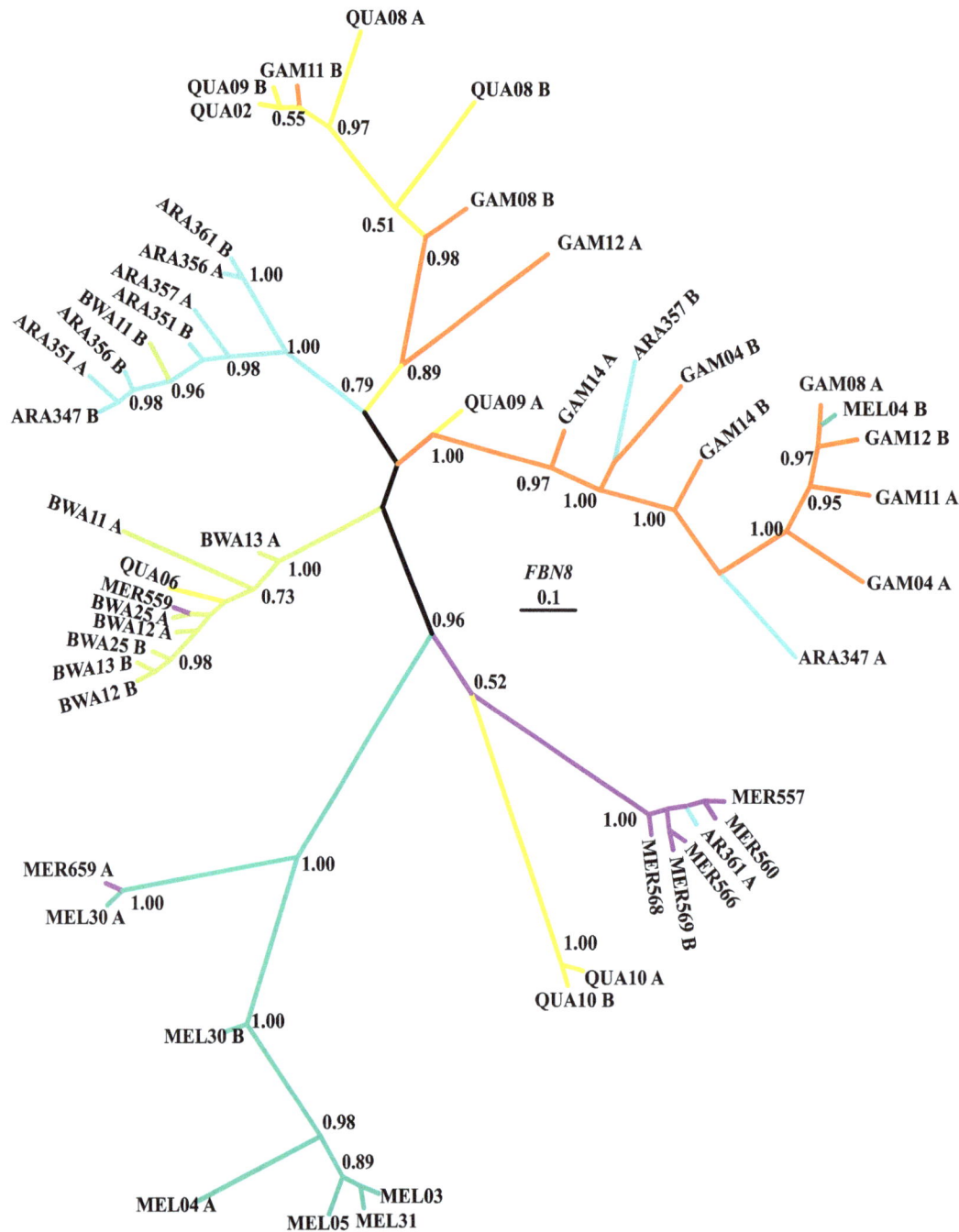

Figure 4. 50% majority-rule consensus Bayesian (unrooted) tree of *FBN8.* Numbers on branches are the posterior probabilities of clades, only values above 0.5 are presented. Species names have been abbreviated as follows: ARA: *An. arabiensis*, BWA: *An. bwambae*, GAM: *An. gambiae*, MEL: *An. melas*, MER: *An. merus*, and QUA: *An. quadriannulatus*. The number following the species abbreviation refers to the individual specimen code, whereas the letters A and B differentiate between the two alleles of a single individual specimen.

In *FBN8* sites 34 and 72 were identified by the BEB method as possibly being under positive selection. However, these sites were not verified by the HyPhy analysis. Site 64, which was identified by the NEB analysis of PAML based on the M3 model (Table 3), was also identified by HyPhy with a dN/dS value of 3.43.

The level of recombination detected in our datasets is below the threshold level suggested by Anisimova *et al.*, (2003), above which recombination may be mistaken for molecular adaptation. Despite this, the PAML analyses for *CLIPB14* and *FBN8*, in which signs of

positive selection were indicated, were re-run after the exclusion of the recombinant sequences. The second series of the PAML analyses, after the exclusion of the recombinant sequences, indicated by the RDP software, verified the results of the initial analyses in both genes. We consider this an analysis scheme that significantly reduces the effect of recombination in the inference of selection patterns acting on the datasets.

From the points just made, we conclude that the data collected and methods of analysis implemented, were adequate to detect

Table 3. Likelihood ratio tests (PAML) in *Anopheles* immunity genes between models that allow positive selection (M3, M2a, M8) and those that do not (M0, M1a, M7) and identification of sites exhibiting dN/dS ratio >1.

	Parameter	M0	M3[b]	M1a	M2a[c]	M7	M8[b]
MDL1	-Ln	-1416.483813	-1408.434119	-1409.626836	-1408.434119	-1411.276475	-1408.462705
	2ΔLn[a]	16.099388		2.385433		5.627539	
	p-value	0.003*		0.303		0.060	
	df	4		2		2	
	[d]Sites exhibiting dN/dS ratio>1	n.a.	72 (A)[e], 139(S)	n.a.	none	n.a.	none
MDL2	-Ln	-989.379352	-978.353695	-978.965428	-978.367537	-979.437982	-978.355848
	2ΔLn[a]	22.051314		1.195782		2.164268	
	p-value	0.000*		0.550		0.339	
	df	4		2		2	
	[d]Sites exhibiting dN/dS ratio>1	n.a.	6 (T)[e]	n.a.	none	n.a.	none
CLIPB14	-Ln	-2401.296114	-2336.814182	-2353.547453	-2338.457621	-2354.454745	-2339.391860
	2ΔLn[a]	128.963864		30.179664		30.125770	
	p-value	0.000*		0.000*		0.000*	
	df	4		2		2	
	[d]Sites exhibiting dN/dS ratio>1	n.a.	4 (C), 10 (K), 46 (V), 52 (Q), 60 (G), **78** (A), 133 (A), **202** (S), 309 (E), 331 (D), 340 (V), 347 (M), 348 (E), 357 (A)	n.a.	**78** (A), **202** (S), 347 (M)	n.a.	4 (C), 60 (G), **78** (A), **202** (S), 347 (M)
FBN8	-Ln	-1958.216880	-1919.582306	-1924.155342	-1919.618536	-1925.833217	-1919.649726
	2ΔLn[a]	77.269148		9.073612		12.366982	
	p-value	0.000*		0.010*		0.002*	
	df	4		2		2	
	[d]Sites exhibiting dN/dS ratio>1	n.a.	34 (L), **64** (V), 72 (T), 82 (D), 93 (Y), 107 (V), 130 (T), 140 (H), 165 (Y)	n.a.	34 (L)	-	34 (L), 72 (T)

*Significant *p-value* at 0.05 significance level; *df*: degrees of freedom.
[a]This quantity is compared to the critical values of a chi-square distribution with the respective degrees of freedom.
[b]Probability>0.95 in the Naive Empirical Bayes (NEB) analyses of PAML. Even though positive selection based on indications of the NEB analysis is questionable, we are reporting the results for within-gene comparative purposes.
[c]Probability>0.99 in the Bayes Empirical Bayes (BEB) analyses of PAML.
[d]Sites refer to amino acid positions of the proteins.
[e]Letters in parentheses refer to the amino acid present at the site.
Sites in bold characters indicate those that were identified by HyPhy as well.

selection for those genes undergoing positive selection. The analyses we used were capable of overcoming problems posed by evolutionary processes such as introgression, ancestral polymorphisms or recombination. It is not surprising, and it is indeed encouraging, that only a minority of the innate immunity genes that have been studied in this way [16,20,22] exhibit signs of positive selection. The "arsenal" of immunity genes is more than 100 [24] known genes and the fact that the approach we used can eliminate several, and yet detect positive signals for a minority of them is to be expected and gives us hope that these are not false positives. That is, the approach followed here has the power to identify negatives and positives between a set of immunity genes that have multiple roles in the defense of *Anopheles* against pathogens. Very strong indications exist for their involvement in the immune response of *Anopheles* against *Plasmodium*, whereas at the same time they are found to be part of an immunity cascade towards bacteria.

Even though specific codons (two in *CLIPB14* and two in *FBN8*), were found to be exhibiting dN/dS ratios greater than one using PAML, we did not detect positive selection acting on specific lineages involving malaria vectors. This may simply reflect the

limitation of the data and the sensitivity of the analytical procedures implemented. Nevertheless, variation at these sites is consistent with an influence on *Plasmodium* infection.

In conclusion, considering only the sites that were consistently identified by all methods applied, two in the *CLIPB14* locus have the most evidence of being adaptively driven. These are sites 78 and 202. Understanding the biological mechanisms underlying this positive selection is beyond the scope of this work. On the other hand, in *FBN8* sites 34 and 72 that were identified by the PAML analyses were not verified by the HyPhy results. Therefore, caution should be exerted regarding this locus and the specific amino acid sites. However, we do believe that these sites could also serve as a starting point for geneticists wishing to genetically manipulate *Anopheles* immunity genes. In most published sequences [25] positively selected sites inferred by the BEB method of PAML were found to be biologically meaningful following a 3D structure study of the proteins. Perhaps a similar approach could be applied to the CLIPB14 and FBN8 proteins and reveal the role of the positively selected sites in the proteins' structures implying function and their possible involvement in the defense against *Plasmodium* and/or other microbes.

Materials and Methods

Mosquitoes Samples

Six species of the *An. gambiae* complex were used: *An. gambiae* sensu stricto, *An. arabiensis*, *An. bwambae*, *An. melas*, *An. merus* and *An. quadriannulatus*. Details on the origin of specimens and DNA extraction methods are provided by [20]. Species names in figures and tables are abbreviated as follows: *An. arabiensis*: ARA, *An.bwambae*: BWA, *An. gambiae*: GAM, *An. melas*: MEL, *An. merus*: MER, *An. quadriannulatus*: QUA/KPN905/SQUA (depending on location of origin).

Analysis of Immunity Genes

A detailed description of the analyzed loci is given in Table 1. Among the analyzed genes are *MDL1* (Ensembl Gene Id: AGAP012352) and *MDL2* (Ensembl Gene Id: AGAP002857). Both genes encode an MD-2-like protein and belong to a 13-member gene family [3]. The expression of both was induced in midgut tissue upon *P. falciparum* ookinete invasion. Furthermore, in RNAi gene silencing assays *MDL1* showed specificity in regulating mosquito resistance in *P. falciparum* but not in *P. berghei*.

CLIPB14, a gene encoding a clip domain serine protease (Ensemble Gene Id: AGAP010833) was also included in the study. This gene is expressed in mosquito hemocytes and is transcriptionally induced by both bacterial and *Plasmodium* challenges [26]. Functional studies applying RNA interference revealed that *CLIPB14* is involved in the elimination of *Plasmodium* ookinetes in *An. gambiae* [26]. Finally, we included a member of the fibrinogen-related protein (FREP) genes, *FBN8* (Ensemble Gene Id: AGAP011223). The fibrinogen-like (FBG) domains in members of this protein family, are predicted to recognize carbohydrates and their derivatives on the surface of microorganisms during the innate immune response [27]. As pointed out by [27], the ability of mosquitoes to recognize parasites in innate immunity and physiologies associated with blood feeding, is probably correlated with the structure of the FBG domains.

Besides the above mentioned reasons for selecting the specific set of immunity genes, we have to note that these loci were also investigated by [3] as well, and scored relatively high regarding their specific involvement in the defense against *Plasmodium*.

Multiple primers were designed for each of the targeted loci based on the *An. gambiae* genome [28]. Primers were manually designed and their characteristics were estimated using FastPCR [29]. This software was also used to investigate potential primer-pair incompatibilities. A nested-PCR protocol was used to amplify *MDL1*, *MDL2* and *CLIPB14*. The sequences of the primers used in the amplification of each locus are shown in Table 1. PCR products were separated electrophoretically on a 1–2% agarose gel, purified using commercially available kits, and were sequenced in both directions in a 3730 ABI capillary sequencer. All individuals that were found to be heterozygous for two or more positions were re-amplified purified and cloned using the TOPO-TA cloning kit for sequencing (Invitrogen). From each individual, a minimum of three transformed colonies were selected, and the size of the DNA insert was determined by PCR using the T3/T7 primer pair of the TOPO-TA vector. In cases where the size of PCR product indicated the presence of the correct insert, this product was sequenced in both directions. To ensure a minimal number of miss-incorporations, Platinum High Fidelity Taq (Invitrogen) was used in all amplifications. Sequence chromatograms were inspected by eye to confirm differences between alleles of the same individual, or within and between species. Sequences were viewed, edited, assembled and aligned using CodonCode Aligner (v.1.6.3 CodonCode Corporation, Dedham, MA, USA).

All sequences were blasted using the BLAST tool of VectorBase (http://www.vectorbase.org/Tools/BLAST) against the *An. gambiae* genome to verify homology to the respective loci. The sequences have been submitted to GenBank under the accession numbers GU432776 to GU432999.

Polymorphism and Divergence

Basic analyses of polymorphism and divergence were performed using the computer program DNAsp [30]. Estimated parameters included the within-species pairwise diversity (Pi) at synonymous and non-synonymous sites, and the average number of nucleotide substitutions per site between species (Dxy). Introgression and/or retention of ancestral polymorphisms have resulted in the sharing of variation between the *An. gambiae* complex members [22,31,32,33] and the calculation of F_{ST} between the members of the complex therefore becomes meaningful [31]. We used DNAsp [30] to calculate F_{ST} values between the six species. F_{ST} values measure the genetic differentiation as a proportion of total diversity that is due to between-group differences. The permutation test (5000 replicates) as implemented in DNAsp, was applied to address the question of whether the observed F_{ST} values are significantly greater than zero.

Detecting Genes Affected by Positive Selection Using PAML

Phylogenies were constructed using both coding and non-coding regions for each of the four genes with MrBayes 3.1 [34], using partitioned or non-partitioned data depending on the dataset. In partitioned datasets a different substitution model was applied to the introns, the first, second, and third codon positions. The substitution models were suggested by Modeltest 3.7 [35] according to the Akaike Information Criterion [36].

These Bayesian trees were used to implement the maximum likelihood methods of the PAML v.4. package [37] aimed at detecting codons that show signs of adaptive evolution. For each locus, datasets were initially analyzed using the M0 (one-ratio) model implemented in the "codeml" program. The M0 model assumes a constant ω value (dN/dS ratio) along all branches in the tree and among all codon sites in the gene [37]. At least two runs of the M0 model were performed on each alignment to check the consistency of the log-likelihood values between the multiple runs. Runs that were not consistent were rerun until the values converged. In the subsequent calculations of the log-likelihood of each tree under the M1a, M2a, M7 and M8 models of PAML, the initial branch lengths were those estimated under the M0 model. Model M1a is a neutral model which divides the codon sites into two categories, one having conserved sites with $\omega_0 = 0$ and the other involving neutral sites with $\omega_1 = 1$. Model M2a allows an additional category of sites with ω_2 estimated from the data, thus accommodating positively selected sites. Models M7 and M8 assume that ω follows a beta distribution with the shape parameters estimated in the interval (0, 1), and M8 includes one additional category to account for positively selected sites [38]. In all these models the rate of synonymous substitutions (dS) is constant among sites, while the rate of non-synonymous substitutions (dN) is variable [39]. According to [37], the site model pairs that appear to be particularly useful for real data analysis, are M1a versus M2a, and M7 versus M8. The significance of positive selection was calculated by comparing twice the log likelihood difference in a chi-square test with two degrees of freedom.

The branch-site 2 test [40,41] as implemented in PAML was used to test for positive selection along specific branches. We tested each of the *Anopheles* clades on the species phylogeny, treating each in turn as the foreground clade. The alternative branch-site model has four codon site categories; two for sites evolving under purifying and neutral selection along branches, and two for sites under positive selection along the foreground branch. The null model restricts sites on the foreground lineage to evolve neutrally. Each branch-site model was run multiple times to ensure convergence of log-likelihood values. The significance of positive selection was calculated by comparing twice the log-likelihood difference in a chi-square test with 1 degree of freedom. Since some species appeared as non-monophyletic in the phylogenetic analyses, two different running schemes were implemented for the branch-site 2 test. In the first scheme all alleles, even those of a different species (non-species alleles), that clustered within a specific *Anopheles* species clade were assigned to the foreground branch. In the second scheme, the non-species alleles were not assigned to the foreground branch.

In PAML the NEB method [25,39] and the BEB method [42] are used to identify sites under positive selection. BEB is implemented under models M2a and M8 only. As suggested in the PAML manual only the results of the BEB method should be considered robust in the identification of sites under selection.

Implementing HyPhy in the Detection of Positive Selection and GARD to Screen for Recombination

To verify whether the codon sites inferred by PAML to be under positive selection are identified by other methods as well, the program HyPhy [43] was implemented using Datamonkey [44], the Web interface of HyPhy. Similarly to PAML, the likelihood methods in HyPhy are based on a codon substitution model [45]. Three different codon-based maximum likelihood methods, SLAC, FEL and REL, can be used to estimate the dN/dS (ω) ratio at every codon in the alignment. A detailed discussion of each approach can be found in Pond & Frost [46].

In HyPhy all methods can take recombination into account, provided that prior to the selection analysis a screening of the sequences for recombination breakpoints is performed. This is done by using the GARD module [47]. In the case that recombination breakpoints have been detected the dataset is partitioned and each partition is allowed to have its own phylogenetic tree. Following that, the selection analysis is performed separately on each tree. The HyPhy approach allowed us to investigate whether the presence of recombination in the datasets was producing false positives in the PAML analyses. In contrast to codeml models, HypHy also estimates the rate of synonymous substitutions (dS) at each codon site, thus taking into account potential synonymous rate variation among sites [48]. Furthermore, the PARRIS method [49] of HyPhy, that extends traditional codon-based likelihood ratio tests to detect if a proportion of sites in the alignment evolve with dN/dS>1, was also applied to the datasets. The PARRIS method also takes recombination and synonymous rate variation into account.

The starting tree of each locus that served as the basis for the HyPhy analyses was inferred by the program itself.

McDonald-Kreitman Test and Positive Selection

A different approach to detect signs of selection involved the McDonald-Kreitman test [50]. This test was applied to our datasets using DNAsp [30]. The McDonald-Kreitman test compares the ratios of fixed to polymorphic substitutions of non-synonymous and synonymous substitutions between species. Under neutrality, the fixation rate of synonymous and non-synonymous substitutions is expected to be equal, but positive selection would increase the rate of fixation in non-synonymous sites. In contrast to the phylogeny-based tests mentioned above,

the McDonald-Kreitman test allows the detection of selection on a whole protein, is bound to be quite conservative in detecting selection [51] and lacks the power of a site by site analysis.

Addressing the Recombination Issue

As already mentioned, within-population recombination can have a confounding effect in the inference of adaptive evolution [52,53]. Patterns of genetic variability created by recombination can closely resemble the effects of molecular adaptation (e.g. [54]). Current codon models of heterogeneous dN/dS ratios among sites assume no recombination, raising concerns about the possibility that the likelihood ratio tests (LRTs) can mistakenly interpret the effects of recombination as evidence for positive selection. However, as [53] have shown using simulated data, when the recombination events are maintained at a low level (fewer than three recombination events in the history of a sample of ten sequences) the positive selection inferring tests, including the LRT, are quite robust. Furthermore, according to the same authors identification of sites under positive selection by the BEB method [42] appears to be less affected than the LRT by recombination.

In this study, two different approaches were applied to account for the effects of recombination. In the first approach the datasets were analyzed (see section above) using the Web interface of HyPhy, namely Datamonkey [44] and applying the GARD algorithm [47]. In the second approach, the datasets were scanned for recombination using the software RDP [55] and implementing all seven tests included in the package. The settings of the scans in RDP were adjusted according to the software's manual (http://darwin.uvigo.es/rdp/rdp.html). Only the statistically significant recombination events detected by any of the tests of RDP, were considered in the consecutive phylogeny-based analyses.

Supporting Information

Table S1 MDL1 protein alignment

Table S2 MDL2 protein alignment

Table S3 CLIPB14 protein alignment

Table S4 FBN8 protein alignmnent

Table S5 MacDonald-Kreitman tests on MDL1 and MDL2 and between species divergence (Dxy)

Table S6 MacDonald-Kreitman tests on CLIPB14 and FBN8 and between species divergence (Dxy)

Figure S1 Within species diversity (coding sequence) in synonymous sites (PiSyn) in each locus

Figure S2 Within species diversity (coding sequence) in non-synonymous sites (PiNonSyn) in each locus

Acknowledgments

We are very grateful to Drs. Anton Cornel, Ralph Harbach and David O'Brochta for providing *Anopheles* specimens. We also wish to express our gratitude to Dr. George Dimopoulos for suggestions on issues relating to the choice of immune genes to be studied. We wish to express our appreciation to three anonymous reviewers that provided comments that greatly improved the manuscript. Furthermore, we would like to thank Dr Sergei L. Kosakovsky Pond that granted us permission to analyze a sequence dataset that exceeded the custom size accepted by the Datamonkey server.

References

1. Capurro MD, Coleman J, Beerntsen BT, Myles KM, Olson KE, et al. (2000) Virus-expressed, recombinant single-chain antibody blocks sporozoite infection of salivary glands in *Plasmodium gallinaceum*-infected *Aedes aegypti*. American Journal of Tropical Medicine and Hygiene 62: 427–433.

2. Riehle MM, Markianos K, Niare O, Xu JN, Li J, et al. (2006) Natural malaria infection in *Anopheles gambiae* is regulated by a single genomic control region. Science 312: 577–579.

3. Dong YM, Aguilar R, Xi ZY, Warr E, Mongin E, et al. (2006) *Anopheles gambiae* immune responses to human and rodent *Plasmodium* parasite species. PLoS Pathogens 2: 513–525.

4. Dong YM, Taylor HE, Dimopoulos G (2006) AgDscam, a hypervariable immunoglobulin domain-containing receptor of the *Anopheles gambiae* innate immune system. PLoS Biology 4: 1137–1146.

5. Waterhouse RM, Kriventseva EV, Meister S, Xi Z, Alvarez KS, et al. (2007) Evolutionary dynamics of immune-related genes and pathways in disease-vector mosquitoes. Science 316: 1738–1743.

6. Collins FH, Sakai RK, Vernick KD, Paskewitz S, Seeley DC, et al. (1986) Genetic selection of a *Plasmodium*-Refractory strain of the malaria Vector *Anopheles gambiae*. Science 234: 607–610.

7. Vernick KD, Collins FH (1989) Association of a *Plasmodium*-refractory phenotype with an esterase locus in *Anopheles-gambiae*. American Journal of Tropical Medicine and Hygiene 40: 593–597.

8. Vernick KD, Collins FH, Gwadz RW (1989) A general system of resistance to malaria infection in *Anopheles gambiae* controlled by 2 main genetic loci. American Journal of Tropical Medicine and Hygiene 40: 585–592.

9. Zheng LB, Cornel AJ, Wang R, Erfle H, Voss H, et al. (1997) Quantitative trait loci for refractoriness of *Anopheles gambiae* to *Plasmodium cynomolgi* B. Science 276: 425–428.

10. Zheng LB, Wang S, Romans P, Zhao HY, Luna C, et al. (2003) Quantitative trait loci in *Anopheles gambiae* controlling the encapsulation response against *Plasmodium cynomolgi* Ceylon. BMC Genetics 4: 16.

11. Feldmann AM, Ponnudurai T (1989) Selection of *Anopheles stephensi* for refractoriness and susceptibility to *Plasmodium falciparum*. Medical and Veterinary Entomology 3: 41–52.

12. Feldmann AM, Ponnudurai T, Meuwissen JHET (1986) The selection of *Anopheles stephensi* for refractoriness and susceptibility to *Plasmodium falciparum*. Tropical and Geographical Medicine 38: 317–318.

13. Tahar R, Boudin C, Thiery I, Bourgouin C (2002) Immune response of *Anopheles gambiae* to the early sporogonic stages of the human malaria parasite *Plasmodium falciparum*. EMBO Journal 21: 6673–6680.

14. Cohuet A, Osta MA, Morlais I, Awono-Ambene PH, Michel K, et al. (2006) *Anopheles* and *Plasmodium*: from laboratory models to natural systems in the field. EMBO Reports 7: 1285–1289.

15. Cohuet A, Krishnakumar S, Simard F, Morlais I, Koutsos A, et al. (2008) SNP discovery and molecular evolution in *Anopheles gambiae*, with special emphasis on innate immune system. BMC Genomics 9: 227.

16. Lehmann T, Hume JCC, Licht M, Burns CS, Wollenberg K, et al. (2009) Molecular evolution of immune genes in the malaria mosquito *Anopheles gambiae*. PLoS ONE 4: e4549.

17. Obbard D, Callister D, Jiggins F, Soares D, Yan G, et al. (2008) The evolution of TEP1, an exceptionally polymorphic immunity gene in *Anopheles gambiae*. BMC Evolutionary Biology 8: 274.

18. Obbard D, Welch J, Little T (2009) Inferring selection in the *Anopheles gambiae* species complex: an example from immune-related serine protease inhibitors. Malaria Journal 8: 117.

19. Obbard DJ, Linton YM, Jiggins FM, Yan G, Little TJ (2007) Population genetics of Plasmodium resistance genes in *Anopheles gambiae*: no evidence for strong selection. Molecular Ecology 16: 3497–3510.

20. Parmakelis A, Slotman M, Marshall J, Awono-Ambene P, Antonio-Nkondjio C, et al. (2008) The molecular evolution of four anti-malarial immune genes in the *Anopheles gambiae* species complex. BMC Evolutionary Biology 8: 79.

21. Simard F, Licht M, Besansky NJ, Lehmann T (2007) Polymorphism at the defensin gene in the *Anopheles gambiae* complex: testing different selection hypotheses. Infection Genetics and Evolution 7: 285–292.

22. Slotman M, Parmakelis A, Marshall J, Awono-Ambene P, Antonio-Nkondjo C, et al. (2007) Patterns of selection in anti-malarial immune genes in malaria vectors: evidence for adaptive evolution in LRIM1 in *Anopheles arabiensis*. PLoS One 2: e793.

23. Besansky NJ (2008) White Paper: Genome analysis of vectorial capacity in major *Anopheles* vectors of malaria parasites. NIH, National Human Genome Research Institute.

24. Christophides GK, Vlachou D, Kafatos FC (2004) Comparative and functional genomics of the innate immune system in the malaria vector *Anopheles gambiae*. Immunological Reviews 198: 127–148.

25. Yang ZH, Swanson WJ, Vacquier VD (2000) Maximum-likelihood analysis of molecular adaptation in abalone sperm lysin reveals variable selective pressures among lineages and sites. Molecular Biology and Evolution 17: 1446–1455.

26. Volz J, Osta MA, Kafatos FC, Muller HM (2005) The roles of two clip domain serine proteases in innate immune responses of the malaria vector *Anopheles gambiae*. Journal of Biological Chemistry 280: 40161–40168.

27. Wang X, Zhao Q, Christensen B (2005) Identification and characterization of the fibrinogen-like domain of fibrinogen-related proteins in the mosquito, *Anopheles gambiae*, and the fruitfly, *Drosophila melanogaster*, genomes. BMC Genomics 6: 114.

28. Holt RA, Subramanian GM, Halpern A, Sutton GG, Charlab R, et al. (2002) The genome sequence of the malaria mosquito *Anopheles gambiae*. Science 298: 129–149.

29. Kalendar R (2007) FastPCR: a PCR primer and probe design and repeat sequence searching software with additional tools for the manipulation and analysis of DNA and protein. Helsinki, Finland.

30. Librado P, Rozas J (2009) DnaSP v5: a software for comprehensive analysis of DNA polymorphism data. Bioinformatics 25: 1451–1452.

31. Besansky NJ, Krzywinski J, Lehmann T, Simard F, Kern M, et al. (2003) Semipermeable species boundaries between *Anopheles gambiae* and *Anopheles arabiensis*: Evidence from multilocus DNA sequence variation. Proceedings of the National Academy of Sciences of the United States of America 100: 10818–10823.

32. Donnelly MJ, Pinto J, Girod R, Besansky NJ, Lehmann T (2004) Revisiting the role of introgression vs shared ancestral polymorphisms as key processes shaping genetic diversity in the recently separated sibling species of the *Anopheles gambiae* complex. Heredity 92: 61–68.

33. Parmakelis A, Russello MA, Caccone A, Marcondes CB, Costa J, et al. (2008) Historical Analysis of a Near Disaster: *Anopheles gambiae* in Brazil. American Journal of Tropical Medicine and Hygiene 78: 176–178.

34. Ronquist F, Huelsenbeck JP (2003) MrBayes 3: Bayesian phylogenetic inference under mixed models. Bioinformatics 19: 1572–1574.

35. Posada D, Crandall KA (1998) MODELTEST: testing the model of DNA substitution. Bioinformatics 14: 817–818.

36. Akaike H (1974) New look at statistical-model identification. IEEE Transactions on Automatic Control Ac19: 716–723.

37. Yang ZH (2007) PAML 4: Phylogenetic analysis by maximum likelihood. Molecular Biology and Evolution 24: 1586–1591.

38. Yang ZH, Nielsen R, Goldman N, Pedersen AMK (2000) Codon-substitution models for heterogeneous selection pressure at amino acid sites. Genetics 155: 431–449.

39. Nielsen R, Yang ZH (1998) Likelihood models for detecting positively selected amino acid sites and applications to the HIV-1 envelope gene. Genetics 148: 929–936.

40. Yang ZH, Nielsen R (2002) Codon-substitution models for detecting molecular adaptation at individual sites along specific lineages. Molecular Biology and Evolution 19: 908–917.

41. Zhang JZ, Nielsen R, Yang ZH (2005) Evaluation of an improved branch-site likelihood method for detecting positive selection at the molecular level. Molecular Biology and Evolution 22: 2472–2479.

42. Yang ZH, Wong WSW, Nielsen R (2005) Bayes empirical Bayes inference of amino acid sites under positive selection. Molecular Biology and Evolution 22: 1107–1118.

43. Pond SLK, Frost SDW, Muse SV (2005) HyPhy: hypothesis testing using phylogenies. Bioinformatics 21: 676–679.

44. Pond SLK, Frost SDW (2005) Datamonkey: rapid detection of selective pressure on individual sites of codon alignments. Bioinformatics 21: 2531–2533.

45. Muse SV, Gaut BS (1994) A Likelihood Approach for Comparing Synonymous and Nonsynonymous Nucleotide Substitution Rates, with Application to the Chloroplast Genome. Molecular Biology and Evolution 11: 715–724.

46. Pond SLK, Frost SDW (2005) Not so different after all: a comparison of methods for detecting amino acid sites under selection. Molecular Biology and Evolution 22: 1208–1222.

Author Contributions

Conceived and designed the experiments: AP AC JRP. Performed the experiments: AP MM NP. Analyzed the data: AP. Contributed reagents/materials/analysis tools: CL MAS JCM PHAA CAN FS. Wrote the paper: AP. Co-ordinated the project and helped draft the manuscript: AC, JRP.

47. Pond SLK, Posada D, Gravenor MB, Woelk CH, Frost SDW (2006) Automated phylogenetic detection of recombination using a genetic algorithm. Molecular Biology and Evolution 23: 1891–1901.

48. Pond SK, Muse SV (2005) Site-to-site variation of synonymous substitution rates. Molecular Biology and Evolution 22: 2375–2385.

49. Scheffler K, Martin DP, Seoighe C (2006) Robust inference of positive selection from recombining coding sequences. Bioinformatics 22: 2493–2499.

50. McDonald JH, Kreitman M (1991) Adaptive protein evolution at the adh locus in *Drosophila*. Nature 351: 652–654.

51. Nielsen R (2001) Statistical tests of selective neutrality in the age of genomics. Heredity 86: 641–647.

52. McVean G, Spencer CCA (2006) Scanning the human genome for signals of selection. Current Opinion in Genetics & Development 16: 624–629.

53. Anisimova M, Nielsen R, Yang ZH (2003) Effect of recombination on the accuracy of the likelihood method for detecting positive selection at amino acid sites. Genetics 164: 1229–1236.

54. McVean GAT (2001) What do patterns of genetic variability reveal about mitochondrial recombination? Heredity 87: 613–620.

55. Martin DP, Williamson C, Posada D (2005) RDP2: recombination detection and analysis from sequence alignments. Bioinformatics 21: 260–262.

12

Incidence of Treatment-Limiting Toxicity with Stavudine-Based Antiretroviral Therapy in Cambodia

Vichet Phan[1]*, **Sopheak Thai**[1], **Kimcheng Choun**[1], **Lutgarde Lynen**[2], **Johan van Griensven**[1,2]

1 Sihanouk Hospital Center of HOPE, Phnom Penh, Cambodia, **2** Institute of Tropical Medicine, Antwerp, Belgium

Abstract

Background: Although stavudine (D4T) remains frequently used in low-income countries in Asia, associated long-term toxicity data are scarce. The aim of this study was to determine the long-term incidence of severe D4T-toxicity (requiring drug substitution) and associated risk factors in HIV-infected Cambodians up to six years on antiretroviral treatment (ART).

Methodology/Principal Findings: This is a retrospective analysis of an observational cohort, using data from an ART program with systematic monitoring for D4T-toxicity. Probabilities of time to D4T substitution due to suspected D4T toxicity (treatment-limiting D4T toxicity) were calculated, a risk factor analysis was performed using multivariate Cox regression modelling. Out of 2581 adults initiating a D4T-containing regimen, D4T was replaced in 276 (10.7%) patients for neuropathy, 14 (0.5%) for lactic acidosis and 957 (37.1%) for lipoatrophy. The main early side effect was peripheral neuropathy (7.0% by 1 year). After the first year, lipoatrophy became predominant, with a cumulative incidence of 56.1% and 72.4% by 3 and 6 years respectively. Older age (aHR 1.8; 95%CI: 1.4–2.3) and lower baseline haemoglobin (aHR 1.7; 95%CI: 1.4–2.2) were associated with the occurrence of neuropathy. Being female (aHR 3.8; 95%CI: 1.1–12.5), a higher baseline BMI (aHR 12.6; 95%CI: 3.7–43.1), and TB treatment at ART initiation (aHR 8.6; 95%CI: 2.7–27.5) increased the likelihood of lactic acidosis. Lipoatrophy was positively associated with female gender (aHR 2.3; 95%CI: 2.0–2.6), an older age (aHR 1.3; 95%CI: 1.1–1.4), and a CD4 count <200 cells/µL (aHR 1.3; 95%CI: 1.1–1.5).

Conclusions: Stavudine-based treatment regimens in low-income countries are associated with significant long-term toxicities, predominantly lipoatrophy. Close clinical monitoring for toxicity with timely D4T substitution is recommended. Phasing-out of stavudine should be implemented, as costs allows.

Editor: Gary Maartens, University of Cape Town, South Africa

Funding: The HIV program was supported by the Belgian Directorate General of Development Cooperation through the framework agreement with the Institute of Tropical Medicine, Antwerp, the Global Fund to fight AIDS, Tuberculosis and Malaria, and Hope World Wide. JvG is supported by the InBev-Baillet Latour Fund. The funders had no role in study design, data collection and analysis, decision to publish, or preparation of the manuscript.

Competing Interests: The authors have declared that no competing interests exist.

* E-mail: phanvichet@yahoo.com

Introduction

HIV is one of the major health problems in low and middle income countries (LMIC), with over 30 million of people infected. Over the last several years, a successful scaling-up of antiretroviral treatment (ART) has occurred, with currently over five million individuals on treatment. Of these, around 14% live in Asia [1]. The availability of a cheap, generic fixed-dose combination (FDC) has been a key issue in achieving this [2]. In line with WHO recommendations at the start of the ART role-out, almost all national programs have implemented first line treatment consisting of a FDC containing stavudine (D4T), lamivudine and nevirapine [3].

Given increasing reports of D4T-related toxicity, including neuropathy, lactic acidosis and lipoatrophy, WHO 2006 guidelines have recommended to use alternative drugs in stead of D4T [4]. Besides the adoption of an alternative first line regimen for those initiating ART, phasing-out of D4T would additionally require the replacement of D4T for the millions of patients currently using this drug. The recommendation to phase-out D4T was reinforced in the 2010 guidelines [5]. However, recent data demonstrate that the vast majority of individuals in LMIC still take D4T-containing regimens [1]. For a number of reasons, including cost and the operational challenges of the complete phasing-out of D4T, frequent use of D4T-containing regimens will most likely remain the reality on the field for the next years to come. In Cambodia, for instance, the use of D4T-based first line treatment continues up to this day.

Despite the ongoing use of D4T, its recognized potential of toxicity and the maturing of many ART programs [6–9], only scarce data on the incidence and timing of its long-term toxicity beyond the first few years on ART are available, particularly from Asian countries. Moreover, studies exploring risk factors of D4T-related toxicity in this region are surprisingly limited. Consequently, it remains unclear which groups might benefit most from any targeted intervention or should be prioritized for phasing-out of D4T. Given the paucity of available data in South-East Asia, including Cambodia, the aim of this study was to determine the long-term incidence of severe D4T-toxicity and associated risk factors in HIV-infected Cambodians. Using data from an ART cohort with systematic monitoring for D4T-toxicity performed from the program-onset in 2003, we provide data on the long-term toxicity associated with D4T by up to six years of treatment.

Methods

Study design and study population

We conducted a retrospective cohort study between March 2003 and December 2010 at the Sihanouk-Hospital-Center-of-Hope (SHCH) in Phnom Penh, Cambodia. Since March 2003, this tertiary care hospital provides comprehensive HIV care at no cost, as part of the national ART program. All adult, ART-naive HIV-infected patients having initiating D4T-based ART at SHCH were included.

Antiretroviral treatment initiation and monitoring

Treatment initiation on ART was according to WHO recommendations: all patients with WHO stage IV, WHO stage III with CD4 cell count <350 cells/μL or with CD4 cell count <200 cells/μL were eligible for ART. First line treatment consisted of a generic FDC containing D4T, lamivudine and nevirapine. Zidovudine or efavirenz was prescribed in case of contraindications to D4T or nevirapine. From 2006 on, D4T was prescribed as 30 mg bid, irrespective of body weight. Prior to that, dosing was done according to body weight with a higher dose (40 mg bid) for individuals with a body weight above 60 kg [4].

Before ART initiation, extensive patient counselling was done, including on the occurrence of toxicities. Patients were seen at monthly visits during the first six months after ART initiation. Subsequently, visits were scheduled less frequently (every 2–3 months) for clinically stable patients. All medical care was provided by physicians, supported by a team of nurses and adherence counsellors. At every clinical encounter, key issues were systematically addressed, including the clinical evolution, evaluation of treatment response and ART-related toxicity. Adherence was evaluated by pill counts at every visit, and using the visual analogue scale (VAS) every six months. Baseline laboratory testing included haematology, liver function tests, hepatitis B/C serology and CD4 cell count determination (FACSCount (Becton Dickinson). After ART initiation, a full blood count and CD4 cell count was done every six months. During the first months of ART, liver function tests were performed more regularly. In case of suspicion of treatment failure, a viral load test was done. Clinical and immunological criteria were used to guide indications for viral load testing. Cotrimoxazole prophylactic treatment was given for all WHO stage II/III/IV patients and all those with a CD4 count <200 cells/μL. All patients with WHO stage 4 disease or a CD4 count <100 cells/μL were started on fluconazole primary prophylaxis. Patients not presenting at their scheduled visit were contacted by phone. Those living in the neighbourhood of the hospital were visited at home. Patients not presenting at the hospital for a period of 6 months without additional information were defined lost to follow-up (LTFU). Additional program details and outcome data of the antiretroviral treatment program in SHCH have been published before [10,11].

Outcome measures

All patients on D4T-containing regimens were routinely screened for associated toxicity using a standardized approach. At every clinic visit, patients were assessed for symptoms suggestive of symptomatic hyperlactatemia or lactic acidosis. Lactate level was measured for suspected cases only. Since no pH determination could be done, cases of symptomatic hyperlactatemia (SH) and lactic acidosis (LA) could not be differentiated and were grouped together as SH/LA. A case of SH/LA was defined as a patient on ART, presenting with compatible symptoms with other mimicking conditions ruled out, and a lactate level $\geq$2.5 mmol/L (capillary blood, Accutrend Lactate). D4T was systematically replaced for these patients. Up to 2005, no lactic acid levels could be measured and diagnosis was clinical. Neuropathy was assessed clinically by the HIV physician, D4T was substituted in case of WHO grade III/IV severity. Patients were assessed for lipoatrophy (loss of subcutaneous fat in the face, arms, legs, cheeks, buttocks) at every encounter by self-report and clinical assessment. Decisions to substitute D4T were guided by the clinical severity of lipoatrophy combined with the patient's preference and perception of the body changes. Consequently, stavudine was essentially replaced for reasons of lipoatrophy if 1) clinically severe or 2) patients perceived this as severe and disturbing, even though clinically it was defined as less pronounced.

Data collection and statistical analysis

Clinical and laboratory data were prospectively collected on a daily basis, using standardized data collection tools and stored in a database. Quality control of the stored data was done at regular intervals.

The primary outcome was time to D4T substitution due to suspected D4T toxicity. We will refer to this in the text as treatment-limiting (or severe) D4T toxicity. The cumulative incidence of D4T substitution due to suspected toxicity was calculated using the Kaplan Meier methodology. Patients were censored at the date of D4T substitution, at the last visit for patients that died, were transferred out or were lost to follow-up, and at December 31, 2010 for the remainder. Patients switched to non-D4T containing second line regimens due to virological failure were censored at the date of switching and defined as having experienced no D4T-related toxicity event. A risk factor analysis was performed using multivariate Cox regression. Collinearity between variables was assessed. We used a backward selection method, retaining those variables with P-values<0.05 in the final model. Data analysis was done using STATA version 11. The level of significance was set at P<0.05.

Ethical issues

Since the launch of the HIV care program, clinical data have been routinely collected for purposes of program monitoring and evaluation, and research activities. Patients were requested to give written informed consent to store and use the data. No linkage of these data with other sources was done. The data collection and informed consent procedure were approved by the Institutional Review Board ITM (Institute of Tropical Medicine, Antwerp) and the Institutional Review Board SHCH (Sihanouk Hospital Center of HOPE). No patient identifiers were included in the dataset used for this analysis.

Results

Characteristics of the study population

By December 2010, 2581 adult patients on D4T-containing regimen were included in analysis, with a median follow-up time of 1.3 years. Of these, 1341 (52%) were female, the median age at the start of treatment was 35 years. Eighty percent were in WHO stage III/IV at treatment initiation. The median baseline CD4 count was 87 cells/μL. The most frequent ART regimen was D4T/lamivudine/nevirapine, with 72% of patients initiating this regimen. In total, 686 (27%) of the patients were on TB treatment at ART initiation (Table 1).

Incidence and timing of D4T-related toxicity

Out of 2581 adult patients initiating a D4T-containing regimen, D4T was replaced in 276 (10.7%) patients for suspected D4T-related neuropathy, 14 (0.5%) for SH/LA and 957 (37.1%) for lipodystrophy. All reported cases of SH/LH were confirmed by lactic acid determination. The main early side effect was peripheral neuropathy (7.0% by 1 year), with a cumulative incidence of 16.6% and 19.0% by 3 and 6 years respectively. SH/LA was mainly seen after the first six months but remained rare overall, with a cumulative incidence of 1% by 6 years. After the first year, lipoatrophy became the predominant side effect, with a cumulative incidence of 56.1% and 72.4% by 3 and 6 years respectively (Table 2; Figure 1).

Risk factors for D4T-related toxicity

In univariate analysis, older age (>40 years), low baseline body mass index (BMI) (<18.5 kg/m²), and low baseline haemoglobin (<10 g/dL) were associated with increased risk of D4T-associated neuropathy (Table 3). Higher baseline BMI (>25 kg/m²), use of efavirenz and being on TB treatment at ART initiation were associated with increased risk of SH/LA. Lipoatrophy was positively associated with older age and female sex. An increased risk was observed with low baseline CD4 cell count (<200 cells/μL) and low baseline haemoglobin. In multivariate analysis, neuropathy remained associated with older age and low baseline haemoglobin. Being female, overweight (BMI>25 kg/m²), and on TB treatment at ART initiation increased the likelihood of SH/LA. Lipoatrophy was positively associated with female gender and

Table 2. Incidence of severe toxicity related to stavudine (N = 2581).

Stavudine-related toxicity	Events (%)	Rate/1000 py	Cumulative incidence (%) – Kaplan-Meier estimates[a]			
			6 m	12 m	36 m	60 m
Neuropathy	276 (10.7)	63.8	2.1	7.0	16.6	19.0
Lactic acidosis	14 (0.5)	3.2	0.1	0.6	0.7	1.0
Lipoatrophy	957 (37.1)	221.1	0.8	7.0	56.1	72.4

[a]Kaplan-Meier estimates: time to first severe toxicity (ie requiring treatment change) at specified months on ART; py:: patient years.

older age. A reduced risk was seen for patients initiating ART with a baseline CD4 count >200 cells/μL (Table 3).

Discussion

This paper is the first to provide estimates of long-term toxicity related to D4T up to six years after treatment initiation from LMICs. By six years on D4T, lipoatrophy was the predominant side-effect, requiring treatment substitution in seven out of ten patients. For each of the different D4T-toxicities, distinct risk factors were identified, indicating which patients might require more close toxicity-monitoring, should avoid D4T altogether or should be prioritized for phasing-out of D4T.

Our findings of older age and female sex as risk factors for lipoatrophy are consistent with other reports from LMIC [12,13]. Regarding baseline CD4 cell count, conflicting data have been reported [12,13]. Our data confirm the reported association of older age and neuropathy [12,14,15]. Whereas most previous studies have reported advanced HIV stage as a risk factor for neuropathy, we observed an increased risk associated with low baseline haemoglobin. Possibly, this is merely a reflection of advanced disease at ART initiation [10,13]. Alternatively, recent studies have observed the strong and independent prognostic information contained in both baseline and time-updated haemoglobin levels, even after adjustment for CD4 cell count

Table 1. Baseline characteristics of adult patients initiating stavudine-containing antiretroviral treatment (N = 2581).

Age (years) - median (IQR)	35 (30–40)
Sex - n (%)	
Male	1240 (48)
Female	1341 (52)
Baseline WHO clinical stage - n (%)	
Stage I	127 (4.9)
Stage II	404 (15.7)
Stage III	1081 (41.9)
Stage IV	969 (37.5)
Baseline body weight (kg) – median (IQR)	49 (43–55)
Baseline body mass index (kg/m²) - median (IQR)	19 (17–21)
Baseline CD4 count (cells/μL) - median (IQR)	87 (25–206)
Baseline haemoglobin (g/dL) - median (IQR)	11.3 (9.9–12.6)
Treatment regimen - n (%)	
Stavudine/lamivudine/nevirapine[a]	1869 (72.5
Stavudine/lamivudine/efavirenz[a]	719 (27.5)
On tuberculosis treatment at ART initiation - n (%)	686 (26.6
Follow-up time with exposure to D4T (years) - median (IQR)	1.3 (0.8–2.3)

IQR: interquartile range, WHO: world health organization, ART: antiretroviral therapy.
[a]From 2006, stavudine was prescribed as 30 mg bid, irrespective of body weight. Prior to that, 40 mg bid was given for individuals with a body weight >60 kg.

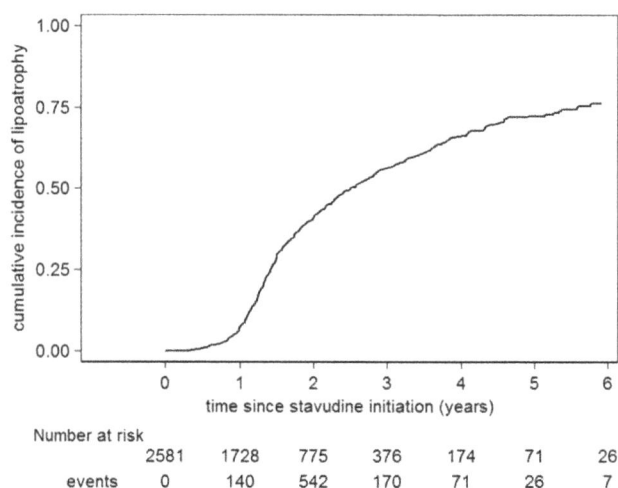

Figure 1. Cumulative incidence of lipoatrophy. Kaplan-Meier curve showing the proportion of patients substituting stavudine due to lipoatrophy.

Number at risk						
	2581	1728	775	376	174	71	26
events	0	140	542	170	71	26	7

Table 3. Risk factors for severe toxicity related to stavudine.

Risk factors	Neuropathy		Lactic acidosis		Lipoatrophy	
	HR (95% CI)	aHR (95% CI)	HR (95% CI)	aHR (95% CI)	HR (95% CI)	aHR (95% CI)
Sex						
Male	1		1	1	1	1
Female	1.1 (0.9–1.4)		2.5 (0.8–8.1)	3.8 (1.1–12.5)	2.2 (1.9–2.5)	2.3 (2.0–2.6)
Age						
≤40 years	1	1	1		1	1
>40 years	1.9 (1.5–2.4)	1.8 (1.4–2.3)	2.8 (1.0–8.1)		1.1 (1.0–1.3)	1.3 (1.1–1.4)
Baseline WHO clinical stage						
I/II	1		1		1	
III/IV	1.4 (1.0–2.0)		1.5 (0.3–6.7)		1.0 (0.9–1.2)	
Baseline BMI						
≤25 kg/m^2	-		1	1	1	
>25 kg/m^2	-		6.4 (2.0–20.5)	12.6 (3.7–43.1)	0.9 (0.7–1.3)	
≥18.5 kg/m^2	1		-	-	-	-
<18.5 kg/m^2	1.3 (1.0–1.7)		-		-	-
Baseline CD4 count						
≥200 cells/µL	1		1		1	1
<200 cells/µL	1.1 (0.8–1.5)		0.8 (0.3–2.6)		1.2 (1.0–1.4)	1.3 (1.1–1.5)
Baseline haemoglobin						
≥10 g/dL	1	1	1		1	
<10 g/dL	1.7 (1.4–2.2)	1.7 (1.4–2.2)	1.3 (0.4–4.3)		1.2 (1.0–1.3)	
NNRTI at start						
EFV	1		1		1	
NVP	0.9 (0.7–1.1)		0.3 (0.1–0.7)		0.9 (0.8–1.1)	
On TB treatment at ART start						
No	1		1	1	1	
Yes	1.1 (0.9–1.5)		5.4 (1.8–16.0)	8.6 (2.7–27.5)	1.0 (0.9–1.2)	

aHR: adjusted hazard ratio, CI: confidence interval, WHO: world health organization, BMI: body mass index, NNRTI: non-nucleoside reverse transcriptase inhibitor; EFV: efavirenz; NVP: nevirapine; TB: tuberculosis; ART: antiretroviral treatment.

values [10,11,16]. In contrast with a South African study [17], we did not find an association of neuropathy with TB treatment. Possible reasons for this could include differences in analytical approach, management of toxicity or timing of ART initiation for patients on TB treatment.

With regards to SH/LA, the association with the use of tuberculosis treatment is somehow surprising and has not been reported yet. In one case-control study, efavirenz was identified as a risk factor for lactic acidosis [18]. Whether this could be the mechanism behind our observed association with tuberculosis treatment, albeit not identified in multivariate analysis, remains to be determined. Alternatively, rapid weight gain after ART initiation, identified as a risk factor for lactic acidosis in a South African study, might be implicated for patients on tuberculosis treatment [12]. Finally, it needs to be pointed out that TB treatment and the use of EFV are closely related variables. Although no clear problem of collinearity was detected during analysis, the problem cannot be entirely ruled out.

Cost has been a major reason for the ongoing use of D4T-containing ART in LMIC. Despite recent cost reductions, tenofovir-based regimens are still more than twice as expensive in terms of drug costs. In Cambodia, the low cost of D4T is a key argument for maintaining this drug within first line treatment

regimens for the next years to come. Our data suggest that the cost-saving effect with D4T-use is limited in time, given the high long-term rates of D4T-replacement. Moreover, its ongoing use continues to expose patients to drug toxicity, with all its negative implications. Whereas our data reinforce the need to phase-out D4T to better tolerated regimens in LMIC, it is clear that this is a major operational undertaking that should be implemented in a phased and controlled manner. In this regard, our experience could be of interest for national programs willing to implement a gradual phasing-out of D4T. By combining patient education, close monitoring for D4T-toxicities, integrating the patient's perception and applying a low threshold for D4T-replacement, a gradual phasing-out of D4T can be expected. Additionally, the occurrence of toxicity could be significantly reduced by prioritizing those at highest risk of D4T toxicity, based on the risk factors identified. Importantly, patient support relative to a uniform and quick D4T replacement strategy might be enhanced with this more targeted approach. A recent study from Cambodia on systematic substitution of zidovudine for D4T highlighted that a fraction of patients preferred to remain on D4T-based HAART [19]. Imposing a treatment change without patient approval might negatively affect on the adherence to the new regimen.

Previous studies have reported on D4T-toxicity up to three years after ART initiation [12,15]. Although incidence of neuropathy in our study was lower, our three-year estimates on lipoatrophy are around twice those recently reported in an African cohort [15]. This could in part relate to the strict criteria for D4T-substitution in this program, relying on a scoring-system of clinical severity of changes in different body sites. In contrast, we also considered the patient's perception and preference. Indeed, recent evidence is consistently pointing out that the subjective experience of ART-related toxicities might be as an important parameter to monitor in ART programs besides the 'objective' changes [20–23]. Self-reported physical and psychological symptoms were identified as strong and independent risk factors for subsequent treatment failure in a recent study [24]. From an operational perspective, the patient's perception is probably an integral part in quantifying the ('subjective') severity of toxicities. Integrating this in therapeutic decisions could contribute towards greater adherence to proposed interventions and towards improvement in the quality of life. This might be especially true for toxicities like body changes, where clear inter-individual differences in perception could exist. The negative impact of perception of body changes on quality of life and adherence has been reported in a number of studies [25–28].

A number of limitations have to be mentioned. This is a retrospective analysis, using data from a treatment program setting. Data on D4T dosing were not recorded in the database. However, given the overall low body weight in this population, few patients initiated high dose D4T (40 mg bid) before revision of the guidelines in 2006. D4T drug changes were driven by suspicion of D4T toxicity by the clinician, hence not necessarily with formal proof of D4T as the culprit drug. Reported data merely demonstrate associations, and not causation. Moreover, this program was probably better resourced with more intensive monitoring compared to other field settings, and this could possibly have resulted in over diagnosis of toxicities. With increasing experience of the program, diagnosis may have been influenced by negative perceptions about D4T by physicians and patients. However, patients were systematically evaluated at each clinical visit, with standard clinical assessment, patient management and reporting. We also note that data were collected prospectively using standardized data collection tools, with continuous monitoring of data quality and clinical management practices. Still, it remains that the unavailability of technical investigations to more rigorously diagnose the different toxicities could have led to misclassification. Moreover, at the start of the program, no lactic acid determination could be done. For lipoatrophy, diagnostic tools such as DEXA-scanning might have allowed to define the exact incidence of lipoatrophy over time. However, our main research question was not to define what happens 'biologically', but rather 'operationally' ie to what extent and for what reasons D4T is replaced over time within a program with close toxicity monitoring.

D4T-based treatment regimens in low-income countries are associated with significant long-term toxicities. With seven out of ten patients developing lipoatrophy by six years of treatment, lipoatrophy represents the major long-term side-effect. Until D4T has been phased-out completely, close monitoring for toxicity combined with the integration of the patient's perspective and a low threshold for D4T-replacement is recommended.

Acknowledgments

We are grateful to the doctors and patients of SHCH for their contribution to the data collection.

Author Contributions

Conceived and designed the experiments: JvG. Performed the experiments: VP KC. Analyzed the data: JvG. Wrote the paper: VP KC LL ST JvG. Assistance in data interpretation: ST LL. Improvement of the intellectual concept of the paper: ST LL.

References

1. World Health Organization (2009) Towards universal access: scaling up priority HIV/AIDS intervention in the health sector: Progress report, September 2009. Available: http://www.who.int/hiv/pub/2009progressreport/en/.

2. Womack J (2009) HIV-related lipodystrophy in Africa and Asia. AIDS Read 19: 131–152.

3. World Health Organization (2004) Scaling up Antiretroviral Therapy in Resource-limited Settings: Treatment Guidelines for a Public Health Approach: 2003 Revision. Available: http://www.who.int/3by5/publications/documents/arv_guidelines/en/.

4. World Health Organization (2006) Antiretroviral therapy for HIV infection in adults and adolescents: Recommendations for a public health approach: 2006 Revision. Available: http://www.who.int/hiv/events/artprevention/gilks.pdf.

5. World Health Organization (2010) Antiretroviral therapy for HIV infection in adults and adolescents, Recommendations for a public health approach, 2010 revision. Available: http://whqlibdoc.who.int/publications/2010/9789241599764_eng.pdf.

6. Gallant JE, Staszewski S, Pozniak AL, DeJesus E, Suleiman JM, et al. (2004) Efficacy and safety of tenofovir DF vs stavudine in combination therapy in antiretroviral-naive patients: a 3-year randomized trial. JAMA 292: 191–201.

7. Mutimura E, Stewart A, Rheeder P, Crowther NJ (2007) Metabolic function and the prevalence of lipodystrophy in a population of HIV-infected African subjects receiving highly active antiretroviral therapy. J Acquir Immune Defic Syndr 46: 451–455.

8. Mercier S, Gueye NF, Cournil A, Fontbonne A, Copin N, et al. (2009) Lipodystrophy and metabolic disorders in HIV-1-infected adults on 4- to 9-year antiretroviral treatment in Senegal: a case-control study. J Acquir Immune Defic Syndr 51: 224–230.

9. Boulle A, Orrel C, Kaplan R, Van CG, McNally M, et al. (2007) Substitutions due to antiretroviral toxicity or contraindication in the first 3 years of antiretroviral therapy in a large South African cohort. Antivir Ther 12: 753–760.

10. Thai S, Koole O, Un P, Ros S, De MP, et al. (2009) Five-year experience with scaling-up access to antiretroviral treatment in an HIV care programme in Cambodia. Trop Med Int Health 14: 1048–1058.

11. Lynen L, An S, Koole O, Thai S, Ros S, et al. (2009) An algorithm to optimize viral load testing in HIV-positive patients with suspected first-line antiretroviral therapy failure in Cambodia. J Acquir Immune Defic Syndr 52: 40–48.

12. Boulle A, Orrel C, Kaplan R, Van CG, McNally M, et al. (2007) Substitutions due to antiretroviral toxicity or contraindication in the first 3 years of antiretroviral therapy in a large South African cohort. Antivir Ther 12: 753–760.

13. van Griensven J, De Naeyer L, Mushi T, Ubarijoro S, Gashumba D, et al. (2007) High prevalence of lipoatrophy among patients on stavudine-containing first-line antiretroviral therapy regimens in Rwanda. Trans R Soc Trop Med Hyg 101: 793–798.

14. Hawkins C, Achenbach C, Fryda W, Ngare D, Murphy R (2007) Antiretroviral durability and tolerability in HIV-infected adults living in urban Kenya. J Acquir Immune Defic Syndr 45: 304–310.

15. van Griensven J, Zachariah R, Rasschaert F, Mugabo J, Atte EF, et al. (2010) Stavudine- and nevirapine-related drug toxicity while on generic fixed-dose antiretroviral treatment: incidence, timing and risk factors in a three-year cohort in Kigali, Rwanda. Trans R Soc Trop Med Hyg 104: 148–153.

16. Kowalska JD, Mocroft A, Blaxhult A, Colebunders R, van IJ, et al. (2007) Current hemoglobin levels are more predictive of disease progression than hemoglobin measured at baseline in patients receiving antiretroviral treatment for HIV type 1 infection. AIDS Res Hum Retroviruses 23: 1183–1188.

17. Westreich DJ, Sanne I, Maskew M, Malope-Kgokong B, Conradie F, et al. (2009) Tuberculosis treatment and risk of stavudine substitution in first-line antiretroviral therapy. Clin Infect Dis 48: 1617–1623.

18. Imhof A, Ledergerber B, Gunthard HF, Haupts S, Weber R (2005) Risk factors for and outcome of hyperlactatemia in HIV-infected persons: is there a need for routine lactate monitoring? Clin Infect Dis 41: 721–728.

19. Isaakidis P, Raguenaud ME, Phe T, Khim SA, Kuoch S, et al. (2008) Evaluation of a systematic substitution of zidovudine for stavudine-based HAART in a program setting in rural Cambodia. J Acquir Immune Defic Syndr 49: 48–54.

20. Santos CP, Felipe YX, Braga PE, Ramos D, Lima RO, et al. (2005) Self-perception of body changes in persons living with HIV/AIDS: prevalence and associated factors. AIDS 19 Suppl 4: S14–S21.

21. Clucas C, Harding R, Lampe FC, Anderson J, Date HL, et al. (2011) Doctor-patient concordance during HIV treatment switching decision-making. HIV Med 12: 87–96.

22. Cooper V, Gellaitry G, Hankins M, Fisher M, Horne R (2009) The influence of symptom experiences and attributions on adherence to highly active anti-retroviral therapy (HAART): a six-month prospective, follow-up study. AIDS Care 21: 520–528.

23. Justice AC, Chang CH, Rabeneck L, Zackin R (2001) Clinical importance of provider-reported HIV symptoms compared with patient-report. Med Care 39: 397–408.

24. Lampe FC, Harding R, Smith CJ, Phillips AN, Johnson M, et al. (2010) Physical and psychological symptoms and risk of virologic rebound among patients with virologic suppression on antiretroviral therapy. J Acquir Immune Defic Syndr 54: 500–505.

25. Guaraldi G, Murri R, Orlando G, Squillace N, Stentarelli C, et al. (2008) Lipodystrophy and quality of life of HIV-infected persons. AIDS Rev 10: 152–161.

26. Burgoyne R, Collins E, Wagner C, Abbey S, Halman M, et al. (2005) The relationship between lipodystrophy-associated body changes and measures of quality of life and mental health for HIV-positive adults. Qual Life Res 14: 981–990.

27. Glass TR, Battegay M, Cavassini M, De GS, Furrer H, et al. (2010) Longitudinal analysis of patterns and predictors of changes in self-reported adherence to antiretroviral therapy: Swiss HIV Cohort Study. J Acquir Immune Defic Syndr 54: 197–203.

28. Nachega JB, Trotta MP, Nelson M, Ammassari A (2009) Impact of metabolic complications on antiretroviral treatment adherence: clinical and public health implications. Curr HIV/AIDS Rep 6: 121–129.

13

Extra-Visual Functional and Structural Connection Abnormalities in Leber's Hereditary Optic Neuropathy

Maria A. Rocca[1,2], **Paola Valsasina**[1,2], **Elisabetta Pagani**[1,2], **Stefania Bianchi-Marzoli**[3], **Jacopo Milesi**[3], **Andrea Falini**[4], **Giancarlo Comi**[2], **Massimo Filippi**[1,2]*

1 Neuroimaging Research Unit, Scientific Institute and University Ospedale San Raffaele, Milan, Italy, **2** Division of Neuroscience, Department of Neurology, Institute of Experimental Neurology, Scientific Institute and University Ospedale San Raffaele, Milan, Italy, **3** Department of Ophthalmology, Scientific Institute and University Ospedale San Raffaele, Milan, Italy, **4** Department of Neuroradiology, Scientific Institute and University Ospedale San Raffaele, Milan, Italy

Abstract

We assessed abnormalities within the principal brain resting state networks (RSNs) in patients with Leber's hereditary optic neuropathy (LHON) to define whether functional abnormalities in this disease are limited to the visual system or, conversely, tend to be more diffuse. We also defined the structural substrates of fMRI changes using a connectivity-based analysis of diffusion tensor (DT) MRI data. Neuro-ophthalmologic assessment, DT MRI and RS fMRI data were acquired from 13 LHON patients and 13 healthy controls. RS fMRI data were analyzed using independent component analysis and SPM5. A DT MRI connectivity-based parcellation analysis was performed using the primary visual and auditory cortices, bilaterally, as seed regions. Compared to controls, LHON patients had a significant increase of RS fluctuations in the primary visual and auditory cortices, bilaterally. They also showed decreased RS fluctuations in the right lateral occipital cortex and right temporal occipital fusiform cortex. Abnormalities of RS fluctuations were correlated significantly with retinal damage and disease duration. The DT MRI connectivity-based parcellation identified a higher number of clusters in the right auditory cortex in LHON vs. controls. Differences of cluster-centroid profiles were found between the two groups for all the four seeds analyzed. For three of these areas, a correspondence was found between abnormalities of functional and structural connectivities. These results suggest that functional and structural abnormalities extend beyond the visual network in LHON patients. Such abnormalities also involve the auditory network, thus corroborating the notion of a cross-modal plasticity between these sensory modalities in patients with severe visual deficits.

Editor: Yi Wang, Cornell University, United States of America

Funding: The authors have no support or funding to report.

Competing Interests: The authors have declared that no competing interests exist.

* E-mail: m.filippi@hsr.it

Introduction

Leber's Hereditary Optic Neuropathy (LHON) is a maternally inherited genetic disease characterised by an acute or subacute bilateral loss of vision, which predominantly affects young men, with a clinical onset between 15 and 35 years [1,2,3]. Pathologically, retinal ganglion cell degeneration and axonal loss in the optic nerve have been described in these patients [4]. These abnormalities are associated with an early and selective damage of the small calibre fibers of the papillomacular bundle. LHON has been linked to three ''primary'' mitochondrial DNA (mtDNA) point mutations, which affect oxidative phosphorylation in mitochondria [5,6].

At present, it is still unclear whether central nervous system (CNS) involvement in patients with LHON is restricted to the optic nerve and visual pathways via chronic damage (i.e., the lateral geniculate nucleus and the visual cortex may be involved by trans-synaptic degeneration phenomena), as has been described in other ocular pathologies, including optic neuritis [7,8], chronic glaucoma [9], retinal degeneration [10], and albinism [11]. Against this view militates the well-known association of LHON with clinical and magnetic resonance imaging (MRI) patterns indistinguishable from those of multiple sclerosis [12], as well as clinical observations which reported neurological disturbances,

such as reflex alterations, cerebellar ataxia, periferic neuropathy and myoclonus in a relatively small percentage of these patients [13]. In addition, MR spectroscopy (MRS) studies of LHON have shown an abnormal mitochondrial energy metabolism in the occipital lobe [14,15,16], and diffuse abnormalities in the normal-appearing white matter have been detected using magnetization transfer MRI [17].

Functional MRI (fMRI) is a non-invasive technique which allows to define how the principal brain systems function in healthy subjects and to interrogate their alterations in patients with CNS pathologies. A method that has been introduced recently for the analysis of functional connections and coherence between different brain neural networks is based on the assessment of low-frequency (<0.1 Hz) fluctuations seen on fMRI scans acquired at rest (i.e., in the absence of any external stimulation). The use of such an approach has demonstrated the presence of a high temporal coherence between spatially distinct, functionally-related brain regions, resembling specific neuroanatomical networks, including the motor, visual, and dorsal and ventral attention systems, which characterise the resting-state networks (RSNs) of the human brain [18,19,20,21]. The main advantage of RSN analysis is that it is not influenced by task performance and clinical impairment, as is the case for task-related fMRI.

In this study, we used fMRI to assess abnormalities within the principal brain RSNs in patients with LHON with the aim to define whether functional CNS abnormalities in this disease are limited to the visual system, or, conversely tend to be more diffuse and involve additional networks. In this latter case, to identify the possible anatomical substrates underlying the observed fMRI changes, an additional analysis was pre-planned, based on the exploitation of structural connectivity profiles of brain regions with significantly different activities between LHON patients and controls, using a connectivity-based analysis of diffusion tensor (DT) MRI data [22,23,24].

Results

Neuro-ophthalmologic assessment

Table 1 summarises the results of the neuro-ophthalmologic assessment in LHON patients. At the time of MRI assessment, all LHON patients had bilateral visual impairment and a variable degree of optic nerve pallor detectable at fundoscopy, which was particularly evident in the temporal sector. Standardised automated perimetry (SAP) showed a central scotoma of variable size in all affected eyes. Optic coherence tomography (OCT) detected a thinning of peripapillary retinal nerve fiber layer thickness (PRNFL) in all affected eyes, especially in the temporal quadrant.

MRI assessment

None of the subjects had T2-hyperintense brain lesions.

a) RS networks. In controls and LHON patients, the analysis of RS data detected 10 networks with potential functional relevance: three RSNs included the primary and secondary visual cortical areas, bilaterally; two the sensorimotor areas, bilaterally; two a set of cortical areas belonging to the default mode network (DMN); two a set of fronto-parietal areas lateralized to the right and the left hemisphere, respectively; and the last the primary and secondary auditory areas, bilaterally. Maps of RS activity for each of these networks, from both healthy controls and LHON patients (one-sample t test), are shown in Figure 1, together with their associated time courses. All these components were stable across multiple runs of IC decomposition, with a stability index assessed by ICASSO ranging from 0.72 to 0.98 for all the components of interest. RS networks of interest derived from the two ICA analyses performed on controls and LHON patients, separately, were very similar to those obtained from ICA performed on the entire study group (spatial correlation coefficients between networks ranging from 0.74 to 0.92).

b) Visual RS networks. Between-group comparisons of the activity over the spatial extent of visual RSNs showed an increase of RS fluctuations in LHON patients *vs.* controls in several areas of the visual cortex in both primary visual RSNs. In detail, foci of increased RS fluctuations in the first visual network were located in the left cuneal cortex (MNI space coordinates: −3, −87, 20; t-value = 3.7; p = 0.05; cluster extent [k] = 5) and right supracalcarine cortex (MNI space coordinates: 3, −87, 12; t-value = 3.6; p = 0.05; k = 5). For the second visual network, the foci of increased RS fluctuations were located in the bilateral occipital pole (MNI space coordinates: 6, −93, −12; t-value = 4.6; p = 0.05; k = 5, and −30, −96, 0; t-value = 4.4; p = 0.05; k = 17), and the left occipital fusiform gyrus (MNI space coordinate: −15, −90, −12; t-value = 4.5; p = 0.05; k = 12) (Figure 2). This analysis also showed decreased RS fluctuations in the right lateral occipital cortex (MNI space coordinates: 45, −63, −8; t-value = 4.1; p = 0.05; k = 7), and right temporal occipital fusiform cortex (MNI space coordinates: 30, −54, −8; t-value = 3.8; p = 0.05; k = 5) for the network of the secondary visual areas (Figure 2).

c) Non visual RS networks. Between-group comparisons of the activity over the spatial extent of the non-visual networks showed significant increased RS fluctuations in the right superior temporal gyrus (including the primary auditory cortex) and the supramarginal gyrus (MNI space coordinates: 60, −33, 12: t-value = 4.6; p = 0.05; k = 11) for the RSN including the primary and secondary auditory areas (Figure 2). Using an uncorrected statistical threshold of 0.01, the same abnormalities were detected also in the left hemisphere. No between-group difference was found for the remaining networks/clusters.

d) Correlations of fMRI abnormalities with clinical and neuro-ophthalmologic measures. In LHON patients, significant correlations were found of disease duration with RS activity of the right lateral occipital cortex (r = −0.77, p = 0.01), left cuneal cortex (r = 0.87, p = 0.003), right occipital pole (r = 0.87, p = 0.003), and right superior temporal gyrus (r = 0.83, p = 0.02). In addition, significant correlations were found of average temporal PRNFL with RS activity of the left cuneal cortex (r = 0.88, p = 0.002) and right superior temporal gyrus (r = 0.79, p = 0.05).

e) DT MRI connectivity-based parcellation. The number of seed points that were used for tractography in each of the considered areas did not differ between controls and LHON patients. However, the number of seed points was significantly different between the left and the right auditory cortices, due to their different representation in the SPM Anatomical Toolbox [25]. The silhouette analysis identified a similar number of clusters in patients and controls for the right V1 (8 clusters in each group), the left V1 (8 clusters in each group), and the left auditory cortex (7 clusters in each group). Conversely, LHON patients had a higher number of clusters in the right auditory cortex compared to controls (4 clusters in patients *vs.* 2 clusters in controls) (Figure 3).

The between-group differences in profile analysis are summarised in Table 2. The cluster-centroid profile analysis showed that the right V1 of LHON patients had a structural connectivity with the temporal fusiform cortex, which was not detected in controls (Figure 4). This analysis also showed that, compared to controls, the right V1 of LHON patients had an increased structural connectivity with the temporal occipital fusiform cortex and a decreased structural connectivity with the lateral occipital cortex and the occipital fusiform gyrus (Figure 4). The left V1 of LHON patients had a structural connectivity with the middle temporal gyrus and inferior temporal gyrus, which were not detected in controls. In addition, compared to controls, the left V1 of LHON patients had an increased structural connectivity with the frontal pole and lateral occipital cortex as well as a decreased structural

Table 1. Results of neuro-ophthalmologic assessment in patients with Leber's hereditary optic neuropathy.

	Left Eye	Right Eye
Mean visual acuity (range)	1.33 (3-0)	1.14 (3-0)
Average mean deviation (range) (dB)	−15.73 (−0.43 to −32.61)	−15.48 (−1.48 to −33.35)
Average PRNFL thickness (range) (μm)	56.9 (33.1–89.3)*	56.5 (38.1–80.4)*
Temporal PRNFL thickness (range) (μm)	36 (31–47)*	49 (19–95)*

Abbreviations: PRNFL = peripapillary retinal nerve fiber layer, SD = standard deviation.
*Below normal (<5th percentile) as compared with a database of age-matched control subjects. See text for further details.

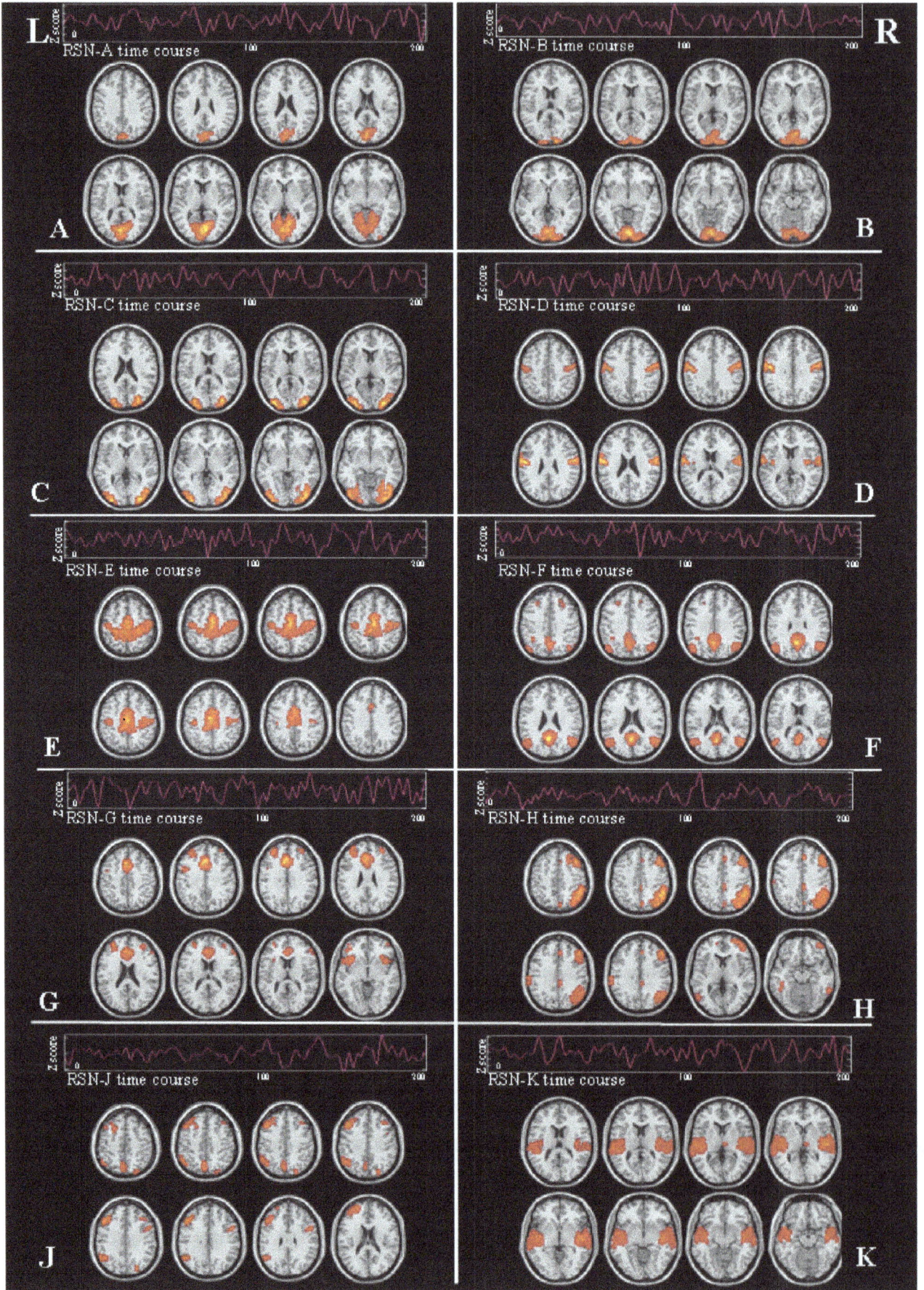

Figure 1. Spatial pattern and corresponding time courses of potentially functionally relevant resting state networks (RSNs) in healthy volunteers and patients with Leber's hereditary optic neuropathy: three RSNs included primary (A, B) and secondary (C) visual cortical areas; two RSNs (D, E) included sensorimotor areas; two RSNs (F, G) included areas that are part of the default mode network; two RSNs included fronto-parietal areas lateralized to the right (H) and left (J) hemispheres; one RSN (K) included primary and secondary auditory areas. See text for further details. Images are in neurologic convention.

connectivity with the temporal pole. The right auditory cortex (Figure 3) of LHON patients had a structural connectivity with the frontal pole, the pallidum, and the supramarginal gyrus, which were not detected in controls. Finally, the left auditory cortex of LHON patients had a structural connectivity with the lateral occipital cortex, which was not detected in controls. Conversely, controls had a structural connectivity with the middle temporal gyrus and inferior temporal gyrus, which was not detected in patients. Compared to controls, LHON patients had a lower number of seeds assigned to cluster 2 in the auditory cortex (Figure 3) (mean numbers of seeds [SD]: 8.1 [4.9] in LHON patients *vs.* 16.7 [5.9] in controls, p<0.001).

In the left auditory cortex, significant correlations were found between:

- the number of seeds assigned to a cluster connected to the superior temporal gyrus *vs.* left temporal PRNFL (r = 0.63, p = 0.02) and average PRNFL (r = 0.61, p = 0.04);

- the number of seeds assigned to a cluster connected to the insular cortex and the parietal operculum cortex *vs.* temporal PRNFL (r = 0.62, p = 0.02).

f) Correspondence between areas of altered functional and structural connectivities. In LHON patients, a correspondence was found between:

- decreased functional connectivity in the right temporal occipital fusiform cortex and increased structural connectivity between the right visual cortex and the right temporal occipital fusiform cortex;

- decreased functional connectivity in the right lateral occipital cortex and decreased structural connectivity between the right V1 and the previous region;

- increased functional connectivity in the right supramarginal gyrus and increased structural connectivity between the right auditory cortex and the previous region.

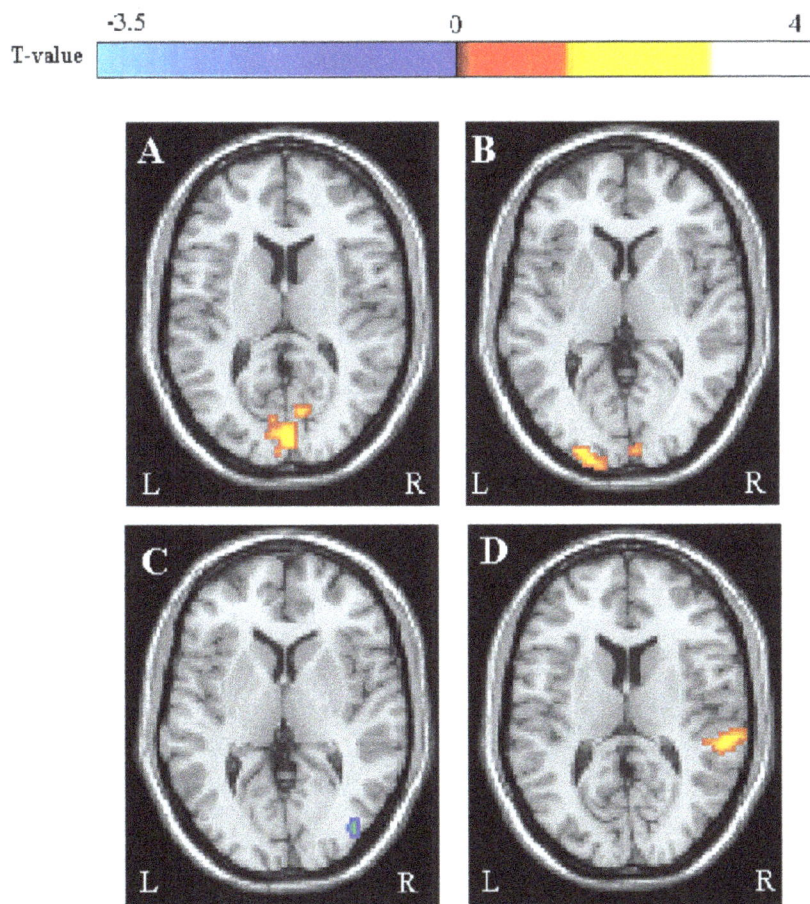

Figure 2. Spatial patterns of between-group differences in resting state (RS) fluctuations of the primary visual network (A, B), the secondary visual network (C) and the auditory network (D) between LHON patients and healthy controls. Clusters of increased RS activity in LHON patients are color-coded with red to yellow T values, while clusters of decreased RS activity in LHON patients are color-coded with dark to light blue T values. Images are in neurologic convention.

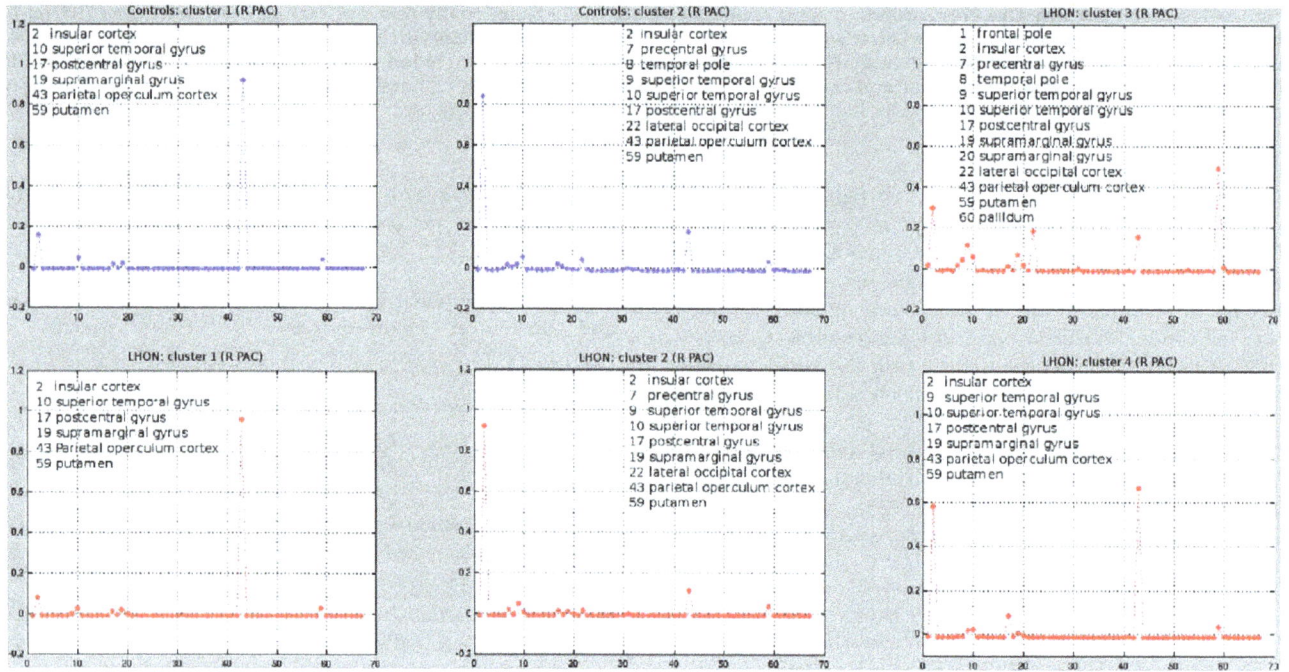

Figure 3. Clusters and cluster-centroids identified in the right (R) primary auditory cortex (PAC) in healthy controls (blue) and Leber's hereditary optic neuropathy (LHON) patients (red). The silhouette analysis identified two clusters in healthy controls and four clusters in LHON patients. The cluster-centroid profile analysis of the R PAC of LHON patients showed a structural connectivity with the frontal pole, the pallidum, and the supramarginal gyrus, which was not detected in controls. X-axis reports brain areas classified according to the Harvard-Oxford cortical and subcortical atlas.

Discussion

We investigated RS fluctuations in patients with LHON to improve our understanding of this disease pathophysiology. The main advantage of the approach we used is that it does not require any active task to be performed, therefore its results are not influenced by possible between-group differences related to impairment and disability or to eye movements (which require an accurate monitoring when dealing with visual stimulations). As a consequence, we believe that these results can be considered representative of the actual cortical reorganization following tissue injury in LHON.

We detected 10 RSNs, which were consistently present in both controls and LHON patients. These RSNs included the sensorimotor areas, the primary and secondary visual systems, the auditory system, as well as attention and memory related networks. The between-group comparisons of the three visual networks showed increased fluctuations in regions that are part of the primary visual cortex, as well as decreased fluctuations in the right lateral occipital cortex and temporal occipital fusiform cortex in LHON patients in comparison to healthy controls, which might reflect a functional disconnection between primary and secondary areas within the visual network. Several studies, in patients with different ocular and retinal conditions have shown consistently

Table 2. Differences in cluster-centroid profiles between patients with Leber's hereditary optic neuropathy and healthy controls.

Areas	R V1	L V1	R Auditory cortex	L Auditory cortex
Temporal fusiform cortex	LHON only	-	-	-
Temporal occipital fusiform cortex	Increased LHON	-	-	-
Lateral occipital cortex	Decreased LHON	Increased LHON	-	LHON only
Occipital fusiform gyrus	Decreased LHON	-	-	-
Middle temporal gyrus	.	LHON only	-	Controls only
Inferior temporal gyrus	-	LHON only	-	Controls only
Frontal pole	-	Increased LHON	LHON only	-
Temporal pole	-	Decreased LHON	-	-
Pallidum	-	-	LHON only	-
Supramarginal gyrus	-	-	LHON only	-

Abbreviations: LHON = Leber's hereditary optic neuropathy, R = right, L = left, V1 = primary visual cortex.

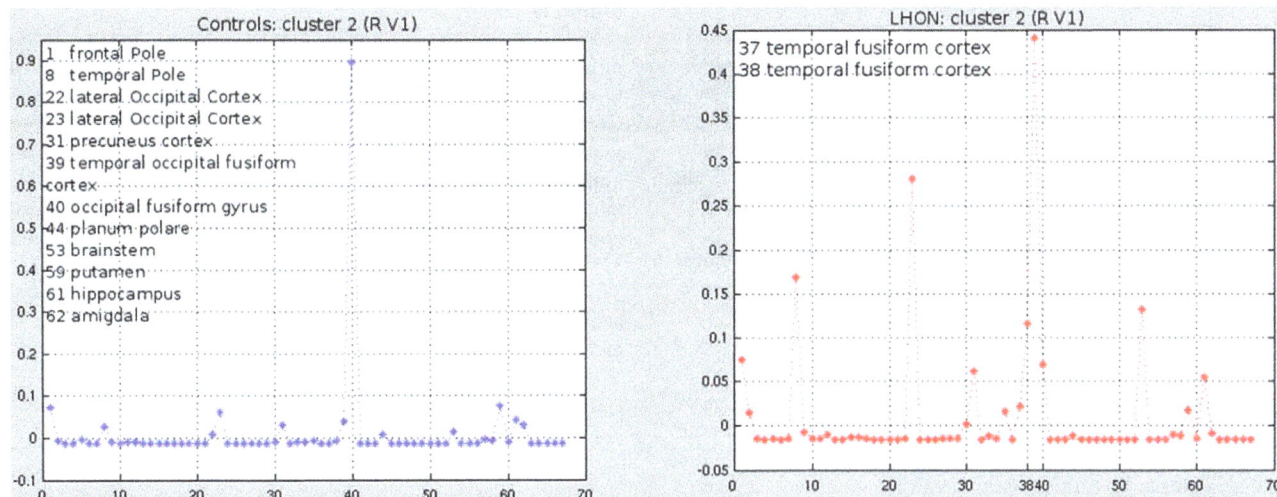

Figure 4. Cluster-centroid profile analysis of the right V1 (cluster II) in healthy controls (blue) and patients with Leber's Hereditary Optic Neuropathy (LHON) (red). The right V1 of LHON patients had a structural connectivity with the temporal fusiform cortex, which was not detected in controls. In addition, compared to controls, the right V1 of LHON patients had an increased structural connectivity with the temporal occipital fusiform cortex and a decreased structural connectivity with the lateral occipital cortex and the occipital fusiform gyrus. X-axis reports areas classified according to the Harvard-Oxford cortical and subcortical atlas.

that damage to the most anterior portions of the visual pathways is associated with functional and structural changes to the striate and extrastriate cortices, which are most likely secondary to trans-synaptic degeneration. A volume reduction of the visual cortical regions has been detected in patients with amblyopia [26], albinism [11], and retinal damage [10,27]. A positron emission tomography study has demonstrated a high level of energy metabolism, at rest, in the visual cortex of early blind adults compared to age-matched blindfolded controls [28]. Our findings, combined with the results of these previous studies, suggest that synapses in the visual cortex of LHON patients are in a hyperactive state. Alternatively, they might reflect a variation of synaptic density. However, such an hypothesis is in contrast with the demonstration of a selective atrophy of the visual cortex in LHON patients [29].

Another important finding of our study is the demonstration that RSN abnormalities in LHON patients are not limited to the visual network, but also involve the auditory network. The coherence of activity between the visual and the auditory networks suggests the existence of an interplay between the two, which corroborates the notion of a cross-modal plasticity involving these sensory modalities in patients with severe visual deficits. Indeed, previous functional imaging studies have demonstrated that visual areas in blind subjects are activated by auditory tasks [30,31]. Using a different method of analysis of low frequency RS fluctuations, based on the assessment of correlation coefficients between a large sets of brain regions, Liu et al. have recently shown decreased functional connectivities in the occipital visual cortex as well as between the visual cortices and the frontal, parietal and temporal cortices in early blind subjects (loss of sight at birth or before one year of age) in comparison to sighted individuals [32]. Differences in the methods of analysis as well as in the clinical and neuro-ophthalmologic characteristics of the patients included (early vs. late blindness) might contribute to explain the discrepancies between our and the previous [32] findings. In detail, we applied spatial ICA, which allowed us to cluster brain RS activity into different networks of spatially independent and temporally coherent brain regions according to

the similarity of the reference time courses. The Z-scores of our spatial RS maps can be thought as a measure of intrinsic RS activity at a given voxel, but they do not give information about the similarity of such an activity with that of voxels from other distant regions belonging to other networks. On the contrary, the functional connectivity approach used by Liu et al. [32] investigated the correlations between pairs of brain regions. Such a method can detect significant couplings between time courses of spatially remote brain regions, but it does not provide any information about the level of RS activity of individual regions. Alternative applications of ICA, such as temporal ICA, might be used to obtain pieces of information more similar to those provided by functional connectivity, but temporal ICA is rarely used is functional neuroimaging literature, probably because of the computational challenges created by the higher data dimensionality [33].

Concerning the age of the onset of blindness, several studies have indicated a dramatic change in density of visual synapses during normal development, characterised by an increase between 2 and 8 months of age, and then by a decline (synaptic revision) to reach the adult level at 11 years [34,35]. This synaptic revision corresponds to the elimination of redundant connections and to the establishment of functional connectivities. Since visual input interruption occurs prior to the stage of synaptic revision in early blind and after its establishment in late blind subjects, this might further contribute to explain the discrepancies between the two studies. Clearly, if confirmed by further work, our findings might have important therapeutic implications because they suggest that LHON patients might benefit from substitutive sensory aids. Remarkably, a recent gene expression profile study has shown that the optic atrophy 1 (OPA1) gene, which is related to autosomal dominant optic atrophy (ADOA), the most common form of hereditary optic neuropathy, is downregulated in some LHON patients [36]. Of note, OPA1 is expressed not only in the optic nerves and in the brain, but also in the inner ear.

To explore possible alterations of structural connections related to the above RS abnormalities, we performed a DT MRI connectivity-based parcellation analysis [22], which allowed us to investigate the structural connections between the primary visual and auditory cortices (which showed significant abnormalities of their functional connections) and other regions of the brain identified using a standard atlas. We choose such an approach, among the different strategies available to investigate the structural architecture of the WM using DT MRI, because the network of anatomical connections linking the neuronal elements of the human brain is still largely unknown, and we did not have strong a priori hypotheses on the possible anatomical connections to be investigated (with the exception of the optic tracts and radiations). A valid alternative strategy would have been the use of fMRI results to guide tractography reconstruction. However, with such a method we would have limited our results to a few WM tracts.

Our DT MRI connectivity-based parcellation analysis results need to be interpreted with caution, but nonetheless provide some important clues to better understand the RS fMRI changes seen in LHON patients. Consistently with the fMRI results which showed abnormalities of function within the auditory network (especially on the right side), the silhouette analysis identified a different number of clusters in healthy controls and LHON patients in the right auditory cortex. Furthermore, subtle differences of cluster-centroid profiles were found between the two groups for all the four seeds analyzed. Noteworthy, similarly to functional connectivity results, also the structural connectivity analysis disclosed areas of increased as well as decreased connectivity in patients *vs.* controls. Intriguingly, for a few of the areas identified by the two analyses, a correspondence was found between abnormalities of functional and structural connectivities. Remarkably, in one of these associations (i.e., decreased functional connectivity in the right temporal occipital fusiform cortex and increased structural connectivity between the right visual cortex and the right temporal occipital fusiform cortex) abnormalities of functional and structural connectivity had an opposite direction. Although we admit that this is only speculative, this observation suggests that structural and functional changes associated to the disease might be dynamic. A "temporal dissociation" between the two phenomena might explain this counter intuitive finding: abnormalities of functional connectivity might be a consequence of retinal damage, and might be then followed by an increased structural connectivity as an adaptive compensatory response.

Clearly, we can not define whether the abnormalities of WM architecture and function we detected in LHON patients are congenital or secondary to damage to the optic nerve. However, the extent of RS and DT MRI abnormalities observed in LHON patients was related to retinal damage (quantified using OCT) and disease duration, supporting the notion that they are likely to be the consequence of their deafferentation, following neuroaxonal damage to the retina and optic nerve.

Future investigations should evaluate whether the abnormalities we observed are stable or, conversely, whether they change over time, the factors influencing these changes, and, finally, whether they are specific of LHON or shared among other forms of hereditary optic neuropathy. This would help to define whether the analysis of RS connectivity might offer clinically relevant biomarkers of disease severity and duration in LHON patients.

Materials and Methods

The study was approved by the Ethics Committee of Scientific Institute and University Ospedale San Raffaele, Milan, Italy and a written informed consent was obtained from all subjects prior to study entry, according to the Declaration of Helsinki.

Subjects

We studied 13 patients with LHON (11 men and 2 women; mean age = 35.6, range = 20–61 years; mean disease duration = 9, range = 2–34 years) recruited from the Neuro-Ophthalmology Clinic at San Raffaele Scientific Institute, Milan, Italy. Inclusion criteria were: (i) presence of one of the three primary mtDNA mutations associated with LHON, (ii) disease duration >12 months, (iii) no history of concomitant neurological, psychiatric, ophthalmological diseases or drug abuse. Eight patients carried the 11778, three the 3460, and two the 14484 mtDNA mutation. Thirteen sex- and age-matched healthy subjects, with no history of neurological and ophthalmological disorders served as controls (11 men and 2 women; mean age 35.2, range 19–59 years).

Neuro-ophthalmologic assessment

LHON patients underwent a complete neuro-ophthalmologic examination at the time of the enrolment. Best-corrected visual acuity was assessed with LogMAR notation performed with high-intensity red-free light. Visual field examination was performed with SAP and mean deviation was quantified (Humphrey Zeiss, 30-2 SITA standard program). Average and temporal PRNFL measurements were obtained using a commercially available optical coherence tomographer as previously described (Stratus OCT, Carl Zeiss Ophthalmic Systems Inc, fast RNFL thickness 3.4) [29].

MRI acquisition

On a 3.0 Tesla Philips Intera scanner, RS fMRI scans were acquired within 24 hours from neuro-ophthalmologic assessment using a T2*-weighted single-shot echo planar imaging (EPI) sequence (repetition time [TR] = 3000 ms, echo time [TE] = 35 ms, flip angle = 90°, field of view [FOV] = 240 mm^2; matrix = 128×128, slice thickness = 4 mm, 200 sets of 30 contiguous axial slices, parallel to the anterior-posterior commissural plane). Total acquisition time was about 10 minutes. During scanning, subjects were instructed to remain motionless, to close their eyes and not to think to anything in particular. All subjects reported they had not fallen asleep during scanning. Movements were minimised using foam padding and ear blocks.

A dual-echo turbo spin echo (TSE), a pulsed-gradient SE EPI (with diffusion gradients applied in 35 non-collinear directions; b factor = 900 mm^2/s and a single b0 image), and a 3D high-resolution T1-weighted fast field echo (FFE) sequence were also obtained, as previously described [37].

RS fMRI analysis

RS fMRI data were first pre-processed using Statistical Parametric Mapping (SPM5). All images were realigned to the first one to correct for subject motion (mean cumulative translations: 1.5 mm, SD = 0.27, and 1.9 mm, SD = 0.19 for controls and LHON patients, p = n.s.; mean rotation <0.2 degrees in both groups). The mean individual motion was calculated for each subject as the average of the six realignment parameters estimated by SPM5. Data were then spatially normalised into the standard Montreal Neurological Institute (MNI) space (with a sub-sampling to 3×3×4 mm^3 resolution, leading to images with a matrix = 53×63×35, and, therefore, a total number [N] of voxels = 116865), using the standard SPM5 EPI template as a reference, and smoothed with a 6-mm, 3D-Gaussian filter. Linear detrending and band-pass filtering between 0.01 and 0.08 Hz were performed using the REST software (http://resting-fmri.sourceforge.net/) to partially remove low-frequency drifts and physiological high-frequency noise.

Independent Component Analysis (ICA) was used to decompose RS fMRI data into spatially independent maps and time courses using the GIFT software (Group ICA of FMRI Toolbox) [33]. GIFT analysis was performed following three main steps: (i) data reduction, (ii) ICA, and (iii) back reconstruction. First, single-subject fMRI data were reduced to a lower temporal dimensionality by using a principal component analysis. The number of independent group components was 40, a dimension determined using the minimum description length criterion [33]. Then, for each time-component of each subject, the 3D fMRI image was flattened to a 1D vector (with dimension N = 116865 voxels) and a single-subject $40 \times N$ matrix was created, containing all flattened images for the 40 temporal components. Finally, the matrices from each of the 26 subjects were vertically concatenated into a $M \times N$ multi-subject matrix ($M = 26 \times 40 = 1040$) containing the fMRI data from all subjects. The group independent components (ICs) were estimated using the Infomax approach [38], and each component was represented by a spatial map and a temporal profile. The group mixing matrix estimated by Infomax, which describes group ICs, can be also thought as made by many side-by-side partitions, each of which is related to ICs of a single subject. Individual subject components maps and time courses were back-reconstructed by subdividing group ICs into the corresponding single subject partitions [33]. Statistical reliability of IC decomposition was tested by using the ICASSO toolbox [39]. Stability of the obtained ICs was assessed by running Infomax 10 times with different initial conditions and bootstrapped datasets, by clustering the results of each run, and by calculating a stability index for each component. Two separate spatial ICAs were also performed in controls and LHON patients to ensure that the resulting components were similar in the two groups. Similarity was assessed by calculating the spatial correlation coefficient between components estimated by each ICA analysis, using the "fslcc" utility included in FSL toolbox (http://www.fmrib.ox.ac.uk/fsl/).

Each individual functional map was converted into Z-scores before entering group statistics, to have voxel values comparable across subjects.

A systematic process was applied to inspect and select the components of interest from the 40 estimated components. The association of each component spatial map with a priori probabilistic maps of gray matter (GM), white matter (WM), and cerebrospinal fluid (CSF) within the MNI space contributed to identify the components with a signal change correlated to the GM. Components with a high correlation to CSF or WM, or with a low correlation with the GM, were excluded. In addition, to identify components with potential functional relevance, a frequency analysis of IC time courses was performed to detect those with a high (50% or greater) spectral power at a low frequency (between 0.01 and 0.05 Hz) [40]. The spatial patterns of the remaining ICs were sorted out on the basis of their matching with relevant RSNs found in previous studies [18,19,20,21].

The magnitude of RS activity within each group, as well as between-group RS activity differences were assessed using SPM5 and a one-sample t test and a two-sample t test, respectively, including the mean subject's motion (calculated as the mean of the six motion parameters estimated by SPM) [41,42] as a confounding covariate. SPMs produced at one-sample t tests were thresholded at p = 0.001 and combined (intersection) in a single image, which was used as mask for the subsequent between-group comparisons. Results of between-group comparisons were then superimposed to the Harvard-Oxford cortical atlas (http://www.fmrib.ox.ac.uk/fsl/fslview/atlas-descriptions.html#ha) to have the results in the same atlas of the structural connectivity results.

In LHON patients, using SPM5 and multiple regression models, a linear regression analysis was performed to assess spatial correlations of RS abnormalities with clinical and neuro-ophthalmologic measures. Clusters exceeding a threshold of p<0.001 (uncorrected for multiple comparisons) underwent a small volume correction (SVC) for multiple comparisons, setting the cut off value for significance at p<0.05 and using a 10-mm radius around the peak derived from the between-group comparisons.

We used a family wise error (FWE) correction at p<0.05 for multiple comparisons at a cluster level as the threshold for statistical significance for between-group comparisons. Only clusters having an extent of $k \geq 5$ were included in this analysis. This extent should not be considered small, because RS data, due to image subsampling to $3 \times 3 \times 4$ mm (= 36 cubic mm volume of each voxel), have a single voxel volume equivalent to that of 4.5 voxels of active fMRI data pre-processed with a standard SPM5 analysis, having usually a dimension of $2 \times 2 \times 2$ mm (= 8 cubic mm volume).

DT MRI connectivity-based parcellation analysis

DT images were first corrected for distortion induced by eddy currents using an in-house software [43]. The DT was then calculated on a pixel-by-pixel basis, using FSL tools (http://www.fmrib.ox.ac.uk/fsl).

Based on the results of RS fMRI analysis (see above), a parcellation analysis was performed on the primary visual (V1) and auditory cortices, bilaterally. They were segmented on 3D T1-weighted images using an atlas-based approach. To this aim, V1 and the auditory cortex (Areas TE 1.0, TE 1.1 and TE 1.2) [44] were selected using the SPM Anatomy Toolbox [25], normalised, using SPM5, to single-subject 3D T1-weighted images (which were previously scalped using the Brain Extraction Tool [BET] [45] and coregistered to the b0 images), and thresholded at 50%. Seeds for tractography were selected as follows: 3D T1-weighted images were segmented into WM, GM and CSF using SPM5 and registered to diffusion space; then, a 2D sobel filter was applied to the GM maps (not binarized) to obtain the boundaries between GM and WM. Finally, the resulting contours were masked with the visual and auditory cortical probability maps derived previously; seeds facing the CSF were removed manually. The resulting seeds were used as starting points for probabilistic tractography [24]. The output of tractography is a file containing the number of visits of tracts in each voxel; this is considered as an index of structural connectivity. Due to computational demands, this output is saved at a 5 mm resolution [23]. Connectivity values from tractography were then summed up within cortical regions identified with the Harvard-Oxford cortical and subcortical atlas available within FSL (http://www.fmrib.ox.ac.uk/fsl/fslview/atlas-descriptions.html#ha). The regions containing the starting seeds were excluded. Connections to the contralateral hemisphere were not considered. Finally, data were reformatted in a matrix layout in which each row is the connectivity profile of a single seed to each of the considered cortical areas, and matrices for all subjects were concatenated in a single matrix, which is the input of the k-means algorithm for clustering. Since the k-means method requires as an input the number of clusters, we used the silhouette method [46,47] to estimate the number of clusters that fitted best. The silhouette method is based on the production of a silhouette profile for each cluster found, which defines how good is the classification of each seed in comparison with its assignment to a second most appropriate cluster. For each seed, the profile plots an index, which is calculated from the ratio between the average similarity of the seed to all other seeds in the cluster and the maximum similarity of the seed to all seeds of other clusters. Index values close to 1 indicate a well-clustered seed, whereas values close to -1 indicate a bad assignment of the seed to a given cluster. Once all silhouettes are combined in a single plot, the average value can be used to select the most appropriate number of clusters.

To do this, we run silhouette for different number of clusters (ranging from 2 to 15) and calculated the average silhouette values for each trial. The optimal number of clusters was that corresponding to the maximum value of the average silhouette profile. During both the optimization and the clustering phase, the control and patient groups were treated separately. The clustering analysis also provided the cluster-centroids, which summarise the structural connectivity profile of each cluster. First, a visual inspection was performed to identify between-group differences in cluster-centroid profile (e.g., presence/absence of a given peak and peak amplitude). Then, for each subject, the number of seeds assigned to each cluster was used as a subject-wise measure to compare patients with controls (t test for independent samples), and to assess correlation with clinical and ophthalmological measures (non parametric correlation, Spearman Rank Correlation Coefficient).

Author Contributions

Conceived and designed the experiments: MAR SB-M AF GC MF. Performed the experiments: MAR JM AF. Analyzed the data: MAR PV EP. Contributed reagents/materials/analysis tools: PV EP. Wrote the paper: MAR PV EP SB-M JM AF GC MF.

References

1. Huoponen K, Vilkki J, Aula P, Nikoskelainen EK, Savontaus ML (1991) A new mtDNA mutation associated with Leber hereditary optic neuroretinopathy. Am J Hum Genet 48: 1147–1153.

2. Newman NJ, Lott MT, Wallace DC (1991) The clinical characteristics of pedigrees of Leber's hereditary optic neuropathy with the 11778 mutation. Am J Ophthalmol 111: 750–762.

3. Wallace DC, Singh G, Lott MT, Hodge JA, Schurr TG, et al. (1988) Mitochondrial DNA mutation associated with Leber's hereditary optic neuropathy. Science 242: 1427–1430.

4. Sadun AA, Win PH, Ross-Cisneros FN, Walker SO, Carelli V (2000) Leber's hereditary optic neuropathy differentially affects smaller axons in the optic nerve. Trans Am Ophthalmol Soc 98: 223–232; discussion 232–225.

5. Johns DR, Smith KH, Miller NR (1992) Leber's hereditary optic neuropathy. Clinical manifestations of the 3460 mutation. Arch Ophthalmol 110: 1577–1581.

6. Mackey D, Howell N (1992) A variant of Leber hereditary optic neuropathy characterized by recovery of vision and by an unusual mitochondrial genetic etiology. Am J Hum Genet 51: 1218–1228.

7. Audoin B, Fernando KT, Swanton JK, Thompson AJ, Plant GT, et al. (2006) Selective magnetization transfer ratio decrease in the visual cortex following optic neuritis. Brain 129: 1031–1039.

8. Ciccarelli O, Toosy AT, Hickman SJ, Parker GJ, Wheeler-Kingshott CA, et al. (2005) Optic radiation changes after optic neuritis detected by tractography-based group mapping. Hum Brain Mapp 25: 308–316.

9. Yucel YH, Zhang Q, Weinreb RN, Kaufman PL, Gupta N (2003) Effects of retinal ganglion cell loss on magno-, parvo-, koniocellular pathways in the lateral geniculate nucleus and visual cortex in glaucoma. Prog Retin Eye Res 22: 465–481.

10. Kitajima M, Korogi Y, Hirai T, Hamatake S, Ikushima I, et al. (1997) MR changes in the calcarine area resulting from retinal degeneration. AJNR Am J Neuroradiol 18: 1291–1295.

11. von dem Hagen EA, Houston GC, Hoffmann MB, Jeffery G, Morland AB (2005) Retinal abnormalities in human albinism translate into a reduction of grey matter in the occipital cortex. Eur J Neurosci 22: 2475–2480.

12. Harding AE, Sweeney MG, Miller DH, Mumford CJ, Kellar-Wood H, et al. (1992) Occurrence of a multiple sclerosis-like illness in women who have a Leber's hereditary optic neuropathy mitochondrial DNA mutation. Brain 115(Pt 4): 979–989.

13. Nikoskelainen EK, Marttila RJ, Huoponen K, Juvonen V, Lamminen T, et al. (1995) Leber's "plus": neurological abnormalities in patients with Leber's hereditary optic neuropathy. J Neurol Neurosurg Psychiatry 59: 160–164.

14. Cortelli P, Montagna P, Avoni P, Sangiorgi S, Bresolin N, et al. (1991) Leber's hereditary optic neuropathy: genetic, biochemical, and phosphorus magnetic resonance spectroscopy study in an Italian family. Neurology 41: 1211–1215.

15. Barbiroli B, Montagna P, Cortelli P, Iotti S, Lodi R, et al. (1995) Defective brain and muscle energy metabolism shown by in vivo 31P magnetic resonance spectroscopy in nonaffected carriers of 11778 mtDNA mutation. Neurology 45: 1364–1369.

16. Lodi R, Carelli V, Cortelli P, Iotti S, Valentino ML, et al. (2002) Phosphorus MR spectroscopy shows a tissue specific in vivo distribution of biochemical expression of the G3460A mutation in Leber's hereditary optic neuropathy. J Neurol Neurosurg Psychiatry 72: 805–807.

17. Inglese M, Rovaris M, Bianchi S, La Mantia L, Mancardi GL, et al. (2001) Magnetic resonance imaging, magnetisation transfer imaging, and diffusion weighted imaging correlates of optic nerve, brain, and cervical cord damage in Leber's hereditary optic neuropathy. J Neurol Neurosurg Psychiatry 70: 444–449.

18. Damoiseaux JS, Beckmann CF, Arigita EJ, Barkhof F, Scheltens P, et al. (2008) Reduced resting-state brain activity in the "default network" in normal aging. Cereb Cortex 18: 1856–1864.

19. Damoiseaux JS, Rombouts SA, Barkhof F, Scheltens P, Stam CJ, et al. (2006) Consistent resting-state networks across healthy subjects. Proc Natl Acad Sci U S A 103: 13848–13853.

20. Beckmann CF, DeLuca M, Devlin JT, Smith SM (2005) Investigations into resting-state connectivity using independent component analysis. Philos Trans R Soc Lond B Biol Sci 360: 1001–1013.

21. Smith SM, Fox PT, Miller KL, Glahn DC, Fox PM, et al. (2009) Correspondence of the brain's functional architecture during activation and rest. Proc Natl Acad Sci U S A 106: 13040–13045.

22. Perrin M, Cointepas Y, Cachia A, Poupon C, Thirion B, et al. (2008) Connectivity-based parcellation of the cortical mantle using q-ball diffusion imaging. Int J Biomed Imaging 2008: 368406.

23. Johansen-Berg H, Behrens TE, Robson MD, Drobnjak I, Rushworth MF, et al. (2004) Changes in connectivity profiles define functionally distinct regions in human medial frontal cortex. Proc Natl Acad Sci U S A 101: 13335–13340.

24. Behrens TE, Johansen-Berg H, Woolrich MW, Smith SM, Wheeler-Kingshott CA, et al. (2003) Non-invasive mapping of connections between human thalamus and cortex using diffusion imaging. Nat Neurosci 6: 750–757.

25. Eickhoff SB, Stephan KE, Mohlberg H, Grefkes C, Fink GR, et al. (2005) A new SPM toolbox for combining probabilistic cytoarchitectonic maps and functional imaging data. Neuroimage 25: 1325–1335.

26. Mendola JD, Conner IP, Roy A, Chan ST, Schwartz TL, et al. (2005) Voxel-based analysis of MRI detects abnormal visual cortex in children and adults with amblyopia. Hum Brain Mapp 25: 222–236.

27. Boucard CC, Hernowo AT, Maguire RP, Jansonius NM, Roerdink JB, et al. (2009) Changes in cortical grey matter density associated with long-standing retinal visual field defects. Brain 132: 1898–1906.

28. De Volder AG, Bol A, Blin J, Robert A, Arno P, et al. (1997) Brain energy metabolism in early blind subjects: neural activity in the visual cortex. Brain Res 750: 235–244.

29. Barcella V, Rocca MA, Bianchi-Marzoli S, Milesi J, Melzi L, et al. (2010) Evidence for retro-chiasmatic tissue loss in Leber's hereditary optic neuropathy. Hum Brain Mapp.

30. Leclerc C, Saint-Amour D, Lavoie ME, Lassonde M, Lepore F (2000) Brain functional reorganization in early blind humans revealed by auditory event-related potentials. Neuroreport 11: 545–550.

31. Poirier C, Collignon O, Scheiber C, Renier L, Vanlierde A, et al. (2006) Auditory motion perception activates visual motion areas in early blind subjects. Neuroimage 31: 279–285.

32. Liu Y, Yu C, Liang M, Li J, Tian L, et al. (2007) Whole brain functional connectivity in the early blind. Brain 130: 2085–2096.

33. Calhoun VD, Adali T, Pearlson GD, Pekar JJ (2001) A method for making group inferences from functional MRI data using independent component analysis. Hum Brain Mapp 14: 140–151.

34. Herschkowitz N (2000) Neuroimaging bases of behavioral development in infancy. Brain Dev 22: 411–416.

35. Herschkowitz N, Kagan J, Zilles K (1997) Neurobiological bases of behavioral development in the first year. Neuropediatrics 28: 296–306.

36. Abu-Amero KK, Jaber M, Hellani A, Bosley TM (2010) Genome-wide expression profile of LHON patients with the 11778 mutation. Br J Ophthalmol 94: 256–259.

37. Rocca MA, Valsasina P, Ceccarelli A, Absinta M, Ghezzi A, et al. (2009) Structural and functional MRI correlates of Stroop control in benign MS. Hum Brain Mapp 30: 276–290.

38. Bell AJ, Sejnowski TJ (1995) An information-maximization approach to blind separation and blind deconvolution. Neural Comput 7: 1129–1159.

39. Himberg J, Hyvarinen A, Esposito F (2004) Validating the independent components of neuroimaging time series via clustering and visualization. Neuroimage 22: 1214–1222.

40. Harrison BJ, Pujol J, Ortiz H, Fornito A, Pantelis C, et al. (2008) Modulation of brain resting-state networks by sad mood induction. PLoS ONE 3: e1794.

41. Rocca MA, Valsasina P, Absinta M, Riccitelli G, Rodegher ME, et al. (2010) Default-mode network dysfunction and cognitive impairment in progressive MS. Neurology 74: 1252–1259.

42. Roosendaal SD, Schoonheim MM, Hulst HE, Sanz-Arigita EJ, Smith SM, et al. (2010) Resting state networks change in clinically isolated syndrome. Brain 133: 1612–1621.

43. Haselgrove JC, Moore JR (1996) Correction for distortion of echo-planar images used to calculate the apparent diffusion coefficient. Magn Reson Med 36: 960–964.

44. Morosan P, Rademacher J, Schleicher A, Amunts K, Schormann T, et al. (2001) Human primary auditory cortex: cytoarchitectonic subdivisions and mapping into a spatial reference system. Neuroimage 13: 684–701.

45. Smith SM (2002) Fast robust automated brain extraction. Hum Brain Mapp 17: 143–155.

46. Kaufman L, Rousseeuw PJ (1990) Finding Groups in Data: An Introduction to Cluster Analysis. Hoboken, NJ: John Wiley & Sons, Inc.

47. Rousseeuw PJ (1986) Silhouettes: a graphical aid to the interpretation and validation of cluster analysis. J Comp and Applied Mathematics 20: 53–65.

14

A Novel Cancer Vaccine Strategy based on HLA-A*0201 Matched Allogeneic Plasmacytoid Dendritic Cells

Caroline Aspord[1,2,3]*, Julie Charles[1,2,3,4], Marie-Therese Leccia[2,3,4], David Laurin[1,2,3], Marie-Jeanne Richard[2,3,5], Laurence Chaperot[1,2,3], Joel Plumas[1,2,3]*

1 Etablissement Français du Sang Rhone-Alpes, R&D Laboratory, La Tronche, France, 2 University Joseph Fourier, Grenoble, France, 3 INSERM, U823, Immunobiology & Immunotherapy of Cancers, La Tronche, France, 4 Centre Hospitalier Universitaire Grenoble, Michallon Hospital, Dermatology, pole pluridisciplinaire de medecine, Grenoble, France, 5 Centre Hospitalier Universitaire Grenoble, Michallon Hospital, Cancerology and Biotherapy, Grenoble, France

Abstract

Background: The development of effective cancer vaccines still remains a challenge. Despite the crucial role of plasmacytoid dendritic cells (pDCs) in anti-tumor responses, their therapeutic potential has not yet been worked out. We explored the relevance of HLA-A*0201 matched allogeneic pDCs as vectors for immunotherapy.

Methods and Findings: Stimulation of PBMC from HLA-A*0201[+] donors by HLA-A*0201 matched allogeneic pDCs pulsed with tumor-derived peptides triggered high levels of antigen-specific and functional cytotoxic T cell responses (up to 98% tetramer[+] CD8 T cells). The pDC vaccine demonstrated strong anti-tumor therapeutic in vivo efficacy as shown by the inhibition of tumor growth in a humanized mouse model. It also elicited highly functional tumor-specific T cells ex-vivo from PBMC and TIL of stage I-IV melanoma patients. Responses against MelA, GP100, tyrosinase and MAGE-3 antigens reached tetramer levels up to 62%, 24%, 85% and 4.3% respectively. pDC vaccine-primed T cells specifically killed patients' own autologous melanoma tumor cells. This semi-allogeneic pDC vaccine was more effective than conventional myeloid DC-based vaccines. Furthermore, the pDC vaccine design endows it with a strong potential for clinical application in cancer treatment.

Conclusions: These findings highlight HLA-A*0201 matched allogeneic pDCs as potent inducers of tumor immunity and provide a promising immunotherapeutic strategy to fight cancer.

Editor: Graham Pockley, University of Sheffield, United Kingdom

Funding: This work was supported by grants from the Institut National du Cancer (ACI-63-04 and canceropole 2004-05) and Etablissement Français du Sang. J. Charles was a recipient of grants from the National Academy of Medicine and canceropole 2004-05. The funders had no role in study design, data collection and analysis, decision to publish, or preparation of the manuscript.

Competing Interests: The authors have declared that no competing interests exist.

* E-mail: carolineaspord@yahoo.com (CA); joel.plumas@wanadoo.fr (JP)

Introduction

The development of effective vaccines for cancer treatment represents a major public health issue [1]. Because cytotoxic T lymphocytes (CTL) are able to recognize and lyse malignant cells, many therapeutic trials have been designed to potentiate CTL responses. Myeloid dendritic cells (mDC)-based vaccines succeeded in inducing specific T cells in patients but without sufficient clinical efficacy [2,3]. Adoptive cellular transfer of anti-tumor effector T cells amplified ex-vivo from TIL induced objective tumor regression [4,5], but the complexity of this strategy has hindered wide development. Therefore, there is a strong need for novel immunotherapeutic strategies to overcome the limitations of current protocols.

Up to now, the induction of specific T cell responses for both adoptive and active immunotherapeutic strategies has been based on mDCs [6–8]. Plasmacytoid dendritic cells (pDC) are however key players in immunity [9,10] with a role in tumor-specific immune responses [11]. pDCs differ from mDCs in many aspects such as TLR expression, migration profile and immune responses triggering. pDC are also capable of antigen capture, processing and presentation [12–15]. Antigen-pulsed pDC can stimulate

specific primary (MelA) and memory (Flu) autologous CD4 and CD8 T cell immune responses in vitro [16–19] and prime functional T cell responses in vivo as shown after vaccination of mice with CpG or virus-activated pDC [20–21]. pDC are found within many tumors in humans [22–26], where they are thought to be immature, tolerogenic or associated with poor prognosis. However, in melanoma, pDC activation by TLR-L could trigger potent anti-tumor effects. In mice, imiquimod application (TLR7-L) [27] or intratumoral injection of CpG (TLR9-L) [28] reversed the functional inhibition of pDC, thereby promoting tumor regression. Moreover local CpG administration in melanoma patients induced the recruitment and activation of pDC in sentinel lymph nodes [29] and subsequent tumor-specific CD8 T cells associated with clinical benefit [30]. The potential of pDC in generating effective tumor-specific immune responses has also been demonstrated in a mouse model [31]. pDC-based approaches and TLR agonists [32] are therefore promising for the treatment of human cancer.

Tumor antigens usually trigger weak responses. In contrast, allogeneic responses directed against non-self MHC are extremely potent. Interestingly, the allogeneic response mediated by MHC

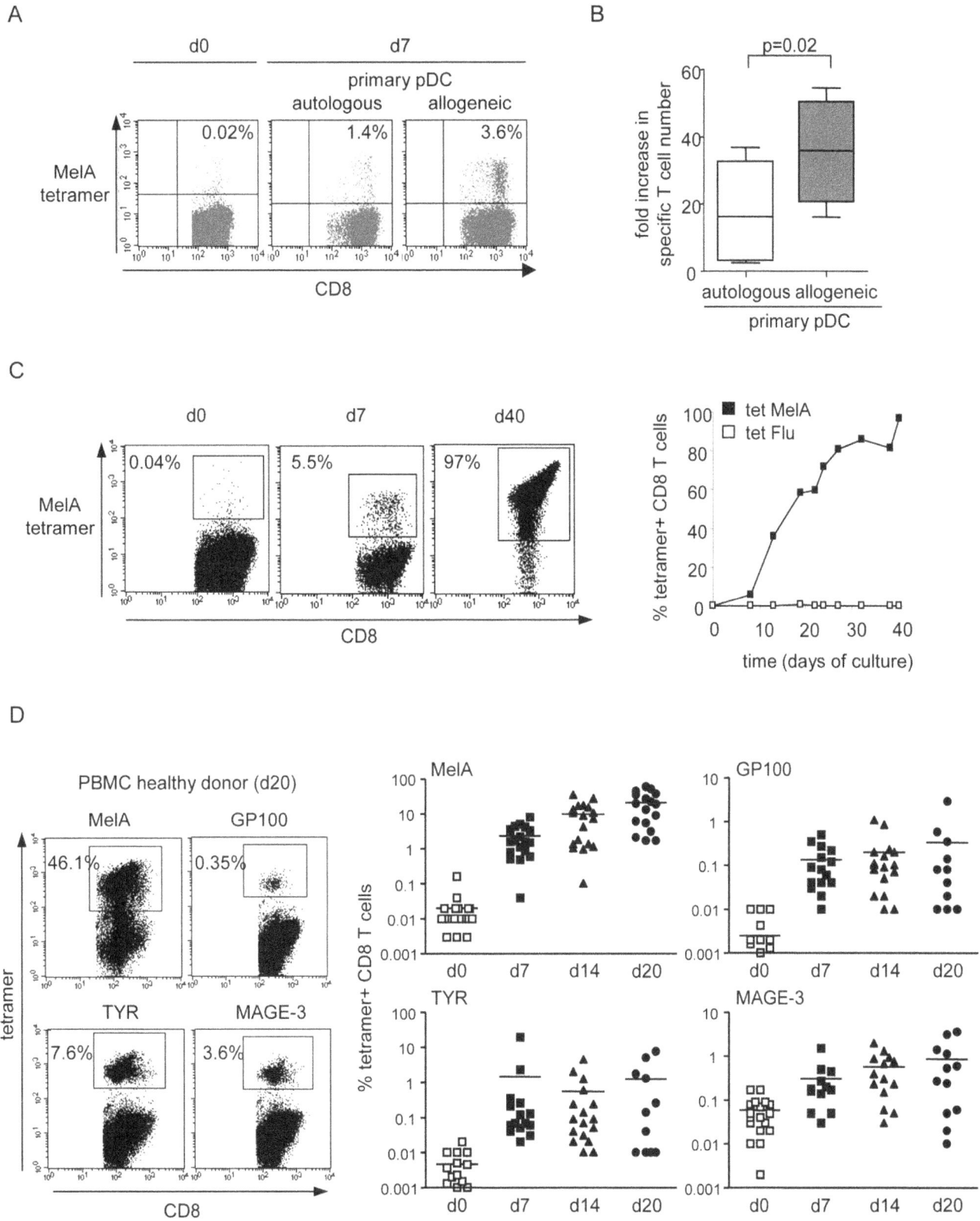

Figure 1. HLA-A*0201 matched allogeneic pDCs induce highly effective tumor-specific T cell responses from HLA-A*0201[+] healthy donors' PBMC in vitro. (A,B) Autologous or allogeneic HLA-A*0201[+] primary pDC sorted from the blood of healthy donors were pulsed with MelA peptide and used to stimulate HLA-A*0201[+] PBMC. The specific T cell response was analyzed at d7 by tetramer labelling. (A) Percentage of MelA specific T cells (gated on CD8+ T cells). One representative experiment is shown. (B) Amplification of the absolute number of specific T cells from d0 to d7 (4 independent experiments performed with 3 different donors). (C,D) allogeneic HLA-A*0201[+] PBMC from healthy donors were stimulated with the irradiated peptide-loaded HLA-A*0201[+] pDC line and weekly restimulated in the presence of IL2. Specificity of the T cells was determined by tetramer labelling and flow cytometry analysis. (C) Representative dotplots gated on CD8+ T cells (left panel) and percentages (right panel) of MelA

tetramer[+] T cells in the culture initially and at different time points after stimulation with the pDC line loaded with MelA peptide. Flu tetramer was used as control. (D) Representative dot plots gated on CD8+ T cells (left panel) and percentages of tetramer[+] CD8+ T cells obtained at days 7, 14 and 20 of the culture towards MelA (n = 18), GP100 (n = 16), TYR (n = 16) and MAGE-3 (n = 16) tumor antigens.

class II-restricted CD4+ T cells promotes bystander specific T cell induction [33,34] as already shown with viral peptides [35] and tumor regression following allogeneic skin graft [36]. Allogeneicity could therefore be exploited to promote immunogenicity towards tumor antigens [37] when considering a partial HLA match between the vaccine and the patient, further referred to as HLA matched allogeneicity.

Because pDCs play a fundamental role in triggering T cell responses, their use could be promising as new immunotherapeutic strategies. However, the use of autologous pDC for cancer immunotherapy is difficult because of the scarcity of these cells [38] and the possible functional alteration of pDCs harvested from tumor-bearing patients. We therefore explored the potential of HLA-A*0201 matched allogeneic pDC to induce HLA-A*0201-restricted anti-tumor immunity. We used a unique human pDC cell line (GEN) established from leukaemic HLA-A*0201[+] pDC with phenotypic and functional features closed to primary pDCs [39,40,41]. The strategy consisted of using the peptide-loaded pDCs to induce HLA-A*0201-restricted antigen-specific CTL. We demonstrate here using tumor and viral model antigens the potential of the irradiated peptide-pulsed human HLA-A*0201 matched allogeneic pDC line (GENiusVac) in vitro, its therapeutic efficacy in vivo in humanized mice, and its clinical relevance ex-vivo with melanoma patients' cells. Our findings highlight HLA-A*0201 matched allogeneic pDCs as potent inducers of anti-tumor immunity and provide a promising new immunotherapeutic strategy to fight cancer.

Materials and Methods

Cell lines and reagents

Cultures were performed in RPMI 1640 Glutamax supplemented with 1% non-essential amino acids, 1 mM sodium pyruvate (Sigma), 100 µg/ml gentamycin and 10% FCS (all from Invitrogen unless notified). Melanoma line Me275 was provided by Pr J-C Cerottini (Ludwig Institute for Cancer Research, Epalinges, Switzerland). Melanoma lines COLO829 and A375, T2 and K562 lines were purchased from ATCC (LGC Standards, Molsheim, France). Melanoma line Mel89 was generated in our laboratory (Figure S1). Anti-human CD45, CD3, CD8 Abs were purchased from Beckman Coulter. Anti-HLA-A2 Abs were purchased from BD Biosciences and anti- human MelA from Sigma.

Peptides and tetramers

We used the following viral- and tumor-derived HLA-A*0201 restricted peptides (NeoMPS) and the corresponding iTag HLA-A*0201 tetramers (Beckman Immunomics): MelA$_{26-35}$ (ELAGIGILTV), GP100$_{209-217}$ (IMDQVPFSV), tyrosinase$_{369-377}$ (YMDGTMSQV), MAGE-3$_{271-279}$ (FLWGPRALV), FluM1$_{58-66}$ (GILGFVFTL), CMVpp65$_{495-503}$ (NLVPMVATV).

PBMC, pDC line, primary pDC isolation and mDCs generation

Human PBMC were obtained from HLA-A*0201[+] healthy donors by Ficoll-Hypaque density gradient centrifugation (Eurobio). The human pDC line GEN2.2 was cultured as previously described [39]. Primary pDC were isolated from the blood of HLA-A*0201[+] healthy donors. DCs were first enriched by

depletion of unwanted cells using the Pan DC pre-enrichment kit (StemCell). Recovered cells were either submitted to BDCA4+ selection (Miltenyi) or labelled with a Lineage cocktail, CD123, HLA-DR and CD11c antibodies (BD) and sorted on a BD FACSAria on the basis of CD123 and HLA-DR expression and lack of Lin and CD11c markers. The purity of pDC after sort was over 98%. mDCs were differentiated from blood monocytes using 500 U/ml GM-CSF and 10 ng/ml IL-4 (TEBU Prepotech, France) for 6 days. This study was conducted under a procedure approved by the French Blood Agency Institutional Review Board. All donors signed informed consent forms.

Melanoma patient samples

Samples were obtained from stage I to IV HLA-A*0201 melanoma patients who signed informed consent forms. We used extra material that was not required for patients' diagnosis or analysis and didn't required supplementary procedures. Therefore in accordance with the French regulation, no ethic approval was required but information and signed consent of the patients. Clinical parameters are shown in Table S1. Blood samples were obtained from 12 patients and PBMC purified by gradient density. Fresh tumor samples were obtained from 6 patients who underwent surgery for in-transit metastasis. Samples were dilacerated and digested in 2 mg/ml collagenase D (Roche Diagnostics) 20 U/ml DNase (Sigma). Then tumor cells were isolated from the cell suspension by adherence and TIL enriched from the non-adherent fraction by density gradient.

Specific T cell response induction in vitro

GEN cells were first loaded with one or several peptide(s) of interest. Briefly, cells were washed 3 times with serum-free RPMI and resuspended at 1.10^6 cells/ml. β2-microglobulin (0.1 µg/ml final) (Sigma) and peptide(s) (1–10 µM final) (NeoMPS) were added. After 3 hours of incubation at 37°C, cells were washed twice, irradiated with 30Gy and resuspended at 2.10^5 cells/ml in RPMI with 10% FCS. Peptide-loaded GEN were then co-cultured with semi-allogeneic HLA-A*0201 PBMC at a 1:10 ratio in RPMI + 10% FCS for at least 7 days. Cultures were weekly restimulated with peptide-loaded GEN and 200 U/ml IL-2 (Proleukine; Chiron). In some experiments, unstimulated primary pDCs or mDCs matured with LPS (1 µg/ml) were used following the same conditions. In some experiments blocking anti-IFNα (50.000 U/ml) and anti-IFNβ (25.000 U/ml) antibodies (PBL Medical laboratories) or control goat IgG were added at day 0 and day 2 of culture. Specific CD8 T cell responses were measured by tetramer labelling of PBMC initially and at different steps of the culture. Cells were resuspended in HBSS with 2% FCS, stained with CD45 FITC, iTag HLA-A*0201 tetramer PE, CD3 PC7, CD8 APC antibodies and analyzed by flow cytometry analysis using a FACSCalibur and Cell Quest software (Becton Dickinson). To determine initial tetramer levels, at least $1–2.10^6$ events were acquired.

In vitro functional assays

IFNγ secretion and CD107 expression by tetramer+ CD8 T cells. T cells were first labelled with iTAg HLA-A*0201 tetramer PE for 30 min at RT, washed and restimulated with peptide-pulsed T2 cells (10:1 ratio) for 5 h30. For IFNγ secretion, 1 µl/ml brefeldin A (BD Biosciences) was added for the last 3 h.

A

MelA specific T cells

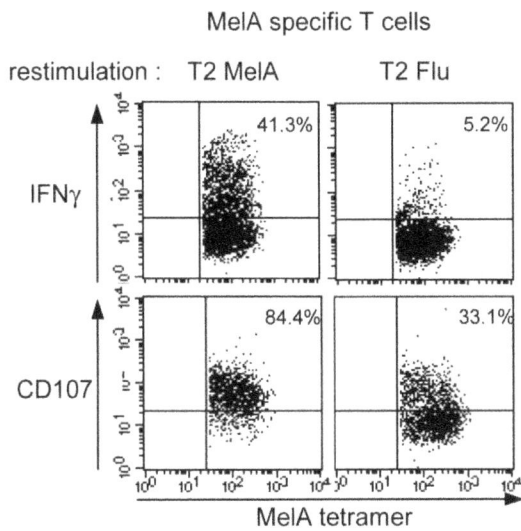

B

MelA specific T cells

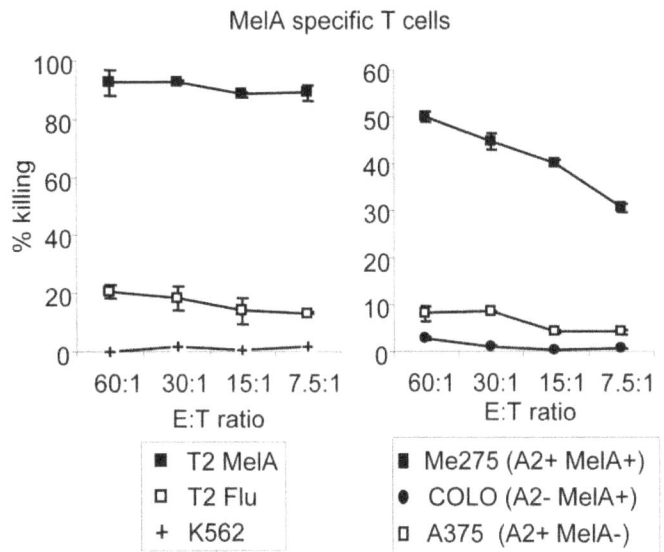

C

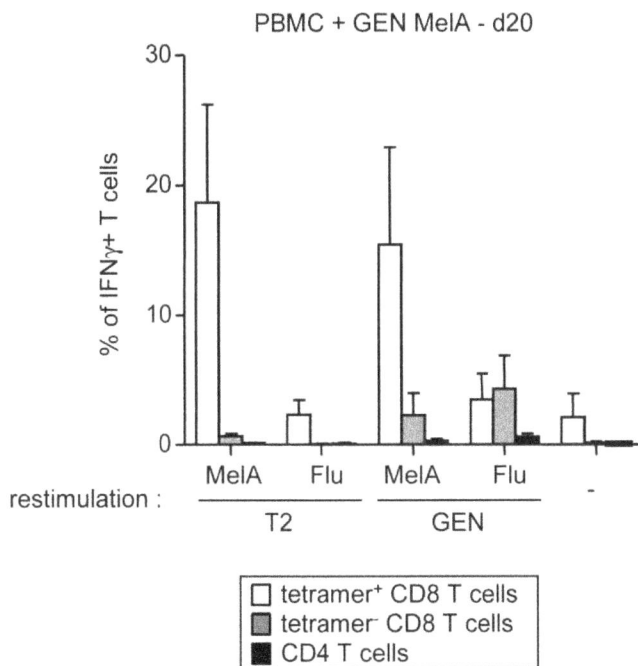

D

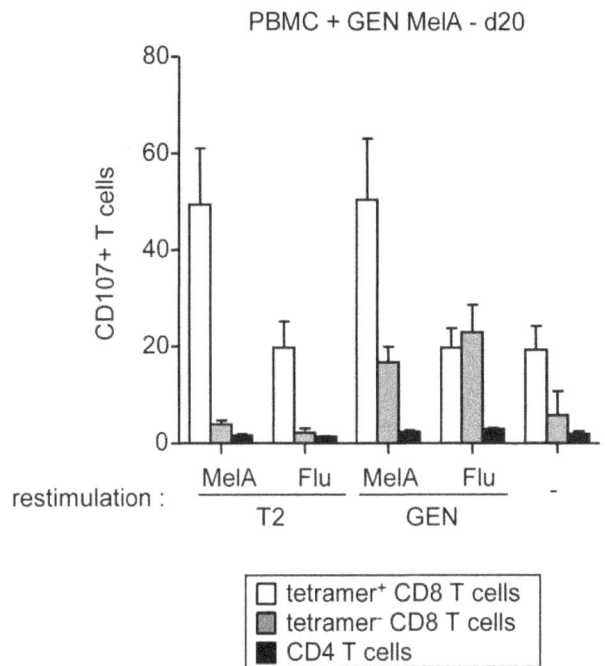

Figure 2. The tumor-specific T cells primed by the HLA-A*0201 matched allogeneic pDC line in vitro exhibited functional antigen- and HLA-A*0201-specific activity. (A) MelA-specific T cells induced by the pDC line secrete IFNγ and express CD107 on the surface upon specific restimulation. Cells from the culture (day 14) were submitted to tetramer labelling and restimulated with T2 cells pulsed with a relevant or control peptide. IFNγ production was assessed by intracellular staining and CD107 expression by adding anti-CD107a+b antibodies during the restimulation. Dotplots are gated on tetramer⁺ CD8+ T cells. Representative of 8 experiments performed with 3 donors at day 8–40 of the culture. (B) MelA-specific T cells induced by the pDC line are cytotoxic. T cells were selected from the culture and submitted to a ⁵¹Cr release assay using peptide-loaded T2 cells and melanoma tumor cells as targets. Representative of 8 experiments performed with 4 donors at d13–40 of the culture. (C,D) IFNγ secretion and CD107 expression were assessed as described in (A) after three stimulations of PBMC and analyzed on the tetramer⁺ CD8+ T cells (white bars) and on the non-specific tetramer⁻ CD8+ T cells (grey bars) and CD4+ T cells (black bars) upon restimulation with peptide-pulsed T2 or GEN cells (4 experiments for each condition).

A

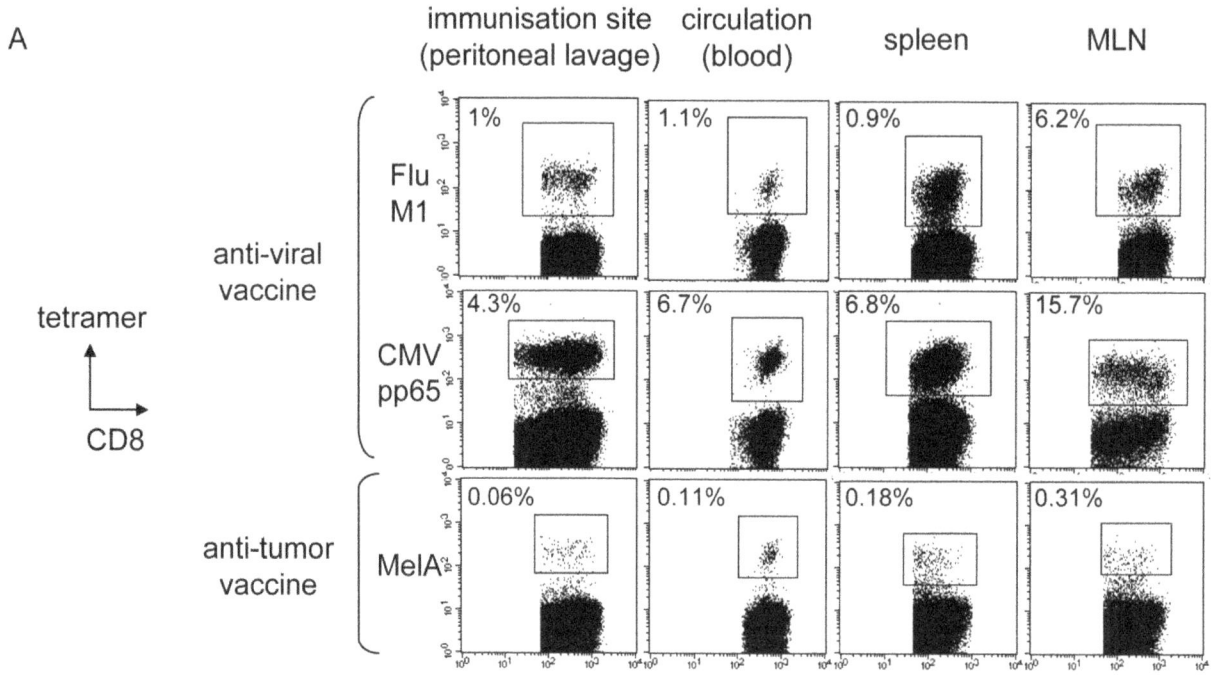

B

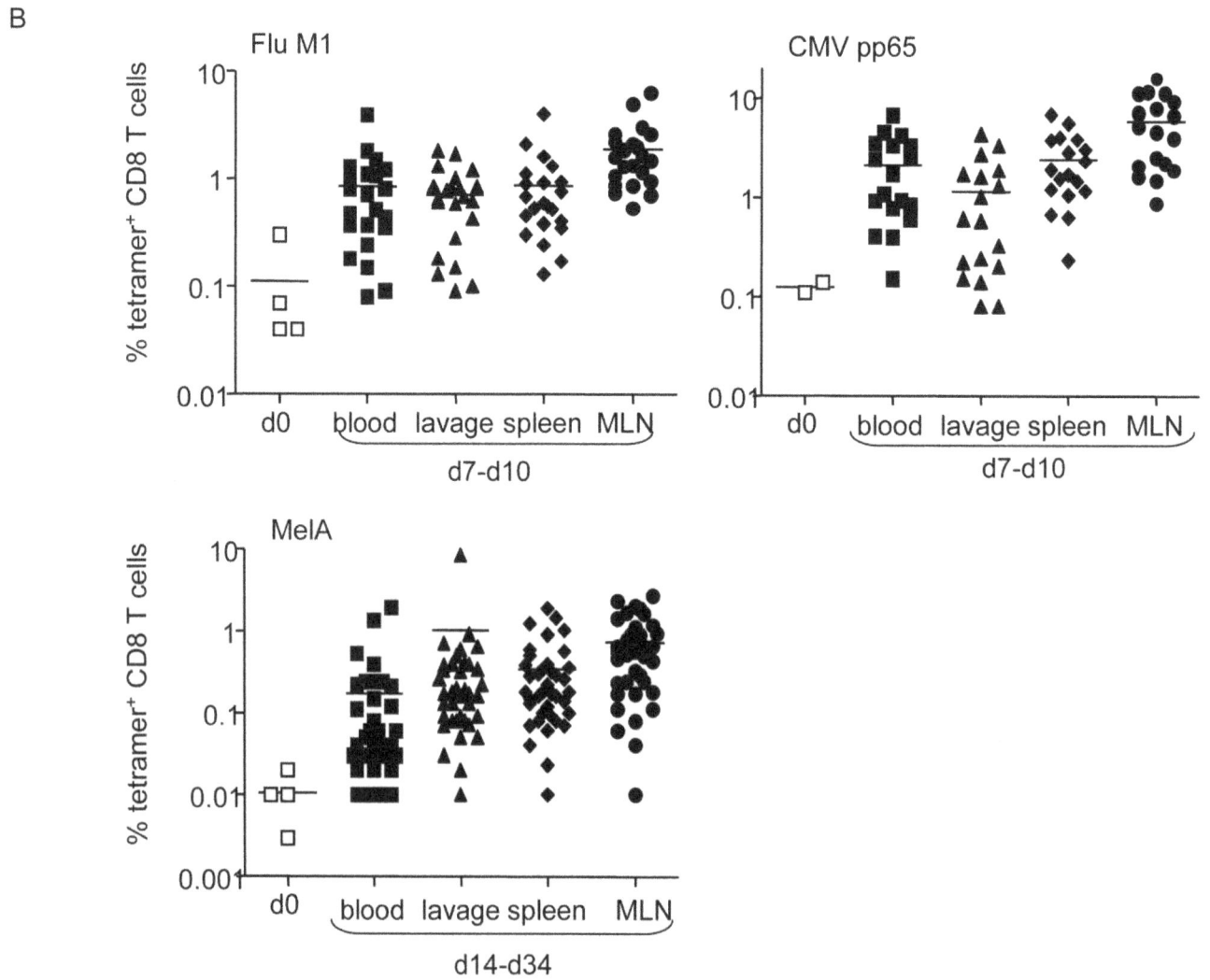

Figure 3. Vaccination with the peptide-loaded HLA-A*0201 matched allogeneic pDC line elicits strong antigen-specific T cell responses in humanized mice. (A-B) Immunodeficient NOD-SCIDβ$_2$m$^{-/-}$ mice were reconstituted intraperitoneally with 50.10^6 human HLA-A*0201$^+$ healthy donors' PBMC and vaccinated by the same route with 5.10^6 irradiated peptide-loaded GEN cells. Specific T cell induction was analyzed at the injection site (lavage), in the circulation (blood) and lymphoid organs (spleen, LN) by tetramer labelling of human T cells in cell suspensions. (A) Vaccination with peptide-loaded GEN cells induced specific T cell responses in vivo. Representative dot plots of tetramer labeled T cells induced after a single vaccination with peptide-loaded GEN cells in different organs at day 8 for anti-viral vaccine (Flu, CMV) and day 10 for anti-tumor vaccine (MelA) (gated on CD8$^+$ T cells). One mice per group is shown. Initial levels of specific T cells within PBMC were 0.04%, 0.14% and 0.003% respectively. (B) Levels of specific T cells before (day 0) and after vaccination with GEN loaded with FluM1 (n = 22 mice, 4 donors, 1 vaccine), CMVpp65 (n = 18 mice, 2 donors, 1 vaccine) and MelA (n = 38 mice, 4 donors, 2–3 vaccines) peptides at the indicated times in different organs. Each dot represents one vaccinated HuPBL mice (bars at mean).

Cells were then surface-labelled with anti-CD3 PC7 and anti-CD8 APC antibodies and submitted to IFNγ intracellular staining (BD Biosciences). For CD107 detection, anti-CD107a and CD107b FITC antibodies (10 µl/1.10^6 cells) (BD Biosciences) were added in the medium at the beginning of the restimulation in presence of Golgi STOP (0.67 µl/ml) for the last 4 h. Cells were then labelled with anti-CD3 PC7 and anti-CD8 APC antibodies. IFNγ and CD107 staining were analyzed on the tetramer$^+$ CD8+ T cells, tetramer$^-$ CD8+ T cells and CD4+ T cells.

Cytotoxicity assay. Antigen-specific cytotoxic activity was measured by performing a standard ^{51}Cr release assay. Effector T cells were sorted from the co-culture using an EasySep human T cell enrichment kit (Stem Cell). Target cells (peptide-pulsed T2 cells, K562, allogeneic or autologous tumor cells) were labeled with 50 µCi for 1 hour at 37°C, washed 3 times and plated with effector T cells at the indicated E:T ratio in round bottom 96-well plates. After 4 hours of incubation, radioactivity was measured on 30 µl of supernatants on a microplate scintillation counter Top Count NXT (Perkin Elmer). The mean of triplicate measurements was expressed as a percentage of specific lysis using the formula: (sample release − spontaneous release)/(maximal release − spontaneous release) ×100.

In vivo functional assays in humanized mice

NOD-SCID β$_2$m$^{-/-}$ immunodeficient mice (NOD.Cg-Prkdc^{SCID}β$_2$m^{Tm1Unc}/J) were purchased from Jackson ImmunoResearch Laboratories (Bar Harbor, USA) and bred at the Plateforme de Haute Technologie Animale (PHTA, La Tronche, France). For active therapy experiments, HuPBL mice were constructed by transplanting intraperitoneally (ip) 50.10^6 PBMC from healthy donors into sublethally irradiated NOD-SCID β$_2$m$^{-/-}$ mice (120–150 cGy). Mice were further vaccinated with 5.10^6 irradiated peptide-pulsed GEN cells by ip or sc routes once a week. Response to vaccination was analysed at different time points in blood, peritoneal lavage, spleen and lymph nodes. Organs were digested 30 min at 37°C with 2 mg/ml collagenase D (Roche Diagnostics). Resultant cell suspensions were washed with HBSS + 2% FCS, stained using the following anti-human antibodies (CD45 FITC, iTAg HLA-A*0201 tetramer PE, CD3 PC7, CD8 APC) and submitted to flow cytometry analysis. To assess therapeutic efficiency, 1.10^6 human tumor cells were implanted subcutaneously into the flank of the humanized mice either 5 days after (prophylactic) or 4 days before (therapeutic) the first vaccination. Vaccination was repeated every week. Tumor size was monitored every 2–3 days and tumor volume calculated using the formula: (short diameter)^2× long diameter/2. To analyse specific T cells at the tumor site and in DLN, tissues were digested as previously described and cell suspensions were submitted to tetramer labelling and flow cytometry analysis. All in-vivo experiments have been approved by the Regional Committee for Animal Ethic Rhone-Alpes (CREEA) affiliated to the CNRS.

Statistical analysis

The statistical analyses were performed by using Mann-Whitney non parametric U test and unpaired t test using Prism software.

Results

Human HLA matched allogeneic pDCs induce antigen-specific T cell responses from healthy donor PBMC with a strong efficacy in vitro

To investigate the potential of HLA matched allogeneic pDC in antigen-specific T cell responses induction, we compared the ability of peptide-loaded primary pDC sorted from healthy donors' blood to induce specific T cell responses in autologous and allogeneic HLA-A*0201-matched settings. pDC led to a significantly higher specific T cell induction in HLA-A*0201 matched allogeneic settings compared to autologous conditions (amplification of the absolute number of MelA-specific T cells in 7 days: 35.6±8.9 vs 17.9±8.7, mean±SEM, p = 0.02) (Figure 1A and 1B, four experiments performed with three different donors). As the scarcity of primary pDC prevents their wide therapeutic use, we used the human pDC cell line (GEN) established from leukaemic HLA-A*0201$^+$ pDC as a source of HLA-A*0201 matched allogeneic pDCs. To assess whether the irradiated HLA-A*0201$^+$ pDC line can induce specific T cell responses like primary pDC in vitro, allogeneic HLA-A*0201$^+$ PBMC from healthy donors were stimulated with the irradiated peptide-loaded GEN cells. For both tumor (MelA) and viral (Flu)-derived peptides, we obtained a massive amplification of specific T cells after only 7 days of culture as detected by tetramer labelling (Figure 1C, Figure S2). This induction was further enhanced by serial stimulations every 7 days with the peptide-loaded pDC line, in combination with IL-2. We routinely obtained 5–25% of tetramer$^+$ CD8 T cells after 7 days, 40–60% after 15 days, and up to 98% after 40 days (Figure 1C). Such high responses were reproduced with cells from 14–20 healthy donors and with various melanoma tumor-derived antigens such as MelA, GP100, TYR, MAGE-3 (Figure 1D) as well as virus-derived antigens (Figure S2). Tumor-specific tetramer$^+$ T cell responses reached averages of 22% for MelA (range 2–60%), 0.3% for GP100 (range 0–3%), 1.2% for TYR (range 0–8%) and 0.84% for MAGE-3 (range 0–4%) in 20 days. Multi-specific responses were also induced using GEN cells loaded with several different peptides (not shown). Thus, HLA matched allogeneic primary pDCs or the pDC line elicit strong primary and memory antigen-specific T cell responses in vitro from healthy donors.

The specific T cells induced by HLA matched allogeneic pDC exhibited in vitro functional HLA-restricted activity

We further examined the functionality of the specific T cells induced by the HLA-A*0201 matched allogeneic pDC line. We first analyzed the ability of tumor-specific T cells to secrete IFNγ and express CD107 upon restimulation. When co-cultured with

A
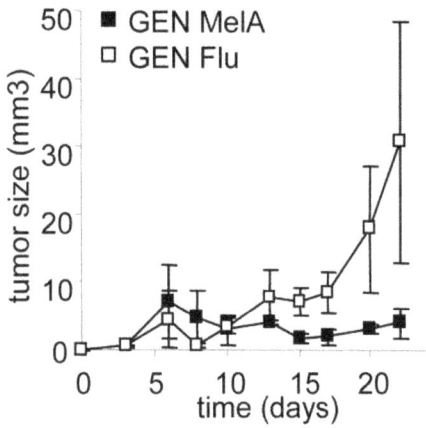

B
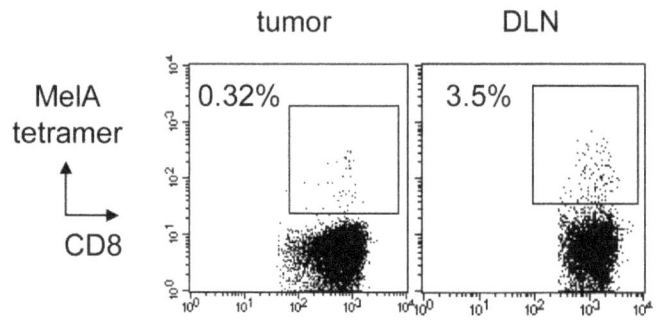

C
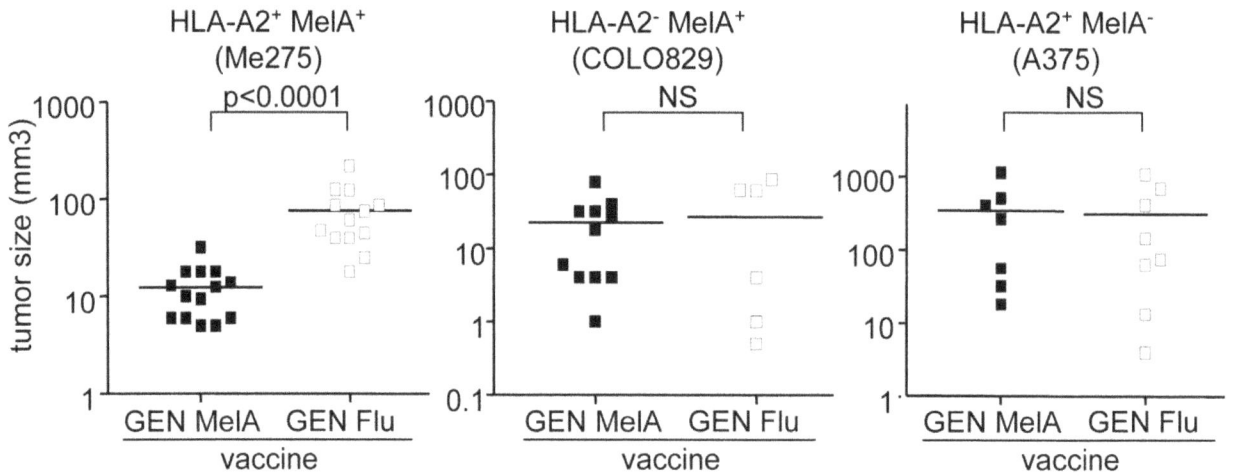

D
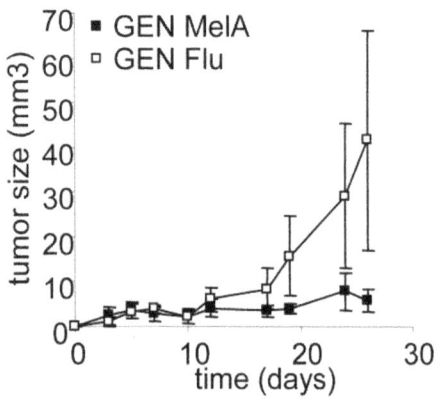

E
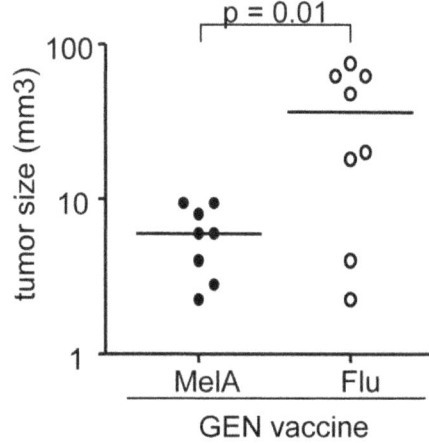

F
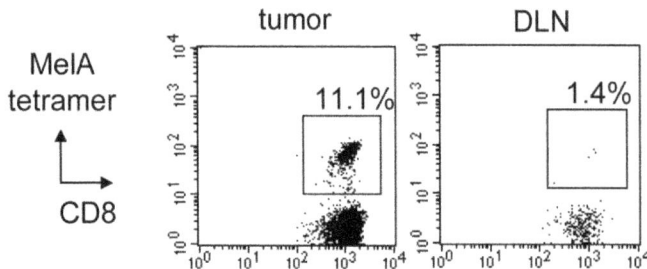

Figure 4. Vaccination with the peptide-loaded HLA-A*0201 matched allogeneic pDC line protect humanized mice from tumor development both prophylactically and therapeutically. (A-C) Immunodeficient NOD-SCID $\beta_2 m^{-/-}$ mice reconstituted intraperitoneally with human HLA-A*0201$^+$ PBMC (HuPBL mice) were weekly vaccinated subcutaneously with irradiated MelA or Flu-loaded GEN cells and challenged 5 days later with melanoma tumor cells in the flank. (A) Follow up of tumor progression. One experiment representative of 5. (B) Tetramer labelling of tumor and draining LN cell suspensions from HuPBL mice vaccinated with MelA-loaded GEN cells showing the presence of MelA-specific T cells (gated on CD8+ T cells). (C) The therapeutic effects of the vaccine are HLA-A*0201-restricted and antigen-specific. Comparative tumor size 27 days after implantation of Me275, COLO829 and A375 melanoma cells into HuPBL mice vaccinated with MelA or Flu-loaded GEN cells (pool of 3 independent experiments for each tumor type performed with 6 to 14 mice per group). (D-F) Immunodeficient NOD-SCID $\beta_2 m^{-/-}$ mice reconstituted intraperitoneally with human HLA-A*0201$^+$ PBMC (HuPBL mice) were first challenged with melanoma Me275 tumor cells in the flank and then vaccinated subcutaneously with irradiated MelA or Flu-loaded GEN cells weekly starting 4 days later. (D) Follow up of tumor progression. One representative experiment out of 2. (E) Comparative tumor size 25 days after tumor implantation (pool of 2 independent experiments, 8 mice/group). (F) Tetramer labelling of tumor and draining LN cell suspensions from HuPBL mice vaccinated with MelA-loaded GEN cells showing the presence of MelA-specific T cells (gated on CD8+ T cells).

peptide-loaded T2 cells, MelA-specific T cells secreted IFNγ and expressed CD107 in the presence of the relevant but not control peptide (Figure 2A). We obtained within tumor-reactive T cells averages of 25% IFNγ$^+$ tetramer$^+$ CD8 T cells upon specific restimulation compared to 5% under control conditions (p = 0.007), and 50% CD107$^+$ tetramer$^+$ CD8 T cells upon specific restimulation compared to 24% under control conditions (p = 0.02) (data not shown). We next tested their cytotoxicity by performing ^{51}Cr release assay using peptide-loaded T2 cells and melanoma tumor lines as targets. MelA-specific T cells exhibited a strong cytotoxic activity towards T2 cells loaded with the relevant but not with control peptide (Figure 2B). We obtained 88% of specific killing versus 13% under control conditions (mean of 8 experiments, p<0.001) (not shown). In addition, MelA-specific T cells were able to lyse HLA-A*0201$^+$MelA$^+$ (Me275) but neither HLA-A*0201$^+$MelA$^-$ (A375) nor HLA-A*0201$^-$MelA$^+$ (COLO829) melanoma tumor cells (Figure 2B, Figure S1) demonstrating the HLA-A*0201-restriction and antigen specificity of this activity. Furthermore, this lysis was inhibited by EGTA-MgCl2 or by CD8 T cell depletion (not shown), which together with CD107 surface expression upon specific restimulation, suggests a mechanism involving cytolytic granule exocytosis from CD8 T cells. Such functional capacities were observed with T cells taken at different timepoints of the 7–40 day culture. Similar analysis performed with virus-specific T cells demonstrated the capacity of Flu tetramer$^+$ T cells to secrete IFNγ and express CD107 upon specific restimulation, and their cytotoxic properties (Figures S3A and S3B). Importantly, we observed only a minor allogeneic response induction as attested by the poor activation of non-specific tetramer$^-$ CD8+ T cells and CD4+ T cells towards GEN cells. This was observed after one stimulation (Flu response) (Figure S3C and S3D) but also after repeated stimulations with the pDC line (MelA response), by measuring IFNγ-secreting (Figure 2C) and CD107-expressing T cells (Figure 2D) upon restimulation with T2 or GEN cells. We also observed the absence of the tetramer$^+$ T cell activity towards GEN cells loaded with an irrelevant peptide. Thus, the pDC line elicits fully functional antigen-specific T cells with minor bystander allogeneic responses.

The peptide-loaded HLA matched allogeneic pDC line elicits strong in vivo antigen-specific T cell responses in humanized mice

The use of HLA matched allogeneic pDCs as a vaccine requires induction of antigen-specific T cell responses in vivo. Therefore we evaluated the vaccine potential of the pDC line in a humanized mouse model [42] constructed by xenotransplanting human PBMC into immunodeficient NOD-SCIDβ2m$^{-/-}$ mice (HuPBL SCID model). Twenty four hours after intraperitoneal transfer, human CD45$^+$ haematopoietic cells were found at the injection site but also in the circulation and lymphoid organs (not

shown). A single intra-peritoneal injection of the irradiated peptide-loaded HLA-A*0201 matched allogeneic pDC line induced strong antigen-specific T cell responses towards viral (FluM1, CMVpp65) and tumor (MelA) antigens in HuPBL mice (Figure 3A). Human tetramer$^+$ CD8 T cells were found not only at the site of immunization (peritoneal lavage) but also in the circulation (blood) and lymphoid organs (spleen, lymph nodes) (Figure 3A). We then evaluated whether several weekly injections of the peptide-pulsed pDC line could enhance the level of the response. Interestingly, viral antigen (Flu) induced a high response that peaked 7 days after the first vaccine and decreased afterwards, whereas response to tumor antigen (MelA) kept increasing upon subsequent restimulations (Figure S4). Within all vaccinated HuPBL mice (n = 22, 18 and 38) reconstituted with human PBMC (baseline levels of tetramer+ CD8+ T cells were 0.11% (FluM1), 0.12% (CMVpp65) and 0.01% (MelA) tetramer$^+$ T cells) levels of specific T cells recovered in the different organs ranged from 0.7 to 1.9% for FluM1, 1.1 to 5.9% for CMVpp65, and 0.2 to 1% for MelA (Figure 3B). Thus, the peptide-pulsed pDC line elicits strong and widespread antigen-specific T cell responses in vivo.

Vaccination with the peptide-loaded HLA matched allogeneic pDC line protect humanized mice from tumor progression in both prophylactic and therapeutic settings

We next investigated the therapeutic potential of this strategy in humanized mice further engrafted with human tumor. NOD-SCIDβ2m$^{-/-}$ mice were reconstituted intra-peritoneally with human HLA-A*0201$^+$ PBMC and weekly vaccinated subcutaneously with irradiated peptide-pulsed GEN cells before or after being challenged with melanoma tumor cells. In a prophylactic setting, injection of HuPBL mice with MelA-loaded GEN cells, compared to Flu-loaded GEN cells, inhibited HLA-A*0201$^+$MelA$^+$ tumor growth (Me275) in five independent experiments (tumor size at day 27 = 12 vs 77 mm^3, p<0.0001) (Figure 4A and 4C). By contrast, the growth of HLA-A*0201$^-$MelA$^+$ (COLO829) and HLA-A*0201$^+$MelA$^-$ (A375) melanoma tumors was not affected after injection of MelA or Flu-loaded GEN cells in three independent experiments (Figure 4C), demonstrating the HLA-A*0201-restriction and antigen specificity of the therapy. Moreover, the peptide-loaded pDC also provoke protective immune responses against already established tumors. Vaccination of tumor-bearing HuPBL mice with MelA-loaded GEN cells inhibited tumor growth compared to Flu-loaded GEN cells (tumor size at day 25 = 6 vs 36mm^3, p = 0.01) (Figure 4D-4F). Notably, tetramer$^+$ CD8+ T cells were found at the tumor site and in the draining LN (Figures 4B and 4F), suggesting that the tumor-reactive T cells induced by the HLA

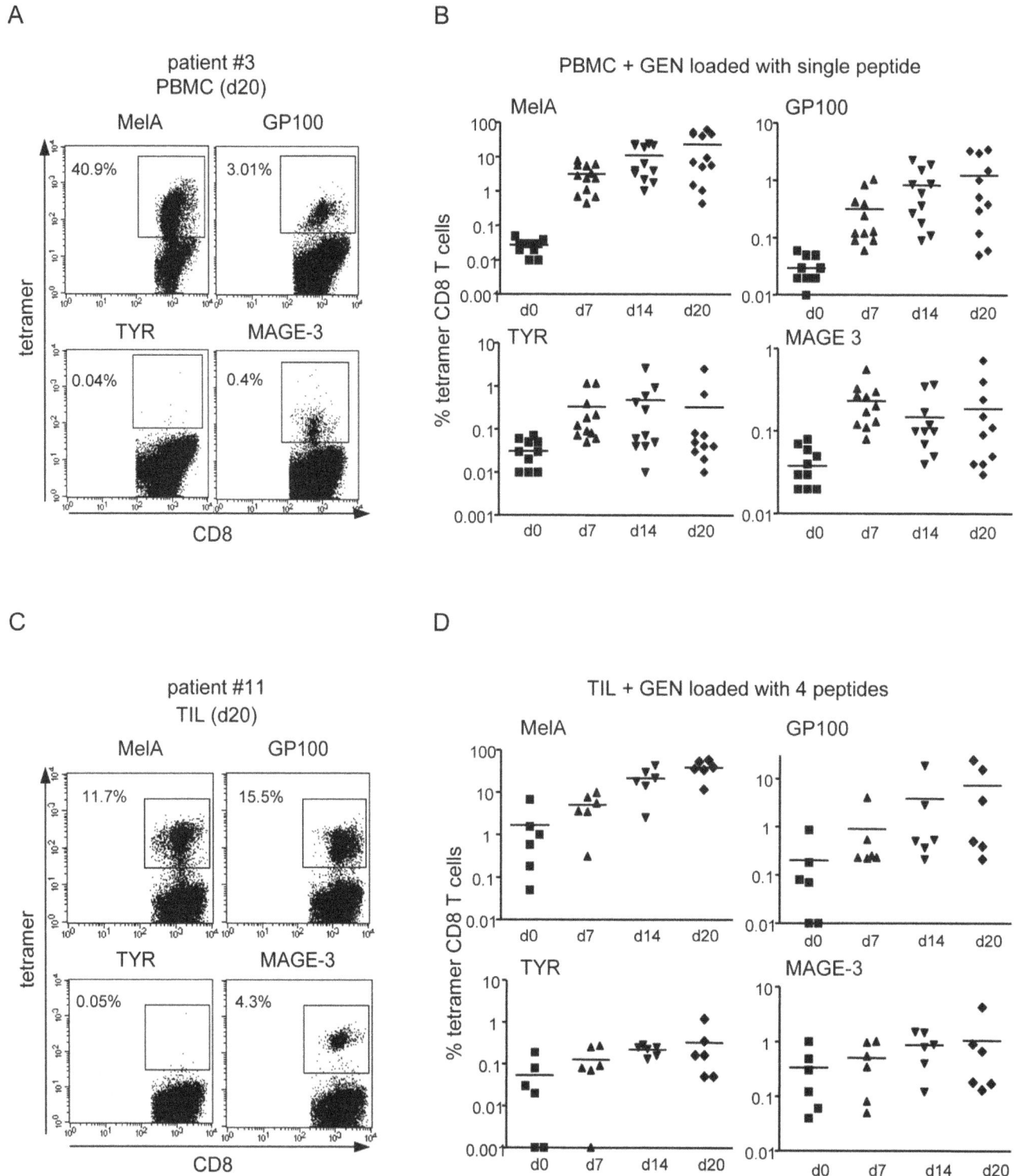

Figure 5. The HLA-A*0201 matched allogeneic pDC line loaded with melanoma-derived peptides induces multi-specific T cell responses ex-vivo from stage I-IV melanoma patients. PBMC (n = 12) and TIL (n = 6) obtained from stage I-IV HLA-A*0201+ melanoma patients were cultured with irradiated GEN cells loaded with MelA, GP100, TYR and/or MAGE-3 derived peptides and restimulated every 7 days. Percentages of specific T cells were determined by tetramer labelling after culture of PBMC with single peptide-loaded GEN cells (A,B) and of TIL with GEN loaded with a mix of the 4 peptides (C,D). Representative experiments with PBMC (A) and TIL (C) are shown at day 20 of the culture. Results from PBMC and TIL cohorts are shown in (B) and (D) at days 0, 7, 14 and 20 of culture. For TYR (D), one patient was excluded due to an extremely intense response (see Figure S5).

A

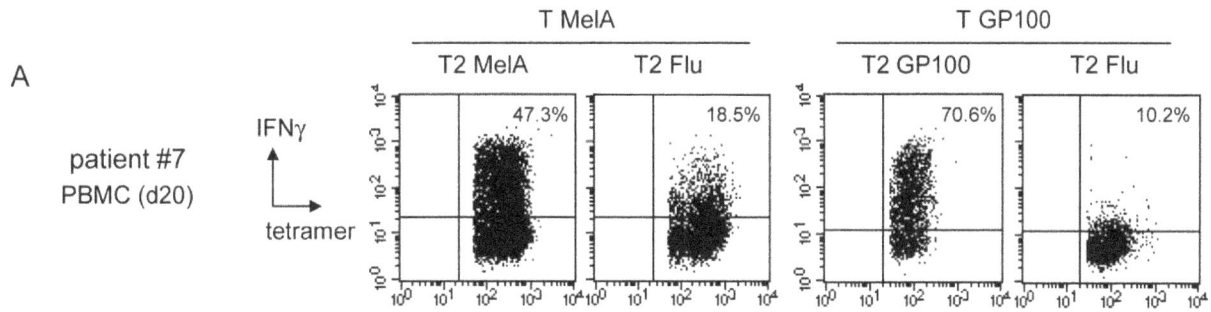

B

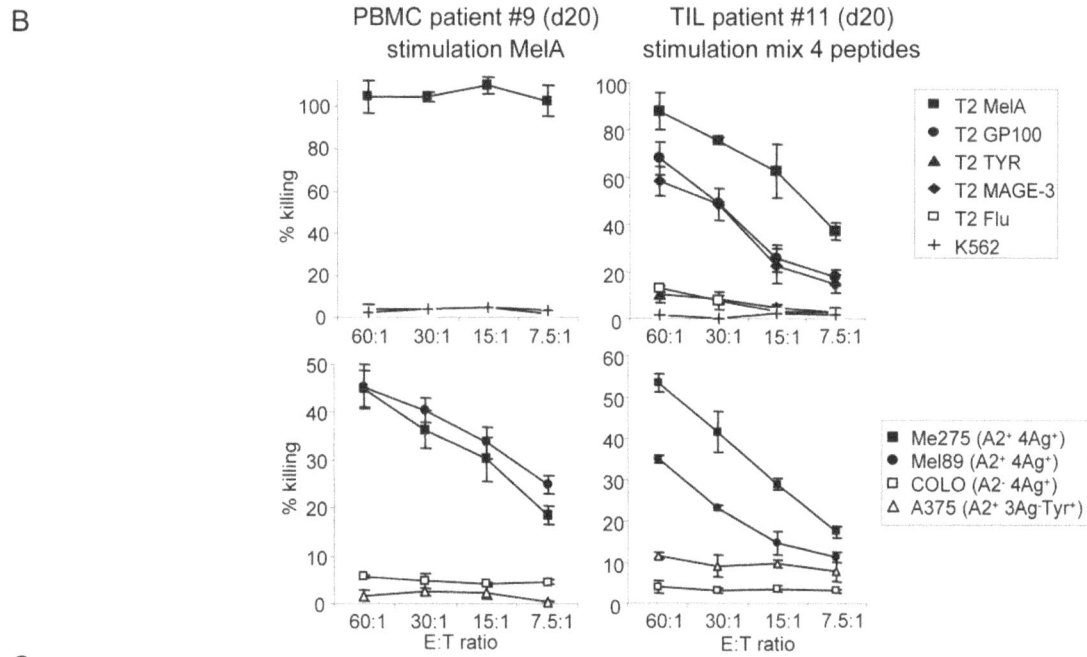

C

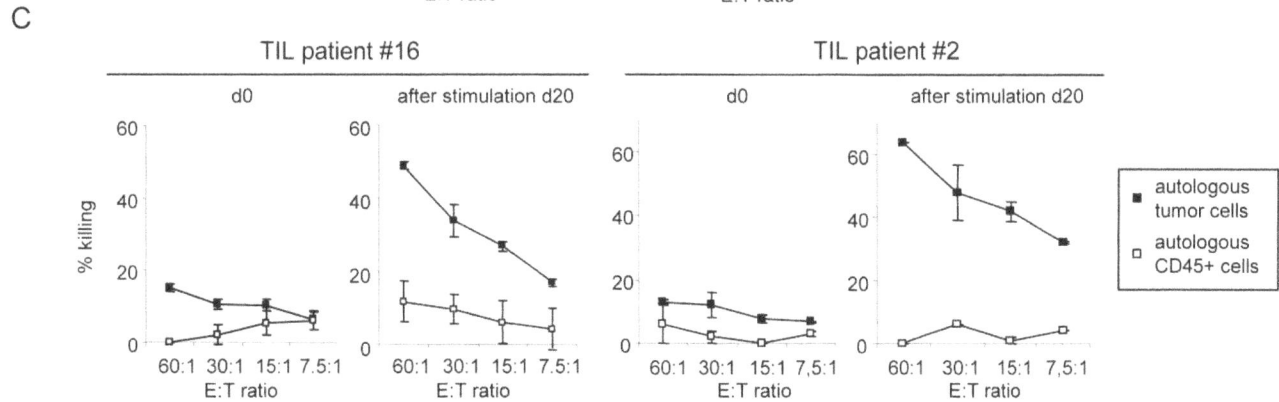

D

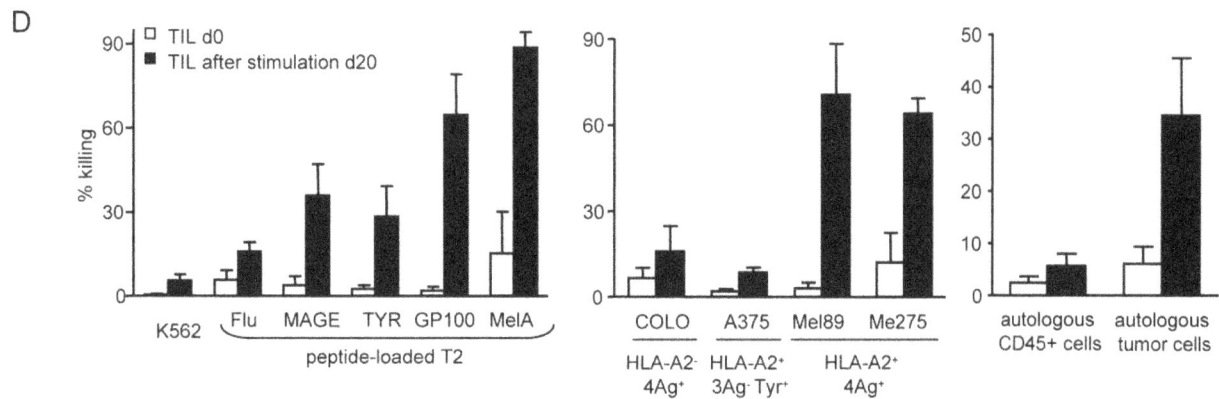

Figure 6. The melanoma patients' tumor-specific T cells induced by the HLA-A*0201 matched allogeneic pDC line are highly cytotoxic and lyse autologous melanoma tumor cells. Tumor-specific T cells induced by the pDC line loaded with melanoma-derived peptides from melanoma patients' PBMC and TIL are highly functional in an HLA-A*0201 and antigen-specific manner. (A) Tetramer[+] T cells specifically secreted IFNγ upon restimulation with T2 cells pulsed with the relevant peptide. Representative of 6 PBMC and 2 TIL samples. (B-D) T cells exhibited cytotoxicity towards allogeneic and autologous melanoma tumor cells and relevant peptide-pulsed T2 cells. T cells induced from PBMC or TIL were purified from days 15–20 cultures and used in a ^{51}Cr release assay against peptide-loaded T2 cells, allogeneic and autologous melanoma tumor cells, and autologous CD45[+] cells. (B) The PBMC sample shown was stimulated with MelA-loaded GEN cells. The TIL sample shown was stimulated with GEN cells loaded with a mixture of 4 peptides and developed a response towards MelA, GP100 and MAGE-3 antigens (see Figure 5C). Representative of 12 PBMC and 6 TIL samples. (C) Percentage of killing of autologous tumor cells compared to autologous CD45[+] cells by TIL before and after stimulation. Representative of 6 TIL samples. (D) Comparison of the killing capacity between unstimulated and stimulated TIL on the indicated targets at a 60:1 ratio. Mean+/-SEM of 6 TIL samples.

matched allogeneic pDC had migrated to the site of antigen expression and the T cells were capable of killing tumor cells.

The HLA matched allogeneic pDC line loaded with melanoma-derived peptides induces multi-specific and highly functional T cell responses ex-vivo from stage I-IV melanoma patients

We next investigated the relevance of this strategy in cancer patients. We tested the capacity of the peptide-pulsed pDC line to trigger ex-vivo tumor-specific responses from PBMC and tumor-infiltrating lymphocytes (TIL) isolated from stage I-V HLA-A*0201[+] melanoma patients (Tables S1 and S2). Weekly stimulations of patients' PBMC with the pDC line pulsed either with MelA, GP100, TYR or MAGE-3 peptide led to the massive amplification of specific CD8+ T cells for at least 2 out of 4 melanoma antigens (Figures 5A and 5B). The tumor-specific tetramer[+] CD8 T cell responses reached averages of 23% for MelA (range 0.4–62%), 1.2% for GP100 (range 0.05–3.5%), 0.3% for TYR (range 0.01–2.5%) and 0.2% for MAGE-3 (range 0.03–0.72%) after 20 days (baseline tetramer+ CD8+ T cells ranged from 0.02 to 0.03% at d0). One patient was excluded from the analysis due to an extremely intense response (85% tetramer[+] T cells at day 14) towards TYR (Figure S5). Furthermore, repeated stimulations of patients'TIL with the pDC line pulsed with a mix of the 4 melanoma peptides led to the massive amplification of specific T cells for at least 3 antigens (Figures 5C and 5D). Tumor-specific tetramer[+] CD8 T cell responses reached averages of 39% for MelA (range 12–59%), 7.4% for GP100 (range 0.2–24%), 0.3% for TYR (range 0.05–1.2%) and 1.1% for MAGE-3 (range 0.1–4.3%) after 20 days with baseline levels format day 0 1.7, 0.2, 0.05 and 0.3%, respectively. The tumor-specific T cells induced from both PBMC (Figure 6A) and TIL (not shown) secreted IFNγ when co-cultured with T2 cells loaded with the relevant but not with a control peptide. We obtained a mean of 42% of IFNγ[+] tetramer[+] CD8 T cells upon specific peptide restimulation compared to 11% in control conditions (n = 12, p = 0.0002, data not shown). Furthermore, these T cells exhibited a strong cytotoxic activity towards T2 cells loaded with relevant but not with control peptides and allogeneic melanoma tumor cells in an HLA-A*0201-restricted and antigen-specific manner (Figure 6B). Strikingly, after stimulation with the pDC line loaded with a mix of four melanoma-derived peptides, TIL acquired the ability to lyse autologous tumor cells but not CD45[+] hematopoietic cells from the patient (Figure 6C). When comparing the killing capacity of unstimulated and stimulated TIL, the pDC line greatly enhanced their cytotoxic activity towards peptide-loaded T2 cells, semi-allogeneic melanoma tumor lines and autologous tumor cells (Figure 6D). Thus, the HLA- matched allogeneic pDC line loaded with melanoma-derived peptides induces multi-specific and highly functional ex-vivo T cell responses from stage I-IV melanoma patients.

The HLA matched allogeneic pDCs are more potent at inducing tumor-specific T cells than conventional autologous or HLA matched allogeneic mDCs

We next compared the T cell stimulatory capacity of the pDC line against conventional mDCs in autologous and semi-allogeneic settings. HLA-A*0201[+] PBMC from healthy donors were stimulated with irradiated peptide-loaded GEN cells, HLA-A*0201[+] allogeneic mDCs or autologous mDCs. The virus-specific (FluM1) and tumor-specific (MelA) responses elicited respectively after a single or three stimulations were higher when using GEN cells compared to allogeneic or autologous mDCs (Figure 7A-7D). Similarly, stimulation of TIL from melanoma patients with GEN cells led to a more potent induction of tumor-specific T cells than semi-allogeneic mDCs in respect to both tetramer+ T cell percentage (Figures 8A and 8B) and fold increase in absolute number of specific T cells (Figure 8C). Notably, the pDC line elicited specific T cells with better functional qualities, as assessed by more potent CTL activity towards autologous tumor cells from melanoma patients, compared to the T cells induced by conventional HLA matched allogeneic mDCs (Figures 8D and 8E). Thus, the induction of specific T cell responses by the pDC line is much more potent compared to that elicited by autologous or HLA matched allogeneic myeloid DCs.

In order to investigate the mechanism of the high efficiency of the pDC line, we analysed changes in the activation level of the pDCs. The 30Gy irradiation provided to the pDC line induced a strong activation of the cells as demonstrated by the upregulation of costimulatory molecules (CD40, CD80, CD86), upregulation of MHC-I molecules (Figure S6). In addition, by using IFNαβ blocking antibodies, we observed that the induction of specific T cell responses by the pDC line was not abrogated, suggesting a type I IFN independent mechanism (Figure S7). We also addressed the comparative avidity of the specific T cells elicited by the pDC line or mDCs by measuring their cytotoxic activity upon stimulation with titrated peptide-MHC complexes. We observed that the specific T cells elicited by the pDCs kept the same level of functionality towards T2 target cells loaded with up to 0.01 μM whereas the specific T cells elicited by allogeneic mDCs displayed a 50% reduced functionality at this peptide concentration (Figure S8). Therefore, the pDCs elicited high avidity specific T cells.

Discussion

pDCs can act as antigen presenting cells and they have been demonstrated to play a role in tumor-specific responses [43]. However, the potential for pDCs in clinical application has not yet been worked out. In this study, we explored the feasibility of peptide-loaded HLA matched allogeneic pDC to induce tumor immunity. We demonstrate here the strong potential of this strategy in inducing multi-specific and highly functional CD8+ T cell responses from healthy donors as well as cancer patients.

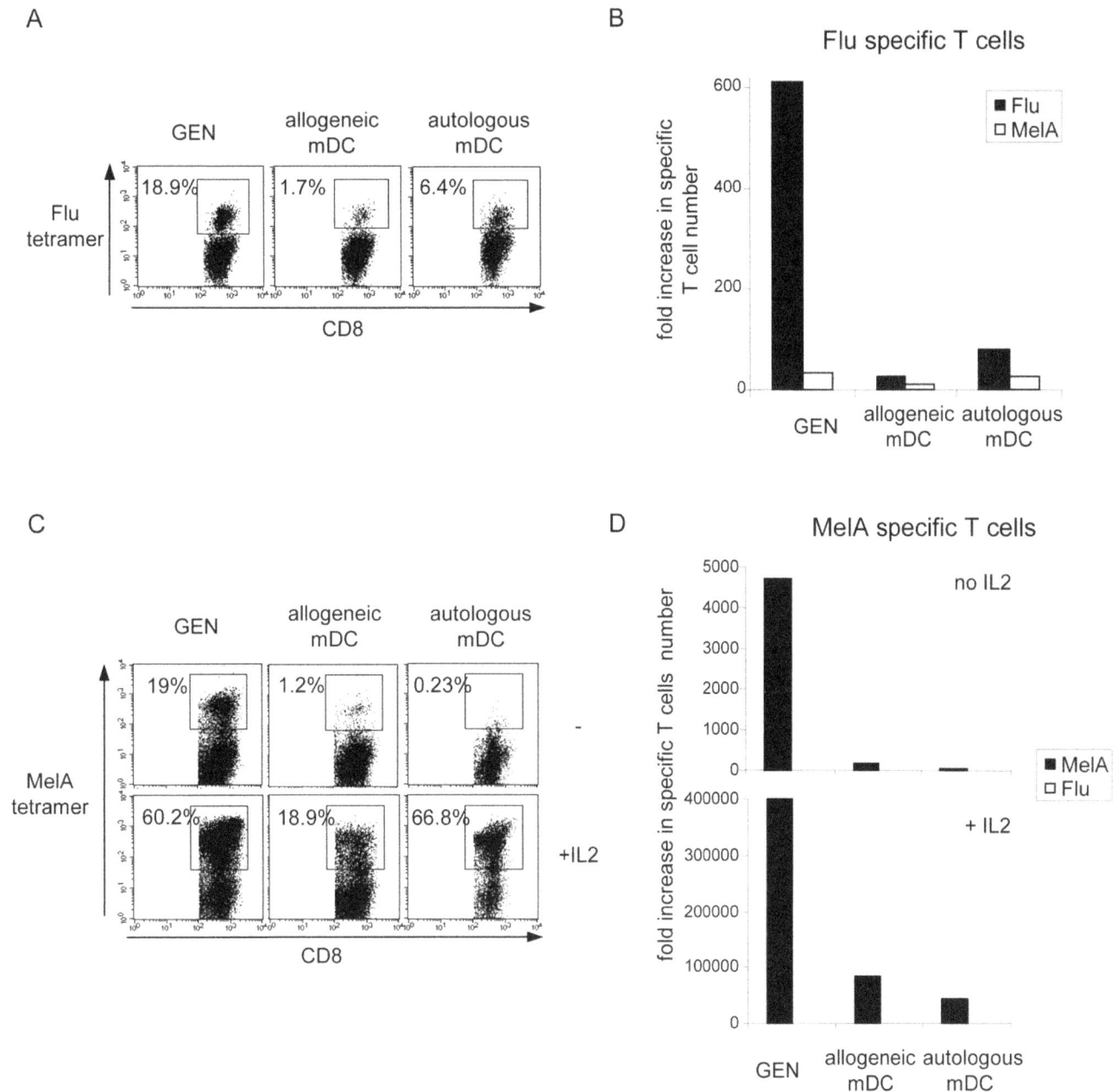

Figure 7. The HLA-A*0201 matched allogeneic pDC line is more effective than conventional mDCs. PBMC from HLA-A*0201[+] healthy donors were stimulated either with the pDC line or with allogeneic or autologous HLA-A*0201[+] mDCs loaded with Flu (A, B) or MelA (C, D) peptide in presence of IL-2 where indicated. (A) Percentages of FluM1 tetramer[+] CD8+ T cells and (B) fold increase in specific T cell number at d7 of culture. MelA tetramer was used as control. (C) Percentages of MelA tetramer[+] CD8+ T cells and (D) fold increase in specific T cell number at d20 of culture. Flu tetramer was used as control.

These findings provide a pre-clinical basis for the use of HLA matched allogeneic pDCs as vectors for cancer immunotherapy.

The use of pDCs to induce T cell responses has already been investigated in vitro and in mouse models of cancer and infection [21,31], but its further development for clinical application was impractical due to the absence of an easy way to generate or purify human pDCs in sufficient number. As peptide-pulsed primary pDCs isolated from the blood induced higher T cell responses in HLA matched allogeneic settings compared to autologous conditions, we further investigated the potential of pDC combined with HLA matched allogeneicity using the HLA-A*0201[+] pDC line. We demonstrated that the irradiated peptide-pulsed pDC line can strongly trigger both primary and memory specific T cell responses more effectively than conventional myeloid DCs. The use of pDC in an allogeneic context with a partial HLA matching between the vaccine and the responding T cells resulted in an enhancement of HLA-A*0201-restricted specific responses, with only minor allogeneic response induction as assessed by the low level of non-specific T cell activation upon restimulation with the vaccine. Thus, there is a strong enhancement induced by HLA matched allogeneicity [37], that is further potentiated by a pDC vaccineThe safety of allogeneic cell therapies has already been

A

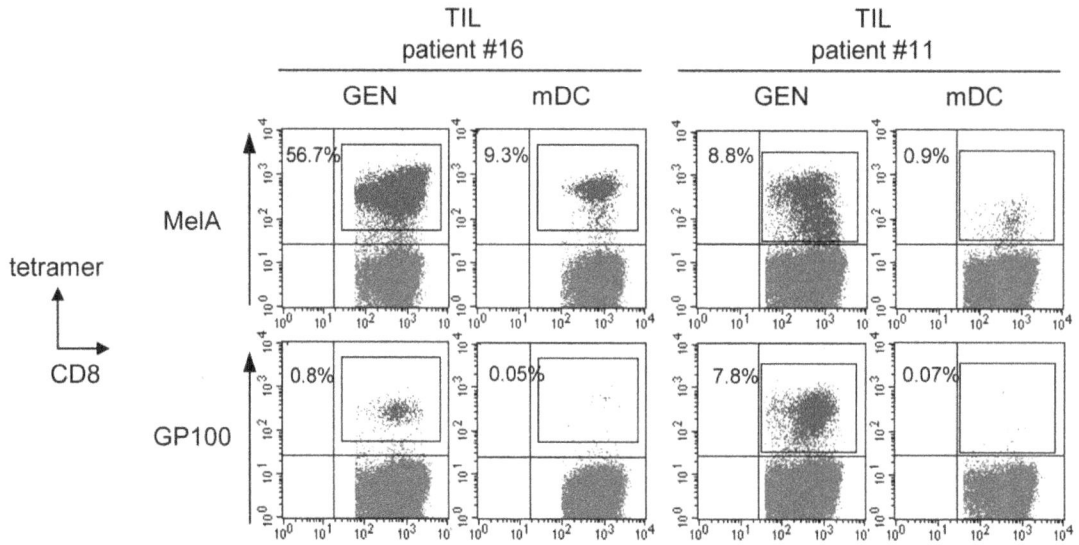

B

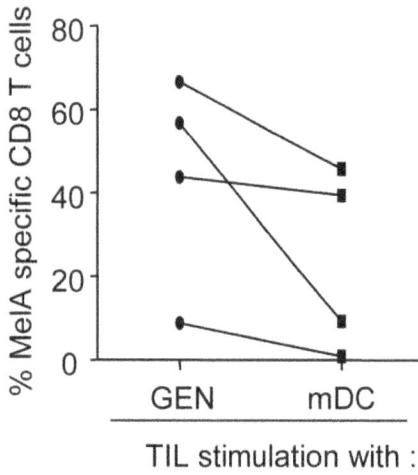

C

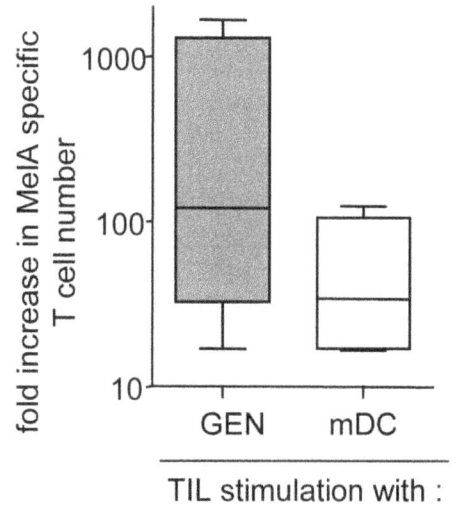

D

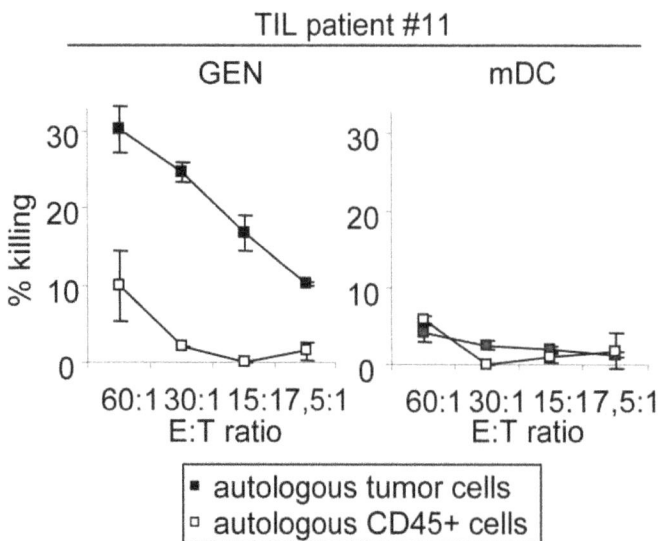

E

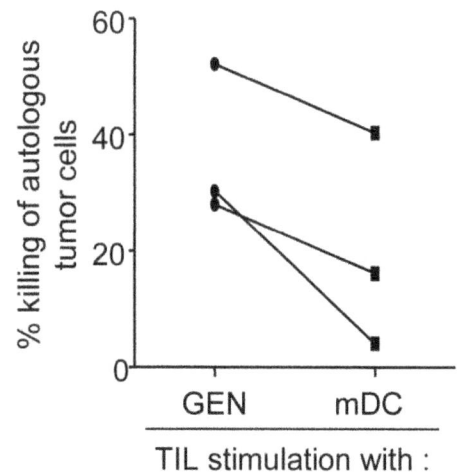

Figure 8. The HLA-A*0201 matched allogeneic pDCs are more potent at inducing tumor-specific T cells from melanoma patients than conventional mDCs. TIL from melanoma patients were cultured either with irradiated GEN cells or allogeneic LPS-matured HLA-A*0201+ mDCs loaded with a mixture of MelA, GP100, TYR and MAGE-3 derived peptides. Percentages of tumor-specific T cells were determined by tetramer labelling after three stimulations at day 20 of culture. (A) Representative dotplots of two cultures. (B) Comparative percentages of MelA-specific T cells and (C) fold increase in specific T cell numbers upon stimulation of TIL with GEN or mDCs (4 patients). (D,E) T cells were purified from the culture and submitted to a ^{51}Cr release assay. (D) Percentage of killing of autologous tumor cells and autologous CD45+ cells after TIL stimulation with GEN or mDCs. One representative patient is shown. (E) Comparative killing efficacy against autologous tumor cells at a 60:1 ratio.

assessed in cancer clinical trials [44–46]. Several trials demonstrated in cancer patients that the use of HLA matched allogeneic mDCs or mDCs/tumor hybrids induced strong anti-tumor immune responses and clinical responses [47,48]. These studies clearly demonstrate the feasibility of generation of tumor-specific T cell responses in vivo on an allo-background. HLA-restricted tumor specific T cell responses are not drowned out by bystander alloresponses.

The use of HLA-matched allogeneic pDCs may explained the relative important HLA-restricted responses over alloresponses induction, and its efficacy. It has been shown that pDCs can induce allogeneic T cell hyporesponsiveness and subsequent prolonged graft survival [49]; this may be due to a high ratio of B7-H1 to B7-1 and B7-2 molecule expression that in turn influence the outcome of their interactions with T cells. It has also been suggested that pDCs are equipped with large "ready-made" intracellular stores of MHC-I molecules than can be rapidly mobilize to the cell surface to initiate antigen-specific CD8 T cell responses [50]. The localization of MHC-I molecules in the recycling endosomal compartment suggests a rapid translocation to the cell surface after stimulation. In addition pDCs cross-present antigens more rapidly and efficiently than do mDCs and this process is IFNα-independent. In line with this, we observed a rapid upregulation of MHC-I molecules on the peptide-loaded pDC line upon activation and the induction of specific T cells was IFNα-independent (not shown). These differences of MHC-I molecules mobilization at early time points between pDCs and mDCs may explain the superiority of pDCs over mDCs. In addition, pDCs and mDCs handle MHC-II molecules differently after activation [51]: pDCs continuously turn over MHC-II molecules after activation whereas mDCs did not which results in sustained surface expression of individual peptide-MHC-II molecules complexes. pDCs display low amounts of MHC-II molecules on their surface and did not upregulate MHC-II synthesis soon after activation [52]. A possible explanation for the selective HLA restricted- over allo-responses triggering by pDCs could be the differential mobilization of MHC-I and MHC-II molecules upon stimulation and the rapid mobilization of MHC-I molecules to the cell surface. We observed that the specific T cell induction by the pDCs was type I IFN independent (not shown). Furthermore, the irradiation of the pDC line induced a strong cell activation as assessed by the upregulation of the costimulatory markers CD40, CD80, CD86 and HLA-A2 molecule and the secretion of pro-inflammatory cytokines (not shown) to similar levels to the one provided by TLR-7 or TLR-9 stimulation. On the contrary mDCs did not upregulate these costimulatory molecules upon irradiation. These unique features of pDCs could allow a preferential MHC-I orientation leading to HLA restricted- over allo-responses induction and contribute to its high HLA-A*0201 restricted CD8 T cell stimulatory capacity.

Tumor-specific T cells induced by the HLA matched allogeneic pDC were highly functional as demonstrated by the capacity of tetramer+ T cells to secrete IFNγ and express CD107 upon specific restimulation, and their strong antigen and HLA-A*0201-specific cytotoxicity. As peptide-loaded T2 cells are more susceptible to lysis than cells expressing the antigen endogenously, we performed each cytotoxicity assay not only on peptide-loaded T2 cells, but also on several allogeneic melanoma cell lines and importantly on autologous melanoma tumor cells from the patients themselves. Our results demonstrate that the specific T cells induced by the pDC line are able to kill tumor cells expressing the antigen endogenously. The phenotype of the effector T cells generated was that of intermediate effectors: CD27+ CD45RO+ CD62L- T cells (not shown), suggesting that they were not terminally differentiated even after serial stimulations. Importantly, intermediate effector cells have been indicated to be optimal for in vivo efficacy [53]. We also observed that the specific T cells elicited by the pDCs had a better affinity and higher avidity compared to specific T cells triggered by allogeneic mDCs, as suggested by a slowest tetramer dissociation rate and a better functionality on titrated peptide-MHC complexes (not shown). These observations suggest that the specific T cells elicited by the pDC vaccine will be able to recognize antigen at the physiological low concentrations. We also demonstrated the strong potential of the peptide-loaded pDC line to induce specific T cell responses in a humanized mouse model, and its efficacy in inhibiting the development of already established tumors.

Importantly, we further provide clinical relevance of this strategy by demonstrating it potently stimulates highly functional tumor-specific T cells from melanoma patients. After stimulation with the pDC line loaded with a mix of four melanoma peptides, T cells from melanoma patients acquired the ability to kill autologous tumor cells. Such results were obtained with PBMC as well as with TIL taken from all tested patients, at different stages of their disease and regardless of their previous treatment, providing the preclinical evidence for the strong potential of our strategy.

We performed a comparison of our strategy with frequently used myeloid derived dendritic cells. As demonstrated for several antigens and with healthy donors' as well as melanoma patients' cells, the pDC line led to a more potent induction of tumor-specific T cells endowed with better functional capacities compared to conventional mDCs. CTL generated by the pDC line are much more effective in killing autologous melanoma tumor cells compared to CTL generated by mDC. Allogeneic leukaemic myeloid cell lines that have DC properties have also been evaluated for their potential to prime tumor-specific CTL [54,55], but our strategy is superior in many aspects including the cell line generation, the settings required for induction of T cell responses, and the efficacy of specific T cells elicited.

The efficacy and design of this immunotherapeutic approach render the strategy very attractive for further clinical developments. Our peptide-pulsed pDC line can be provided directly as a ready-to-use GMP secured frozen vaccine. Notably, it represents a multi-usage flexible strategy, as the same vaccine can be used for every HLA-A*0201+ patient, and by utilizing target antigens it can be suitable for various pathologies. Regarding clinical use, we have already addressed a number of biosafety issues, in accordance with regulatory requirements.

This work demonstrates that HLA matched allogeneic pDCs are promising vectors for cancer immunotherapy. GENiusVac represents a real advancement in the challenging area of cancer immunotherapy with broad clinical applications.

Supporting Information

Figure S1 HLA-A2 and tumor antigen expression by melanoma tumor cell lines. (A) Analysis by flow cytometry of surface HLA-A2 (top panels) and intracellular MelA (lower panels) expression by Me275, Mel89, COLO829 and A375 melanoma tumor cell lines. (B) Analysis by real time PCR of MelA, GP100, tyrosinase and MAGE-3 gene expression by Me275, Mel89, COLO829 and A375 melanoma tumor cell lines.

Figure S2 The HLA-A*0201 matched allogeneic pDC line induces highly effective virus-specific T cell responses from HLA-A*0201$^+$ healthy donors' PBMC in vitro. Allogeneic HLA-A*0201 PBMC from healthy donors were stimulated with the irradiated peptide-loaded HLA-A*0201$^+$ pDC line. Specificity of the T cells was determined by tetramer labelling and flow cytometric analysis. (A) Representative dot plot of Flu M1 tetramer labelling at d0 and d7 of culture (gated on CD8+ T cells). (B) Percentages of Flu M1 tetramer$^+$ CD8+ T cells determined at d0 and d7 of culture (n = 20). (C) Representative dot plot of CMVpp65 tetramer labelling at d0 and d7 of culture (gated on CD8+ T cells). (D) Percentages of CMV pp65 tetramer$^+$ CD8+ T cells determined at d0 and d7 of culture (n = 14). Anti-viral tetramer$^+$ T cell responses reached averages of 11% for FluM1 (range 0.1–49) and 12% for CMVpp65 (range 0.04–76) in 7 days starting from respectively 0.23 and 0.18%.

Figure S3 The virus-specific T cells induced in vitro by the HLA-A*0201 matched allogeneic pDC line exhibited functional HLA-A*0201- and antigen-specific activity. (A) Flu-specific T cells induced by the pDC line secrete IFNγ and express CD107 on the surface upon restimulation. Cells from the culture (day 8) were tetramer labeled and restimulated with T2 cells pulsed with a relevant or control peptide. IFNγ production was assessed by intracellular staining and CD107 expression by adding anti-CD107a+b antibodies during the restimulation. Dotplots are gated on tetramer$^+$ CD8+ T cells. Representative of 4 experiments performed with 3 donors at day 8-10 of the culture. (B) Flu-specific T cells induced by the pDC line are cytotoxic. T cells were selected from the culture and submitted to a ^{51}Cr release assay using peptide-loaded T2 cells as targets. T cells killed T2 cells loaded with the relevant but not the control peptide. Representative of 7 experiments performed with 4 donors at d7-10 of the culture. (C,D) IFNγ secretion and CD107 expression were assessed as described in (A) after a single stimulation of PBMC and analyzed on the tetramer$^+$ CD8+ T cells (white bars) and on the non-specific tetramer$^-$ CD8+ T cells (grey bars) and CD4+ T cells (black bars) upon restimulation with peptide-pulsed T2 or GEN cells (4 experiments for each condition).

Figure S4 Response kinetics to vaccination with peptide-loaded GEN cells in humanized mice. Immunodeficient NOD-SCID β$_2$m$^{-/-}$ mice were reconstituted intraperitoneally with 50.10^6 human HLA-A*0201 PBMC and weekly vaccinated by the same route with 5.10^6 irradiated peptide-loaded GEN cells. Specific T cell induction was analyzed at different timepoints after vaccination at the injection site (lavage), in the circulation (blood) and lymphoid organs (spleen, MLN) by tetramer labelling of human T cells in cell suspensions. (A) Tumor-specific response to MelA-loaded GEN vaccination and (B) virus-specific response to Flu-loaded GEN vaccination. Each dot represents one vaccinated HuPBL mice.

Figure S5 TYR-specific T cells induction. Percentage of TYR-specific T cells determined at different timepoints of the PBMC culture from a melanoma patient (#4) with TYR-loaded GEN cells (gated on CD8+ T cells).
Found at: doi:10.1371/journal.pone.0010458.s005 (4.49 MB TIF)

Figure S6 The 30Gy irradiation induced activation of the pDC line. pDCs were either untreated or submitted to a 30Gy irradiation. Twenty four hours later, the expression of costimulatory and HLA-A2 molecules were analysed by flow cytometry (representative of three experiments).

Figure S7 The induction of specific T cells by the pDC line is type I IFN independent. Allogeneic HLA-A*0201$^+$ PBMC from healthy donors were stimulated with the irradiated Flu- or MelA-peptide loaded HLA-A*0201$^+$ pDC line in the presence of anti-IFNα and anti-IFNβ antibodies or control goat IgG. The level of specific T cells was determined at day 7 of the culture by tetramer labelling and flow cytometry analysis.

Figure S8 Comparative avidity of the specific T cells elicited by the pDC line and allogeneic mDCs. Allogeneic HLA-A*0201$^+$ PBMC from healthy donors were stimulated with the irradiated Flu-peptide loaded HLA-A*0201$^+$ pDC line or HLA-A*0201$^+$ mDC. At day 7 of the culture, the cytotoxic activity of the specific T cells was evaluated by a ^{51}Cr release assay on T2 cells loaded with decreasing concentrations of Flu peptide (1 μM to 0.0001 μM), irrelevant peptide or unloaded. Data are expressed as a percentage of the maximum lysis measured for a E:T ratio of 30:1.

Table S1 Melanoma patients' samples and clinical parameters description.

Table S2 Initial levels of tetramer$^+$ CD8 T cells within melanoma patients' samples.

Acknowledgments

We are grateful to C. Morand, I. Michaud, P. Drillat, F. Bernard and their staff from EFS Rhone-Alpes for providing blood samples, F. Blanquet and R. Balouzat of the Plateforme de Haute Technologie Animale for expert animal care, and Francis Herodin from the CRSSA for animal irradiation. We thank F. De Fraipont, the surgeons and the medical staff of the Dermatology and Anatomopathology Departments from the CHU of Grenoble specially D. Salameire for providing patients blood samples and tumor exeresis. We thank Pr J-C. Cerottini for providing Me275 cell line and J-P. Molens for technical assistance. We are grateful to C. Caux and Davor Frleta for expert critical review of the manuscript, and K. Palucka for helpful discussions. We thank the healthy volunteers and melanoma patients who consented to participate in this study.

Author Contributions

Conceived and designed the experiments: CA JC LC JP. Performed the experiments: CA JC DL. Analyzed the data: CA JC DL LC JP. Contributed reagents/materials/analysis tools: JC MTL DL MJR. Wrote the paper: CA LC JP. Recruited patients: JC MTL.

References

1. Finn OJ (2008) Cancer immunology. N Engl J Med 358: 2704–2715. Review.

2. Thurner B, Haendle I, Röder C, Dieckmann D, Keikavoussi P, et al. (1999) Vaccination with mage-3A1 peptide-pulsed mature, monocyte-derived dendritic

cells expands specific cytotoxic T cells and induces regression of some metastases in advanced stage IV melanoma. J Exp Med 190: 1669–1678.

3. Palucka AK, Dhodapkar MV, Paczesny S, Ueno H, Fay J, et al. (2005) Boosting vaccinations with peptide-pulsed CD34+ progenitor-derived dendritic cells can expand long-lived melanoma peptide-specific CD8+ T cells in patients with metastatic melanoma. J Immunother 28: 158–168.

4. Gattinoni L, Powell DJ, Jr., Rosenberg SA, Restifo NP (2006) Adoptive immunotherapy for cancer: building on success. Nat Rev Immunol 6: 383–393. Review.

5. Dudley ME, Wunderlich JR, Yang JC, Sherry RM, Topalian SL, et al. (2005) Adoptive cell transfer therapy following non-myeloablative but lymphodepleting chemotherapy for the treatment of patients with refractory metastatic melanoma. J Clin Oncol 23: 2346–2357.

6. Banchereau J, Palucka AK (2005) Dendritic cells as therapeutic vaccines against cancer. Nat Rev Immunol 5: 296–306. Review.

7. Fajardo-Moser M, Berzel S, Moll H (2008) Mechanisms of dendritic cell-based vaccination against infection. Int J Med Microbiol 298: 11–20. Review.

8. Melief CJ (2008) Cancer immunotherapy by dendritic cells. Immunity 29: 372–383.

9. Colonna M, Trinchieri G, Liu YJ (2004) Plasmacytoid dendritic cells in immunity. Nat Immunol 5: 1219–1226.

10. Liu YJ (2005) IPC: Professional Type 1 Interferon-Producing Cells and Plasmacytoid Dendritic Cell Precursors. Annu Rev Immunol 23: 275–306.

11. Kim R, Emi M, Tanabe K, Arihiro K (2007) Potential functional role of plasmacytoid dendritic cells in cancer immunity. Immunology 121(2): 149–57.

12. Marañón C, Desoutter JF, Hoeffel G, Cohen W, Hanau D, et al. (2004) Dendritic cells cross-present HIV antigens from live as well as apoptotic infected CD4+ T lymphocytes. Proc Natl Acad Sci U S A 101: 6092–6097.

13. Siegal FP, Kadowaki N, Shodell M, Fitzgerald-Bocarsly PA, Shah K, et al. (1999) The nature of the principal type 1 interferon-producing cells in human blood. Science 284: 1835–1837.

14. Villadangos JA, Young L (2008) Antigen-presentation properties of plasmacytoid dendritic cells. Immunity 29: 352–361.

15. Lui G, Manches O, Angel J, Molens JP, Chaperot L, et al. (2009) Plasmacytoid dendritic cells capture and cross-present viral antigens from influenz-virus infected cells. Plos One - In press.

16. Cella M, Facchetti F, Lanzavecchia A, Colonna M (2000) Plasmacytoid dendritic cells activated by influenza virus and CD40L drive a potent TH1 polarization. Nat Immunol 1: 305–310.

17. Fonteneau JF, Gilliet M, Larsson M, Dasilva I, Münz C, et al. (2003) Activation of influenza virus-specific CD4+ and CD8+ T cells: a new role for plasmacytoid dendritic cells in adaptive immunity. Blood 101: 3520–3526.

18. Salio M, Cella M, Vermi W, Facchetti F, Palmowski MJ, et al. (2003) Plasmacytoid dendritic cells prime IFN-gamma-secreting melanoma-specific CD8 lymphocytes and are found in primary melanoma lesions. Eur J Immunol 33: 1052–1062.

19. Rothenfusser S, Hornung V, Ayyoub M, Britsch S, Towarowski A, et al. (2004) CpG-A and CpG-B oligonucleotides differentially enhance human peptide-specific primary and memory CD8+ T-cell responses in vitro. Blood 103: 2162–2169.

20. Sapoznikov A, Fischer JA, Zaft T, Krauthgamer R, Dzionek A, et al. (2007) Organ-dependent in vivo priming of naive CD4+, but not CD8+, T cells by plasmacytoid dendritic cells. J Exp Med 204: 1923–1933.

21. Schlecht G, Garcia S, Escriou N, Freitas AA, Leclerc C, et al. (2004) Murine plasmacytoid dendritic cells induce effector/memory CD8+ T-cell responses in vivo after viral stimulation. Blood 104: 1808–1815.

22. Vermi W, Bonecchi R, Facchetti F, Bianchi D, Sozzani S, et al. (2003) Recruitment of immature plasmacytoid dendritic cells (plasmacytoid monocytes) and myeloid dendritic cells in primary cutaneous melanomas. J Pathol 200: 255–268.

23. Hartmann E, Wollenberg B, Rothenfusser S, Wagner M, Wellisch D, et al. (2003) Identification and functional analysis of tumor-infiltrating plasmacytoid dendritic cells in head and neck cancer. Cancer Res 63: 6478 6487.

24. Zou W, Machelon V, Coulomb-L'Hermin A, Borvak J, Nome F, et al. (2001) Stromal-derived factor-1 in human tumors recruits and alters the function of plasmacytoid precursor dendritic cells. Nat Med 7: 1339–1346.

25. Treilleux I, Blay JY, Bendriss-Vermare N, Ray-Coquard I, Bachelot T, et al. (2004) Dendritic cell infiltration and prognosis of early stage breast cancer. Clin Cancer Res 10: 7466–7474.

26. Perrot I, Blanchard D, Freymond N, Isaac S, Guibert B, et al. (2007) Dendritic cells infiltrating human non-small cell lung cancer are blocked at immature stage. J Immunol 178: 2763–2769.

27. Palamara F, Meindl S, Holcmann M, Lührs P, Stingl G, et al. (2004) Identification and characterization of pDC-like cells in normal mouse skin and melanomas treated with imiquimod. J Immunol 173: 3051–3061.

28. Furumoto K, Soares L, Engleman EG, Merad M (2004) Induction of potent antitumor immunity by in situ targeting of intratumoral DCs. J Clin Invest 113: 774–783.

29. Molenkamp BG, van Leeuwen PA, Meijer S, Sluijter BJ, Wijnands PG, et al. (2007) Intradermal CpG-B activates both plasmacytoid and myeloid dendritic cells in the sentinel lymph node of melanoma patients. Clin Cancer Res 13: 2961–2969.

30. Molenkamp BG, Sluijter BJ, van Leeuwen PA, Santegoets SJ, Meijer S, et al. (2008) Local administration of PF-3512676 CpG-B instigates tumor-specific CD8+ T-cell reactivity in melanoma patients. Clin Cancer Res 14: 4532–4542.

31. Liu C, Lou Y, Lizée G, Qin H, Liu S, et al. (2008) Plasmacytoid dendritic cells induce NK cell-dependent, tumor antigen-specific T cell cross-priming and tumor regression in mice. J Clin Invest 118: 1165–1175.

32. Krieg AM (2007) Development of TLR9 agonists for cancer therapy. J Clin Invest. 117(5): 1184–94. Review.

33. Mitchison NA, O'Malley C (1987) Three-cell-type clusters of T cells with antigen-presenting cells best explain the epitope linkage and noncognate requirements of the in vivo cytolytic response. Eur J Immunol 17: 1579–1583.

34. Medzhitov R, Janeway CA, Jr. (1998) Innate immune recognition and control of adaptive immune responses. Semin Immunol 10: 351–353. Review.

35. Gjertsen HA, Lundin KE, Hansen T, Thorsby E (1993) T cells specific for viral antigens presented by HLA-Dw4 recognize DR13 on allogeneic cells: a possible mechanism for induction of rejection. Transpl Immunol 1: 126–131.

36. Muir G, Rajbabu K, Callen C, Fabre JW (2006) Preliminary evidence that the allogeneic response might trigger antitumour immunity in patients with advanced prostate cancer. BJU Int 98: 989–995.

37. Fabre JW (2001) The allogeneic response and tumor immunity. Nat Med 7: 649–652. Review.

38. Blom B, Ho S, Antonenko S, Liu YJ (2000) Generation of interferon alpha-producing predendritic cell (Pre-DC)2 from human CD34(+) hematopoietic stem cells. J Exp Med 192: 1785–1796.

39. Chaperot L, Blum A, Manches O, Lui G, Angel J, et al. (2006) Virus or TLR agonists induce TRAIL-mediated cytotoxic activity of plasmacytoid dendritic cells. J Immunol 176: 248–255.

40. Di Domizio J, Blum A, Gallagher-Gambarelli M, Molens JP, Chaperot L, et al. (2009) TLR7 stimulation in human plasmacytoid dendritic cells leads to the induction of early IFN-inducible genes in the absence of type I IFN. Blood 114(9): 1794–802.

41. Lui G, Manches O, Angel J, Molens JP, Chaperot L, et al. (2009) Plasmacytoid dendritic cells capture and cross-present viral antigens from influenza-virus exposed cells. PLoS One 4(9): e7111.

42. Aspord C, Yu CI, Banchereau J, Palucka AK (2007) Humanized Mice for Development and Testing of Human Vaccines. Expert Opin Drug Discov 2: 949–960. Review.

43. Schettini J, Mukherjee P (2008) Physiological role of plasmacytoid dendritic cells and their potential use in cancer immunity. Clin Dev Immunol;DOI: 10.1155/2008/106321.

44. Newton DA, Romano C, Gattoni-Celli S (2000) Semiallogeneic cell hybrids as therapeutic vaccines for cancer. J Immunother 23: 246–254.

45. Höltl L, Ramoner R, Zelle-Rieser C, Gander H, Putz T, et al. (2005) Allogeneic dendritic cell vaccination against metastatic renal cell carcinoma with or without cyclophosphamide. Cancer Immunol Immunother 54: 663–670.

46. Hus I, Roliński J, Tabarkiewicz J, Wojas K, Bojarska-Junak A, et al. (2005) Allogeneic dendritic cells pulsed with tumor lysates or apoptotic bodies as immunotherapy for patients with early-stage B-cell chronic lymphocytic leukemia. Leukemia 19: 1621–1627.

47. Tamir A, Basagila E, Kagahzian A, Jiao L, Jensen S, et al. (2007) Induction of tumor-specific T-cell responses by vaccination with tumor lysate-loaded dendritic cells in colorectal cancer patients with carcinoembryonic-antigen positive tumors. Cancer Immunol Immunother 56(12): 2003–16.

48. Trefzer U, Herberth G, Wohlan K, Milling A, Thiemann M, et al. (2004) Vaccination with hybrids of tumor and dendritic cells induces tumor-specific T-cell and clinical responses in melanoma stage III and IV patients. Int J Cancer 110(5): 730–40.

49. Abe M, Wang Z, de Creus A, Thomson AW (2005) Plasmacytoid dendritic cell precursors induce allogeneic T-cell hyporesponsiveness and prolong heart graft survival. Am J Transplant 5(8): 1808–19.

50. Di Pucchio T, Chatterjee B, Smed-Sörensen A, Clayton S, Palazzo A, et al. (2008) Direct proteasome-independent cross-presentation of viral antigen by plasmacytoid dendritic cells on major histocompatibility complex class I. Nat Immunol 9(5): 551–7.

51. Young LJ, Wilson NS, Schnorrer P, Proietto A, ten Broeke T, et al. (2008) Differential MHC class II synthesis and ubiquitination confers distinct antigen-presenting properties on conventional and plasmacytoid dendritic cells. Nat Immunol 9(11): 1244–52.

52. van den Hoorn T, Neefjes J (2008) Activated pDCs: open to new antigen-presentation possibilities. Nat Immunol 9(11): 1208–10.

53. Gattinoni L, Klebanoff CA, Palmer DC, Wrzesinski C, Kerstann K, et al. (2005) Acquisition of full effector function in vitro paradoxically impairs the in vivo antitumor efficacy of adoptively transferred CD8+ T cells. J Clin Invest 115: 1616–1626.

54. Masterson AJ, Sombroek CC, De Gruijl TD, Graus YM, van der Vliet HJ, et al. (2002) MUTZ-3, a human cell line model for the cytokine-induced differentiation of dendritic cells from CD34+ precursors. Blood 100(2): 701–3.

55. Santegoets SJ, Schreurs MW, Masterson AJ, Liu YP, Goletz S, et al. (2006) In vitro priming of tumor-specific cytotoxic T lymphocytes using allogeneic dendritic cells derived from the human MUTZ-3 cell line. Cancer Immunol Immunother 55(12): 1480–90.

15

Management of Metformin-Associated Lactic Acidosis by Continuous Renal Replacement Therapy

Geoffray Keller[1,2], Martin Cour[1,2], Romain Hernu[1], Julien Illinger[1], Dominique Robert[1,2], Laurent Argaud[1,2]*

1 Hospices Civils de Lyon, Groupement Hospitalier Edouard Herriot, Service de Réanimation Médicale, Lyon, France, 2 Université de Lyon, Université Lyon 1, Faculté de médecine Lyon-Est, Lyon, France

Abstract

Background: Metformin-associated lactic acidosis (MALA) is a severe metabolic failure with high related mortality. Although its use is controversial, intermittent hemodialysis is reported to be the most frequently used treatment in conjunction with nonspecific supportive measures. Our aim was to report the evolution and outcome of cases managed by continuous renal replacement therapy (CRRT).

Methodology and Principal Findings: Over a 3-year period, we retrospectively identified patients admitted to the intensive care unit for severe lactic acidosis caused by metformin. We included patients in our study who were treated with CRRT because of shock. We describe their clinical and biological features at admission and during renal support, as well as their evolution. We enrolled six patients with severe lactic acidosis; the mean pH and mean lactate was 6.92 ± 0.20 and 14.4 ± 5.1 mmol/l, respectively. Patients had high illness severity scores, including the Simplified Acute Physiology Score II (SAPS II) (average score 63 ± 12 points). Early CRRT comprised either venovenous hemofiltration ($n = 3$) or hemodiafiltration ($n = 3$) with a mean effluent flow rate of 34 ± 6 ml/kg/h. Metabolic acidosis control and metformin elimination was rapid and there was no rebound. Outcome was favorable in all cases.

Conclusions and Significance: Standard use of CRRT efficiently treated MALA in association with symptomatic organ supportive therapies.

Editor: Jeffrey A. Gold, Oregon Health and Science University, United States of America

Funding: The authors have no support or funding to report.

Competing Interests: The authors have declared that no competing interests exist.

* E-mail: laurent.argaud@chu-lyon.fr

Introduction

Metformin is the recommended first-line treatment for overweight patients with type 2 diabetes mellitus [1]. The incidence of metformin-associated lactic acidosis (MALA) is rare, estimated at 2–9 patients per 100,000 patients receiving metformin per year; MALA accounts for approximately 1% of total patients admitted to intensive care units (ICU) [2]. This life-threatening complication is usually associated with a mortality rate of 30%–50% [2,3]. The etiology of lactic acidosis is multifactorial and uncertain. Briefly, metformin increases the redox potential from aerobic to anaerobic metabolism, and inhibits gluconeogenesis by reducing hepatic lactate reuptake [4]. This situation is worsened by circulatory failure and altered tissue perfusion, both of which increase lactate production.

The optimal treatment modality for MALA is controversial and relies on nonspecific supportive measures. The use of intermittent hemodialysis may be protective, and it is recommended by many intensivists [2,5,6]. Despite potential advantages, continuous renal replacement therapy (CRRT) to treat MALA is poorly documented with only a few case reports available, and it has only been considered as a rescue therapy under exceptional circumstances [7–9]. We report on six cases of severe MALA that were successfully managed with CRRT and discuss the safety and effectiveness of CRRT when it is used for this purpose.

Materials and Methods

The ethics committee of the Hospices Civils de Lyon approved this retrospective noninterventional study. This institutional review board waived the need for consent given the retrospective design of the project. The study was performed in compliance with the ethical standard of the Helsinki Declaration and according to the French laws.

From November 2005 to October 2008, we identified all of the patients who were admitted to our ICU for severe MALA and treated with CRRT because of hemodynamic instability. Patients were included if they met the two following criteria: blood pH<7.20 and arterial lactate >5 mmol/l [10]. An abdominal ultrasound exploration and/or a computerized tomography scanner was systematically performed to eliminate mesenteric infarction.

The following clinical features were collected at admission: age, sex, MacCabe and Knaus scores (used to assess the severity of comorbidities and functional status, respectively), Charson index (to evaluate comorbidity), preexisting chronic renal failure, use of

Table 1. Patient characteristics.

	Case 1	Case 2	Case 3	Case 4	Case 5	Case 6	Mean ± SD
Demographics							
Age (years)	81	81	72	54	63	64	69±11
Gender	F	F	F	M	F	F	-
Coexisting medical conditions							
McCabe scale	0	0	0	1	0	0	-
Knaus score	B	B	B	C	D	A	-
Charlson comorbidity index	3	5	1	2	2	1	2.3±1.5
Chronic renal failure	No	No	Yes	Yes	No	No	-
Nephrotoxic drugs							
Diuretics	No	Yes	No	Yes	Yes	Yes	-
Angiotensin converter inhibitors	Yes	No	No	Yes	No	Yes	-
Nonsteroidal anti-inflammators	No	No	No	No	No	No	-
Aspirin	No	No	No	Yes	No	Yes	-
Metformin							
Daily dose (mg)	2250	3000	1700	1000	3000	3000	2375±842

F, female; M, male; McCabe scale (life expectancy), 0: none or nonfatal underlying disease, 1: ultimately fatal disease (death≤5 years), 2: rapidly fatal disease (death≤1 year); Knaus score (functional status), A: no daily activity limitation, the patient was in good health, B: moderate limitation of activity because of a chronic medical problem, C: strong limitation of activity due to disease, D: severe limitation and/or restriction of activity due to disease; Charlson comorbidity index, components (weights): myocardial infarct (1), congestive heart failure (1), peripheral vascular disease (1), cerebrovascular disease (1), dementia (1), chronic pulmonary disease (1), connective tissue disease (1), ulcer disease (1), mild liver disease (1), diabetes (1), hemiplegia (2), moderate or severe renal disease (2), diabetes with end-organ damage (2), any tumor (2), leukemia (2), lymphoma (2), moderate or severe liver disease (3), metastatic solid tumor (6), AIDS (6).

Table 2. Illness severity.

	Case 1	Case 2	Case 3	Case 4	Case 5	Case 6	Mean ± SD
Admission vitals							
Heart rate (beats/min)	104	101	83	82	78	120	95±16
Mean arterial blood pressure (mmHg)	44	41	48	38	55	54	47±7
Respiratory rate (breaths/min)	32	20	30	30	29	40	30±7
Body temperature (°C)	33.0	34.5	33.0	35.8	35.9	30.9	33.9±1.9
Diuresis (ml/h)	4	9	0	88	8	0	18±34
Glasgow coma score	15	11	8	15	11	12	12±3
Multiple organ failure							
Cardiovascular dysfunction	Yes	Yes	Yes	Yes	Yes	Yes	-
Renal dysfunction	Yes	Yes	Yes	Yes	Yes	Yes	-
Respiratory dysfunction	No	Yes	No	Yes	Yes	Yes	-
Neurological dysfunction	No	Yes	Yes	No	No	No	-
Hepatic dysfunction	No	No	Yes	No	No	No	-
Hematological dysfunction	No	No	No	No	No	No	-
Number of organ dysfunctions	2	4	4	3	3	3	3.2±0.8
SOFA score	9	14	15	8	12	14	12±3
Symptomatic intensive therapies							
Renal replacement therapy (days)	7	12	15	2	3	5	7±5
Mechanical ventilation (days)	0	19	0	5	15	9	8±8
Vasoactive drugs (days)	3	9	4	1	2	5	4±3
Norepinephrine (μg/kg/min)	0.3	1.3	0.8	0.2	0.2	0.9	0.6±0.5
SAPS II	66	74	73	51	46	66	63±12

SOFA, Sequential-related Organ Failure Assessment; SAPS II, Simplified Acute Physiology Score II.

medication potentially responsible for renal impairment, daily dose of metformin, Simplified Acute Physiology Score II (SAPS II), hemodynamics, body temperature, Glasgow coma score, number of organ failures according to Fagon *et al.*, Sequential-related Organ Failure Assessment (SOFA score), type and intensity of renal support, mechanical ventilation and vasopressor requirement, and ICU length of stay and outcome [11–17]. Biological data recorded at admission were pH and lactate, bicarbonate, partial oxygen pressure (PaO_2) and partial carbon dioxide pressure ($PaCO_2$) from arterial samples, and sodium, potassium, aminotransferase ALAT, creatine kinase, troponin I, creatinine, urea, glucose, hemoglobin and C-reactive protein (CRP) concentrations, as well as anion gap, prothrombin index, white blood cell and platelets counts from venous samples. The presence of metformin was identified, and both plasmatic and erythrocyte concentrations were quantified in a venous blood sample by high performance liquid chromatography (HPLC).

CRRT (i.e., continuous venovenous hemofiltration [CVVH] or hemodiafiltration [CVVHDF]) was performed with a Prismaflex device (Hospal, Meyzieu, France). We used polysulfone hollow-fiber hemofilters with a surface area of 1.2 m². Blood flow rate was maintained between 150 and 250 ml/min according to the targeted ultrafiltration rate. Bicarbonate-based replacement solutions to maintain fluid balance were infused so that the predilution was equal to 30%. Anticoagulation was performed with 5000 IU unfractionated heparin, added to the priming solution and followed by a continuous infusion, with a targeted systemic activated partial

thromboplastin (aPTT) at 1.5 time control. CRRT was discontinued as soon as clinical condition and renal function had improved.

Data are expressed as mean values and standard deviation (SD). Comparisons between time-based measurements were performed with two-way ANOVA with repeated measures on one factor using GraphPad Prism 5 (GraphPad Software, La Jolla, CA, USA). Statistical significance was defined at a value of $p < 0.05$.

Results

Patient clinical characteristics at admission are shown in both Table 1 and Table 2. There was one man and five women. In all cases, acute renal failure was present and associated with clinically and biologically profound extracellular dehydration. Patients 3 and 4 had previous chronic renal insufficiency without a requirement for renal replacement therapy. Except for patient 3, all of the patients took at least one of the following potentially nephrotoxic medications: diuretics, angiotensin converter enzyme inhibitors, nonsteroidal anti-inflammatory drugs, or aspirin (Table 1).

All of the patients presented with clinical nonspecific symptoms such as malaise, myalgia, drowsiness, or abdominal pain, as well as hemodynamic failure which required fluid challenge and vasopressive support (Table 2). Hypothermia was systematically present; four patients required mechanical ventilation (Table 2).

Biological characteristics at admission are presented in Table 3. None of the patients experienced severe hypoglycemia (Table 3). Inflammatory syndrome, if present, was minor since CRP level was always below 30 mg/l.

Table 3. Biological data at admission.

	Case 1	Case 2	Case 3	Case 4	Case 5	Case 6	Mean ± SD
Arterial blood gases							
Arterial pH	7.04	6.81	6.71	7.09	7.15	6.72	6.92±0.20
Arterial lactate (mmol/l)	16.2	19.1	15.6	9.8	6.6	19.0	14.4±5.1
Bicarbonate (mmol/l)	5	2	1	7	15	1	5±5
Anion gap (mmol/l)	51	42	51	52	36	54	48±7
$PaCO_2$ (mmHg)	16.5	15.0	24.8	23.3	43.5	9.0	21.8±12.0
PaO_2/FiO_2 (mmHg)	250	238	194	181	233	313	235±47
Standard biochemistry							
Sodium (mmol/l)	140	135	131	139	136	133	136±3
Potassium (mmol/l)	5.0	6.2	7.5	6.7	7.6	7.2	6.7±1.0
Glycemia (mmol/l)	12.5	2.2	9.3	13.0	8.7	6.3	8.7±4.0
Urea (mmol/l)	26	26	39	24	21	31	28±7
Creatinine (μmol/l)	670	416	841	585	372	723	601±181
Aminotransferase ALAT (IU/l)	12	29	128	40	13	15	39±45
Creatine kinase (IU/l)	150	63	554	124	43	484	236±224
Troponin I (ng/ml)	0.18	<0.1	1.33	<0.1	<0.1	1.14	0.9±0.6
Hematology							
Hemoglobin (g/l)	81	116	93	100	128	86	101±18
Platelets (10^9/l)	160	161	350	251	363	401	281±106
White blood cell (10^9/l)	18	25	27	17	13	39	23±9
Prothrombin index (%)	50	48	24	60	41	28	42±14
Metformin concentration							
Plasma (mg/l), N<1 mg/l	80.0	125	74.4	36.4	54.9	61.9	72.1±30.1
Erythrocyte (mg/l), N<0.81 mg/l	25.8	26.8	22.5	14.7	51.8	20.6	27.0±12.9

N, laboratory level limit; $PaCO_2$, partial carbon dioxide pressure in arterial blood; PaO_2, partial oxygen pressure in arterial blood; FiO_2, inspiratory fraction of oxygen.

Continuous renal replacement management, as well as outcomes, are shown in Table 4. CVVH and CVVHDF were each used in three patients. Metabolic acidosis, as well as metformin plasma concentrations, were dramatically reduced in the first 24 h and/or normalized on the second day in every case (Figure 1). There was no rebound in acidosis. The mean individual rates of metformin elimination, from the blood compartment, in the first 24 hours after admission was estimated from 1.5 to 4.0%/h (Table 4). CRRT was well tolerated in our patients. There was no occurrence of CRRT-associated complications such as bleeding. Renal replacement was not necessary after discharge for any of the patients, and kidney function recovered prior levels in each case. All of the patients were transferred to a medical ward before they were discharged to their homes.

Discussion

To our knowledge, this study represents the largest case series of MALA managed by early CRRT. All six patients had a favourable outcome despite severe initial metabolic disorders associated with multiple organ failure.

MALA is strictly defined by arterial lactate >5 mmol/l and blood pH<7.35 within the context of recent metformin exposure [10,18]. It is the most frequent pattern of lactic acidosis related to metformin use [10]. This confusing term of MALA, shared by many different nosologic entities, is caused by an acute metformin accumulation [10]. Because metformin normally undergoes rapid and unchanging glomerular filtration and tubular excretion, MALA occurs only if renal function is altered or in rare cases of

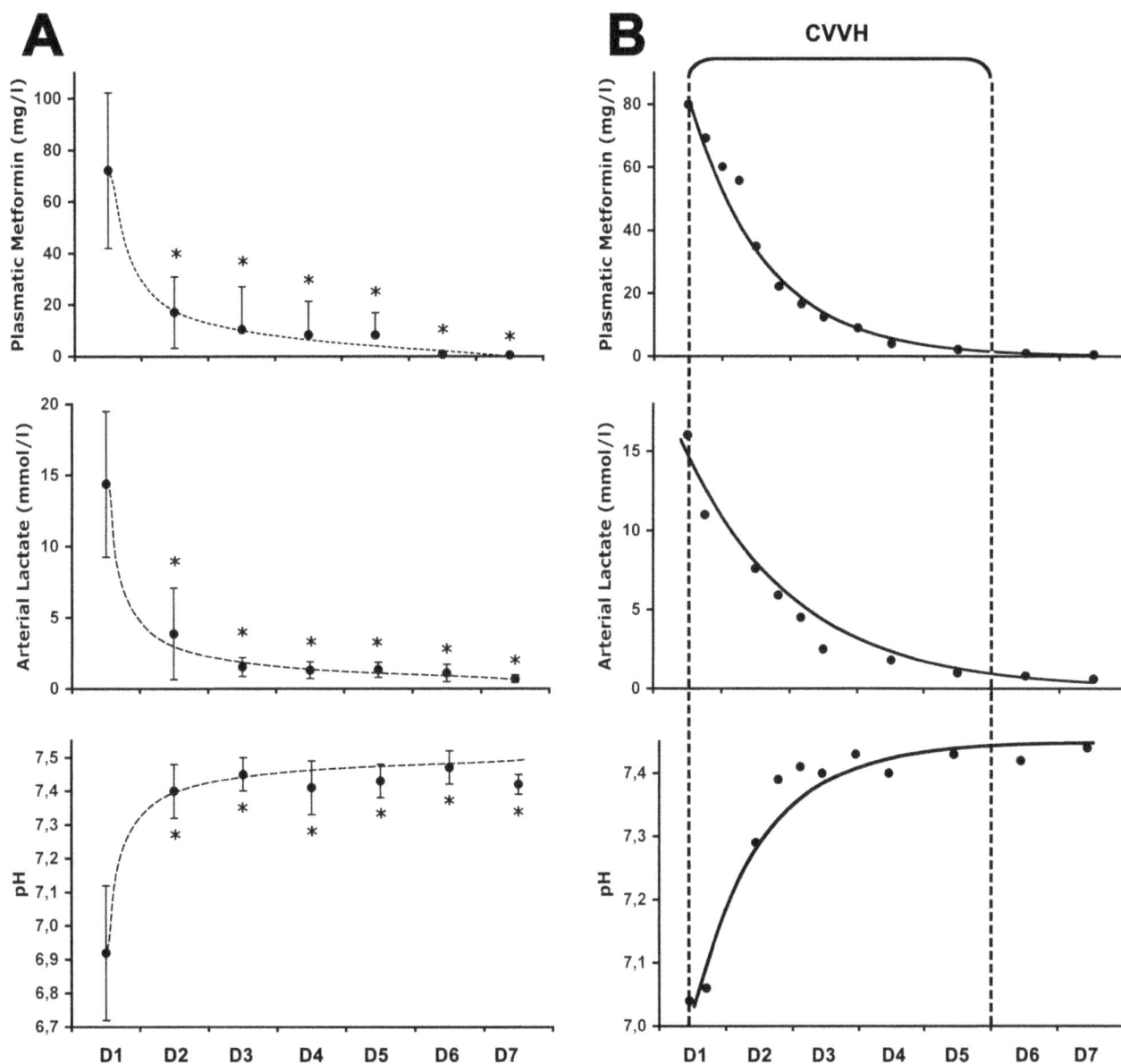

Figure 1. Acidosis, lactate and metformin levels under continuous renal replacement therapy. Panel A: Data from all patients, expressed as mean ± SD, showing that metabolic acidosis, as well as the excessive dose of metformin observed at admission (day 1, D1), were dramatically reduced from day 2 (D2). * p<0.01 versus D1. Panel B: Typical evolution in case patient 1 of both metformin plasma concentrations and metabolic disorders, which were controlled within 2 days of initiating continuous venovenous hemofiltration (CVVH), i.e. without dialysate.

Table 4. Continuous renal replacement therapy and outcomes.

	Case 1	Case 2	Case 3	Case 4	Case 5	Case 6	Mean ± SD
Type							
CVVH or CVVHDF	CVVH	CVVH	CVVHDF	CVVH	CVVHDF	CVVHDF	-
Therapy parameters							
Blood flow rate (ml/min)	200	180	150	200	180	250	193±33
Effluent rate (ml/kg/h)	34	33	39	22	38	36	34±6
Dialysate rate (ml/h)	0	0	2500	0	2000	500	1250±1215
Replacement fluid rate (ml/h)	1600	2500	2000	2500	2500	2800	2317±436
Filtration fraction (%)	13	30	22	29	17	19	22±7
Initial fluid removal (ml/h)	0	50	0	0	100	0	25±42
Length (days)	5	12	15	1	3	5	7±5
Metformin clearance							
Rate of elimination (%/h)	2.7	4.0	1.5	1.6	2.1	2.3	2.4±0.9
Outcomes							
ICU length of stay (days)	11	26	17	8	22	9	16±7
Survival to discharge	Yes	Yes	Yes	Yes	Yes	Yes	-
Discharge at home	Yes	Yes	Yes	Yes	Yes	Yes	-

CVVH, continuous venovenous hemofiltration; CVVHDF, continuous venovenous hemodiafiltration.

massive metformin ingestion [8,10]. Dehydration was the precipitating factor responsible for acute renal failure in our patients. In addition, the use of nephrotoxic drugs and/or chronic renal failure may have favoured the development of MALA.

Our patients presented with classical symptoms of MALA within a context that suggested metformin accumulation [2,10]. However, the diagnosis of MALA was made only once other causes of lactic acidosis (e.g., mesenteric infarction or septic shock) were excluded. Plasma metformin concentrations, ideally measured in the emergency room, helped us to ensure the correct diagnosis. These measurements are usually performed to eliminate metformin as the cause of lactic acidosis in patients with low plasma levels. However, the concentration of metformin in erythrocytes may be more useful, since it better reflects tissue accumulation [19]. Thus, as reported in this case series of metformin-treated patients, severe lactic acidosis associated with acute renal failure and/or other sepsis-like symptoms should systematically lead physicians to request metformin assays. Using this restrictive approach, we were able to generate a report on a rare, albeit small, series of MALA-only patients.

There are some concerns about using renal replacement therapy to manage MALA. For example, it is not certain whether rapid metformin elimination, either by intermittent hemodialysis or CRRT, is an appropriate endpoint in studies of MALA therapy [10]. Indeed, as previously reported by Lalau and Race, metformin (and also lactate) concentrations are not closely associated with prognosis [20]. In addition, increased levels of both metformin and lactate could even have beneficial cardiovascular, metabolic, and cytoprotective properties [21,22]. With regard to lactate management, it is now well established that lactate is not an acidogenic substance; the amount removed by replacement therapy with dialysis using bicarbonate-buffered fluids is negligible when compared to the overall plasma lactate clearance [23]. In the same way, the CRRT that was used in this case series is considered by some authors to be a supportive measure only to buffer metabolic acidosis and control volemia [10].

Even if there is also no consensus as to the best replacement therapy, hemodialysis appears to be the first-line treatment in association with symptomatic organ failure treatment [2,4–6,24]. In contrast, CRRT to manage MALA has only received attention in a few case reports [7–9,25,26]. Surprisingly, it usually appears to have been used as a rescue therapy either when high flow rates are set or in combination with hemodialysis [8,25,26]. In our practice, we began CRRT as early as possible after patients were admitted to the ICU. Using unfractionated heparin as anticoagulation, we did observe in the present study any of the classical CRRT-associated complications such as bleeding or extracorporeal circuit clotting [27]. We chose to use of CVVHDF, rather than CVVH, in cases of severe and threatening hyperkalemia. We used also a flow rate of the total effluent (the sum of the dialysate and ultrafiltrate) averaging 34±6 ml/kg/h; i.e., a "standard" dose of replacement solution when compared to the very high flow rates (50 to 80 ml/kg/h) sometimes proposed to treat MALA [25,26]. As classically reported, renal recovery (urine output increase and spontaneous urea/creatinine decrease), metabolic state improvement, fluid overload correction, as well as hemodynamic stability were the mean criteria to decide cessation of CRRT [28].

CRRT seems more physiologically appropriate than intermittent hemodialysis in this setting for several reasons. First, because of the drug's low molecular weight and lack of protein binding, conventional modalities of treatment (i.e., dialysis and/or ultrafiltration) can perform high plasma clearance of metformin [24]. Second, metformin has a large volume of distribution (3.1 l/kg) secondary to intracellular penetration [29]. Seidowsky *et al.* determined recently that 15 cumulative hours of hemodialysis were needed to return patients to therapeutic levels of metformin [5]. CRRT can be used for extended durations and maximizes metformin removal, with a rate of metformin elimination from the blood compartment averaging 2.4±0.9%/h. If prolonged renal therapy is required, initiation of CRRT upon patient admission may be a fast and convenient treatment. Third, all of our patients had circulatory failure upon admission. Because of this, we needed to avoid the detrimental impact of highly intermittent dialysis on hemodynamics, which is caused by major variations in solutes, bicarbonate, electrolytes, pH, and volemia. Thus, CRRT may be a superior choice for MALA, because it gradually removes solutes and places patients in a prolonged physiologically steady state [30].

The reported mortality in patients with MALA was initially very high, nearing 50% [3,18]. More recently, Peters *et al.* reported a 30% death rate in patients admitted to the ICU with MALA [2]. Awareness of metformin complications, as well as better organ failure treatment in ICUs may be the reasons for this decrease in mortality. Indeed, symptomatic management of organ failure (e.g., mechanical ventilation and/or vasoactive drugs) at admission was our priority even before ensuring diagnosis and starting CRRT as a specific treatment. Furthermore, in the present study, in addition to CRRT, we aggressively corrected both the precipitating and the underlying conditions of metformin accumulation by nonspecific therapeutic measures, which could also explain the favourable outcomes we observed.

In summary, early CRRT appears to be a safe and effective means of managing MALA in patients with hemodynamic instability and its use should become more widespread. This modality of replacement therapy, in conjunction with other symptomatic intensive therapies, rapidly corrects metabolic disorders and efficiently eliminates metformin when the standard guidelines for use are followed. However, further studies are needed to determine the most adequate ways of administering this CRRT in patients with MALA.

Author Contributions

Conceived and designed the experiments: LA DR GK. Performed the experiments: GK MC RH JI. Analyzed the data: GK. Contributed reagents/materials/analysis tools: GK LA. Wrote the paper: GK DR LA.

References

1. UK Prospective Diabetes Study (UKPDS) Group (1998) Effect of intensive blood-glucose control with metformin on complications in overweight patients with type 2 diabetes (UKPDS 34). Lancet 352: 854–865.
2. Peters N, Jay N, Barraud D, Cravoisy A, Nace L, et al. (2008) Metformin-associated lactic acidosis in an intensive care unit. Crit Care 12: R149.
3. Misbin RI, Green L, Stadel BV, Gueriguian JL, Gubbi A, Fleming GA (1998) Lactic acidosis in patients with diabetes treated with metformin. N Engl J Med 338: 265–6.
4. Kruse JA (2001) Metformin-associated lactic acidosis. J Emerg Medicine 20: 267–272.
5. Seidowsky A, Nseir S, Houdret N, Fourrier F (2009) Metformin-associated lactic acidosis: a prognostic and therapeutic study. Crit Care Med 37: 2191–2196.
6. Lalau JD, Westeel PF, Debussche X, Dkissi H, Tolani M, et al. (1987) Bicarbonate haemodialysis: an adequate treatment for lactic acidosis in diabetics treated by metformin. Intensive Care Med 13: 383–387.
7. Bruijstens LA, van Luin M, Buscher-Jungerhans PM, Bosch FH (2008) Reality of severe metformin-induced lactic acidosis in the absence of chronic renal impairment. Neth J Med 66: 185–190.
8. Galea M, Jelacin N, Bramham K, White I (2007) Severe lactic acidosis and rhabdomyolysis following metformin and ramipril overdose. Br J Anaesth 98: 213–215.
9. Arroyo AM, Walroth TA, Mowry JB, Kao LW (2010) The MALAdy of metformin poisoning: is CVVH the cure? Am J Ther 17: 96–100.
10. Lalau JD, Race JM (2000) Metformin and lactic acidosis in diabetic humans. Diabetes Obes Metab 2: 131–137.
11. Jackson GG, Arana Sialer JA, Andersen BR, Grieble HG, McCabe WR (1962) Profiles of pyelonephritis. Arch Intern Med 110: 63–75.
12. Knaus WA, Zimmerman JE, Wagner DP, Draper EA, Lawrence DE (1981) APACHE-acute physiology and chronic health evaluation: a physiologically based classification system. Crit Care Med 9: 591–597.
13. Charlson ME, Pompei P, Ales KL, MacKenzie CR (1987) A new method of classifying prognostic comorbidity in longitudinal studies: development and validation. J Chronic Dis 40: 373–383.
14. Le Gall JR, Lemeshow S, Saulnier F (1993) A new Simplified Acute Physiology Score (SAPS II) based on a European/North American multicenter study. JAMA 270: 2957–2963.
15. Teasdale G, Murray G, Parker L, Jennett B (1979) Adding up the Glasgow Coma Score. Acta Neurochir Suppl 28: 13–16.
16. Fagon JY, Chastre J, Novare A, Medioni P, Gibert C (1993) Characterization of intensive care unit patients using a model based on the presence or absence of organ dysfunctions and/or infection: the ODIN model. Intensive Care Med 19: 137–144.
17. Vincent JL, Moreno R, Takala J, Willatts S, De Mendonca A, et al. (1996) The SOFA (Sepsis-related Organ Failure Assessment) score to describe organ dysfunction/failure. On behalf of the Working Group on Sepsis-Related Problems of the European Society of Intensive Care Medicine. Intensive Care Med 22: 707–710.
18. Stades AM, Heikens JT, Erkelens DW, Hollememan F, Hoekstra JB (2004) Metformin and lactic acidosis: cause or coincidence? A review of case reports. J Intern Med 255: 179–187.
19. Lalau JD, Lacroix C (2003) Measurement of metformin concentration in erythrocytes: clinical implications. Diabetes Obes Metab 5: 93–98.
20. Lalau JD, Race JM (1999) Lactic acidosis in metformin-treated patients. Prognostic value of arterial lactate levels and plasma metformin concentrations. Drug Saf 20: 377–384.
21. Kirpichnikov D, McFarlane SI, Sowers JR (2002) Metformin: an update. Ann Intern Med 137: 25–33.
22. Leverve XM (2005) Lactate in the intensive care unit: pyromaniac, sentinel or fireman? Crit Care 9: 588–593.
23. Levraut J, Ciebiera JP, Jambou P, Ichai C, Labib Y, et al. (1997) Effect of continuous venovenous hemofiltration with dialysis on lactate clearance in critically ill patients. Crit Care Med 25: 58–62.
24. Guo PY, Storsley LJ, Finkle SN (2006) Severe lactic acidosis treated with prolonged hemodialysis: recovery after massive overdoses of metformin. Semin Dial 19: 80–83.
25. Pan LT, MacLaren G (2009) Continuous venovenous haemodiafiltration for metformin-induced lactic acidosis. Anaesth Intensive Care 37: 830–83.
26. Panzer U, Kluge S, Kreymann G, Wolf G (2004) Combination of intermittent haemodialysis and high-volume continuous haemofiltration for the treatment of severe metformin-induced lactic acidosis. Nephrol Dial Transplant 19: 2157–2158.
27. Finkel KW, Podoll AS (2009) Complications of continuous renal replacement therapy. Semin Dial 22: 155–159.
28. Uchino S, Bellomo R, Morimatsu H, Morgera S, Schetz M, et al. (2009) Discontinuation of continuous renal replacement therapy: a posthoc analysis of a prospective multicenter observational study. Crit Care Med 37: 2576–2582.
29. Sambol NC, Chiang J, O'Conner M, Liu CY, Lin ET, et al. (1996) Pharmacokinetics and pharmacodynamics of metformin in healthy subjects and patients with noninsulin-dependent diabetes mellitus. J Clin Pharmacol 36: 1012–1021.
30. Ronco C, Ricci Z (2008) Renal replacement therapies: physiological review. Intensive Care Med 34: 2139–2146.

16

Mitochondrial DNA Variant Discovery and Evaluation in Human Cardiomyopathies through Next-Generation Sequencing

Michael V. Zaragoza[1]*, Joseph Fass[2], Marta Diegoli[3], Dawei Lin[2], Eloisa Arbustini[3]

1 Genetics & Metabolism Division, Pediatrics Department and Center for Mitochondrial and Molecular Medicine and Genetics (MAMMAG), University of California Irvine, Irvine, California, United States of America, 2 Bioinformatics Core, UC Davis Genome Center, University of California Davis, Davis, California, United States of America, 3 Centre for Inherited Cardiovascular Diseases, IRCCS Foundation Policlinico San Mateo, Pavia, Italy

Abstract

Mutations in mitochondrial DNA (mtDNA) may cause maternally-inherited cardiomyopathy and heart failure. In homoplasmy all mtDNA copies contain the mutation. In heteroplasmy there is a mixture of normal and mutant copies of mtDNA. The clinical phenotype of an affected individual depends on the type of genetic defect and the ratios of mutant and normal mtDNA in affected tissues. We aimed at determining the sensitivity of next-generation sequencing compared to Sanger sequencing for mutation detection in patients with mitochondrial cardiomyopathy. We studied 18 patients with mitochondrial cardiomyopathy and two with suspected mitochondrial disease. We "shotgun" sequenced PCR-amplified mtDNA and multiplexed using a single run on Roche's 454 Genome Sequencer. By mapping to the reference sequence, we obtained 1,300× average coverage per case and identified high-confidence variants. By comparing these to >400 mtDNA substitution variants detected by Sanger, we found 98% concordance in variant detection. Simulation studies showed that >95% of the homoplasmic variants were detected at a minimum sequence coverage of 20× while heteroplasmic variants required >200× coverage. Several Sanger "misses" were detected by 454 sequencing. These included the novel heteroplasmic 7501T>C in tRNA serine 1 in a patient with sudden cardiac death. These results support a potential role of next-generation sequencing in the discovery of novel mtDNA variants with heteroplasmy below the level reliably detected with Sanger sequencing. We hope that this will assist in the identification of mtDNA mutations and key genetic determinants for cardiomyopathy and mitochondrial disease.

Editor: Wenjun Li, Duke University Medical Center, United States of America

Funding: Financial support was provided by the National Institutes of Health K08 award HL081222 from National Heart, Lung, and Blood Institute to MVZ and by grants "Cariplo" and RC from the Ministry of Health for Inherited Cardiomyopathies and EC INHERITANCE project 241924, Health-2009-2.4.2-3 awarded to EA. The funders had no role in study design, data collection and analysis, decision to publish, or preparation of the manuscript.

Competing Interests: The authors have declared that no competing interests exist.

* E-mail: mzaragoz@uci.edu

Introduction

Mitochondrial DNA and inheritance

Human mitochondrial DNA (mtDNA) is a circular, 16,569 base sequence that encodes for 13 proteins, 22 transfer RNAs (tRNAs) and 2 ribosomal RNAs [1]. MtDNA is essential for mitochondrial energy production through oxidative phosphorylation, and hundreds to thousands of mtDNA molecules may be found per cell depending upon the energy requirements of the tissue [2].

In contrast to nuclear genes (nDNA), mtDNA is inherited only from the mother [3]; therefore, mtDNA mutations associated with inherited mitochondrial diseases follow the maternal lineage with no transmission from the father [4]. Along the maternal lineage, different amounts of a pathogenic and normal mtDNAs may be inherited due to a genetic bottle neck during oogenesis and/or by purifying selection of severe mtDNA mutations [5–7]. Homoplasmy describes the state where only mutant or variant mtDNAs exist; whereas, in heteroplasmy there is a mixture of normal and mutant or variant mtDNAs. Depending on the inheritance (maternally-derived or *de novo*), segregation and postnatal selection, an affected individual may have different ratios of mutant and normal mtDNA in different tissues that result in mitochondrial disease.

Mitochondrial DNA analysis by capillary and next generation sequencing

Traditionally, the most comprehensive method used to detect variants is Sanger capillary sequencing of whole mtDNA [8,9]. However, limitations prevent the routine use of whole mtDNA studies by Sanger sequencing including the amount of labor and time to manually inspect data for heteroplasmic mutations. Thus, large scale efforts have been lacking to critically evaluate the role of mtDNA mutations in human disease and to investigate the scope of normal mtDNA variation in populations.

Recently, advances in microfluidics, digital imaging systems and bioinformatics have lead to new sequencing methods or Next Generation Sequencing (NGS) that may overcome these limitations. NGS methods can generate vast amounts of sequencing data in less time and overall costs compared to traditional methods [10]. So, many people believe that NGS may replace the traditional methods to detect pathogenic mutations in patients. However, a major problem is the lack of patient studies to evaluate NGS for mutation detection in comparison to Sanger sequencing [11]. In addition, few NGS studies have focused on mtDNA [12,13] and the detection of heteroplasmy [14,15] with only one study on patients with known or suspected mitochondrial disease [16].

The goal of this study was to explore NGS as a method to detect mtDNA mutations in patients. Our aims were: (1) to identify all mtDNA variants and potential mutations; (2) to evaluate variant detection performance by comparing Roche 454 pyrosequencing and Sanger sequencing technologies; and (3) to estimate the amount of sequence coverage needed to detect homoplasmic and heteroplasmic mtDNA mutations or variants. In this report, we provide the results of mtDNA analysis for 20 patients with mitochondrial cardiomyopathy or suspected mitochondrial disease.

Results

Study population

We studied the mtDNA for 20 cases: 18 with mitochondrial cardiomyopathy and 2 with suspected mitochondrial disease. For each case, general features and the numbers of mtDNA variants detected by Sanger and 454 sequencing are listed in Table 1.

MtDNA variant calls based on bioinformatics analysis of 454 sequences

For Sanger sequencing, we made 330,979 (99.9%) of 331,380 possible base calls (20 mtDNAs ×16,569 bases/mtDNA). Compared to the reference, we identified 460 mtDNA variants that consisted of 414 single nucleotide substitutions, 410 homoplasmic and 4 heteroplasmic variants (Table 1). For each case, we found 10 to 41 variants for an average of 23 variants per mtDNA; details for the Sanger mtDNA variants will be in a separate report (unpublished data).

For 454 sequencing, the results are provided in Table 1 for total coverage and read length; Table S1 for detailed results for all variants; and Table S2 for the mapping statistics. Using a single 454 run, we obtained approximately 440 Mb of raw sequencing data from 1.2 million sequence reads. On average, 97.1% of the reads and 98.4% of the bases mapped to the reference sequence for each case (Table S2) which corresponded to an average coverage (redundant and non-redundant sequences) of 1,300×

Table 1. Summary of mtDNA mapping and sequencing results for 20 cases.

Case	Cardiac	454 Mapping Ave.[b]		454 Variants[c]				Sanger Variants[a,c]			
No.[a]	Feature	Depth	Length	Total	Subst	Indel	Repeat	Total	Subst	Indel	Repeat
1[d]	HCM, HF	463	355	39	34	3	2	37	33	0	4
3	HCM	1,148	377	23	14	9	0	15	14	0	1
5	SCD, HF	944	373	33	31	2	0	32	30	0	2
6	DCM	1,542	374	28	17	11	0	18	17	0	1
7	HCM	1,561	372	25	17	8	0	18	17	0	1
8	HCM	1,294	381	24	15	8	1	18	15	0	3
9	HCM	1,506	374	20	12	7	1	15	13	0	2
10	HCM	1,635	377	19	10	8	1	12	10	0	2
11	HCM	1,393	373	25	10	14	1	14	10	1	3
12	HCM	1,442	379	17	10	6	1	13	11	0	2
13	DCM	1,042	373	39	32	6	1	36	32	1	3
14	DCM	1,498	372	35	25	7	3	28	25	0	3
15	DCM	2,140	376	35	25	10	0	26	25	0	1
16	DCM	1,823	381	15	9	6	0	10	9	0	1
17	DCM	1,134	375	38	30	8	0	30	29	0	1
18	DCM	1,431	369	45	36	8	1	41	36	1	4
19	DCM	1,147	368	17	7	9	1	10	7	0	3
20	DCM	2,054	380	51	40	11	0	41	39	0	2
NonCM1	ECHO nl	57[e]	363	30	29	1	0	31	29	0	2
NonCM2	ECHO nl	716	376	23	14	9	0	15	13	0	2
	AVE:	1,299	373	29	21	8	1	23	21	0	2
	TOTAL:	–	–	581	417	151	13	460	414	3	43

Abbreviations: HCM = hypertrophic cardiomyopathy; HF = heart failure; DCM = dilated cardiomyopathy; SCD = sudden cardiac death; ECHO nl = echocardiograms normal.
[a]Additional case information and Sanger data analysis for haplotype and potential mutations are described in a separate report (unpublished data); cases 2 and 4 were not included in the present study.
[b]454 mapping statistics: depth = average number of mapped sequences (non-redundant and redundant sequences) at each base position; length = average base length of mapped sequences.
[c]Mitochondrial DNA variants compared to NCBI Reference (NC_012920); Variant types: subst = single nucleotide substitutions; indel = insertion or deletion; repeat = polymorphic repeats at positions: 303–315, 522–523, 574, 16180–16193 and 16519 (www.mitomap.com).
[d]From previously reported HCM family with MYH7 mutation [17].
[e]Decreased reads for NonCM1 possibly due to a pre-sequencing technical error.

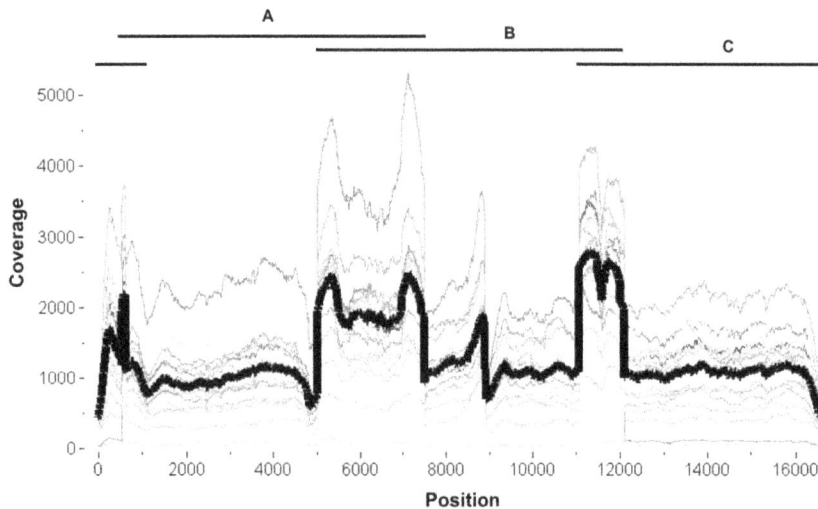

Figure 1. Variability in 454 sequence coverage. Total read coverage (redundant and non-redundant) is plotted at each mtDNA position (1 to 16569) and graphed as a continuous thin gray trace for each case (different shades for each case). The mean coverage for all 20 cases is represented by a thick dark black trace. The shape of the traces shows coverage variability both between cases and along the same mtDNA. The black horizontal lines (A, B & C) above the graph represent the three mtDNA PCR fragments used for 454 sequencing. Greater coverage was noted in the regions in which the PCR fragments overlap compared to coverage in non-overlapping regions.

and to an average mapped read length of 373 bases (range: 355 to 380 bases) (Table 1).

Similar to previous studies on 454 sequencing, we found variability in the depth of coverage between multiplexed cases and along the same mtDNA molecule (Figure 1) [11,12,18]. We attributed the lowest coverage due to a technical error in sample preparation for NonCM1. When this case was excluded, we still found that the read depth varied between cases up to ten-fold (Figure 1). For coverage along the same mtDNA, we observed a significant increase in the average coverage per base within the regions where the PCR fragments overlap (mean = 1,947, SD = 991) compared to the average coverage in non-overlapping regions (mean = 1,072, SD = 543), $p<0.0001$. Overall, these findings suggest that uniform coverage might be achieved by

single or two fragment LR-PCR instead of three fragments [12,19].

We mapped the reads using the Roche GS Mapper software and identified "high confidence" differences (HCDiffs) between each mtDNA contig and the reference (Table 1). For the 20 cases, all 331,380 possible base calls were made. These included 581 HCDiffs with 417 single nucleotide substitutions, 411 homoplasmic and 6 heteroplasmic variants (Table 2 and Table S1). For each case, we found 15 to 51 HCDiffs for an average of 29 variants per mtDNA.

Comparison of 454 and Sanger results indicated high concordance for substitutions

We first compared the numbers and types of variants (substitutions, indels and repeats) detected by 454 and Sanger

Table 2. Discordant and/or heteroplasmic substitution mtDNA variants.

| Type | Method[a] | | Case No. | Position | 454 depth | Type of error | Reason for |
	Sanger	454			(% variant) [b]		discordance
Homoplasmic	+	−	9	8473T>C	231 (83%)	454 false -	Homopolymer
	+	−	12	16566G>A	352(100%)	454 false -	Software miscall
	−	+	17	3010G>A	350 (100%)	Sanger false -	Miscall
	−	+	20	15326A>G	405 (100%)	Sanger false -	Miscall
	−	+	1	13967C>T	244 (100%)	Sanger false -	Poor data
Heteroplasmic	−	+	NonCM2	16093T>C	246 (14%)	Sanger false -	Miscall
	−	+	5	7501T>C	298 (18%)	Sanger false -	Miscall
	+	+	6	3243A>G	340 (19%)	N/A	N/A
	+	+	20	9854T>G	344 (39%)	N/A	N/A
	+	+	7	3645T>C	382 (47%)	N/A	N/A
	+	+	NonCM1	15222A>G	45 (64%)	N/A	N/A

[a]Sequencing method: variant detected = "+", variant not detected = "−".
[b]454 depth = total number of non-redundant reads with percentage of variant reads in parentheses.

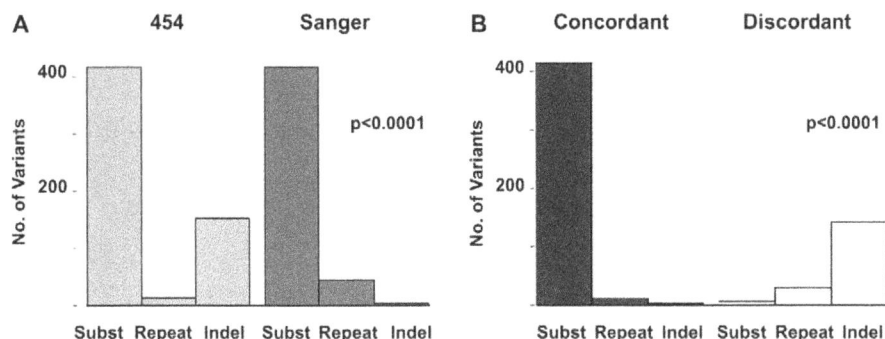

Figure 2. Comparison of 454 and Sanger sequencing results. Histograms show the distribution of variants by type: single nucleotide substitutions (subst), repeats and insertion/deletions (indel). **A. Sequencing method.** Results are separated by detection using 454 (left panel, light gray) or Sanger (right panel, dark gray). **B. Concordance.** Results are separated by concordant detection using 454 and Sanger sequencing (left panel, dark gray) or by discordant detection, 454 or Sanger sequencing only (right panel, light gray). We observed high concordance between the two methods for mtDNA substitutions and significant discordance for indels.

sequencing (Table 1). There was a significant difference due to a greater number of indels detected by 454, X^2 (2, N = 1041) = 146.2, p<0.0001 (Figure 2A). In total, 614 mtDNA variants were identified by 454 or Sanger sequencing (Table S1). These included 427 (70%) concordant variants (detected by both platforms) and 187 (30%) discordant variants (initially detected by a single method). The 427 concordant variants consisted of: 412 of 419 (98%) substitutions, 12 of 44 (27%) repeats and 3 of 151 (2%) indels (Figure 2B). Compared to the concordant variants, the distribution of 187 discordant variants was significantly different and included: 7 of 419 (2%) substitutions, 32 of 44 (73%) repeats and 148 of 151 (98%) indels, X^2 (2, N = 614) = 526, p< 0.0001 (Figure 2B).

Discordant variants include a potential, novel mtDNA mutation missed by Sanger

Next, we wanted to determine the possible sources of error for the seven discordant substitution variants, two (8473T>C and 16566G>A) detected by Sanger and five identified by 454 (Table 2). We first reviewed the Sanger chromatograms and 454 reads that mapped to these positions and concluded that all seven discordant results were false negative errors. For 8473T>C, the discordance may be from masking of variant reads by erroneous 454 reads due to the formation of a six base homopolymer (Table S1). For 16566G>A, we found the variant in all mapped reads at that position; however, it was not identified as a high confidence variant.

For the five discordant variants detected by 454 (Table 2), retrospective review of the initial chromatograms and repeat Sanger sequencing confirmed the presence of each variant. From this, we concluded that four false negative errors resulted from miscalled Sanger sequences, and the fifth Sanger "miss" to the lack of coverage. We found that the most significant miscall was a heteroplasmic variant, 7501T>C in *MT-TS1* for tRNA serine 1 (Figure 3).

Analysis of heteroplasmic mtDNA variants

We next compared the results of 454 and Sanger sequencing for the detection of heteroplasmic variants defined as having 80% or less variant read frequency after excluding erroneous reads from a homopolymer. We evaluated all substitution and indel variants detected by 454 and excluded repeat polymorphisms because of the possibility of false positive errors from PCR amplification [20].

Based on these criteria, we found six heteroplasmic variants of 419 total substitutions. These included four of 412 concordant substitutions (3243A<G, 9854T<G, 3645T<C and 15222A<G) with variant read frequencies of 19% to 64% and two of seven discordant substitutions (16093T>C and 7501T>C) with frequencies of 14% and 18% (Table 2). Similar to 7501T>C, we failed to identify 16093T>C by our initial Sanger analysis and detected the variant first by 454 sequencing.

We continued our evaluation to determine the presence of heteroplasmy for the 151 indels detected by 454 sequencing. Based on our criteria, indels had a significantly higher proportion of variants with read frequencies of 80% or less (148 of 151 indels) compared to substitutions (6 of 419), X^2 (1, N = 570) = 520, p<0.0001. However, after reviewing all 454 reads for the 148 indels, we found that each indel was associated with a homopolymer (4 to 8 bases) at or within four bases of the variant position (Table S1). So, we concluded that all 148 indels were most likely homopolymer-associated false positive errors and were not true heteroplasmic variants, findings consistent with the Sanger data for these positions.

Performance metrics for 454 and Sanger sequencing

As another means of comparison, we used performance metrics [11] that we modified to reflect mtDNA genotypes with heteroplasmy (Table S3). We calculated 454 sequence accuracy as 99.95% and variant accuracy as 99.5% excluding repeat polymorphisms. Next, we calculated the error rates and found no significant difference in the false negative rate for 454 (2 of 421 = 0.5%) and Sanger (4 of 421 = 1%), X^2 (1, N = 842) = 0.168, p = 0.6820. However, we found a significantly greater false positive rate for 454 (148 of 329938 = 0.044%) compared to Sanger in which we did not find false positive errors (0 of 329938 = 0%), X^2 (1, N = 659876) = 148.033, p<0.0001, as we expected from homopolymer-associated 454 indels.

Simulation studies- variant detection at different coverages

After our comparisons between 454 and Sanger sequencing, we estimated the minimum 454 sequence coverage for detection of heteroplasmy (Figure 4 and Table S4). We simulated nine levels of coverage from 2× to 500× and then calculated the variant detection rate for 419 total substitution variants: 6 heteroplasmic variants and 413 homoplasmic variants. In this analysis, we excluded repeat polymorphisms and indels because nearly all

A

B 454   7501T>C, *tRNA ser1*

54
variant
reads

GG---CCC---CC---A-T

244
reference
reads

GG---CC-T--CC---A-T

C Sanger

G G C C C C C A T
G G C C T C C A T

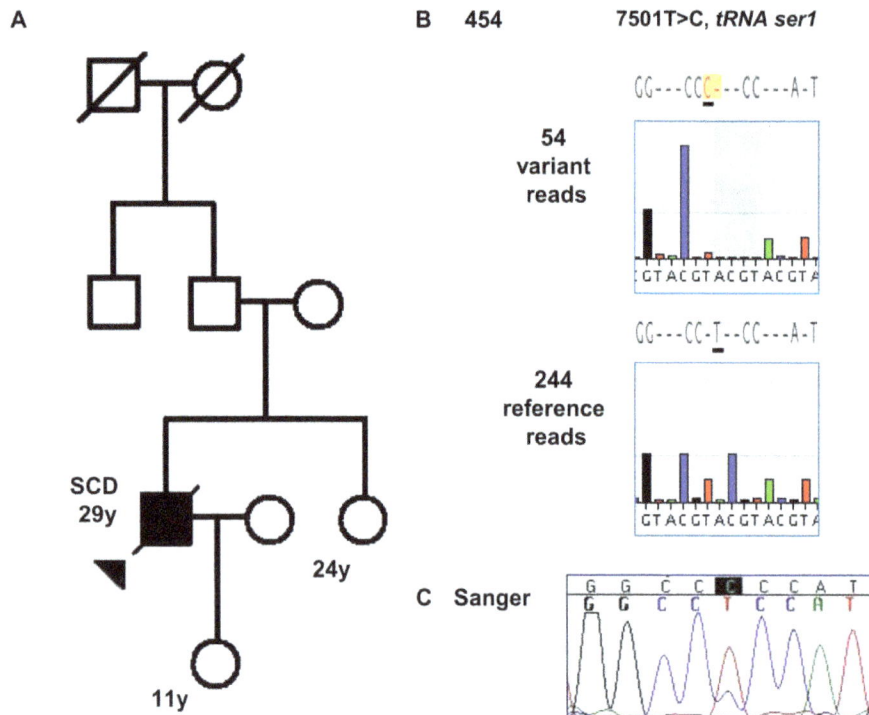

Figure 3. Novel, potential mtDNA mutation 7501T>C detected by 454 sequencing. A. Case 5 pedigree. Circles represent females and squares represent males; solid shapes are affected individuals; an arrow indicates the proband that died from sudden cardiac death (SCD). **B. 454 sequencing.** Shown are representative 454 data flowgrams. We obtained 298 total unique reads, 54 reads had the 7501T>C variant (top) and 244 reads had the reference sequence (bottom). **C. Sanger sequencing.** Retrospective analysis of Sanger data revealed the missed variant. As shown in the chromatogram, two peaks are found at position 7501 consistent with a low level of heteroplasmy.

indels were homopolymer-associated false positive errors and the possibility of the repeats being PCR artifacts. From these simulations, we estimated that to detect >95% of mtDNA variants by 454 sequencing, read coverages of at least >20× for

homoplasmy and >200× for heteroplasmy (range: 10%–80%) were needed.

Discussion

Roche 454 versus Sanger sequencing for whole mtDNA analysis

Our results showed that 454 sequencing was comparable to Sanger sequencing in the detection of single nucleotide substitutions. High concordance (98%) was obtained for the detection of over 400 single nucleotide substitutions including four heteroplasmic variants previously detected by Sanger sequencing. A previous 454 sequencing study of a 110 kb nDNA region supports this finding; the study found 98.5% agreement for nearly 400 SNPs at 30× average coverage [21].

This high concordance, in addition, is reflected in the high 454 sequencing (99.95%) and variant accuracies (99.5%) in our study. The 454 sequencing accuracy is consistent with the NGS study that also directly compared results to Sanger analysis; they obtained >99.9% 454 sequencing accuracy for a 266 kb nDNA region in 4 samples with 43× average coverage [11]. Our variant accuracy, however, was significantly greater than the 454 variant accuracy (93.9%) [11]. Since variant accuracy only includes Sanger detected variants, one possible explanation for this difference was our exclusion of repeat polymorphisms—identified commonly by Sanger but not by 454 sequencing. To confirm these repeats are real variants (and thus, true 454 false negatives), non-amplification and single molecule analysis may be possible using the next wave of sequencing technologies [22].

For our discordant results, not surprisingly, we found 454 indels consistent with false positive errors from homopolymers in

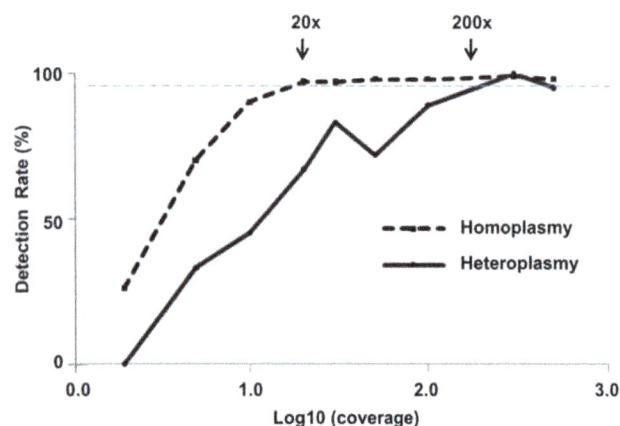

Figure 4. Coverage simulations and variant detection rate for mtDNA variants. By subsampling all mapped 454 reads, we simulated nine levels of coverage (2× to 500×) for 419 mtDNA substitution variants. Graph shows the variant detection rate by the log10 (coverage) for homoplasmy (black solid line, n = 413) and heteroplasmy (black dashed line, n = 6). We estimated that the minimum coverages to detect 95% of the variants (gray dashed horizontal line) are >20× for homoplasmy and >200× for heteroplasmy.

previous reports [23–25]; however, we found, in addition, two 454 false negative errors that resulted in an ~0.5% false negative rate. This rate was less than the 3% 454 false negative rate previously reported [11], possibly again due our exclusion of repeat polymorphisms. For SNP calling, previous 454 studies reported no false negatives with average coverages at 30× [21] and 43× [11].

Including the results of our studies, we concluded that false negative errors for SNP calling were rare for 454 sequencing. For one of the 454 false negatives 8473T>C, we concluded it was from the unusual creation of a new homopolymer with the variant. The T>C base change created a six cytosine homopolymer (position 8471–8476) by linking adjacent cytosine bases. The resulting indel reads (frequency = 17%) associated with the homopolymer may have masked the call of 8473T>C as a high confidence variant. The second 454 false negative, 16566G>A, likely resulted from a software error. Although 16566G>A was found in all mapped sequences (352 unique reads) of the contig, 16566G>A was not called as a 454 variant. In support, we found the updated Roche GS Mapper software (version 2.3) correctly called the variant (data not shown).

Taken together, these results show that 454 sequencing was reliable as Sanger sequencing in the SNP detection. Still, one concern may be the decreased ability to resolve homopolymeric regions by 454 sequencing that potentially may mask a mutation at or adjacent to the region. It is possible that this may have little impact on the ability to detect mtDNA mutations. We found that the 148 homopolymer-associated indels involved only 23 nucleotide positions (Table S1). The vast majority were located in coding regions; however, mutations associated with mitochondrial disease have not been reported at any of these positions (www.MITOMAP.org).

Detection of missed heteroplasmy by 454 sequencing

With the remaining discordant results, we provide evidence that 454 sequencing may detect variants missed by Sanger analysis—mtDNA variants with roughly less than 20% heteroplasmy. We first noted, overall, five Sanger false negatives that resulted in a 1% Sanger false negative rate. Our estimated rate was less than the 3% Sanger false negative rate previously reported [11]; we speculate this difference may be from improved variant detection by duplicate mtDNA analyses in two laboratories. Still, we had five Sanger false negatives including two mtDNA variants with low levels of heteroplasmy (read frequency = 14%–18%) and three homoplasmic variants initially missed by manual inspection or not identified due to a sequence gap. When we included the four heteroplasmic concordant variants, our results suggest that 454 sequencing may detect heteroplasmy at the level reliably detected by Sanger sequencing (above ~20%) [26] but also below that limit [14].

Of the two heteroplasmic variants missed by Sanger analysis, 7501T>C is a novel, potential mutation in the mtDNA tRNA serine 1 gene (MT-TS1). Mutations in tRNA serine 1 have been described in patients with mitochondrial disease [27] but no one with cardiomyopathy or sudden cardiac death as for our patient (Case 5). However, although 7501T>C was not found in the mtDNA databases with more than 5,000 sequences [28,29], it is possible that 7501T>C is only a benign polymorphism not found in the specific mtDNA haplogroups comprising the databases. As another possible explanation, 7501T>C may be one of many heteroplasmic variants detectable in normal individuals at low levels [14]. Therefore, we emphasize that we cannot conclude that 7501T>C is truly a mutation until we obtain additional evidence through family studies, functional studies of 7501T>C for

mitochondrial defects and population studies to investigate the amount of normal mtDNA variation within this patient's haplogroup.

Sequence coverage needed to detect mtDNA variants

In addition to our 454 and Sanger comparisons, we used the deep 454 sequence coverage (average 1300×) and computer simulations to estimate the minimum amounts of coverage needed to detect homoplasmic and heteroplasmic mtDNA variants. The results suggest that 20× coverage was needed for homoplasmy and at least 200× coverage for heteroplasmy greater than 10%, the limit of this study. This is consistent with the observed 10-20× coverage sufficient for the detection of homoplasmy in a previous 454 study of 14 mtDNAs [13] and the ≥200× coverage selected as criteria for potential heteroplasmy in an Illumina GAII sequencing study of three mtDNAs [16]. Thus, detection of heteroplasmic mtDNA variants at frequencies above 10% requires greater 454 coverage than the >30× coverage estimated for the detection of heterozygous nDNA variants [21,30], and detection of heteroplasmic variants at lower frequencies may require deeper sequencing, coverages estimated to be at least 1,500× for ≥5% [15] and 15,000× to 100,000× for as low as 2% [14,31].

In summary, our results support the potential use of 454 sequencing for detection of mtDNA substitutions with heteroplasmy of greater than 10%. Using this data, we also estimate a single 454 GS FLX run would obtain sufficient coverage (20×) to detect homoplasmic mtDNA variants in 300 mtDNAs. These results, thus, support high-throughput population studies on mtDNA variation as another potential use of 454 sequencing [12,13]. As the performance and output for sequencing technologies continue to improve, we may anticipate higher accuracies and deeper coverages that will enable low cost global analysis of mtDNA variation and highly sensitive mtDNA mutation detection. We hope that this will identify key genetic determinants for heart failure, cardiomyopathy and mitochondrial disease leading to the personalized understanding of disease mechanisms and personalized treatments.

Materials and Methods

Study population/ethics statement

We evaluated 20 patients referred to Dr. Eloisa Arbustini at Center for Inherited Cardiovascular Diseases in Pavia, Italy (Table 1). This included 18 patients with mitochondrial cardiomyopathy and two suspected of mitochondrial disease. The 20 cases were a subset of 29 cases to be reported on a web-based bioinformatics approach to identify potential mtDNA mutations by Sanger sequencing (unpublished data). Case 1 was from previously reported HCM family with an MYH7 mutation and possible mtDNA mutation 9957T>C [17]. We obtained informed written consent of all participants; the study was approved by the bioethics committee of the IRCCS Foundation Policlinico San Matteo in Pavia and by the UC Irvine Institutional Review Board for de-identified DNA samples (#2009-6931).

Mitochondrial DNA sequencing

We extracted genomic DNA from blood except for Case 7 in which we used heart tissue. Sanger sequencing method (costs ~$130 per mtDNA) and mtDNA data analyses are described in a separate report (unpublished data).

For Roche 454 sequencing (Figure 5), we first PCR amplified mtDNA from genomic DNA using Roche Expand Long Range PCR dNTPack (Roche Applied Science, Indianapolis, IN). Using three pairs of mtDNA-specific primers, we produced three

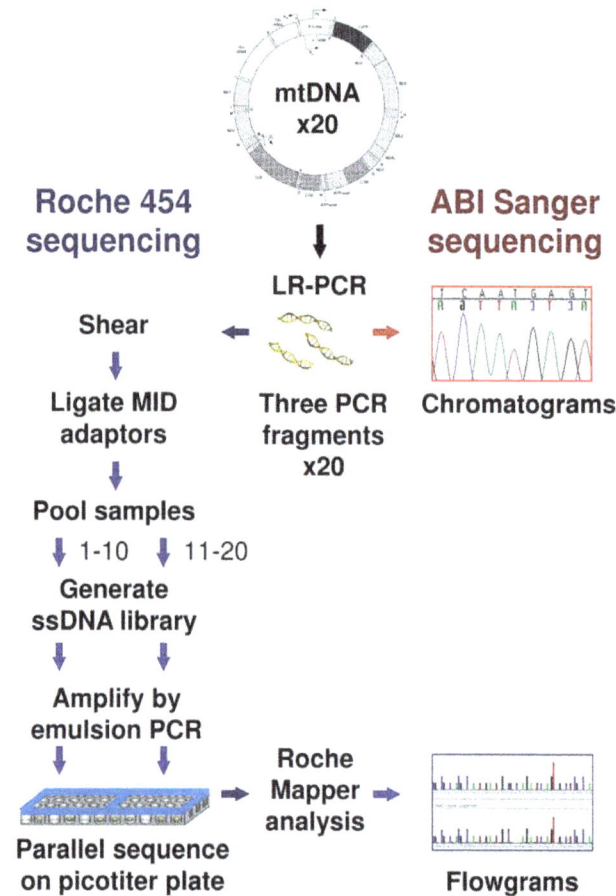

Figure 5. Mitochondrial DNA sequencing approach. Schematic depicts steps in ABI Sanger and Roche 454 sequencing [23]. We isolated DNA from 20 cases and amplified mitochondrial DNA (mtDNA) by long range PCR (LR-PCR). We sequenced the PCR fragments using standard Sanger and 454 sequencing methods. For 454, the fragments were sheared and then ligated to Multiplex Identifier (MID) adaptors. Next, we made two pooled samples by combining the tagged fragments for cases 1–10 and cases 11–20. Single-stranded DNA (ssDNA) libraries were made from each pooled sample and clonally amplified by emulsion PCR. Parallel sequencing was done on a single picotiter plate divide into two regions. The final data, represented as a Sanger chromatogram and 454 flowgrams, are shown.

overlapping PCR fragments; A: 6929 bp, position 569–7497; B: 7050 bp, position 5061–12111; C: 6866 bp, 11107–1405 (Figure 1). We purified each fragment using Roche High Pure PCR Product Purification Kit. Primer sequences and PCR conditions are available upon request.

We conducted Roche 454 FLX sequencing for the 20 cases at the Genotyping & Sequencing Core/Orphan Disease Testing Center at the University of California, Los Angeles. Using standard protocols [23], we "shotgun" sequenced the three mtDNA PCR fragments for each of the 20 cases (costs ~$835 per mtDNA). First, the three fragments were quantified by fluorimetry using the PicoGreen Assay, and 2 micrograms of each fragment were combined. Each of the 20 resulting samples was sheared using the Covaris system (Covaris, Inc., Woburn, MA) and the sizes of the DNA fragments were checked using the Agilent 2100 Bioanalyzer system (Agilent Technologies, Inc., Santa Clara, CA). Roche's 10-base Multiplex Identifier (MID) Adaptors were added, and equimolar quantities of the tagged fragments for the first 10 cases and the last 10 cases were pooled together. For each of the two pooled samples, single-stranded DNA libraries were made and amplified by emulsion PCR. We conducted a single 454 sequencing run using one PicoTiterPlate divided into two regions, each with 10 MID tagged samples.

Bioinformatics analysis

We used the Roche 454 GS Mapper software (version 2.0.01) to assemble and compare the sequencing reads to the mtDNA reference sequence [GenBank: NC_012920] [32]. After standard image and signal processing, we sorted the sequencing reads from the Standard Flowgram Format (SFF) files using the distinct MID for each case. Reads were mapped to the reference sequence which produced a consensus sequence and identified "high-confidence differences" (HCDiffs). The criteria for HCDiffs were defined by GS Mapper: variants detected in at least three unique (non-duplicate) sequencing reads of high quality with both forward and reverse reads and found in >10% of the total unique sequencing reads.

We categorized each HCDiff by the variant type (single nucleotide substitution, insertion/deletion (indel) or repeat polymorphism) and by the presence or absence of heteroplasmy. HCDiffs at positions 303–315, 522–523, 574, 16180–16193 and 16519 were considered repeat polymorphisms [33,34]. For assessment of heteroplasmy, we developed criteria based on variant frequency, the number of variant reads divided by the total number of unique sequencing reads. We also carefully reviewed the variant and non-variant reads in the HCDiff text files to identify results most likely due to homopolymers, a known false positive source because of the technical limitations in 454 pyrosequencing [11,23–25]. We classified an HCDiff as heteroplasmic if: (1) the variant frequency was between 0.10 and 0.80 and (2) all non-variant reads contained only the reference allele, and as homoplasmic if: (1) variant frequency was ≥0.80 and (2) all non-variant reads may be explained by a homopolymer error that occurred at or adjacent to the nucleotide position. Since a variant had to be detected in >10% of unique reads to be considered an HCDiff, we did not evaluate variants with ≤0.10 frequencies.

All new sequence data for the 20 cases has been deposited in GenBank [accession numbers HM765456-HM765475].

Simulation studies

To estimate the minimal coverage for variant detection, we calculated the detection rate at different levels of simulated read coverage. We estimated from an average read length of ~375 bases that $1\times$ coverage of the ~16.5 kb mitochondrial sequence would be ~50 reads. Therefore, to simulate nine coverage levels ($2\times$, $5\times$, $10\times$, $20\times$, $30\times$, $50\times$, $100\times$, $300\times$ and $500\times$), we generated random subsamples of 100, 250, 500, 1000, 1500, 2500, 5000, 15000 and 25000 sequencing reads, respectively for each of the 20 cases. Three simulations were done for each coverage level. As before, we used Roche's GS Mapper to call HCDiffs and then filtered for single nucleotide polymorphisms. For each coverage level, we calculated the variant detection rate, the proportion of HCDiffs called out of the total number variants detected with full coverage.

Performance metrics and statistical analysis

To compare the mtDNA sequencing performances of the 454 and Sanger platforms, we used defined metrics [11]. We used JMP 7.0 (SAS Institute, Cary, NC) for statistical analysis and graphs. We considered p<0.05 as a significant difference.

To calculate performance metrics, we defined annotations that represented genotype differences between 454 and Sanger platforms [11] but modified to take heteroplasmy into account for mtDNA analysis (Table S3). For this analysis, we excluded the results for 31 nucleotide positions that had repeat polymorphisms: 303–315, 522–523, 574, 16180–16193 and 16519. When multiple Sanger sequence peaks are found staggered at these positions, it is unclear whether this finding resulted from true heteroplasmy or possibly an artifact due to polymerase error [20,35].

For 454 sequencing, we calculated sequencing and variant accuracies (Table S3). We defined sequencing accuracy (SA) as the percentage of the genotype calls that were concordant between 454 and Sanger vs. the sum of numbers of concordant and discordant calls; it can be also expressed as the symbols defined in Table S3. SA = (A1 + B2 + C3) / (A1 + A2 + A3 + B1 + B2 + B3 + C1 + C2 + C3). We defined variant accuracy (VA) as the percentage of homoplasmic and heteroplasmic variant calls by Sanger that were concordant with 454 vs. total number of variants found by both technologies; we calculated variant accuracy as VA = (B2 + C3) / (A2 + A3 + B2 + B3 + C2 + C3).

Finally, we calculated the false positive and false negative rates for both platforms (Table S3). The false positive rates were the proportion of reference genotypes (i.e., confirmed genotypes with false positive or true negative results) that were called as variants by each sequencing platform. The false negative rates were the proportion of variant genotypes (i.e., confirmed genotypes with false negative or true positive results) that were not called as variants by each sequencing platform.

Supporting Information

Table S1   Mitochondrial DNA variants identified by 454 and/or Sanger sequencing, n = 614.

Table S2   454 Mapping Statistics.

Table S3   Sequencing performance metrics: data tables (A) and calculations (B).

Table S4   Coverage simulations for heteroplasmic and homoplasmic mtDNA substitutions.

Acknowledgments

We thank the patients and families that participated in this study. The authors gratefully acknowledge Dr. W. Grody at the UCLA Orphan Disease Testing Center and Dr. J. Papp, U. Dandekar and H. Wijesuriya at the UCLA Genotyping & Sequencing Core for sharing their knowledge on next-generation sequencing.

Author Contributions

Conceived and designed the experiments: MVZ JF DL EA. Performed the experiments: MVZ JF MD. Analyzed the data: MVZ JF MD DL EA. Contributed reagents/materials/analysis tools: MVZ JF MD DL EA. Wrote the paper: MVZ.

References

1. Anderson S, Bankier AT, Barrell BG, de Bruijn MH, Coulson AR, et al. (1981) Sequence and organization of the human mitochondrial genome. Nature 290: 457–465.

2. Wallace DC (2007) Why do we still have a maternally inherited mitochondrial DNA? Insights from evolutionary medicine. Annu Rev Biochem 76: 781–821.

3. Giles RE, Blanc H, Cann HM, Wallace DC (1980) Maternal inheritance of human mitochondrial DNA. Proc Natl Acad Sci U S A 77: 6715–6719.

4. Cree LM, Samuels DC, Chinnery PF (2009) The inheritance of pathogenic mitochondrial DNA mutations. Biochim Biophys Acta 1792: 1097–1102.

5. Cao L, Shitara H, Horii T, Nagao Y, Imai H, et al. (2007) The mitochondrial bottleneck occurs without reduction of mtDNA content in female mouse germ cells. Nat Genet 39: 386–390.

6. Cree LM, Samuels DC, de Sousa Lopes SC, Rajasimha HK, Wonnapinij P, et al. (2008) A reduction of mitochondrial DNA molecules during embryogenesis explains the rapid segregation of genotypes. Nat Genet 40: 249–254.

7. Fan W, Waymire KG, Narula N, Li P, Rocher C, et al. (2008) A mouse model of mitochondrial disease reveals germline selection against severe mtDNA mutations. Science 319: 958–962.

8. Sanger F, Nicklen S, Coulson AR (1977) DNA sequencing with chain-terminating inhibitors. Proc Natl Acad Sci U S A 74: 5463–5467.

9. Schrijver I, Pique LM, Traynis I, Scharfe C, Sehnert AJ (2009) Mitochondrial DNA analysis by multiplex denaturing high-performance liquid chromatography and selective sequencing in pediatric patients with cardiomyopathy. Genet Med 11: 118–126.

10. Voelkerding KV, Dames SA, Durtschi JD (2009) Next-generation sequencing: from basic research to diagnostics. Clin Chem 55: 641–658.

11. Harismendy O, Ng PC, Strausberg RL, Wang X, Stockwell TB, et al. (2009) Evaluation of next generation sequencing platforms for population targeted sequencing studies. Genome Biol 10: R32.

12. Meyer M, Stenzel U, Myles S, Prüfer K, Hofreiter M (2007) Targeted high-throughput sequencing of tagged nucleic acid samples. Nucleic Acids Res 35: e97.

13. Meyer M, Stenzel U, Hofreiter M (2008) Parallel tagged sequencing on the 454 platform. Nat Protoc 3: 267–278.

14. He Y, Wu J, Dressman DC, Iacobuzio-Donahue C, Markowitz SD, et al. (2010) Heteroplasmic mitochondrial DNA mutations in normal and tumour cells. Nature 464: 610–614.

15. Tang S, Huang T (2010) Characterization of mitochondrial DNA heteroplasmy using a parallel sequencing system. BioTechniques 48: 287–296.

16. Vasta V, Ng SB, Turner EH, Shendure J, Hahn SH (2009) Next generation sequence analysis for mitochondrial disorders. Genome Med 1: 100.

17. Arbustini E, Fasani R, Morbini P, Diegoli M, Grasso M, et al. (1998) Coexistence of mitochondrial DNA and beta myosin heavy chain mutations in hypertrophic cardiomyopathy with late congestive heart failure. Heart 80: 548–558.

18. Jex AR, Hall RS, Littlewood DT, Gasser RB (2010) An integrated pipeline for next-generation sequencing and annotation of mitochondrial genomes. Nucleic Acids Res 38: 522–533.

19. Hu M, Jex AR, Campbell BE, Gasser RB (2007) Long PCR amplification of the entire mitochondrial genome from individual helminths for direct sequencing. Nat Protoc 2: 2339–2344.

20. Clarke LA, Rebelo CS, Gonçalves J, Boavida MG, Jordan P (2001) PCR amplification introduces errors into mononucleotide and dinucleotide repeat sequences. Mol Pathol 54: 351–353.

21. Bordoni R, Bonnal R, Rizzi E, Carrera P, Benedetti S, et al. (2008) Evaluation of human gene variant detection in amplicon pools by the GS-FLX parallel Pyrosequencer. BMC Genomics 9: 464–471.

22. McCaughan F, Dear PH (2010) Single-molecule genomics. J Pathol 220: 297–306.

23. Margulies M, Egholm M, Altman WE, Attiya S, Bader JS, et al. (2005) Genome sequencing in microfabricated high-density picolitre reactors. Nature 437: 376–380.

24. Moore MJ, Dhingra A, Soltis PS, Shaw R, Farmerie WG, et al. (2006) Rapid and accurate pyrosequencing of angiosperm plastid genomes. BMC Plant Biol 6: 17.

25. Huse SM, Huber JA, Morrison HG, Sogin ML, Welch DM (2007) Accuracy and quality of massively parallel DNA pyrosequencing. Genome Biol 8: R143.

26. Hancock DK, Tully LA, Levin BC (2005) A Standard Reference Material to determine the sensitivity of techniques for detecting low-frequency mutations, SNPs, and heteroplasmies in mitochondrial DNA. Genomics 86: 446–61.

27. Zifa E, Giannouli S, Theotokis P, Stamatis C, Mamuris Z, et al. (2007) Mitochondrial tRNA mutations: clinical and functional perturbations. RNA Biol 4: 38–66.

28. Brandon MC, Ruiz-Pesini E, Mishmar D, Procaccio V, Lott MT, et al. (2009) MITOMASTER: a bioinformatics tool for the analysis of mitochondrial DNA sequences. Hum Mutat 30: 1–6.

29. Pereira L, Freitas F, Fernandes V, Pereira JB, Costa MD, et al. (2009) The diversity present in 5140 human mitochondrial genomes. Am J Hum Genet 84: 628.

30. Bentley DR, Balasubramanian S, Swerdlow HP, Smith GP, Milton J, et al. (2008) Accurate whole human genome sequencing using reversible terminator chemistry. Nature 456: 53–59.

31. Thomas RK, Nickerson E, Simons JF, Janne PA, Tengs T, et al. (2006) Sensitive mutation detection in heterogeneous cancer specimens by massively parallel picoliter reactor sequencing. Nat Med 12: 852–855.

32. Andrews RM, Kubacka I, Chinnery PF, Lightowlers RN, Turnbull DM, Howell N (1999) Reanalysis and revision of the Cambridge reference sequence for human mitochondrial DNA. Nat Genet 23: 147.

33. Ruiz-Pesini E, Lott MT, Procaccio V, Poole J, Brandon MC, et al. (2007) An enhanced MITOMAP with a global mtDNA mutational phylogeny. Nucleic Acids Research 35 (Database issue):D823-D828. URL: http://www.mitomap.org.

34. van Oven M, Kayser M (2009) Updated comprehensive phylogenetic tree of global human mitochondrial DNA variation. Hum Mutat 30:E386-E394. http://www.phylotree.org.

35. Szibor R, Plate I, Heinrich M, Michael M, Schöning R, et al. (2007) Mitochondrial D-loop (CA)n repeat length heteroplasmy: frequency in a German population sample and inheritance studies in two pedigrees. Int J Legal Med 121: 207–213.

17

Mitochondrial Diabetes in Children: Seek and You will Find it

Cristina Mazzaccara[1,2,♪], Dario Iafusco[3,♪], Rosario Liguori[1,2], Maddalena Ferrigno[4], Alfonso Galderisi[3], Domenico Vitale[1], Francesca Simonelli[5], Paolo Landolfo[5], Francesco Prisco[3], Mariorosario Masullo[2,6], Lucia Sacchetti[1,2]*

1 CEINGE – Advanced Biotechnologies S. C. a R. L., Naples, Italy, 2 Department of Biochemistry and Medical Biotechnologies, University of Naples Federico II, Naples, Italy, 3 Department of Pediatrics, Second University of Naples, Naples, Italy, 4 SDN Foundation, Naples, Italy, 5 Department of Ophthalmology, Second University of Naples, Naples, Italy, 6 Department of Study of the Institutions and Territorial Systems, University of Naples "Parthenope", Naples, Italy

Abstract

Maternally Inherited Diabetes and Deafness (MIDD) is a rare form of diabetes due to defects in mitochondrial DNA (mtDNA). 3243 A>G is the mutation most frequently associated with this condition, but other mtDNA variants have been linked with a diabetic phenotype suggestive of MIDD. From 1989 to 2009, we clinically diagnosed mitochondrial diabetes in 11 diabetic children. Diagnosis was based on the presence of one or more of the following criteria: 1) maculopathy; 2) hearing impairment; 3) maternal heritability of diabetes/impaired fasting glucose and/or hearing impairment and/or maculopathy in three consecutive generations (or in two generations if 2 or 3 members of a family were affected). We sequenced the mtDNA in the 11 probands, in their mothers and in 80 controls. We identified 33 diabetes-suspected mutations, 1/33 was 3243A>G. Most patients (91%) and their mothers had mutations in complex I and/or IV of the respiratory chain. We measured the activity of these two enzymes and found that they were less active in mutated patients and their mothers than in the healthy control pool. The prevalence of hearing loss (36% vs 75–98%) and macular dystrophy (54% vs 86%) was lower in our mitochondrial diabetic adolescents than reported in adults. Moreover, we found a hitherto unknown association between mitochondrial diabetes and celiac disease. In conclusion, mitochondrial diabetes should be considered a complex syndrome with several phenotypic variants. Moreover, deafness is not an essential component of the disease in children. The whole mtDNA should be screened because the 3243A>G variant is not as frequent in children as in adults. In fact, 91% of our patients were mutated in the complex I and/or IV genes. The enzymatic assay may be a useful tool with which to confirm the pathogenic significance of detected variants.

Editor: Katriina Aalto-Setala, University of Tampere, Finland

Funding: This work was supported by CEINGE Regione Campania (DGRC 1901/2009). The funders had no role in study design, data collection and analysis, decision to publish, or preparation of the manuscript.

Competing Interests: The authors have declared that no competing interests exist.

* E-mail: sacchett@unina.it

♪ These authors contributed equally to this work.

Introduction

Maternally Inherited Diabetes and Deafness (MIDD) is a rare form of diabetes that accounts for up to 1% of all diabetes cases in Europeans and is due to defects in mitochondrial DNA (mtDNA) [1,2]. In addition to maternal transmission of diabetes, the clinical features of MIDD are mainly neurosensorial deafness, followed by other mitochondrial disorders, myopathies, and macular dystrophy [1]. MIDD is often misdiagnosed as type 1, type 2 or monogenic diabetes [1,3]. The absence of autoimmunity and obesity and the presence of maternal heritability, respectively, distinguish the latter three forms of diabetes from MIDD [1,3]. Besides the frequently reported mtDNA 3243A>G mutation, whose functional significance has been evaluated [4], several other mtDNA variants have been associated with a diabetic phenotype suggestive of MIDD [5,6]. However, few studies have explored the mitochondrial efficiency associated with detected mtDNA variants [7,8]. Consequently, the pathogenic significance of many newly identified variants remains to be established.

The aim of this study was to look for DNA variants in the mitochondrial genome of a pediatric cohort with suspected mitochondrial diabetes from Southern Italy. Patients were selected for investigation based on stringent diagnostic criteria. The pathogenic role of the detected mutations was investigated using an informatics approach. We also spectrophotometrically evaluated the enzyme activity of the respiratory chain complexes I and IV mutated in the mtDNA of most of our patients and their mothers.

Results

The clinical and metabolic characteristics of the 11 patients with suspected mitochondrial diabetes are listed in Table 1 and their family pedigrees are shown in Figure 1. Median age at diabetes onset was 11 years (age range 5–14 years). Maternal inheritance of diabetes or IFG was documented in all but 1 patient: patient 6 who was affected by hypoacusia and had a maternal history of hypoacusia. All 11 patients needed insulin therapy and most were

Table 1. Clinical and metabolic characteristics of pediatric patients from Southern Italy with suspected mitochondrial diabetes (n = 11)[a].

Age at onset (years)	11.0 (5.0–14.0)
Ophthalmic diseases	
-Macular dystrophy	54%
-Cataract	18%
Hearing impairment	36%
Normal weight	82%
BMI (z score)[b]	1.4 (−0.9–2.4)
Insulin therapy	100%
Fasting Plasma glucose (mmol/L)	13.0 (8.0–21.2)
HbA$_{1c}$ at diagnosis (%)	9.5 (6.3–14.0)
HbA$_{1c}$ at diagnosis (mmol/mol)	80.33 (45.3–129.5)
Fasting C peptide at diagnosis (nmol/l)	0.06 (0.033–0.495)
CK (>174 U/L) and/or LDH (>190 U/L)	64%
Presence of HLA DQ2 and/or DQ8 alleles	100%
Thyroiditis	36%
Presence of celiac disease	27%
Maternal[c] history of:	
-Deafness	45%
-Maculopathy	9%
-Thyroiditis	45%

[a]Continuous variables are reported as median (2.5th-97.5th percentiles) and categorical variables as percentages;
[b]BMI z score = Body mass index z score;
[c]Mother and/or maternal relatives.

of normal weight (median z score 1.4). Macular dystrophy was the most frequent diabetes-associated disease (54%), but no patient had diabetic retinopathy, whereas neurosensorial hearing impairment was observed only in one-third of patients. Seven patients (64%) showed alterations of the muscle enzymes CK and/or LDH, 4 patients (36%) were affected by thyroiditis, and 9 patients had a maternal history of deafness and/or macular dystrophy and/or thyroiditis. Particularly, in addition to the clinical characteristics described in Fig. 1, we detected: high CK levels in patient 2; high CK, LDH and ALP levels in patients 4$_1$, 4$_2$, 4$_3$; high LDH levels in patient 6; high ALP levels in patient 9; muscle pain in patient 14; and high CK levels and lactic acidosis in patient 15. Interestingly, HLA gene typing in the 11 patients revealed HLA-DQ2 and/or DQ8 molecules, and 3 were also affected by celiac disease (27%).

We sequenced the entire mitochondrial genome of the 11 patients, their mothers and 80 controls. The results were compared to the Revised Cambridge Reference Sequence (rCRS:NC_012920) [14]. We identified a total of 416 variants, among which 325 were detected only in controls, 58 were present in both controls and cases (Table S3), and 33 suspected mutations (4/33 novel) (Table 2) were present only in cases and their mothers. Among the suspected mutations detected only in patients, 22/33 were in the coding region (50% synonymous and 50% caused an amino acid change). Table 2 shows the main features (i.e.,the nucleotide variation, the relative amino acid substitution and its conservation across species, together with the bioinformatic-predicted role of the changed amino acid in the structure and/or function of the relative protein) of the variants

detected in each patient. Each patient had from one to seven suspected mtDNA mutations. Table 2 also shows previously reported variants.

The 3243A>G variant in tRNA leucine, which is the mutation most frequently associated with MIDD, was present in only one of our patients (patient 5) at heteroplasmic level. The level of heteroplasmy was higher in the DNA of patient 5 than in his mother's DNA, in both swab and blood samples (Figure S1). qRT-PCR confirmed a higher level of heteroplasmy in the patient than in his mother (respectively 34% and 3%). The distribution (percentage) of suspected mutations in the non-coding and in the coding regions of mtDNA is reported in Figure 2. Most suspected mutations (67%) were in the coding region and those with the highest frequencies occurred in complex I (46%) (ND1: 4024A>G, 4086C>T; ND2:5093T>C, 5300C>T; ND3: 10373G>A; ND4: 11253T>C, 11447G>A, 11928A>G; ND4L:10685G>A; ND5:12346C>T, 13135G>A, 14002A>G; ND6:14365C>T, 14502T>C, 14582A>G), in complex-IV (15%) (CO2:7762G>A; CO3:9803A>G, 9935T>C, 9947G>A, 9548G>A) of the respiratory chain enzymes followed by complex III (3%) (CYB:15530T>C) and complex V (3%) (ATP8:8562C>G). Within the non-coding region, the highest suspected mutation frequency was in the D-Loop (18%) (HVI: 16048G>A, 16137A>G, 16354C>T, 16526G>A; HVII:293T>C, 385A>G), followed by RNRs (951G>A, 960delC) and tRNAs (TV:1664G>A; TL1:3243A>G) both 6%, and by the NC7 region (3%) (8289_8290insCCCCCTCTA).

Because almost all patients (10/11 = 91%) had suspected mutations in complex I and/or in complex IV, we measured the enzymatic activities of these two complexes to investigate if the variants identified were associated with impaired mitochondrial function in patients and in their mothers when samples were available (i.e., patients 2, 6, 9, 10 and 15). Patient 5 carried mutation 3243A>G and was not further investigated because the functional significance of this mutation has been well established (4). Table 3 shows the enzyme activities recorded in patients and their mothers after normalization first vs citrate synthase and then vs the healthy control pool. Residual complex I and/or complex IV enzyme activities were lower (below the detected biological variability of 40%) than in the control pool (set at 100%) in 4/5 patients and borderline in 1/5 patients. The enzyme activities in mothers were similar to those measured in their offspring except in mother 2 (a subject bearing 2 variants in complex IV, one of which at heteroplasmic level), in whom the residual enzyme activity was higher than in her son.

Discussion

Potentially pathogenetic mtDNA mutations have been identified in more than 5% of patients affected by type 2 diabetes [6], which suggests that the true prevalence of mitochondrial diabetes could be higher than usually reported in Europeans subjects 1% [1]. In our geographic area, the global incidence of diabetes, in the population under 15 years of age, is 6.4/100,000/year [19]. In our pediatric diabetology unit we diagnosed mitochondrial diabetes in 11/1600 children with a diabetic phenotype observed from 1989 to 2009, which corresponds to a prevalence of 0.6% of the diabetes. The study population included a "historical" case of 1972.

Most MDD studies [1,20] started with the search for mutation 3243A>G in patients affected by both diabetes and deafness. Identification of the mutation prompted the investigation of the other common features (i.e., maculopathy and maternal heritability). Our approach was first to test all the diabetic patients of our Pediatric Diabetology Unit for maculopathy. Second, we carried

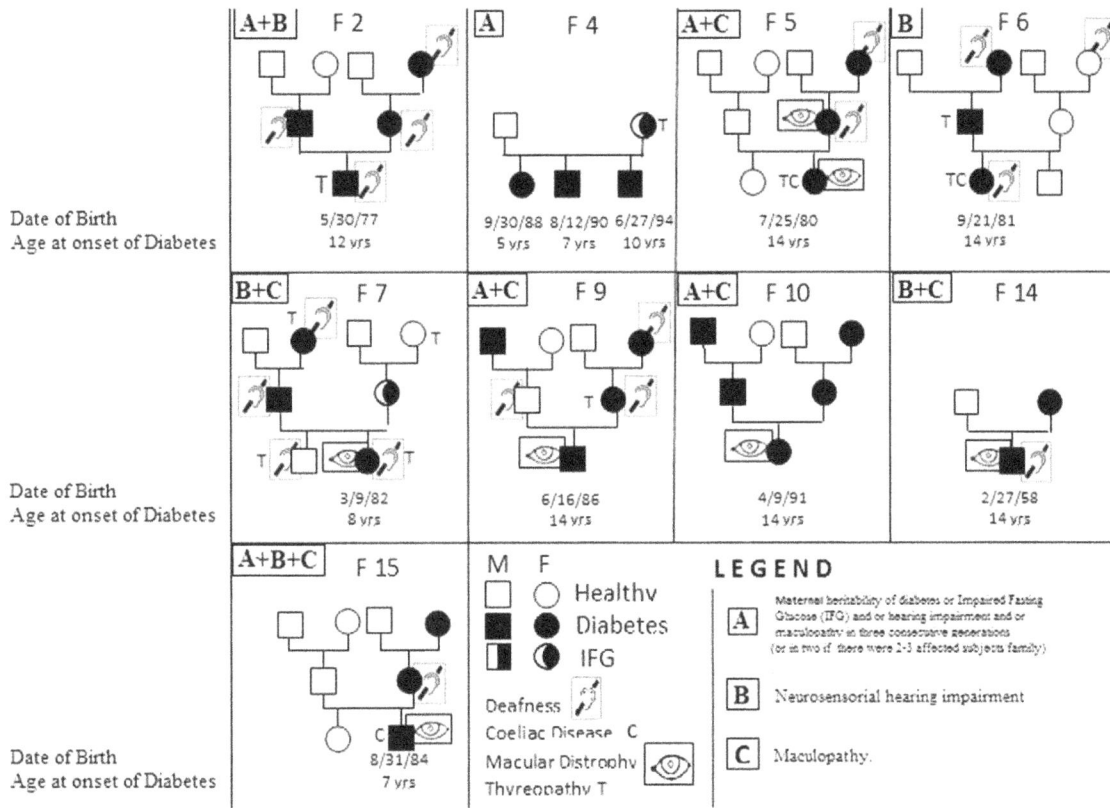

Figure 1. Familial (F) pedigrees of the suspected mitochondrial diabetes patients enrolled in the study. The inclusion criteria were: Diabetes+at least one of the following: A) maternal heritability of diabetes or Impaired Fasting Glucose (IFG) and/or hearing impairment and/or maculopathy in three consecutive generations (or in two if there were 2–3 affected subjects/family); B) neurosensorial hearing impairment; and C) maculopathy. In each square it's reported the presence of the criteria (A, B and/or C) in the probands.

out an audiometric examination of all patients positive for maculopathy or, if negative, in patients presenting maternal heritability of diabetes or IFG and/or hearing impairment and/or maculopathy in three consecutive generations (or in two generations if 2–3 members of the family were affected). This approach resulted in a lower incidence of deafness (36%) than previously reported, namely from 75% to 98% in 3243A>G-carriers with diabetes, with or without a maternal history of diabetes [1,20], and 58% in type 2 diabetic patients bearing mtDNA variations [6]. The low incidence of deafness in our patients suggests that the designation of deafness as the main diagnostic criterion for mitochondrial diabetes may result in underestimation of the real prevalence of the disease. This is why, in our patients, we call the disorder "mitochondrial diabetes" rather than MIDD.

Macular dystrophy was present in 54% of our patients, which is also lower than the 86% reported in carriers of mutation 3243A>G [1,20]. All our patients had DQ2 and/or DQ8 molecules that predispose to type 1 diabetes and to celiac disease. Intriguingly, celiac disease was detected in 27% (3/11 patients) of our suspected mitochondrial diabetic patients versus 1% of the general population [21] and versus 3%–6% of patients with type 1 diabetes [22]. As far as we are aware, this is the first report of an association between celiac disease and mitochondrial diabetes. Further investigations of mitochondrial function in celiac patients are required to verify the involvement of mtDNA variants in the pathogenesis or progression of the celiac disease. Notably, one-third of our mitochondrial diabetic patients had secondary

thyroiditis, which has been previously reported in 3243A>G carriers in the presence of diabetes or other mitochondrial diseases [1,23].

To our knowledge, there are no previous studies of mitochondrial diabetes in pediatric cohorts. In studies conducted in adults, young adults, in family case reports and in the MIDD 1 form, diabetes was usually diagnosed in patients aged between 16 and 43 years [1,6,24,25]. The age at MIDD onset is also related to the heteroplasmy level of the mutations. In fact, in 3243A>G carriers with heteroplasmy levels of 34.5%, 14.9%, 14.6% and 5.9%, the age of MIDD onset was 15, 41, 44 and 65 years, respectively [26]. In agreement with these data, the age of diabetes onset was 14 years in our mitochondrial diabetic patient (patient 5) who had a heteroplasmy 3243A>G level of 34%. The heteroplasmic level of the mutation was higher in patient 5 than in his mother in both buccal cells and blood leucocytes, which is in agreement with previous reports [27]. This finding supports the concept that the heteroplasmy load in blood of 3243A>G declines with age [1,28].

As mentioned above, the genetic analysis of MIDD usually focuses on the search for the 3243A>G mutation in selected diabetic patients affected by hearing loss; the entire mitochondrial genome is rarely screened [29,30]. Sequence analysis of the whole mtDNA in our suspected mitochondrial diabetic pediatric patients and controls resulted in a high rate of mtDNA polymorphisms (a total of 383/416 variants, present also in controls). Consequently, it is important to ascertain the pathogenic significance of newly identified variants. Among the 33 suspected mutations, 11/22 (50%) of those occurring in the coding region caused an amino

Table 2. Characteristics of suspected mtDNA mutations detected by sequence analysis in mitochondrial diabetic patients and their bioinformatic analysis.

Patient	Gene	Variant position	Amino acid change	ClustalW Conservation[a]	SIFT Score[b]	Poliphen prediction[c]	References[d]
2	NC7	8289–8290 insCCCCCTCTA					Novel Variant
	CO3	9803A>G	syn				Novel Variant
	CO3	9947G>A[e]	syn				31
4₁, 4₂, 4₃	ND3	10373G>A	syn				-
	ND4	11447G>A	V230M	C	T/0.11	Benign	-
5	TL1	3243A>G[e]					32
6	HVII	293T>C					-
	ND5	12346C>T	H4Y	N	T/0.17	Benign	-
	CYB	15530 T>C	syn				-
7	HVII	385A>G					-
	TV	1664G>A					-
	ND2	5093T>C	syn				-
	ND2	5300C>T	syn				Novel Variant
	ATP8	8562C>G	P66R	N	T/0.44	Possibly Damaging	Novel Variant
	ND4	11928A>G	N390S	H	A/0.00	Benign	-
	ND1	4086C>T	syn				33
9	ND5	13135G>A	A267T	N	T/0.50	Benign	34
10	RNR1	960delC					35
	ND1	4024A>G	T240A	N	T/0.12	Benign	-
	ND6	14365C>T	V103M	C	A/0.01	Benign	-
	ND6	14582A>G	V31A	N	T/1	Benign	-
	HVI	16048G>A					-
14	CO3	9935T>C	syn				-
	CO3	9548G>A	syn				36
	ND4L	10685G>A	syn				-
	HVI	16137A>G					-
	HVI	16526G>A					-
15	RNR1	951G>A					-
	CO2	7762G>A	syn				-
	ND4	11253 T>C[e]	I165T	C	A/0.01	Possibly Damaging	37
	ND5	14002A>G	T556A	N	T/0.42	Benign	-
	ND6	14502T>C	I58V	C	T/0.36	Benign	-
	HVI	16354C>T					-

[a]Amino acid conservation evaluated with the ClustalW program, C: conserved/semi-conserved, N: not conserved, H: highly conserved.
[b]Score: T (tolerated: Score >0.05): The substitution is predicted to be functionally neutral, A (affected: score <0.05): The substitution is predicted to affect protein function.
[c]Evaluated with the Poliphen program (see Materials and Method for details). Benign: changes most likely lack a phenotypic effect; Possibly damaging: reflects a likelihood of affecting protein function or structure.
[d]When there is no reference, the variant was reported in MITOMAP, which is a human mitochondrial genome database http://www.mitomap.org.
[e]Heteroplasmic variants.

acid change. Using informatics we predicted a benign change by SIFT and/or Polyphen programs for 10/11 variants; however, contrasting results were generated for 4/11 variants. Only one of the four novel suspected mutations (8562C>G) detected in our population caused an amino acid change (P66R: a not conserved amino acid) in the ATP8 gene, the others being synonymous (2 variants) or present in the control region (1 variant).

Most of the suspected mutations detected in our cohort have been described previously, often in a single patient or family, in association with diabetes, with other mitochondriopathies (mito-chondrial encephalomyopathy, lactic acidosis and stroke-like episodes: MELAS, Leber's hereditary optic neuropathy: LHON), with hearing loss [31–37], with cancer and with Parkinson disease or in population studies (MITOMAP: A Human Mitochondrial Genome Database:http://www.mitomap.org). However, the true clinical significance of these suspected mutations, apart from 3243A>G [4], has been scarcely investigated [7,8]. Given the highly polymorphic patterns detected in our patients, each usually bearing more than one variant (range: 1–7), and each variant being present once in the cohort, we measured the enzyme

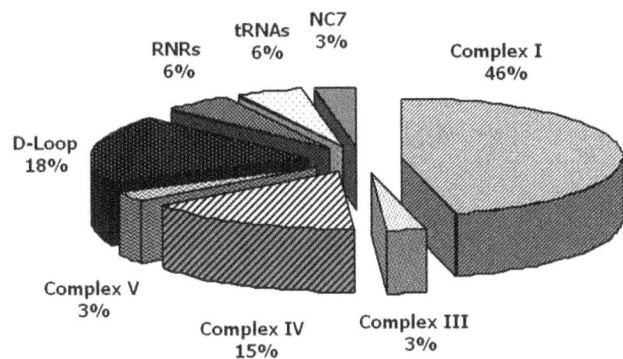

Figure 2. Percentage distribution in mitochondrial genome of suspected mutations detected in pediatric mitochondrial diabetic patients. Most diabetic associated variants (67%), detected by sequencing analysis, occurred in the coding region. The highest variant frequencies were observed in complex I (46%) and in complex IV (15%). In the non-coding region, the highest variant frequency was in the D-Loop (18%).

activities of complexes I and IV, where most of the variants occurred. The residual enzyme activity of the relative complex was lower in mitochondrial diabetic patients (5 patients) and in their mothers (complex I 12–65% and complex IV 46–76%) than in the healthy control pool set at 100%, although there was no correlation between the diabetic phenotype and the level of the residual enzyme activity in our patients. Intriguingly, patient 6 was affected by diabetes and deafness, her grandmother was affected by deafness and her father by diabetes. Although we detected some potentially pathogenic mtDNA variants and a reduced enzyme activity of complex I in both patient 6 and her mother, we cannot exclude that other genetic factors could have contributed to the diabetic phenotype of this patient. In fact, the phenotype of a pathogenic mtDNA mutation, or the severity of an mtDNA mutation that may not be pathological in some cases, could be influenced by the mitochondrial DNA haplogroup [38]. In addition, the genetic instability of mtDNA heteroplasmic mutations in the patient's somatic tissues [39], or the nuclear background, by nuclear modifiers, may also play a role in determining mtDNA mutation pathogenicity [40].

In conclusion, mitochondrial diabetes should be considered a complex syndrome with several phenotypic variants. Deafness is not an essential component of the disease in children. Investigations of patients should include the study of the entire mtDNA because the 3243A>G variant is not as frequent in children as in adults. In fact, 91% of our patients were mutated in the complex I and/or IV genes. The enzymatic assay may be a useful tool with

which to measure the mitochondrion dysfunction associated with detected mtDNA variants.

Materials and Methods

Patients and controls

Sixteen patients (including 3 brothers), with suspected mitochondrial diabetes were enrolled from among the diabetic population attending the Department of Pediatrics of the Second University of Naples (Italy) (15/16 from 1989 to 2009 and 1/16, a historical case in 1972). Controls (10 affected by type 1 diabetes and 70 healthy controls) were recruited at DASMELAB/CEINGE–Advanced Biotechnology/University of Naples Federico II. All patients (54% males), their mothers, and controls had lived in Southern Italy for at least 2–3 generations. All the diabetic children were screened for maculopathy by ophtalmoscopic examination. Inclusion criteria for suspected mitochondrial diabetes, in addition to the presence of diabetes defined according to the American Diabetes Association (ADA) [9], were: 1) maternal heritability of diabetes or impaired fasting glucose (IFG) and/or hearing impairment and/or maculopathy in three consecutive generations (or in two generations if 2 or 3 members of the family were affected); 2) neurosensorial hearing impairment; and 3) maculopathy. At least one or more of these criteria were required for enrollment in the study (Figure 1). Audiometric examination was performed in all patients with maculopathy, and in patients without maculopathy if they fulfilled one of the above-indicated clinical criteria. A cut-off point of 250 Hz with a slope of 24 dB/oct was considered diagnostic of hearing impairment [10]. The ophthalmoscopic examinations were performed according to standardized procedures [11,12]. Age at disease onset, need of insulin therapy, levels of fasting C peptide, and type 1 diabetes autoantibodies were also recorded. All pedigrees were verified from the patients' records by expert pediatricians and in cooperation with the family doctor. Patients with suspected mitochondrial diabetes were also typed for Human Leukocyte Antigen (HLA) -DRB1(*03/*04/*07/*11), DQA1 (*02/*03/*05), and DQB1(*02–*06) alleles (Histotype Special Medium Resolution and Histotype DQB Low SSP Kits- BAG Healthcare) to identify HLA alleles predisposing to type 1 diabetes and/or to other autoimmune diseases. To determine whether our patients were affected by the autoimmune diseases most frequently associated with type 1 diabetes (thyroiditis and celiac disease), we carried out the following immunofluorometric or immunoenzymatic assays: free triiodothyronine (FT3), free thyroxine (FT4), thyroid-stimulating hormone (TSH), thyroglobulin (TG), anti-thyroglobulin (Anti-TG), anti-peroxidase (Anti-TPO) antibodies and IgA-IgG anti-gliadin antibodies (AGA) and IgA transglutaminase (TGase) antibodies. The presence of celiac disease in serology-positive

Table 3. Enzyme activities of the respiratory chain complexes I and IV evaluated in lymphocytes from mitochondrial diabetic patients (pt) and their mothers (m) bearing mtDNA variants in these complexes.

Sample ID	Pool[a]	pt2	m2	pt6	m6	pt9	m9	pt10	m10	pt15	m15
Mutated Complex		IV	IV	I	I	I	I	I	I	I,IV	I,IV
Complex I residual activity %[b](nmol NADH oxidized min^{-1} mU^{-1} citrate synthase)	100	90	ND	39	12	64	65	32	33	52	20
Complex IV residual activity %[b] (nmol Cytc oxidized min^{-1}mU^{-1}citrate synthase)	100	51	76	ND	ND	ND	ND	99	ND	46	56

[a]Pool is relative to 12 healthy control subjects.
[b]Residual activity (%) was obtained by normalization of the enzyme activity firstly vs citrate synthase and then vs the healthy cont rol pool. ND: Not determined.

participants was confirmed by total or subtotal villous atrophy at biopsy examination. We also screened our patients for myopathy (muscle enzymes alterations) by measuring creatine kinase (CK)>174 U/L and/or lactate dehydrogenase (LDH)>190 U/L) levels. A detailed family history, and anthropometric and clinical data were collected on a standard case-record form.

The presence of hypertension, defined as blood pressure in excess of the $90°$ percentile in children [13] was also explored. A fasted blood sample was collected from all patients at the first clinical examination for routine biochemical investigations: glucose, C-peptide, glycated hemoglobin (HbA$_{1C}$), islet cell antibody (ICA), Anti-glutamate decarboxylase (GAD), protein tyrosine phosphatase (IA2), insulin auto antibody (IAA), CK, LDH, creatinine, which were determined with routine procedures. Based on biochemical findings, five of 16 suspected mitochondrial diabetic patients were diagnosed as type 1 diabetes (high positivity for all the tested diabetes type 1 autoimmune markers), and were excluded from the study. Although autoimmune markers do not rule out a mitochondrial form of diabetes, in this preliminary study we preferred to avoid any factor that could interfere with the pathogenetic mechanism of a supposed "mitochondrial form". A peripheral blood+EDTA sample was also collected from patients, their mothers and controls to obtain DNA samples for mtDNA sequence analysis. The mtDNA analysis was also performed in patients with suspected mitochondrial diabetes and their mothers on buccal cells collected by swab. Written informed consent was obtained from all recruited subjects, in the case of children, consent was obtained from their parents, and the study was approved by the Ethics Committee of the Faculty of Medicine of the Second University of Naples (Italy). The study was performed according to the Helsinki declaration.

DNA extraction and mtDNA sequencing

Genomic DNA was extracted with the Kit-Nucleon-BACC2 (Illustra DNA-Extraction Kit-BACC2-GE Healthcare, UK) and stored at +4°C. The primers used to amplify by PCR the mtDNA were chosen by the PRIMER 3 program (http://frodo.wi.mit.edu/primer3/) and were selected to generate two overlapping fragments encompassing the whole mitochondrial genome. Primers are listed in Table S1. The mtDNA was amplified by long PCR using GeneAmp PCR System 9700 (Applied-Biosystems, Foster City, CA, USA). The long PCR mixture and conditions are detailed in Methods S1. The PCR fragments were examined by electrophoresis to assess yield and purity, then amplicons were purified over affinity spin columns (Qiaquick-PCR purification Kit, Qiagen Hilden, Germany). The whole mitochondrial genome was then sequenced with the BigDye Terminator v3.1 cycle sequencing method on the ABI-Prism 3730 Genetic Analyzer (Applied-Biosystems) by using 32 forward primers, summarised in Table S2, and analyzed using the SeqScape program (v2.5 Applied-Biosystems) to compare the mtDNA sequences of patients and controls with the revised Cambridge Reference Sequence (rCRS) [14].

Real-time quantitative PCR

We used the TaqMan system (7900HT Fast-Real-Time-system; Applied-Biosystems) to evaluate by real-time quantitative PCR (qRT-PCR) the level of heteroplasmic 3243A>G mutation detected in one patient and his mother. Primers and Real-time quantitative PCR conditions were detailed in Methods S2. To quantify total and mutant mtDNA, standard curves were constructed using plasmids with the wild-type (WT) and the mutant mtDNA fragments respectively. The ratio between total mtDNA and mutant mtDNA was calculated in each sample.

Bioinformatic analysis

We used the Sorting Intolerant from Tolerant (SIFT) (http://sift.jcvi.org/), Polymorphism Phenotyping (PolyPhen) (http://genetics.bwh.harvard.edu/pph) and ClustalW http://www.ebi.ac.uk/Tools/clustalw2/index.html) programs to predict the pathogenicity of the detected missense suspected mutations. The evaluation included amino acid conservation across species and the role of the changed amino acid in the structure and/or in the function of the relative protein.

Evaluation of the enzyme activities of complexes I and IV of the respiratory chain

Lymphocytes from mitochondrial diabetic patients, their mothers, and 12 healthy controls were first isolated from fresh peripheral blood+EDTA (10 ml) and then separated on Ficoll medium using Ficoll Paque plus reagent (GE Healthcare, Waukesha, WI, USA) as previously described [15]. Briefly, the blood was diluted by the addition of an equal volume of PBS (Sigma-Aldrich Corp., St. Louis, MO, USA), then aliquots of 7 mL of this mixture were layered over 3 mL of Ficoll Paque and centrifuged at 400 g, at 18°C for 30 min. The mononuclear cell fraction was removed, diluted in PBS (1:10) and centrifuged. The pellet was washed with 5 mL of PBS and lymphocytes were counted with the automated Analyzer Coulter LH 750 (Beckman Coulter Inc., Fullerton, CA, USA) and finally aliquots of 2.5×10^6 lymphocytes were resuspended in an ice-cold buffer (SHE-PIM) containing 250 mmol/l sucrose, 10 mmol/l HEPES pH 7.4 and 1 mmol/l EDTA (SHE) supplemented with a protease inhibitor mixture (PIM) (Complete, EDTA-free, Roche Diagnostics, Mainheim, Germany). These aliquots of lymphocytes were rapidly frozen in liquid nitrogen and stored at −80°C.

Sample preparation for the enzyme assays. Cells were permeabilized by four freeze/thawing cycles. The protein content of the aliquots of lymphocytes was determined by the Bio-Rad Protein Assay (Biorad Laboratories, GmbH, Munchen, Germany) using BSA as standard.

NADH: Ubiquinone-oxidoreductase (Complex-I) Activity: Complex-I activity was measured as previously described [16] by monitoring the oxidation of NADH to NAD$^+$ at 340 nm at 37°C, using a Cary 1E Spectrophotometer (Varian), equipped with an electronic temperature controller, and a molar extinction coefficient of 6220 $M^{-1}cm^{-1}$. The baseline absorbance variation was determined by adding an appropriate amount of permeabilized lymphocytes (usually 2.5×10^6–5.0×10^6). Therefore, the reaction started with the addition of 50 μmol/l Coenzyme-Q (CoQ1) in the absence or in the presence of 5 μmol/l rotenone, a specific complex I inhibitor, and was monitored for an additional 3–5 min. Under these conditions, the rate of NADH oxidation measured in the absence of rotenone corresponded to the total NADH-CoQ oxidoreductase activity, whereas that measured in its presence reflected the rotenone-insensitive NADH-CoQ oxidoreductase activity (RINQ), which is not associated to complex I activity. Therefore, the activity of complex I can be derived subtracting the rate of RINQ from the total activity and is expressed as nmol of NADH oxidized min^{-1} mg^{-1} of protein.

Cytochrome c oxidase (complex IV) activity. Complex IV activity was determined by monitoring the oxidation of reduced cytochrome-c (rCyt-c) at 550 nm (molar extinction coefficient 29500 M^{-1} cm^{-1}). rCyt-c was prepared from commercially available oxidised Cytochrome c (Sigma Aldrich) by reduction with dithiothreitol (DTT) and quantification as indicated by the manufacturer. The assay mixture, prepared in 10 mmol/l potassium phosphate, pH 7.4, contained 1.5% n-dodecyl-β-D-maltoside, which is required to maximize complex IV activity [17], and

25 µmol/l rCyt-*c*. After reading the baseline activity, the reaction was started by adding appropriate amounts of permeabilized lymphocytes (usually 2.0×10^4–3.0×10^4 cells), and followed by measuring the decrease of the absorbance at 550 nm for an additional 2–3 min. Complex IV activity was expressed as nmol Cyt-*c* oxidized min^{-1} mg^{-1} of protein. Both complex I and complex IV activities were normalized to citrate synthase activity, which is an index of mitochondrial mass, as previously reported [17], to correct for any differential mitochondrial content due to mitochondrial dysfunction [18]. Finally, the residual percent activities of complex I and complex IV in both mitochondrial diabetic patients and their mothers were obtained by comparing their activities with that measured in a healthy control pool set at 100%. The biological variability of enzyme activities in the samples used for the control pool was 40%, in agreement with the previously reported value [16]. To check the quality of our assay, we also verified the enzyme activity of two un-mutated complexes in two patients (patients 2 and 10) and in the father of a diabetic patient (data not shown). The residual enzyme activities in these controls ranged from 87% to 99%.

Statistical analysis

The statistical analysis of biochemical and general data from patients was carried out using PASW 18.0 software version (SPSS Inc., Chicago, IL, USA). The Kolmogorov-Smirnov test was used to evaluate the distribution of continuous variables (age at onset, BMI Z score, fasting plasma glucose, glycated haemoglobin, fasting C peptide at diagnosis) that were expressed as median (2.5^{th}–97.5^{th} percentiles). The categorical variables were reported as percentage.

Supporting Information

Figure S1   Detection of 3243A>G mitochondrial mutation by sequence analysis. Sequence analysis of swab and blood mtDNA from patient 5 (pt5) and from her mother (m5) showing the heteroplasmic 3243A>G mutation. Levels of heteroplasmy were higher in mtDNA from pt5 than in mtDNA from m5 in both swab and blood samples.

Methods S1   Mixture and conditions for Long PCR of mtDNA.

Methods S2   Primers and Real-time quantitative PCR conditions.

Table S1   Primers sequence for Long PCR of mtDNA. Table shows the two primers pair used for the amplification of the entire mtDNA.

Table S2   Primers sequence for mtDNA sequencing. Table shows the primers used for the sequencing of the mtDNA amplification products.

Table S3   MtDNA Variants detected in control subjects or both in control subjects and patients. Table reports the 325 mtDNA variants detected only in our controls subjects and the 58 variants detected both in control subjects and patients. For each variant is reported the mitochondrial region, the nucleotide and amino acid change and the relative frequency.

Acknowledgments

We thank Jean Ann Gilder (Scientific Communication srl) for revising and editing the manuscript. We thank our mitochondrial diabetic patients and their families for their kind cooperation in this study.

Author Contributions

Conceived and designed the experiments: DI CM LS. Performed the experiments: CM RL MF DI AG DV MM LS. Analyzed the data: CM RL MF DI AG MM LS. Contributed reagents/materials/analysis tools: LS. Wrote the paper: DI CM LS. Ophthalmoscopic examination: FS PL. Performed the critical revision of the article for important intellectual content: FP MM. Final approval of the article: LS.

References

1. Murphy R, Turnbull DM, Walker M, Hattersley AT (2008) Clinical features, diagnosis and management of maternally inherited diabetes and deafness (MIDD) associated with the 3243A>G mitochondrial point mutation. Diabet Med 25: 383–399.

2. Maassen JA, Jahangir Tafrechi RS, Janssen GM, Raap AK, Lemkes HH, et al. (2006) New insights in the molecular pathogenesis of the maternally inherited diabetes and deafness syndrome. Endocrinol Metab Clin North Am 35: 385–396.

3. Murphy R, Ellard S, Hattersley AT (2008) Clinical implications of a molecular genetic classification of monogenic β–cell diabetes. Nat Clin Pract Endocrinol Metab 4: 200–213.

4. Maassen JA, 'T Hart LM, Van Essen E, Heine RJ, Nijpels G, et al. (2004) Mitochondrial diabetes: molecular mechanisms and clinical presentation. Diabetes 53(Suppl 1): S103–S109.

5. Maechler P, Wollheim CB (2001) Mitochondrial function in normal and diabetic beta–cells. Nature 414: 807–812.

6. Crispim D, Estivalet AA, Roisenberg I, Gross JL, Canani LH (2008) Prevalence of 15 mitochondrial DNA mutations among type 2 diabetic patients with or without clinical characteristics of maternally inherited diabetes and deafness. Arq Bras Endocrinol Metab 52: 1228–1235.

7. Mariotti C, Tiranti V, Carrara F, Dallapiccola B, Di Donato S, et al. (1994) Defective respiratory capacity and mitochondrial protein synthesis in transformant cybrids harboring the tRNA(Leu(UUR)) mutation associated with maternally inherited myopathy and cardiomyopathy. J Clin Invest 93: 1102–1107.

8. Malfatti E, Bugiani M, Invernizzi F, de Souza CF, Farina L, et al. (2007) Novel mutations of ND genes in complex I deficiency associated with mitochondrial encephalopathy. Brain 130: 1894–1904.

9. American Diabetes Association (2010) Diagnosis and Classification of Diabetes Mellitus. Diabetes Care 33(Suppl 1): S62–S69. Erratum in: Diabetes Care. 2010 33:e57.

10. Sawada S, Takeda T, Kakigi A, Saito H, Suehiro T, et al. (1997) Audiological findings of sensorineural deafness associated with a mutation in the mitochondrial DNA. Am J Otol 18: 332–335.

11. Massin P, Virally-Monod M, Vialettes B, Paques M, Gin H, et al. (1999) Prevalence of macular pattern dystrophy in Maternally Inherited Diabetes and Deafness. GEDIAM Group. Ophthalmology 106: 1821–1827.

12. Massin P, Guillausseau PJ, Vialettes B, Paquis V, Orsini F, et al. (1995) Macular pattern dystrophy associated with a mutation of mitochondrial DNA. Am J Ophthalmol 120: 247–248.

13. Chobanian AV, Bakris GL, Black HR, Cushman WC, Green LA, et al. (2003) Seventh report of the Joint National Committee on Prevention, Detection, Evaluation, and Treatment of High Blood Pressure. Hypertension 42: 1206–1252.

14. Andrews RM, Kubacka I, Chinnery PF, Lightowlers RN, Turnbull DM, et al. (1999) Reanalysis and revision of the Cambridge reference sequence for human mitochondrial DNA. Nat Genet 23: 147.

15. Fuss IJ, Kanof ME, Smith PD, Zola H (2009) Isolation of whole mononuclear cells from peripheral blood and cord blood. Curr Protoc Immunol 85: 7.1.1–7.1.8.

16. de Wit LE, Spruijt L, Schoonderwoerd GC, de Coo IF, Smeets HJ, et al. (2007) A simplified and reliable assay for complex I in human blood lymphocytes. J Immunol Methods 326: 76–82.

17. Kirby DM, Thorburn DR, Turnbull DM, Taylor RW (2007) Biochemical assays of respiratory chain complex activity. In: Pon LA, Schon EA, eds. Methods in cell biology, 2nd ed, Elsevier Press, San Diego, USA. pp 93–119.

18. Boushel R, Gnaiger E, Schjerling P, Skovbro M, Kraunsoe R, et al. (2007) Patients with type 2 diabetes have normal mitochondrial function in skeletal muscle. Diabetologia 50: 790–796.

19. Prisco F, Vicedomini D, Iafusco D, De Felice E, Amodeo BM, et al. (1996) Incidence of IDDM in the Campania Region, Italy. Diabetes Care 19: 1454–1455.

20. Guillausseau PJ, Massin P, Dubois-LaForgue D, Timsit J, Virally M, et al. (2001) Maternally inherited diabetes and deafness: a multicenter study. Ann Intern Med 134: 721–728.
21. Kagnoff MF (2007) Celiac disease: pathogenesis of a model immunogenetic disease. J Clin Invest 117: 41–49.
22. Dubé C, Rostom A, Sy R, Cranney A, Saloojee N, et al. (2005) The prevalence of celiac disease in average-risk and at-risk Western European populations: a systematic review. Gastroenterology 128(Suppl 1): S57–S67.
23. Balestri P, Grosso S (2000) Endocrine disorders in two sisters affected by MELAS syndrome. J Child Neurol 15: 755–758.
24. Hosszúfalusi N, Karcagi V, Horváth R, Palik E, Várkonyi J, et al. (2009) A detailed investigation of maternally inherited diabetes and deafness (MIDD) including clinical characteristics, C- peptide secretion, HLA-DR and –DQ status and autoantibody pattern. Diabetes Metab Res Rev 25: 127–135.
25. Guillausseau PJ, Dubois-Laforgue D, Massin P, Laloi-Michelin M, Bellanné-Chantelot C, et al. (2004) GEDIAM, Mitochondrial Diabetes French Study Group. Heterogeneity of diabetes phenotype in patients with 3243 bp mutation of mitochondrial DNA (Maternally Inherited Diabetes and Deafness or MIDD). Diabetes Metab 30: 181–186.
26. Zhang S, Tong AL, Zhang Y, Nie M, Li YX, et al. (2009) Heteroplasmy level of the mitochondrial tRNaLeu (UUR) A3243G mutation in a Chinese family is positively associated with earlier age-of onset and increasing severity of diabetes. Chin Med Sci J 24: 20–25.
27. Maassen JA, Janssen GM, 't Hart LM (2005) Molecular mechanisms of mitochondrial diabetes (MIDD). Ann Med 37: 213–221.
28. Laloi-Michelin M, Meas T, Ambonville C, Bellanné-Chantelot C, Beaufils S, et al. (2009) Mitochondrial Diabetes French Study Group. The clinical variability of maternally inherited diabetes and deafness is associated with the degree of heteroplasmy in blood leukocytes. J Clin Endocrinol Metab 94: 3025–3030.
29. Choo-Kang AT, Lynn S, Taylor GA, Daly ME, Sihota SS, et al. (2002) Defining the importance of mitochondrial gene defects in maternally inherited diabetes by sequencing the entire mitochondrial genome. Diabetes 51: 2317–2320.
30. Alcolado JC, Laji K, Gill-Randall R (2002) Maternal transmission of diabetes. Diabet Med 19: 89–98.
31. Hanna MG, Nelson IP, Morgan-Hughes JA, Wood NW (1998) MELAS: a new disease associated mitochondrial DNA mutation and evidence for further genetic heterogeneity. J Neurol Neurosurg Psychiatry 65: 512–517.
32. Howes T, Madden C, Dasgupta S, Saeed S, Das V (2008) Role of mitochondrial variation in maternally inherited diabetes and deafness syndrome. J Laryngol Otol 122: 1249–1252.
33. Chen J, Yang L, Yang A, Zhu Y, Zhao J, et al. (2007) Maternally inherited aminoglycoside-induced and nonsyndromic hearing loss is associated with the 12S rRNA C1494T mutation in three Han Chinese pedigrees. Gene 401: 4–11.
34. Qian Y, Zhou X, Hu Y, Tong Y, Li R, et al. (2005) Clinical evaluation and mitochondrial DNA sequence analysis in three Chinese families with Leber's hereditary optic neuropathy. Biochem Biophys Res Commun 332: 614–621.
35. Elstner M, Schmidt C, Zingler VC, Prokisch H, Bettecken T, et al. (2008) Mitochondrial 12S rRNA susceptibility mutations in aminoglycoside-associated and idiopathic bilateral vestibulopathy. Biochem Biophys Res Commun 377: 379–383.
36. Horváth R, Reilmann R, Holinski-Feder E, Ringelstein EB, Klopstock T (2008) The role of complex I genes in MELAS: a novel heteroplasmic mutation 3380G>A in ND1 of mtDNA. Neuromuscul Disord 18: 553–556.
37. Leo-Kottler B, Luberichs J, Besch D, Christ-Adler M, Fauser S (2002) Leber's hereditary optic neuropathy: clinical and molecular genetic results in a patient with a point mutation at np T11253C (isoleucine to threonine) in the ND4 gene and spontaneous recovery. Graefes Arch Clin Exp Ophthalmol 240: 758–764.
38. Gutiérrez Cortés N, Pertuiset C, Dumon E, Börlin M, Herbert-Chatelain E, et al. (2012) Novel mitochondrial DNA mutations responsible for maternally inherited non-syndromic hearing loss. Hum MutatIn press.
39. Bannwarth S, Abbassi M, Valéro M, Fragaki K, Dubois N, et al. (2011) A novel instable mutation in mitochondrial DNA responsible for maternally inherited diabetes and deafness. Diabetes Care 34(12): 2591–3.
40. Carelli V, Giordano C, d'Amati G (2003) Pathogenic expression of homoplasmic mtDNA mutations needs a complex nuclear-mitochondrial interaction. Trends Genet 19(5): 257–62.

18

Liver as a Source for Thymidine Phosphorylase Replacement in Mitochondrial Neurogastrointestinal Encephalomyopathy

Elisa Boschetti[1,2], Roberto D'Alessandro[3], Francesca Bianco[1], Valerio Carelli[2], Giovanna Cenacchi[2], Antonio D. Pinna[1], Massimo Del Gaudio[1], Rita Rinaldi[4], Vincenzo Stanghellini[1], Loris Pironi[1], Kerry Rhoden[1], Vitaliano Tugnoli[2], Carlo Casali[5], Roberto De Giorgio[1]*

1 Department of Surgical and Medical Sciences, University of Bologna, Bologna, Italy, **2** Department of Biomedical and Neuromotor Sciences, University of Bologna, Bologna, Italy, **3** Institute of Neurological Sciences, University of Bologna, Bologna, Italy, **4** Neurology Unit, St. Orsola-Malpighi Hospital, Bologna, Italy, **5** Department of Medico-Surgical Sciences and Biotechnologies, University 'La Sapienza', Rome, Italy

Abstract

Mitochondrial neurogastrointestinal encephalomyopathy (MNGIE) is a rare autosomal recessive mitochondrial disease associated with mutations in the nuclear *TYMP* gene. As a result, the thymidine phosphorylase (TP) enzyme activity is markedly reduced leading to toxic accumulation of thymidine and therefore altered mitochondrial DNA. MNGIE is characterized by severe gastrointestinal dysmotility, neurological impairment, reduced life expectancy and poor quality of life. There are limited therapeutic options for MNGIE. In the attempt to restore TP activity, allogenic hematopoietic stem cell transplantation has been used as cellular source of TP. The results of this approach on ~20 MNGIE patients showed gastrointestinal and neurological improvement, although the 5-year mortality rate is about 70%. In this study we tested whether the liver may serve as an alternative source of TP. We investigated 11 patients (7M; 35–55 years) who underwent hepatic resection for focal disorders. Margins of normal liver tissue were processed to identify, quantify and localize the TP protein by Western Blot, ELISA, and immunohistochemistry, and to evaluate *TYMP* mRNA expression by qPCR. Western Blot identified TP in liver with a TP/GAPDH ratio of 0.9 ± 0.5. ELISA estimated TP content as 0.5 ± 0.07 ng/µg of total protein. TP was identified in both nuclei and cytoplasm of hepatocytes and sinusoidal lining cells. Finally, *TYMP* mRNA was expressed in the liver. Overall, our study demonstrates that the liver is an important source of TP. Orthotopic liver transplantation may be considered as a therapeutic alternative for MNGIE patients.

Editor: Paul A. Cobine, Auburn University, United States of America

Funding: This work was partly supported by grants from the Italian Ministry of Health (Ricerca Finalizzata 2009 RF2009) and funds from University of Bologna (R. De G.). R. De G., V. T. and E. B. were the recipients of grants from "Fondazione Del Monte di Bologna e Ravenna", Bologna, Italy. The funders had no role in study design, data collection and analysis, decision to publish, or preparation of the manuscript.

Competing Interests: The authors have declared that no competing interests exist.

* E-mail: roberto.degiorgio@unibo.it

Introduction

Mitochondrial neurogastrointestinal encephalomyopathy (MNGIE) is a rare autosomal recessive mitochondrial disease due to mutations in the nuclear *TYMP* gene encoding thymidine phosphorylase (TP). This enzyme converts the nucleosides thymidine (dThd) and deoxyuridine into thymine and uracil, respectively [1]. *TYMP* mutations lead to a marked reduction (or virtual absence) of TP activity [2] resulting in a toxic accumulation of nucleosides in plasma of MNGIE patients. This biochemical imbalance leads to secondary mitochondrial DNA (mtDNA) point mutations, multiple deletions and, more importantly, mtDNA depletion [3,4]. The nucleotide pool for mtDNA replication depends on the salvage pathway. In MNGIE, excess dThd enters mitochondria and competes with deoxycytidine for thymidine kinase 2, becoming its predominant substrate and causing mtDNA abnormalities [5,6]. In tissues with high cell turnover and active proliferation, such as bone marrow or liver, dThd accumulation is prevented with a rapid equilibration of nucleotides between the cytosol and the mitochondrial matrix. On the opposite, post-mitotic, high-energy dependent tissues, such as brain, skeletal and smooth muscle, rely only on the nucleotide salvage pathway and are therefore the target for MNGIE [5,6,7,8]. Since nuclear and mitochondrial nucleotide pools originate from different pathways, *TYMP* mutations do not influence nuclear DNA turnover [5].

From a clinical standpoint, MNGIE is characterized by severe gastrointestinal symptoms and frequent intestinal sub-occlusive episodes (i.e. chronic intestinal pseudo-obstruction) [9] due to marked impairment of gut motility; in addition, other common features include ptosis and ophthalmoparesis, cachexia, peripheral neuropathy, myopathy, leukoencephalopathy (detectable by MRI), and lactic acidosis [10,11]. Clinical manifestations differ depending on the degree of the TP defect. Indeed, typical MNGIE patients have ~5% residual TP activity, experience major symptoms from the second decade, and their overall life expectancy is limited to the fourth decade. In contrast, patients with a partial loss of TP function (~10–15% residual TP activity) manifest symptoms later at an adult age and their life expectancy is beyond the fifth decade. Notably, MNGIE relatives carrying heterozygous *TYMP* mutations never manifest the syndrome. Since TP is a homodimer, the presence of a mutant allele leads to the formation of only 25% wild-type TP molecules, while 75% of dimers contain at least one dysfunctional monomer. Asymptomatic heterozygous subjects have ~25–35% residual TP activity and this threshold may represent the target for therapeutic purposes [12,13].

So far, there are no established therapeutic options for patients with MNGIE. Peritoneal dialysis is a commonly used approach to lower plasma concentrations of toxic nucleosides in order to reduce the clinical manifestations of the disease, and in particular the gastrointestinal symptoms (e.g. vomiting, abdominal pain, and weight loss). This approach, however, produces only a transient benefit since clearance lasts for only a few hours [14,15]. Another strategy is based on the replacement of TP activity using cells containing adequate levels of the enzyme. Platelet infusion has been used to this end although with limited success [16], and erythrocyte encapsulated TP is under clinical development [17]. Gene therapy may be also a valuable option. TP-deficient B-lymphoblastoid cells from MNGIE patients and partially myeloablated double *TYMP/UPP1* knockout mice have been transfected with lentiviral or adeno-associated virus (AAV) vectors carrying the *TYMP* coding sequence with a reduction in nucleoside concentrations [18,19]. The effectiveness of *TYMP* gene therapy, however, still awaits confirmation in *ad hoc* clinical trials. Finally, allogenic hematopoietic stem cell transplantation (AHSCT) has been performed to provide a permanent cellular source of TP in MNGIE patients [20]. So far, the worldwide experience has shown some positive results characterized by symptomatic improvement, increased TP activity and reduced dThd and deoxyuridine blood levels [21]. However, AHSCT is dramatically limited by an overall mortality, that has been demonstrated to be ~70% [22], (Hirano et al., Child Neurology Society's annual meeting, 2013, Austin, TX).Based on this experience, organ transplantation, other than AHSCT, may represent an alternative option for treating patients with MNGIE. Since the liver is the main organ for protein biosynthesis and the transplantation success is estimated at ~90% of cases [23], the present study has been designed to test whether the liver can be proposed as a source of TP. Herein we provide evidence that liver is a good source of TP and suggest that MNGIE patients might benefit from orthotopic liver transplantation.

Materials and Methods

Tissue Sampling

Hepatic tissue samples (1×1 cm), were obtained from eleven subjects (7M, 32–67 years), undergoing open surgery for neoplastic (primary hepato-cellular carcinoma) liver disease. Tissue samples were harvested in a macroscopically normal area and the histopathological analysis confirmed a normal liver histology. Collected specimens were processed as follows: a) five samples were immediately frozen in RNA*later* RNA Stabilization Reagent (Sigma Aldrich, Milan, Italy) and stored at −80°C; b) six samples were formalin fixed and paraffin embedded.

Ethical Considerations

The Institutional Review Board of the St. Orsola-Malpighi University Hospital Ethics Committee approved this research project (31/2013/U/OssN Prot.nr.1380/2013), which complied with the Declaration of Helsinki. A written informed consent was obtained from each participant and anonymized samples were collected as 'MNGIE-(consecutive number)-age-sex' or 'NON-MNGIE-(consecutive number)-age-sex'.

Protein extraction

Total protein was extracted from five liver tissue samples (0.5 g) (3 M) using tissue protein extraction reagent in the presence of a protease inhibitor cocktail (Thermo Scientific, Milan, Italy) according to the manufacturer's instructions. Protein fractions were quantified for total protein content using a NanoDrop 2000 spectrophotometer (Thermo Scientific, Milan, Italy), and were stored at −80°C. Total protein extracts from our laboratory archive (obtained with the same technique) served as controls. Specifically, total protein was extracted from bone marrow (n = 3, 2 M; 40–65 years), duodenal mucosa (n = 3, 1 M; 38–57 years), skeletal muscles (n = 3, 2 M; 33–61 years), and non-MNGIE (n = 3, 1 M; 33–61 years) and MNGIE buffy coats (n = 1, female aged 29 years).

Western blot (WB) analysis

Protein separation was carried out on 50 μg samples of total protein in a 12% tris-glycine gel (Thermo Scientific, Milan, Italy). Protein was transferred onto nitrocellulose membrane (Macherrey-Nagel, Düren, Germany) overnight at 12 mV. Membranes were blocked with a buffer containing 5% fat-free milk and then incubated overnight at 4°C with a mouse anti-TP primary antibody (Thermo Scientific, Milan, Italy) at a final concentration of 2 μg/ml. Membranes were washed three times and incubated with an anti-mouse peroxidase-conjugated secondary antibody (Sigma Aldrich, Milan, Italy). Immunoreactive bands were visualized by enhanced chemiluminescence (GE Healthcare, Buckinghamshire, UK) on a ChemiDoc MP System and quantified by Image Lab software version 4.0 (Bio-Rad Laboratories, Hercules, CA, USA). Band intensities were expressed relative to total protein and/or to the intensity of GAPDH detected on the same membrane following stripping with Restore Plus Western Blot Stripping Buffer (Thermo Fisher Scientific, Pittsburgh, PA, USA) and overnight incubation with GAPDH antibody at 4°C at a 1:1000 dilution (Abcam, Cambridge, UK). Each assay was conducted in technical triplicate.

ELISA TP quantification

TP amount was measured on total protein extracts from the same 5 subjects included in the WB separation, using an ELISA Kit for human TP (Uscn Life Science Inc., Wuhan, China) according to the manufacturer's instructions. A quantity of 10 μl of protein extract (5 μg/μl of total protein) for each sample was assayed in triplicate. When reactions were complete, multi-well ELISA pre-coated plates were read in an Infinite M200 multi plate reader (TECAN, Männedorf, Switzerland) at λ 450 nm. TP concentrations in each sample were estimated from a TP standard curve. Assays were performed in duplicate.

Immunohistochemical analysis

Anti-TP immunohistochemical analysis was performed on formalin-fixed, paraffin-embedded liver samples from 6 subjects. Sections of normal liver tissue, obtained from the laboratory histology archive, were used as controls. Additionally, duodenum (n = 3) and skeletal muscles (n = 3) (from 6 different subjects, 4 M; 32–67 years) were processed as positive and negative controls, respectively. Moreover, paraffin-fixed liver, duodenum, and skeletal muscle tissue samples from one MNGIE patient (male; 37 years) were included.

a

b

c

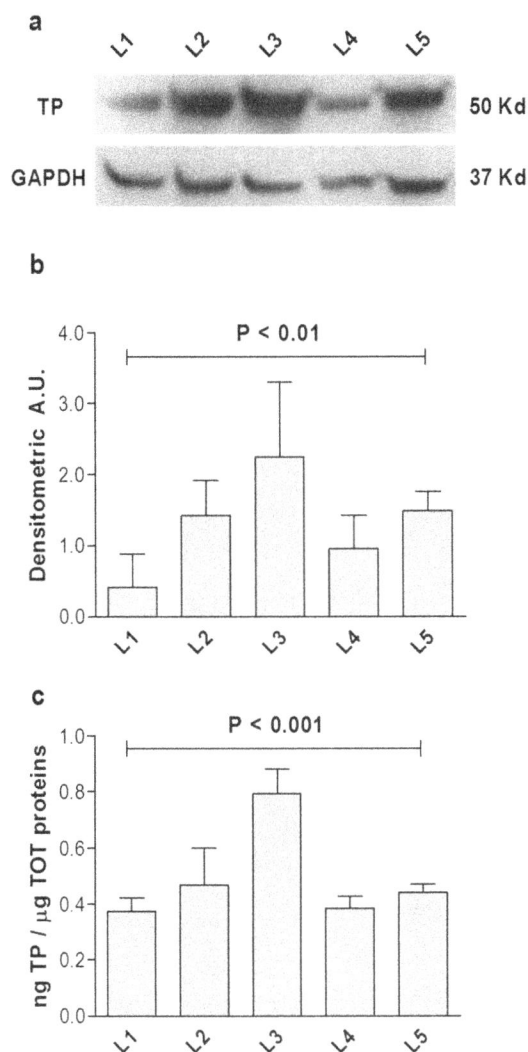

Figure 1. TP occurrence and concentration in control liver.
Figure 1A shows an example of a WB separation of 50 ng total protein from healthy liver. TP and reference protein GAPDH chemiolumines-cence are reported from liver L1 to L5. Figure 1B illustrates the densitometric arbitrary units (A.U.) calculated normalizing TP chemio-luminescent signal on the internal reference protein GAPDH ± SD and showing a significant variability among non-MNGIE subjects (P< 0.01, one way non parametric test ANOVA). The graph in Figure 1C reports the TP concentration measured by ELISA and expressed as ng TP/µg total proteins for the 5 liver tissue samples ± SD and showing a significant variability among non-MNGIE subjects (P< 0.001, one way non parametric test ANOVA).

Tissue sections were deparaffinized in xylene and rehydrated through graded ethanol (Carlo Erba, Milan, Italy). Antigen retrieval was carried out by heating sections in a 90°C water for 25 min in the presence of 10 mmol/l sodium citrate buffer pH 6.0 (Carlo Erba, Milan, Italy). Sections were treated with an endogenous peroxidase blocking kit (Gene Tex, Aachen, Germany). Subsequent steps were performed using a commercial kit (Millipore, Milan, Italy) following the manufacturer's instructions. Sections were incubated with mouse primary anti-TP antibody at a final concentration of 0.002 µg/µl (Abcam, Cambridge, UK), in a humidified chamber overnight at 4°C. After dehydration slides were cover-slipped using DPX (Sigma-Aldrich, Milan, Italy).

RNA Extraction

Liver tissue samples (30 mg) (n = 6, 3M, aged 32–67 years) were mechanically disrupted with sterile scissors and homogenized using QIAshredder according to the manufacturer's instructions. RNA was extracted using RNeasy mini kit (Qiagen, Hilden, Germany) and eluted in a final volume of 60 µl. Sample purity was assessed with a NanoDrop 2000 spectrophotometer (Thermo Scientific, Milan, Italy). Total RNA extracts from healthy donors, used as controls, were purchased from BioChain (Milan, Italy) and included: bone marrow (n = 6, 3 M, aged 27–65 years), duodenal mucosa (n = 6, 4 M aged 31–63 years), and skeletal muscle (n = 6, 3 M aged 24–65 years).

Reverse Transcription (RT)

RT was performed on 500 ng of total RNA in a 20 µl total reaction volume using Quantitect reverse transcription kit (Qiagen, Hilden, Germany). Samples were incubated for 2 min at 42°C with gDNA Wipeout Buffer to avoid possible genomic DNA contamination. RT conditions were: 15 min 45°C, 3 min 95°C and 5 min 4°C. Each sample was reverse transcribed twice and the obtained cDNA stored at −20°C.

qPCR assay

Relative gene expression analysis was performed on an Applied Biosystem 7500 Fast real time PCR system (Life Technologies, Milan, Italy) by two step qPCR assays using Quanti Fast Probe Assay Duplex Detection (Qiagen, Hilden, Germany) and following MIQE guidelines [24]. Amplification was performed in a 25 µl final volume including 2 µl of cDNA as template. Each sample was assayed in triplicate and the analysis was duplicated using cDNA from two independent RT reactions. The PCR Master Mix was prepared according to the manufacturer's instructions in the presence of High-ROX dye Solution. Amplification conditions were: 5 min at 95°C followed by 40 cycles (95°C for 30 sec, 60°C for 30 sec). Amplicon length was assessed using 2% agarose gel electrophoresis using SYBR green 1X (Invitrogen, Paisley, UK). Primer probes (Qiagen, Hilden, Germany), optimized for use with the Quanti Fast Probe Assay Duplex Detection Kit, were Hs_TYMP_1_FAM (QF00274225) for TYMP and Hs_ACTB_2_MAX (QF00531209) for $actin$-β Data were reported as $\Delta\Delta C_T$ using $actin$-β as a reference since the mRNA transcript for this gene was similar among the selected human tissues. Bone marrow was the calibrator tissue at unit value.

Statistical analysis

Differences between samples analyzed by WB, ELISA and qPCR, were detected by the One Way ANOVA non-parametric test followed by Tukey's post-test.

Results

TP analysis and quantification

The presence and the amount of TP in healthy human liver tissues were assessed by WB and ELISA (Figure 1). To avoid artifacts assays were performed using independent protein extractions as starting material from five subjects and the results obtained with the two techniques were concordant. Figure 1A shows that TP protein is expressed in all samples. The densitometric arbitrary units (AU), obtained normalizing TP chemioluminescent signal on the internal reference protein GAPDH, is illustrated in Figure 1B. The mean densitometric ratio TP/GAPDH is 0.9±0.5 AU and TP expression varies

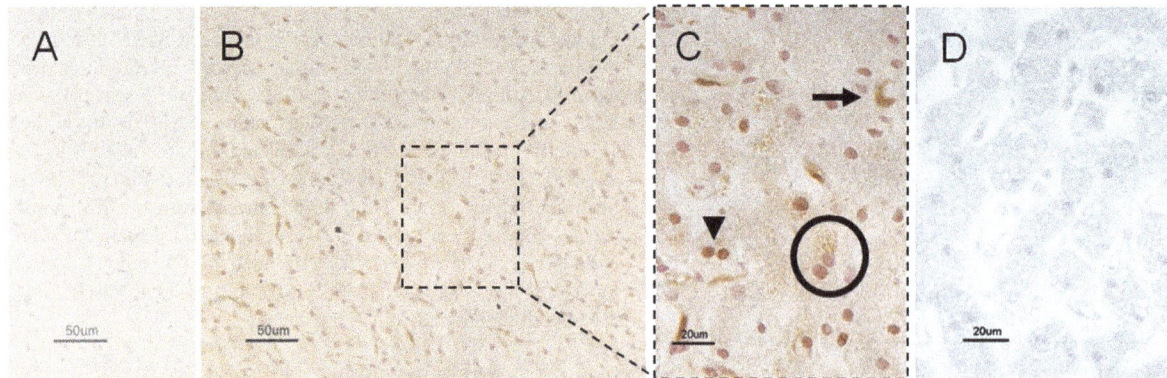

Figure 2. Representative photomicrographs showing TP immunoreactivity in control and MNGIE liver. Figure 2A demonstrates the lack of TP immunolabeling in a normal liver section in which the primary antibody was omitted (negative control). Figure 2B (low magnification) and 2C (high magnification) illustrate TP immunoreactivity in a normal liver section. In Figure 2C, the arrowhead and circle, (Figure 2C) point to TP immunostained nuclei and cytoplasm of hepatocytes, while the arrow indicates non-hepatocytic cells with features of bile duct elements. Also, note the lack of any TP immunolabeling in a MNGIE liver section (Figure 2D). Calibration bars = 20 μm and 50 μm in 2C, 2D and 2A, 2B, respectively.

significantly among subjects (P<0.01). TP quantification, expressed as ng TP/μg total protein, is obtained with ELISA (Figure 1C). The average of TP content is 0.5 ng/μg total protein, ranging from 0.4 to 0.75 ng/μg total protein. The variation in TP expression among subjects is confirmed by ELISA (P<0.001).

TP localization in liver and in a selected human tissue panel

Figure 2 demonstrates the TP immunoreactivity in liver tissues of controls (A-C) and in a MNGIE patient (D). Compared to MNGIE liver tissue, which lacked TP immunostaining (Figure 2D), TP immunoreactivity was clearly detected in the cytoplasm as well

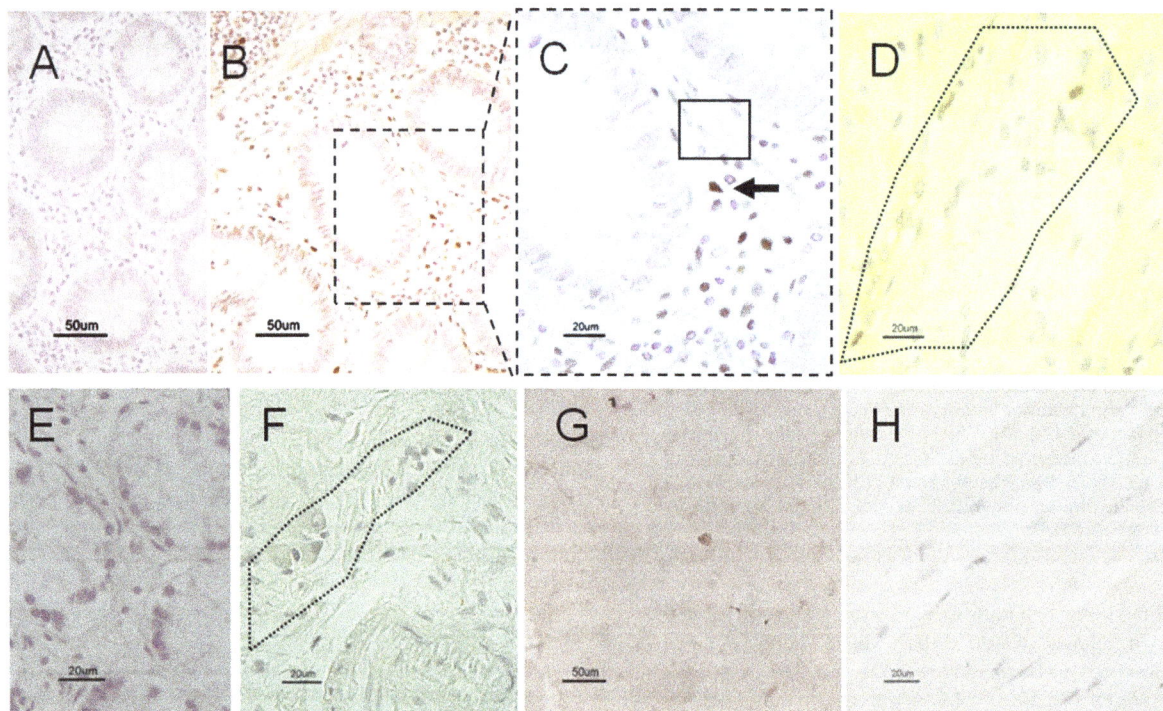

Figure 3. TP immunoreactivity in the duodenum and skeletal muscle of control and in a MNGIE patient. TP immunolabeling is lacking in a tissue section of normal duodenal mucosa in which primary antibody was omitted (negative control) (Figure 3A). Figure 3B (low magnification) and 3C (high magnification) show TP immunolabeling in the control mucosa. The black arrow indicates TP immunolabeled cells with features of immunocytes distributed throughout the *lamina propria*; the rectangle shows a less intense TP immunostaining in the cytoplasm of cells with features of fibroblasts. The dotted line area in figure 3D indicates a myenteric plexus displaying TP immunolabelling in non-neuronal cells (likely glial cells). Note the lack of TP immunolabeling in the mucosal *lamina propria* (Figure 3E) and myenteric plexus (dotted line) of a MNGIE patient (Figure 3F). The TP immunolabeling was negative also in normal (Figure 3G) and MNGIE (Figure 3H) skeletal muscle. Calibration bars = 20 μm and 50 μm in 3C, 3D, 3E, 3F, 3H and 3A, 3B, 3G respectively.

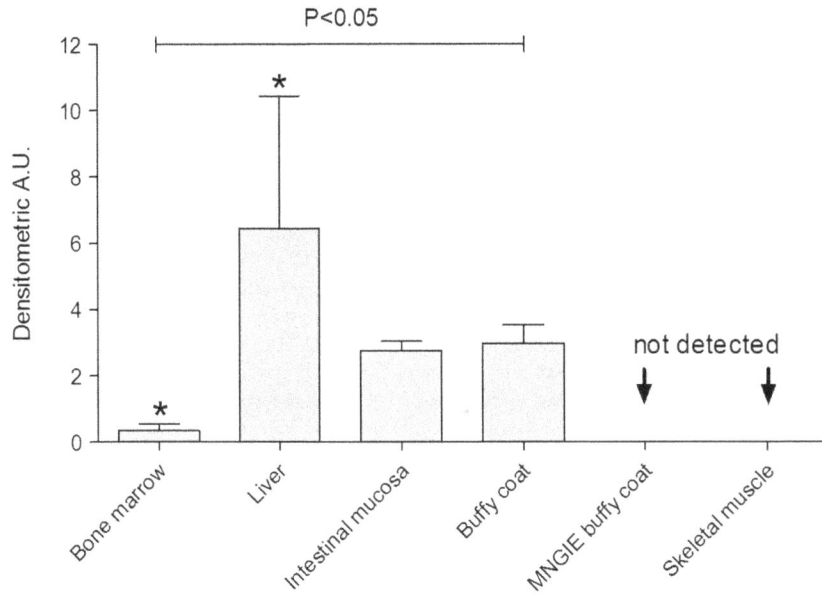

Figure 4. TP concentration and distribution in a panel of selected human tissues. The graph reports the A.U. calculated normalizing TP chemioluminescent signal on total proteins. Data are reported as mean ± SD using bone marrow as calibrator tissue. The TP concentrations vary significantly among different tissues (P< 0.05 one way ANOVA non-parametric test; *P< 0.05 Tukey's post-test).

as nuclei of hepatocytes in control tissues (Figures 2B-C). In addition, some sinusoidal lining cell resembling Kupffer cells showed TP immunolabeling (Figures 2B-C).

TP localization was also identified in a panel of selected human tissues (Figure 3). In the duodenal mucosa, TP immunoreactivity was revealed in the cytoplasm of cells reminiscent of immunocytes normally distributed throughout the *lamina propria* (Figures 3 A-C). Also, TP immunolabeling was detected in the duodenal neuro-muscular compartment, specifically in non-neuronal cells (likely glial cells) of the myenteric plexus (Figure 3 D). As expected, TP immunolabeling was not identified in any cell of the duodenal

mucosal *lamina propria* and myenteric plexus of a MNGIE patient (Figures 3 E, F). Finally, both normal (Figure 3 G) (negative control) and MNGIE skeletal muscle (Figure 3 H) lacked TP immunolabeling.

TP abundance in a selected human tissue panel

Quantitative TP expression in human liver was compared to that of other tissues based on previously published animal models (Figure 4) [25]. Control liver samples have TP densitometric values six times higher than bone marrow samples (P<0.05), whereas normal buffy coats and intestinal mucosa have TP levels intermediate between liver and bone marrow (neither reached statistical significance). As expected, TP is not detectable in negative controls, i.e. normal skeletal muscle, or buffy coat of a patient with MNGIE. TP concentrations vary significantly among tissues containing the enzyme (P<0.05).

qPCR screening

TYMP mRNA levels in bone marrow, liver, duodenum, and skeletal muscle were investigated by qPCR (Figure 5). Bone marrow, liver, and duodenum expressed *TYMP* at a comparable level, whereas skeletal muscle did not express any *TYMP* mRNA.

Discussion

In this study, we assessed the expression of TP in normal human liver in comparison with a number of other control as well as MNGIE tissues. The results unequivocally demonstrate that the normal liver expresses *TYMP* and markedly synthesizes TP, suggesting that this organ is a possible option for transplantation in MNGIE patients.

So far, two main non-invasive strategies have been attempted to reduce circulating toxic levels of dThd, i.e. peritoneal dialysis [3] and platelet infusion [16]. These therapeutic approaches, however, have demonstrated only short term beneficial effects in MNGIE patients, paving the way for tissue transplantation as a permanent source of TP. Long term TP replacement is thought to reduce

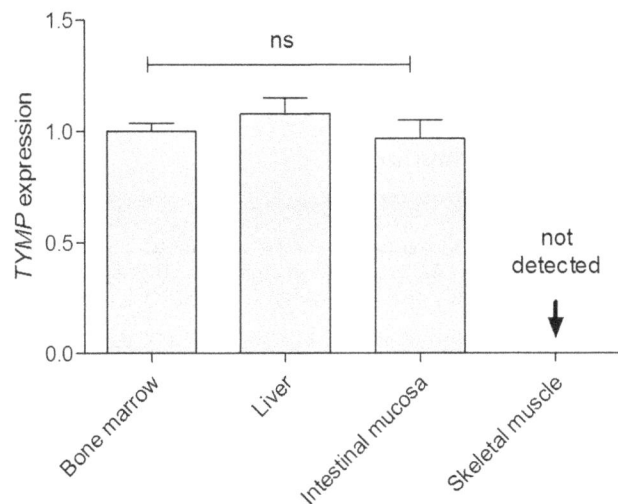

Figure 5. *TYMP* mRNA transcription in a panel of healthy human tissues. The amount of *TYMP* mRNA has been reported ± SD. Bone marrow was used as a calibrator tissue. *TYMP* mRNA expression did not vary significantly in bone marrow, liver, and duodenal mucosa. No *TYMP* transcript was found in skeletal muscle.

dThd accumulation in plasma and tissues thereby preventing the progression of MNGIE-related clinical manifestations. In support of this concept, heterozygous subjects for *TYMP* mutations have ~30% of TP residual activity which is sufficient to avoid the MNGIE phenotype [26]. AHSCT has proven to be valuable to permanently restore TP function, reduce dThd and mitigate symptoms in MNGIE patients. So far ~20 cases of MNGIE have undergone AHSCT, although the 5-year overall mortality is the ~50% [22] and increasing up to ~70% in recently presented results (Hirano et al., Child Neurology Society's annual meeting, 2013, Austin, TX).

In order to find a new permanent source of TP, possibly with a lower risk of mortality associated with transplantation, we considered the liver as a potentially useful tissue because of its physiological roles and transplantation outcome. First of all, the liver is the prototype organ for protein biosynthesis, trafficking and release; secondly, orthotopic liver transplantation has been found to be successful in 90% of cases [23]. Another important aspect is that AHSCT is associated with quite a high mortality which seems likely the consequence of immunosuppression, usually more pronounced than that required for liver transplantation [27]. Recently, cirrhosis has been documented as a rare complication in a patient with MNGIE likely due to the accumulation of toxic intermediates in the liver [28]. Based on this case report, liver transplantation would be indicated not only as a source of TP, but also to prevent nucleoside-induced injuries [28].

The first quantification of TP activity has been obtained in animal models in the early 50's by Friedkin and Roberts [25,29]. Using the rabbit, they found that TP expression in the liver was less abundant than only that of the small intestinal mucosa, although greater than bone marrow > kidney > spleen. Heart, lung, skeletal muscle, and brain showed negligible activity [29]. Notably, the two authors demonstrated that liver TP activity was ~6 times higher than those of the bone marrow (liver 10.0 ± 2.9 vs. bone marrow 1.77 ± 1.6 μM TP released h^{-1} g tissue^{-1}) [29], the only tissue that has so far been proposed for transplantation in MNGIE patients. Friedkin and Roberts also demonstrated that TP is highly expressed in most mammalian (horse, cow, and rat) and non-mammalian (chicken) liver [25,29]. Interestingly, in chicken embryos (5 to 18 days) most of the TP activity was found in the liver as compared to other tissues, suggesting that TP production during chicken embryogenesis is mainly dependent on the liver [29].

In this study, we have extensively characterized TP in human liver and demonstrated that TP is present in independent tissue protein extracts using both WB and ELISA. The WB approach provided evidence that TP is expressed in all analyzed samples, while the ELISA quantification revealed that TP content was 0.5 ng/μg total protein and varied significantly among subjects, confirming and expanding previous data by Yoshimura et al. [30]. Further immunohistochemical results demonstrated TP localiza-

tion throughout the liver. Indeed, TP immunolabeling was detected not only (as expected) in the cytoplasm of hepatocytes, but also in the nuclei. This latter finding is interesting because it provides a morphological correlate for the well-known TP-mediated regulatory role in tissue proliferation and angiogenesis [31,32]. TP activity was not measured in the investigated tissues as it is well known that TP protein expression correlates with its activity [33]. Furthermore, TYMP, formerly known as platelet-derived endothelial cell growth factor" (PD-ECGF), may exert a role in different types of tumors. In particular, TP expression has been found to be elevated in various solid tumors where it is likely involved in mechanisms that regulate cell proliferation, apoptosis, and angiogenesis [34,35]. Finally, TP immunolabeling was also identified in sinusoidal lining Kupffer-like cells (i.e. possibly belonging to the mononuclear phagocyte system) [36]. However, the role exerted by TP in these specialized cells is still largely unknown.

Using WB we also compared TP levels in a number of normal tissues and found that the amount of TP measured in the duodenal mucosa was between that of liver and bone marrow. These findings are in line with finding of a dense infiltrate of TP immunopositive cells distributed mainly throughout the *lamina propria* and displaying features of immunocytes and fibroblasts. Normal buffy coats showed TP levels similar to the duodenal mucosa, but was not detectable in MNGIE buffy coats (used as negative control). Finally, TP immunoreactivity was undetectable in skeletal muscle, a finding that has previously been referred to as the 'muscle paradox' since this tissue is known to be a target of disease in MNGIE patients but does not contain TP [29,30,37,38]. The explanation for the 'muscle paradox' remains unclear and this intriguing topic clearly requires further study.

Our data on TYMP transcript indicate endogenous synthesis and discard the possibility of TP uptake by the liver. TYMP mRNA is expressed in comparable amounts in bone marrow, liver and duodenal mucosa. No transcript was detected in skeletal muscle confirming the 'muscle paradox'. Since TP protein concentrations vary in different tissues but is not associated with TYMP mRNA changes, it is conceivable that specific post-transcriptional regulation may occur.

In conclusion, our study demonstrates that the liver is a useful source of TP, six times higher than bone marrow. Thus, we propose orthotopic liver transplantation as a therapeutic alternative for MNGIE patients with a possible better outcome in terms of survival rate.

Author Contributions

Conceived and designed the experiments: EB RDA FB VC GC ADP MDG RR VS LP KR VT CC RDG. Performed the experiments: EB FB GC VT. Analyzed the data: EB RDA FB VC GC RR VS VT RDG. Contributed reagents/materials/analysis tools: GC ADP MDG LP KR VT RDG. Wrote the paper: EB RDA VC GC VS KR VT CC RDG.

References

1. DiMauro S, Schon EA (2003) Mitochondrial respiratory-chain diseases. N Engl J Med 348: 2656–2668.
2. Nishino I, Spinazzola A, Hirano M (1999) Thymidine phosphorylase gene mutations in MNGIE, a human mitochondrial disorder. Science 283: 689–692.
3. Spinazzola A, Marti R, Nishino I, Andreu AL, Naini A, et al. (2002) Altered thymidine metabolism due to defects of thymidine phosphorylase. J Biol Chem 277: 4128–4133.
4. Marti R, Nishigaki Y, Hirano M (2003) Elevated plasma deoxyuridine in patients with thymidine phosphorylase deficiency. Biochem Biophys Res Commun 303: 14–18.
5. Ferraro P, Pontarin G, Crocco L, Fabris S, Reichard P, et al. (2005) Mitochondrial deoxynucleotide pools in quiescent fibroblasts: a possible model for mitochondrial neurogastrointestinal encephalomyopathy (MNGIE). J Biol Chem 280: 24472–24480.
6. Gonzalez-Vioque E, Torres-Torronteras J, Andreu AL, Marti R (2011) Limited dCTP availability accounts for mitochondrial DNA depletion in mitochondrial neurogastrointestinal encephalomyopathy (MNGIE). PLoS Genet 7: e1002035.
7. Song S, Wheeler LJ, Mathews CK (2003) Deoxyribonucleotide pool imbalance stimulates deletions in HeLa cell mitochondrial DNA. J Biol Chem 278: 43893–43896.
8. Pontarin G, Ferraro P, Valentino ML, Hirano M, Reichard P, et al. (2006) Mitochondrial DNA depletion and thymidine phosphate pool dynamics in a cellular model of mitochondrial neurogastrointestinal encephalomyopathy. J Biol Chem 281: 22720–22728.
9. Giordano C, Sebastiani M, De Giorgio R, Travaglini C, Tancredi A, et al. (2008) Gastrointestinal dysmotility in mitochondrial neurogastrointestinal encephalomyopathy is caused by mitochondrial DNA depletion. Am J Pathol 173: 1120–1128.

10. Hirano M, Silvestri G, Blake DM, Lombes A, Minetti C, et al. (1994) Mitochondrial neurogastrointestinal encephalomyopathy (MNGIE): clinical, biochemical, and genetic features of an autosomal recessive mitochondrial disorder. Neurology 44: 721–727.

11. Papadimitriou A, Comi GP, Hadjigeorgiou GM, Bordoni A, Sciacco M, et al. (1998) Partial depletion and multiple deletions of muscle mtDNA in familial MNGIE syndrome. Neurology 51: 1086–1092.

12. Marti R, Verschuuren JJ, Buchman A, Hirano I, Tadesse S, et al. (2005) Late-onset MNGIE due to partial loss of thymidine phosphorylase activity. Ann Neurol 58: 649–652.

13. Lara MC, Valentino ML, Torres-Torronteras J, Hirano M, Marti R (2007) Mitochondrial neurogastrointestinal encephalomyopathy (MNGIE): biochemical features and therapeutic approaches. Biosci Rep 27: 151–163.

14. la Marca G, Malvagia S, Casetta B, Pasquini E, Pela I, et al. (2006) Pre- and post-dialysis quantitative dosage of thymidine in urine and plasma of a MNGIE patient by using HPLC-ESI-MS/MS. J Mass Spectrom 41: 586–592.

15. Yavuz H, Ozel A, Christensen M, Christensen E, Schwartz M, et al. (2007) Treatment of mitochondrial neurogastrointestinal encephalomyopathy with dialysis. Arch Neurol 64: 435–438.

16. Lara MC, Weiss B, Illa I, Madoz P, Massuet L, et al. (2006) Infusion of platelets transiently reduces nucleoside overload in MNGIE. Neurology 67: 1461–1463.

17. Fairbanks LD, Levene M, Bax BE (2013) Validation of a HPLC method for the measurement of erythrocyte encapsulated thymidine phosphorylase (EE-TP) activity. J Pharm Biomed Anal 76: 8–12.

18. Torres-Torronteras J, Gomez A, Eixarch H, Palenzuela L, Pizzorno G, et al. (2011) Hematopoietic gene therapy restores thymidine phosphorylase activity in a cell culture and a murine model of MNGIE. Gene Ther 18: 795–806.

19. Torres-Torronteras J, Viscomi C, Cabrera-Perez R, Camara Y, Di Meo I, et al. (2014) Gene Therapy Using a Liver-targeted AAV Vector Restores Nucleoside and Nucleotide Homeostasis in a Murine Model of MNGIE. Mol Ther. e-Pub

20. Halter J, Schupbach WM, Casali C, Elhasid R, Fay K, et al. (2011) Allogeneic hematopoietic SCT as treatment option for patients with mitochondrial neurogastrointestinal encephalomyopathy (MNGIE): a consensus conference proposal for a standardized approach. Bone Marrow Transplant 46: 330–337.

21. Hirano M, Marti R, Casali C, Tadesse S, Uldrick T, et al. (2006) Allogeneic stem cell transplantation corrects biochemical derangements in MNGIE. Neurology 67: 1458–1460.

22. Filosto M, Scarpelli M, Tonin P, Lucchini G, Pavan F, et al. (2012) Course and management of allogeneic stem cell transplantation in patients with mitochondrial neurogastrointestinal encephalomyopathy. J Neurol 259: 2699–2706.

23. O'Mahony CA, Goss JA (2012) The future of liver transplantation. Tex Heart Inst J 39: 874–875.

24. Bustin SA, Benes V, Garson JA, Hellemans J, Huggett J, et al. (2009) The MIQE guidelines: minimum information for publication of quantitative real-time PCR experiments. Clin Chem 55: 611–622.

25. Friedkin M, Roberts D (1954) The enzymatic synthesis of nucleosides. II. Thymidine and related pyrimidine nucleosides. J Biol Chem 207: 257–266.

26. Hirano M, Nishigaki Y, Marti R (2004) Mitochondrial neurogastrointestinal encephalomyopathy (MNGIE): a disease of two genomes. Neurologist 10: 8–17.

27. Wu SL, Pan CE (2013) Tolerance and chimerism and allogeneic bone marrow/stem cell transplantation in liver transplantation. World J Gastroenterol 19: 5981–5987.

28. Finkenstedt A, Schranz M, Bosch S, Karall D, Burgi SS, et al. (2013) MNGIE Syndrome: Liver Cirrhosis Should Be Ruled Out Prior to Bone Marrow Transplantation. JIMD Rep 10: 41–44.

29. Friedkin M, Roberts D (1954) The enzymatic synthesis of nucleosides. I. Thymidine phosphorylase in mammalian tissue. J Biol Chem 207: 245–256.

30. Yoshimura A, Kuwazuru Y, Furukawa T, Yoshida H, Yamada K, et al. (1990) Purification and tissue distribution of human thymidine phosphorylase; high expression in lymphocytes, reticulocytes and tumors. Biochim Biophys Acta 1034: 107–113.

31. Miyadera K, Sumizawa T, Haraguchi M, Yoshida H, Konstanty W, et al. (1995) Role of thymidine phosphorylase activity in the angiogenic effect of platelet derived endothelial cell growth factor/thymidine phosphorylase. Cancer Res 55: 1687–1690.

32. Akiyama S, Furukawa T, Sumizawa T, Takebayashi Y, Nakajima Y, et al. (2004) The role of thymidine phosphorylase, an angiogenic enzyme, in tumor progression. Cancer Sci 95: 851–857.

33. van Triest B, Pinedo HM, Blaauwgeers JL, van Diest PJ, Schoenmakers PS, et al. (2000) Prognostic role of thymidylate synthase, thymidine phosphorylase/platelet-derived endothelial cell growth factor, and proliferation markers in colorectal cancer. Clin Cancer Res 6: 1063–1072.

34. Bonotto M, Bozza C, Di Loreto C, Osa EO, Poletto E, et al. (2013) Making capecitabine targeted therapy for breast cancer: which is the role of thymidine phosphorylase? Clin Breast Cancer 13: 167–172.

35. Toi M, Atiqur Rahman M, Bando H, Chow LW (2005) Thymidine phosphorylase (platelet-derived endothelial-cell growth factor) in cancer biology and treatment. Lancet Oncol 6: 158–166.

36. Baffy G (2009) Kupffer cells in non-alcoholic fatty liver disease: the emerging view. J Hepatol 51: 212–223.

37. Waltenberger J, Usuki K, Fellstrom B, Funa K, Heldin CH (1992) Platelet-derived endothelial cell growth factor. Pharmacokinetics, organ distribution and degradation after intravenous administration in rats. FEBS Lett 313: 129–132.

38. Fox SB, Moghaddam A, Westwood M, Turley H, Bicknell R, et al. (1995) Platelet-derived endothelial cell growth factor/thymidine phosphorylase expression in normal tissues: an immunohistochemical study. J Pathol 176: 183–190.

19

Participation in Mass Gatherings can Benefit Well-Being: Longitudinal and Control Data from a North Indian Hindu Pilgrimage Event

Shruti Tewari[1], Sammyh Khan[2], Nick Hopkins[2]*, Narayanan Srinivasan[1], Stephen Reicher[3]

1 Centre of Behavioural and Cognitive Sciences, University of Allahabad, Allahabad, Uttar Pradesh, India, **2** School of Psychology, University of Dundee, Dundee, Scotland, United Kingdom, **3** School of Psychology, University of St Andrews, St Andrews, Scotland, United Kingdom

Abstract

How does participation in a long-duration mass gathering (such as a pilgrimage event) impact well-being? There are good reasons to believe such collective events pose risks to health. There are risks associated with communicable diseases. Moreover, the physical conditions at such events (noise, crowding, harsh conditions) are often detrimental to well-being. Yet, at the same time, social psychological research suggests participation in group-related activities can impact well-being positively, and we therefore investigated if participating in a long-duration mass gathering can actually bring such benefits. In our research we studied one of the world's largest collective events – a demanding month-long Hindu religious festival in North India. Participants (comprising 416 pilgrims who attended the gathering for the whole month of its duration, and 127 controls who did not) completed measures of self-assessed well-being and symptoms of ill-health at two time points. The first was a month before the gathering commenced, the second was a month after it finished. We found that those participating in this collective event reported a longitudinal increase in well-being relative to those who did not participate. Our data therefore imply we should reconceptualise how mass gatherings impact individuals. Although such gatherings can entail significant health risks, the benefits for well-being also need recognition. Indeed, an exclusive focus on risk is misleading and limits our understanding of why such events may be so attractive. More importantly, as our research is longitudinal and includes a control group, our work adds robust evidence to the social psychological literature concerning the relationship between participation in social group activities and well-being.

Editor: Petter Holme, Umeå University, Sweden

Funding: This work was supported by an ESRC (UK) research grant entitled "Collective participation and social identification: A study of the individual, interpersonal and collective dimensions of attendance at the Magh Mela" (RES-062-23-1449). The funders had no role in study design, data collection and analysis, decision to publish, or preparation of the manuscript.

Competing Interests: The authors have declared that no competing interests exist.

* E-mail: n.p.hopkins@dundee.ac.uk

Introduction

There is an increasing recognition that our well-being is shaped by social factors such as our social relationships [1–3]. Various processes have been posited to explain this relationship. Some of these concern the beliefs and practices of particular groups. Others concern the more general features of group life.

For example, being religious has a positive impact on well-being. In part, this is because religious beliefs provide cognitive schemas or encourage meditative practices relevant to the appraisal of life events and coping [4,5]. In part, it is also because of one's participation in a congregation and the fact that one acts alongside others [6–11]. In similar vein, research on work groups operating in stressful environments shows that the more one feels a part of the team, the better one's well-being [12,13], and evidence from studies of the elderly living in residential homes reveals that a range of activities (from drinking water to avoid dehydration to reminiscing about the past) bring about benefits because they are done in groups [14,15].

The underlying psychological process that link group membership with well-being is argued to derive from a sense of shared identity ('we-ness') that develops in groups. This leads people to experience mutual trust, respect and cooperation [16,17]. It can also lead people to expect support from their fellow group members and develop greater resilience [18]. Building upon such insights it has been argued that since we spend most of our time in the company of others, we should study health in group settings [19].

To date, though, research in this tradition has been done principally upon small and organized groups. Our focus here is on a very different type of collectivity – a long-duration mass gathering. When it comes to such gatherings (e.g., pilgrimage events such as the *Hajj*) a very different viewpoint tends to prevail. They are viewed as posing significant risks to well-being and health [20,21]. Some risks concern the dangers posed by communicable diseases [22]. Some relate to the rudimentary living and sanitary facilities at such events [23]. Still other risks arise from the presence of others. These latter include the dangers of crushing and the stresses of living in crowded and noisy conditions. For example, the dense crowding characteristic of collective events can increase stress and blood pressure [24]. So too, the loud noise levels that characterise mass gatherings, can increase stress and mental health symptoms [25].

However, an exclusive focus on the risks of participation may lead us to overlook the potential benefits that participation in mass gatherings can have. Although not specifically focussed on well-being, social anthropological theory has long argued that mass gatherings (e.g., carnivals and religious festivals) can be joyous occasions and involve a sense of intimacy even between people who do not know each other [26,27]. Moreover, such theory has spoken of the ways in which mass gatherings revivify social bonds and re-establish group identities. However, as several researchers lament, these more positive features of collective events are routinely overlooked in much contemporary academic research [28]. Indeed as Getz shows, even researchers interested in the tourism associated with mass events (e.g., sports events, cultural festivals, etc.) tend to overlook how participation may impact positively on participants' well-being [29,30]. Instead, such research typically focuses on the economic and environmental impacts of these events or on issues of safety management.

In the research reported here we seek to rebalance the situation by addressing the neglected benefits of collective participation. Specifically we investigate how participation in one of the world's largest collective events - the *Magh Mela* at Allahabad in Northern India – impacts participants' well-being [31]. Our data are quantitative and derived from an orally-administered question-naire concerning well-being. These self-report data were obtained before and after the collective event, and from a sample attending the event and from a sample of controls (comparable others who did not attend). Before elaborating on our design and measures, we describe the context and nature of the event more fully.

Setting

Every year, in the Hindu month of *Magh* (mid-January to mid-February), pilgrims gather at the confluence of the Ganges and Yamuna rivers to perform a series of sacred rituals - notably to bathe in the rivers. The event is on a 12-year cycle. In the twelfth year (the *Maha Kumbh Mela*) it is claimed that up to 50 million people attend and over 10 million can be present on a single bathing day. Every six years (the *Ardh Kumbh Mela*), somewhere in the region of 20 million participate. Yet, even for the 'routine' yearly gatherings – the *Magh Mela* - millions attend, and hundreds of thousands undertake to remain for the full month.

Those pilgrims who stay for the whole month (known as *Kalpwasis*) live in conditions that are more difficult than those they experience at home. They live in rudimentary tents without heating, often without sanitary facilities, sleeping on the ground and experiencing night-time temperatures approaching zero centigrade. The event is also very crowded, and again this contrasts with life in the villages from which the pilgrims come. The crowds make walking to the bathing areas difficult and on days that bathing is judged particularly auspicious in terms of Hindu traditions, it can take several hours to walk a kilometre or so. Another striking feature of the event is its noise level. A vast array of competing loudspeakers broadcast religious discourses, songs, announcements and other administrative information throughout the day (and into the night). Our measurements show that on an ordinary day the noise level rarely falls below 75 dB and is often 80–85 dB. It is noteworthy that, according to the US National Institute on Deafness and Other Communication Disorders, exposure to 85 dB or more will cause hearing damage after 8 hours. Again, the contrast between this aspect of the environment and that of the pilgrims' home villages is striking. All in all, life in the Mela is difficult and demanding.

Even if enduring hardship is integral to the act of pilgrimage [32] and even if such hardships do not deter pilgrims from attending, these various circumstances - unsanitary conditions,

severe cold, dense crowding and intense noise - are all those that would be expected to be bad for well-being. But are they? We ask if, in the light of social psychological research identifying associations between involvement in social group-related activities and well-being, participation in this mass gathering could impact well-being positively. To find that participation in such an arduous mass gathering impacts well-being positively would be striking, and would underline the wider relevance and applicability of psychological research concerning the benefits associated with social participation in group activities.

Methods

We recruited a sample of those who participated in the Magh Mela for the full month-long festival (Kalpwasis) and a sample of comparable others who did not attend at all (Controls), and asked both about their well-being and their experience of various symptoms of ill-health. We gathered these data one month before the 2011 Magh Mela (Time 1 - T1) and one month after it had ended (Time 2 - T2), and explored the degree to which the Kalpwasis sample showed a longitudinal increase in reported well-being compared to the Controls.

Participants

The sample consisted of 543 respondents providing data at two time points: before (T1) and after (T2) the Mela. Of these, 416 were Kalpwasis who attended the Mela and 127 Control others who did not. In the first round of data collection (pre-Mela), the sample comprised a total of 792 respondents (604 planning to attend the Mela and 188 not). With attrition, 249 (31.44%) participants were lost giving an overall completion rate of 68.56%. Attrition was equivalent amongst those planning to attend (188 or 31.13%) and the controls (61 or 32.45%). Analyses of the pre-mela data show no differences in the socio-demographic attributes (age, gender, marital-status, educational level, and caste) of our final sample and those lost through attrition.

The final samples of Kalpwasis and Controls were comparable in their socio-demographic attributes: Age (Kalpwasis $M = 64.38$ years, $SD = 9.32$; Controls $M = 60.90$, $SD = 13.44$ years); Gender (Kalpwasis: 57.0% female; Controls 50.4% female); Caste (Kalpwasis: 92.3% *General Caste*, 7.7% *Other Backward Caste* ; Controls: 85.8% *General Caste*, 14.2% *Other Backward Caste*). In all analyses involving comparisons between Kalpwasis and Controls, age, gender, caste, marital and educational-status were employed as covariates.

Ethics statement

This study was approved by the Ethics Committees of the University of Dundee and the University of Allahabad. When approaching potential participants, the researchers gave an overview of the questions to be asked. Participants gave informed consent to participate. As many were unable to read and write, this consent was oral. The decision to seek oral rather than written consent was approved by the above Ethics Committees. The procedure for documenting that oral consent was given was as follows. After explaining the research, participants were asked a formal consent question: 'Do we have your consent to participate in this survey study?' The researcher registered the answer as 'Yes' or 'No' on the response sheet. The researcher also signed their name on this response sheet.

Procedure

Data were gathered with a questionnaire administered orally in Hindi by a trained team of 10 Hindi-speaking field investigators at participants' homes which were within a radius of 100–120 KMs from Allahabad, India. As a sample from rural India has little (if any) experience of questionnaire surveys, and still less experience of using 5-point scales, we took considerable care to conduct the research in a manner that was intelligible. For example, to convey the concept of a 5-point scale, we showed participants drawings of five glasses containing increasing levels of water (ranging from empty to full) and used these to explain to participants how they could communicate their level of well-being and the degree to which they experienced symptoms of ill-health (see Figure 1). The survey took approximately 30 minutes to complete. To ensure the translation was conceptually appropriate, the questionnaire was translated and back-translated (English-Hindi-English) by two independent groups of translators. Any differences between the translations were resolved by improving the questionnaire items. Before the survey was administered, the scales were piloted amongst both illiterate and literate Hindi-speaking participants. This ensured the items were clear and intelligible to participants of widely varying educational backgrounds.

The T1 survey was administered between December 1st and 15th, 2010 - one month before the beginning of the 2011 Magh Mela. The T2 survey was administered between March 3rd and 15th, 2011 - one month after the Mela's conclusion. The average time difference between T1 and T2 was 90 days ($SD = 3$ days). An independent samples t-test revealed no significant difference between the Kalpwasis and Controls in the number of days between T1 and T2, $t(541) = 1.23$, $p = .20$, Cohen's $d = .11$.

Measures

Well-being. Reports of well-being were obtained with three items from the core module of the Centers for Disease Control and Prevention Health Related Quality of Life Measure (CDC HRQOL-14) [33]: "Over the last week, how would you describe your physical health", "Over the last week, how would you describe your state of mind", "Over the last week, how would you describe your energy levels." Responses were gathered on a 5-point scale illustrated with glasses containing varying levels of water. The empty glass (scored '1') was anchored, "Very Poor", the full glass (scored '5') was anchored, "Very Good". Item scores were averaged together such that a higher score indicated better well-being. The reliability (Cronbach's alpha) of this scale was excellent (T1 Participants = .77; T2 Participants = .86; T1 Controls = .81; T2 Controls = .91).

Symptoms of Ill-health. Participants' reported well-being was also measured with six items concerning symptoms of ill-health taken from a scale specifically developed for use in the Indian Subcontinent [34,35]. Three items concerned psychological well-being: "Over the last week, to what extent have you felt anxious without any reason", "Over the last week, to what extent have you felt restless without any reason", "Over the last week, to what extent have you felt irritable without any reason?" Three concerned physical well-being: "Over the last week, to what extent have you suffered from body-aches and pains", "Over the last week, to what extent have you suffered from breathlessness", "Over the last week, to what extent have you suffered from headaches?" Again responses were gathered on a 5-point scale illustrated with glasses

containing varying levels of water and anchored: 1 = "Not at all", 5 = "A lot" (in Hindi the word used translates literally as "Completely"). Item scores were averaged together such that a lower score indicated less symptoms of ill-health. The reliability (Cronbach's alpha) of this scale was excellent (T1 Participants = .81; T2 Participants = .85; T1 Controls = .84; T2 Controls = .84).

Results

Average levels of self-assessed Well-being and Symptoms of ill-health are reported for Kalpwasis and Controls before and after the Mela in Table 1.

Well-being

Participants' levels of Well-being were inspected in a 2 (Condition: Kalpwasis/Controls) ×2 (Time: T1/T2) Mixed Factorial ANCOVA (in which age, gender, caste, marital and educational-status featured as covariates). This showed no effect of Time, $F(1, 533) = .01$, $p = .93$, $\eta_p^2 < .001$, and that Kalpwasis reported better well-being than Control participants, $F(1,533) = 6.05$, $p = .014$, $\eta_p^2 = .011$. However, and most importantly, interpretation of this effect was qualified by an interaction, $F(1, 533) = 6.23$, $p = .013$, $\eta_p^2 = .012$. The relevant Estimated Marginal Means and Standard Errors are plotted in Figure 2. Decomposing this interaction shows that whereas there was no difference in well-being between Kalpwasis and Controls at T1 (Kalpwasis $EMM = 3.35$, $SE = .04$; Controls $EMM = 3.30$, $SE = .08$), $F(1, 533) = .40$, $p = .53$, $\eta_p^2 = .001$, at T2 Kalpwasis reported better Well-being ($EM = 3.62$, $SE = .04$) than Controls ($EMM = 3.30$, $SE = .08$), $F(1, 533) = 11.71$, $p = .001$, $\eta_p^2 = .021$. Moreover, inspecting the Kalpwasis' data revealed an improvement in Well-being from T1 ($EMM = 3.35$, $SE = 04$) to T2 ($EMM = 3.62$, $SE = .04$), $F(1, 415) = 31.25$, $p < .001$, $\eta_p^2 = .07$. In contrast, there was no such improvement amongst Controls (T1: $EMM = 3.30$; $SE = .08$; T2 $EMM = 3.30$, $SE = .08$), $F(1, 126) = .001$, $p = .98$, $\eta_p^2 < .001$.

Symptoms of ill-health

Participants' reported symptoms of ill-health were inspected in a similar 2 (Condition: Kalpwasis/Controls) ×2 (Time: T1/T2) Mixed Factorial ANCOVA (with age, gender, caste, marital and educational-status featuring as covariates). This showed a similar pattern. There was no main effect of Time, $F(1, 533) = 1.48$, $p = .23$, $\eta_p^2 = .003$, and Kalpwasis reported less symptoms than Controls, $F(1,533) = 9.45$, $p = .002$, $\eta_p^2 = .017$. However, interpretation of this main effect was again qualified by the predicted interaction, $F(1, 533) = 4.23$, $p = .04$, $\eta_p^2 = .008$. The relevant Estimated Marginal Means and Standard Errors are plotted in

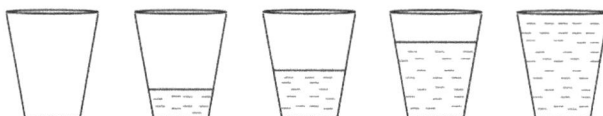

Figure 1. Visual representation of 5-point scale employing glasses with varying levels of water. The anchoring of the empty and full glasses varied according to the questions asked (see text).

Table 1. Well-being and Symptoms of Ill-health amongst Kalpwasis and Controls at T1 and T2.

		Kalpwasis		Controls	
		T1	**T2**	**T1**	**T2**
Well-being	EMM	3.35	3.62	3.30	3.30
	SE	.04	.04	.08	.08
Symptoms of ill-health	EMM	2.04	1.66	2.16	1.96
	SE	.04	.04	.07	.07

Estimated Marginal Means (EMM) and Standard Errors (SE).

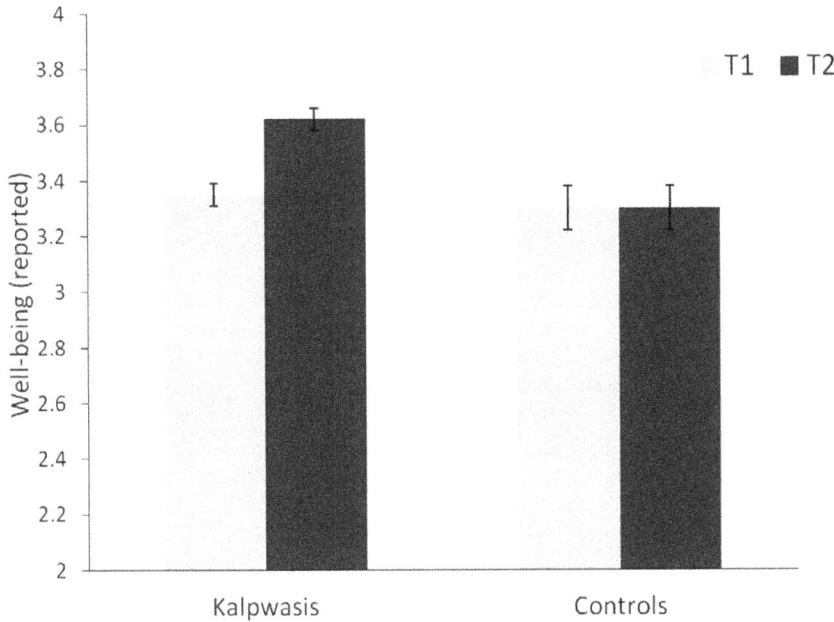

Figure 2. Well-being amongst Kalpwasis and Controls at T1 and T2. Estimated Marginal Means and Standard Errors.

Figure 3. Decomposing this interaction shows that whereas there was no difference between the two groups at T1 (Kalpwasis $EMM = 2.04$, $SE = .04$; Controls $EMM = 2.16$, $SE = .07$), F (1, 533) = 2.03, $p = .16$, $\eta_p^2 = .004$, at T2 Kalpwasis reported significantly fewer symptoms ($EMM = 1.66$, $SD = .04$) than Controls ($EMM = 1.96$, $SE = .07$), F (1, 533) = 15.02, $p < .001$, $\eta_p^2 = .027$. Moreover, for the Kalpwasis there was a sharper decrease in their reporting of symptoms from T1 ($EMM = 2.04$, $SE = .04$) to T2 ($EMM = 1.66$, $SE = .04$), F (1, 415) = 88.35, $p < .001$, $\eta_p^2 = .176$, than amongst the Controls (T1 $EMM = 2.16$, $SE = .07$; T2 $EMM = 1.96$, $SE = .07$), F(1, 126) = 6.67, $p = .011$, $\eta_p^2 = .05$.

Discussion

Our results reveal that whilst Kalpwasis and Controls had comparable pre-Mela scores on both of our measures (Well-being and Symptoms of Ill-health), their post-Mela scores diverge to show the Kalpwasis doing better. With regards to the Well-being measure, the Kalpwasis showed an improvement from before to after the Mela whereas the Controls did not. With regards to their reporting of Symptoms of Ill-health, the pattern is similar. Whilst there is some evidence that both groups improved (perhaps because the first measure was taken in the winter and the second

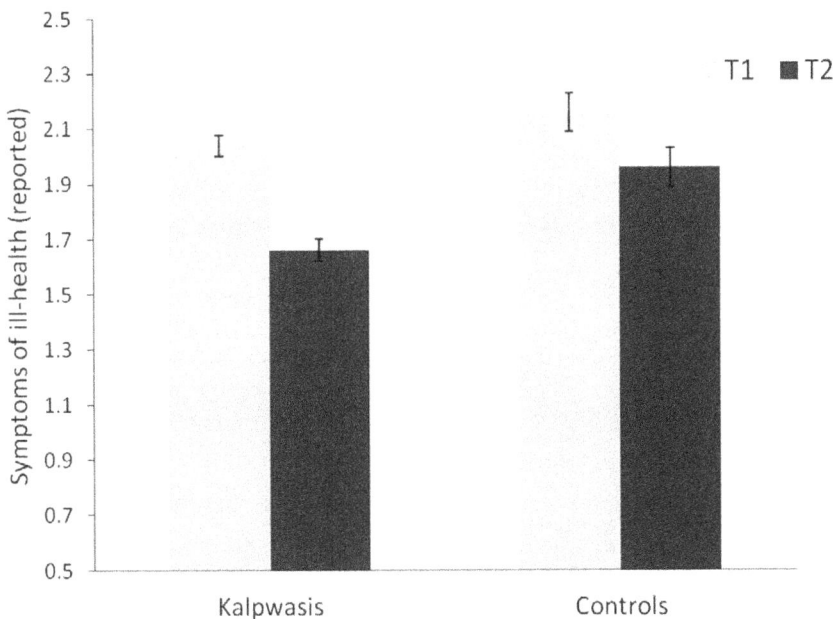

Figure 3. Symptoms of Ill-health amongst Kalpwasis and Controls at T1 and T2. Estimated Marginal Means and Standard Errors.

was taken in spring) the improvement was greater for the Kalpwasis.

Based on the findings obtained with these two measures we have good grounds for believing that taking part in this demanding collective event did indeed have beneficial effects. These are all the more striking for the fact that we set out to study a crowded, noisy and physically-testing mass gathering.

The next obvious question is why, and hence when, participation may result in such outcomes. Being able to follow one's religious beliefs and enact religious rituals is likely to be identity-affirming and this may contribute to a sense of well-being. Moreover, the collective nature of this enactment is also likely to be important [36]. As discussed in the introduction, there is good evidence that a key ingredient in the association between well-being and religious belief/practice concerns the collective dimension to religious activity. This underlines the importance of considering how participation in group activities can be beneficial through leading people to feel supported by others and hence better able to control their everyday lives.

Our findings require that we reappraise the way we look at mass gatherings. Such gatherings are judged as posing a variety of risks. Certainly these risks are serious and should not be underplayed: planning for the control of disease and the through-flow of people at such events is important. However, we also need to consider the benefits associated with such events. Such benefits may be diverse [29,30]. Here we show they can include well-being. Moreover, we

found such benefits obtained even where the physical conditions are harsh (as they are in the collective event studied here). Recognizing the potential for such benefits is important. They help explain some of the attractions of such events and hence why people may be so determined to participate (of obvious importance for event-management). More generally our data provide distinctive evidence for the idea that participation in the social life of a group membership impacts well-being positively. As much work addressing the relationship between social group processes and well-being is cross-sectional in nature (rather than longitudinal) and derived from research conducted in Europe and North America, our data are particularly significant.

Acknowledgments

We gratefully acknowledge the input of Dr. Kavita Pandey, Dr. Shail Shankar, Dr Tushar Singh, (all at the Centre of Behavioural and Cognitive Sciences, Allahabad), Prof. Mark Levine, (Exeter, England), Dr. Gozde Ozakinci (St Andrews, Scotland) and Dr. Clifford Stevenson (Limerick, Ireland).

Author Contributions

Conceived and designed the experiments: ST SK NH NS SR. Performed the experiments: ST . Analyzed the data: SK. Wrote the paper: NH SR NS SK ST.

References

1. Helliwell J F, Putnam R D (2004) The social context of well-being. Philos Trans R Soc Lond B 359: 1435–1446.
2. Cohen S (2004) Social relationships and health. Am Psychol 59: 676–684.
3. Walton G M, Cohen G L (2011) A brief social-belonging intervention improves academic and health outcomes of minority students. Science 331: 1447–1451.
4. James A, Wells A (2003) Religion and mental health: Towards a cognitive-behavioural framework. Br J Health Psychol 8: 359–376.
5. Seeman T E, Dubin L F, Seeman M (2003) Religiosity/spirituality and health: A critical review of the evidence for biological pathways. Am Psychol 58: 53–63.
6. George LK, Larson D B, Koening H G, McCullogh M E (2000) Spirituality and Health: What We Know, What We Need to Know. J Soc Clin Psych 19: 102–116.
7. Green M, Elliott M, Religion (2010) Religion, health and psychological well-being. J Rel Health 2010; 49: 149–163.
8. George L K, Ellison C G, Larson D B (2002) Explaining the relationship between religious involvement and health. Psychol Inq 13: 190–200.
9. Lim C, Putnam R D (2010) Religion, social networks and life satisfaction. Am Sociol Rev 75: 914–933.
10. Salsman J M, Brown T L, Brechting E H, Carlson C R (2005) The link between religion and spirituality and psychological adjustment: The mediating role of optimism and social support. Pers Soc Psychol Bull 31: 522–535.
11. Powell L H, Shahabi L, Thorsen C E (2003) Religion & spirituality: Linkages to physical health. Am Psychol 58: 36–52.
12. Haslam S A, O'Brien A, Jetten J, Vormedal K, Penna S (2005) Taking the strain: Social identity, social support, and the experience of stress. Br J Soc Psychol 44: 355–370.
13. Wegge J, Van Dick R, Fisher G K, Wecking C, Moltzen K (2006) Work motivation, organizational identification, and well-being in call centre work. Work Stress, 20: 60–83.
14. Gleibs I H, Haslam C, Jones J, Haslam S A, McNeill J, Connolly H (2011) No country for old men? The role of a "Gentlemen's Club" in promoting social engagement and psychological well-being in residential care. Ageing Mental Health, 15: 456–467.
15. Haslam C, Haslam S A, Jetten J, Bevins A, Ravenscroft S, Tonks J (2010) The social treatment: The benefits of group interventions in residential care settings. Psych Aging, 25: 157–167.
16. Tyler T R, Blader S L (2000) Cooperation in Groups: Procedural Justice, Social Identity, and Behavioral Engagement. New York: Psychology Press.
17. Haslam S A, Jetten J, Postmes T, Haslam C (2009) Social Identity, health and well-being: An emerging agenda for applied psychology. App Psychol – Int Rev, 58: 1–23.
18. Drury J, Cocking C, Reicher S D (2009) The nature of collective resilience: Survivor reactions to the 2005 London bombings. Int J Mass Emerg and Disasters 27: 66–95.
19. Peterson P, Park N, Sweeney P J (2008) Group well-being: Morale from a positive psychology perspective. Appl Psychol - Int Rev 57: 19–36.
20. Memish Z A, Stephens G M, Steffen R, Ahmed Q A (2012) Emergence of medicine for mass gatherings: lessons from the Hajj. Lancet Infect Dis 12: 56–65.
21. Tam J S, Barbeschi M, Shapovalova N, Briand S, Memish Z A (2012) Research agenda for mass gatherings: a call to action. Lancet Infect Dis 12: 231–239.
22. Abubakar I, Gautret P, Brunette G V, Blumberg L, Johnson D, et al. (2012) Global perspectives for prevention of infectious diseases associated with mass gatherings. Lancet Infect Dis 12: 66–74.
23. Steffen R, Bouchama A, Johansson A, Dvorak J, Isla N, et al. (2012) Non-communicable health risks during mass gatherings. Lancet Infect Dis 12: 142–149.
24. Paulus P, McCain G, Cox V (1978) Death rates, psychiatric commitments, blood pressure and perceived crowding as a function of institutional crowding. Environ Psychol Non-Verbal Behav 3: 107–116.
25. Ising H, Kruppa B (2004) Health effects caused by noise: Evidence in the literature from the past 25 years. Noise Health 6: 5–13.
26. Durkheim E (1912, 1995) The Elementary Forms of Religious Life. Translated by K.E. Fields. New York: Free Press.
27. Turner V (1969) The Ritual Process: Structure and Anti-Structure. New York: Aldine De Gruyter.
28. Ehrenreich B (2006) Dancing in the streets. New York: Metropolitan.
29. Getz D (2008) Event tourism: Definition, evolution, and research. Tourism Manage 29: 403–428.
30. Getz D (2010) The nature and scope of festival studies. Int J Event Manage 5: 1–47.
31. Tully M (2002) The Kumbh Mela. London: Indica Books.
32. Nordin A (2011) The Cognition of Hardship Experience in Himalayan Pilgrimage. Numen 58: 632–673.
33. Measuring Healthy Days. Atlanta, Center for Disease Control and Prevention, 2000.
34. Ruback R B, Begum H A, Tariq N, Kamal A, Pandey J (2002) Reactions to environmental stressors: Gender differences in the slums of Dhaka and Islamabad. J Cross-Cult Psychol 33: 100–119.
35. Ruback R B, Pandey J, Begum H A (1997) Urban stressors in South Asia: Impact on male and female pedestrians in Delhi and Dhaka. J Cross-Cult Psychol 28: 23–43.
36. Graham J, Haidt J (2010) Beyond beliefs: Religions bind individuals into moral communities. Pers Soc Psychol Rev 14: 140–150.

20

Rickettsia Species in African *Anopheles* Mosquitoes

Cristina Socolovschi[1], Frédéric Pages[2], Mamadou O. Ndiath[3], Pavel Ratmanov[1], Didier Raoult[1]*

1 Aix Marseille Université, URMITE, UM63, CNRS 7278, IRD 198, Inserm 1095, Marseille, France, **2** CIRE/ARS Océan Indien, La Réunion, France, **3** IRD, Laboratoire de Paludologie, UMR 198 URMITE, Dakar, Sénégal

Abstract

Background: There is higher rate of *R. felis* infection among febrile patients than in healthy people in Sub-Saharan Africa, predominantly in the rainy season. Mosquitoes possess a high vectorial capacity and, because of their abundance and aggressiveness, likely play a role in rickettsial epidemiology.

Methodology/Principal Findings: Quantitative and traditional PCR assays specific for *Rickettsia* genes detected rickettsial DNA in 13 of 848 (1.5%) *Anopheles* mosquitoes collected from Côte d'Ivoire, Gabon, and Senegal. *R. felis* was detected in one *An. gambiae* molecular form S mosquito collected from Kahin, Côte d'Ivoire (1/77, 1.3%). Additionally, a new *Rickettsia* genotype was detected in five *An. gambiae* molecular form S mosquitoes collected from Côte d'Ivoire (5/77, 6.5%) and one mosquito from Libreville, Gabon (1/88, 1.1%), as well as six *An. melas* (6/67, 9%) mosquitoes collected from Port Gentil, Gabon. A sequence analysis of the *glt*A, *omp*B, *omp*A and sca4 genes indicated that this new *Rickettsia* sp. is closely related to *R. felis*. No rickettsial DNA was detected from *An. funestus, An. arabiensis,* or *An. gambiae* molecular form M mosquitoes. Additionally, a BLAST analysis of the *glt*A sequence from the new *Rickettsia* sp. resulted in a 99.71% sequence similarity to a species (JQ674485) previously detected in a blood sample of a Senegalese patient with a fever from the Bandafassi village, Kedougou region.

Conclusion: *R. felis* was detected for the first time in *An. gambiae* molecular form S, which represents the major African malaria vector. The discovery of *R. felis,* as well as a new *Rickettsia* species, in mosquitoes raises new issues with respect to African rickettsial epidemiology that need to be investigated, such as bacterial isolation, the degree of the vectorial capacity of mosquitoes, the animal reservoirs, and human pathogenicity.

Editor: Kristin Michel, Kansas State University, United States of America

Funding: These authors have no support or funding to report.

Competing Interests: The authors have declared that no competing interests exist.

* E-mail: Didier.Raoult@univmed.fr

Introduction

Mosquitoes, of the family Culicidae, are blood-sucking arthropods with a global distribution that have played a destructive role in human history. Although their bites are widely considered a nuisance, they are today, as in the past, likely the most dangerous vector to the health of humans in terms of morbidity or mortality. Their infectivity is linked to their ability to transmit a wide variety of pathogens, such as filarial parasites, plasmodium, and arboviruses [1]. Due to climatic conditions in tropical and subtropical regions, the aggressiveness of anthropophagic mosquitoes may be high both in urban and rural settings, which helps to explain the burden of mosquito-borne diseases [2,3]. Most of the mosquito vectors able to cause human disease belong to three genera: *Anopheles*, *Aedes* and *Culex*. These three genera can transmit arboviruses, human filariasis and dirofilariasis, although only anopheline mosquitoes can transmit the five parasites known to cause human malaria. Despite intense research into mosquito-borne infections [4–6], no study has focused on the potential transmission of *Rickettsiae* by mosquitoes in humans.

In 1924, the presence of intracellular *Rickettsia*-like microorganisms in the cells of the ovary and testes in *Culex pipiens* mosquitoes was reported [7]. Later, this bacterium was described as *Wolbachia pipientis*, a member of the family Anaplasmataceae

within the order Rickettsiales. In addition, in 1975, Yen [4] using electron microscopy described a second transovarially transmitted *Rickettsia* species. Thus, we have hypothesized that additional, unidentified *Rickettsia* species likely exist in mosquitoes. Recently, *Rickettsia felis* was considered a rare emerging pathogen transmitted to date by fleas. Recently, it has been detected in 3.1% of *Aedes albopictus* mosquitoes collected from Libreville, Gabon [8]. Two teams investigating the etiology of unexplained fevers in Senegal and Kenya reported a high incidence of *R. felis* infection among the indigenous populations [9–12]. Moreover, *R. felis* DNA has also been found in blood samples of healthy people [12]. Moreover, no *R. felis* specimens were detected in fleas from Senegal, but the presence of a new *Rickettsia* species closely related to *R. felis* was detected and shown to have a high rate of infection (91.4%) [13].

Ae. albopictus was first described in Gabon in 2006 and has not yet been described in Senegal or Kenya; therefore, other alternative mosquito species need to be considered. Anopheline mosquitoes are present throughout Africa and exist primarily in rural settings but can also be found in urbanized areas. Due to their abundance and anthropophily, the potential role of malaria vectors in the epidemiology of rickettsial diseases in Africa should not be underestimated. In this work, different species of

Anopheline mosquitoes from West and Central Africa were screened for the presence of *Rickettsia* species, particularly *R. felis*.

Materials and Methods

Mosquito Collection and Identification

The mosquitoes were sampled using human landing catches both indoors and outdoors during malaria transmission surveys conducted by French forces in rural or urban areas of Côte d'Ivoire, Gabon and Senegal [2,14–16]. Additional details concerning the sampling methodology are available in the reference papers [2,14–16]. The mosquitoes were sorted by genus, and the anopheline mosquitoes were identified morphologically according to the Gillies and Coetzee keys [17]. From these African countries, 772 unfed mosquitoes stored individually in numbered vials containing a desiccant (silica gel 13767 Sigma-Aldrich) preserved at −20°C were chosen until processing at the Medical Entomology Unit of the Institute for Tropical Medicine (IMTSSA) in Marseille, France. From Dielmo, Senegal, 76 unfed mosquitoes were collected and stored under identical conditions at the Malaria Laboratory in Dakar, Senegal. The choice of using non-engorged mosquitoes was done to ensure that the presence of rickettsia in mosquitoes was not due to the presence of blood from a bacteriemic host. Females of the *An. gambiae* complex and the M and S molecular forms of *An. gambiae* were identified by PCR-RFLP [18].

Ethics Statement

The collectors gave prior informed written consent and received anti-malaria prophylaxis and yellow fever immunizations. The study protocol was approved by the Marseille II Ethics Committee (Advice N. 02/81, 12/13/2002). In addition, an authorization of medical research was obtained also for a period of two years with the Ministry of Health and Public Hygiene in charge of Family and Women Promotion, Gabon (Decision No. 001085 of September 2008).

Rickettsia Detection by Real-time PCR

Each mosquito was directly dissected in the tube. A new needle was used for each mosquito. The DNA was extracted in the incoming year after the capture and conserved at −20°C. Total mosquito DNA was extracted using the Qiagen BioRobot 8000 (QIAGEN group) and the QIAamp Media MDX kit at the IMTSSA (772 specimens) and the WHO Collaborative Center for Rickettsial Diseases and Arthropod-Borne Bacterial Disease (URMITE) in Marseille (76 specimens), according to the manufacturer's instructions. The dried DNA pellets from one mosquito were resuspended in 120 µl elution buffer. For each PCR reaction, 5 µl mosquito DNA was added in 15 µl mix. A negative control, which consisted of DNA extracted from an uninfected laboratory tick free of *Rickettsia*, *Ehrlichia*, *Anaplasma*, *Bartonella* and *Coxiella burnetii*, was included in each test. In 2010–2011, all of the DNA samples were tested for the presence of the *Rickettsia* spp. citrate synthase (*glt*A) gene and the *R. felis* biotin synthase (*bio*B) gene at URMITE, as described previously [10]. All real-time PCR reactions for the rickettsial screening were performed according to the manufacturer's protocol using a 7900HT Fast Real-Time PCR system (Applied Biosystems, Foster City, USA). All rickettsial- and *R. felis*-positive samples were confirmed with the detection of the RC0338 and *orf*B genes, respectively, using the CFX96™ Real-Time PCR System (Bio-Rad) [8,10]. Specificity of the qPCR for 4 genes (*glt*A, RC0338, *bio*B and *orf*B genes) was cheked in silico and on the 31 *Rickettsia* spp. from our laboratory. The analytical sensitivities of the real-

time PCR targeted these genes were determined in triplicate reactions with ten-fold serial dilutions of a known titration of *R. felis* cell culture. Based on these results we extrapolated the mean copies of each gene by mosquito sample. The quality of DNA extraction was verified using standard PCR targeting the mitochondrial cytochrome oxidase subunit II (COII) gene with the COII-2a and COII-9b primers from several randomly selected samples [19] and of DNA handling using same standart methods conducted in *Rickettsia* spp. detection studies [13,20–23] and in mosquitoes [15,24].

Rickettsia Characterization: Traditional PCR and Sequencing

All mosquito *Rickettsia*-positive samples were subjected to a traditional PCR analysis targeting the outer membrane protein (r*omp*A) gene with the primer set 190-70 and 190–701 (Eurogentec, Seraing, Belgium), which amplifies a 629–632-bp fragment, as previously described [25]. The complete *glt*A gene was amplified from one *An. gambiae* molecular form S mosquito from Côte d'Ivoire (N.101731) and one *An. melas* from Gabon (N.10244) using a battery of primers that amplify a 1234-bp sequence, as previously described [26]. In addition, for *An. gambiae* N.101731 free of *R. felis* DNA, three additional PCR reactions were performed: (i) a PCR using a battery of primers to amplify a 4346-bp fragment of the rickettsial *omp*B gene [27]; (ii) a PCR using a battery of primers to amplify a 2783-bp fragment of the *sca*4 gene [28]; and (iii) a PCR using a battery of primers to amplify a 1500-bp fragment of the 16S rRNA gene [29]. These amplicons are commonly used to characterize *Rickettsiae* at both the genus and species levels [30]. A positive control, which consisted of *R. montanensis* DNA, was included in each test.

The *glt*A fragment from the RKND03 system (*Rickettsia*-specific real-time PCR), the *bio*B and *orf*B fragments from the *R. felis*-specific real-time PCRs, and the *omp*A, *glt*A, *omp*B, sca4, and 16S rDNA PCR products from the traditional PCRs were purified and sequenced as previously described [25,30]. All of the sequences were analyzed using ChromasPro Version 2.31 and compared to those of the *Rickettsiae* sequences present in GenBank using the BLAST search tool. Multiple sequence alignments have been done with *glt*A sequences obtained from this study and of the nearest *Rickettsia* spp. sequences from GenBank using the ClustalX program (ftp://ftp.ebi.ac.uk/pub/software/clustalw2). Phylogenetic tree was constructed using the test minimum-evolution tree algorithm, MEGA program. The support for the tree nodes was calculated with 100 bootstrap replicates.

Results

Entomological Investigation

In Côte d'Ivoire. The catches were conducted in 2004 at the Kahin site. This area was selected because it was known to contain the three main malarial vectors for this country: *An. gambiae* s.s., *An. funestus* and *An. nili*. A total of 84 *An. funestus*, 96 *An. nili* and 96 *An. gambiae* s.s. mosquitoes were screened for the presence of *Rickettsia* spp. (Table 1). In this rural area, the aggressiveness of *Ae. aegypti* was low, and only a small number of specimens were caught at dusk or dawn.

In Gabon. The catches were conducted in 2007 at the two main towns within the country, Libreville and Port Gentil. In Port Gentil, the study site was situated in a peri-urban area, which was surrounded on its west and south sides by forested or deforested areas that were liable to flooding during the rainy season and on the other sides by a few modern and traditional habitations. *An. gambiae* molecular form S and *An. melas* were the only two members

Table 1. Rickettsial detection in different mosquito species collected in Côte d'Ivoire, Gabon, and Senegal.

Country	Mosquito species	DNA samples	Rickettsial detection			
			Positive samples, SFG *Rickettsiae*		Positive samples, *R. felis*-specific	
			*glt*A gene	RC0338 gene	*bio*B gene	*orf*B gene
Kahin, **Côte d'Ivoire** (06.91°N, 07.63°W)	*Anopheles funestus*	84	0/84	-	0/84	-
	An. nili	96	0/96	-	0/96	-
	An. gambiae molecular form S	77	**6/77 (7.8%)**	6/6[CI]	**1*/77 (1.3%)**	1/6
	An. gambiae molecular form M	19	0/19	-	0/19	-
Libreville, **Gabon** (0°23'24"N 9°26'59"E)	*An. gambiae* molecular form S	88	**1/88 (1.1%)**	1/1[GL]	0/88	0/1
Port Gentil, **Gabon** (0°43'11"N 8°46'47"E)	*An. gambiae* molecular form S	21	0/21	-	0/21	-
	An. melas	67	**6/67 (9%)**	6/6[GPG]	0/67	0/6
Dielmo, **Senegal** (13°43'N, 16°24'W)	*An. gambiae*	76	0/76	-	0/76	-
	An. arabiensis	120	0/120	-	0/120	-
Dakar, **Senegal** (14°40'20"N, 17°25'22"W)	*An. arabiensis*	200	0/200	-	0/200	-
Total	**One genus, five mosquito species**	**848**	**13/848 (1.5%)**	**13**	**1/848 (0.1%)**	**1**

*One sample (N.101761) was positive for a *Rickettsia*-specific real-time PCR that targeted two different genes and for an *R. felis*-specific real-time PCR that targeted two species-specific genes.
[CI]Number of positive samples: 101761*; 101731; 101729; 101733; 101722; 101728.
[GL]Number of positive sample: 12942.
[GPG]Number of positive samples: 10244; 10109; 10251; 10111; 10296; 10110.

of the *An. gambiae* complex to be identified, and these types represented 25.5% and 74.5%, respectively, of the total *An. gambiae* complex population (Table 1). *Ae. albopictus* was not caught during the study period at this site, and only a few *Ae. aegypti* mosquitoes were caught.

In Senegal. The catches were conducted from 2005 to 2007 in two urban areas of Dakar, as well as in Dielmo, a rural area in the south of Senegal. *An. arabiensis* was identified in the two areas of Dakar over this three-year period. In Dielmo, the molecular forms M and S of *An. gambiae* and *An. arabiensis* were identified (Table 1).

Rickettsia Detection in Mosquito Samples

A total of 13 mosquito samples (13/848, 1.5%) were tested positive for the *glt*A and RC0338 genes, according to the *Rickettsia*-specific real-time PCR analysis. The mean of the cycle thresholds (Ct) value and standard deviation [±SD] of rickettsial DNA for the *glt*A and RC0338 fragments in these samples were 33.28±6.694 (mean copies/mosquito 7×10^4, max: 13×10^9, min: 3×10^2) and 33.45±6.9 (mean copies/mosquito 28×10^4, max: 12×10^{10}, min: 2×10^3), respectively. The positive samples included the following mosquito types: six *An. gambiae* molecular form S mosquitoes (6/77, 7.8%) from Kahin, Côte d'Ivoire (N. 101761; 101731; 101729; 101733; 101722; 101728); six *An. melas* (6/67, 9%) mosquitoes from Port Gentil, Gabon (N.10244; 10109; 10251; 10111; 10296; 10110); and one *An. gambiae* molecular form S mosquito (1/88, 1.1%) from Libreville, Gabon (N.12942) (Table 1). We considered the mosquito samples as positive only if the real-time PCR results for both rickettsial genes were positive and the subsequent traditional PCR and sequencing analyses produced the rickettsial fragment. When we analyzed our data with the previously published data [2,14–16], all Rickettsia positive mosquitoes were

negative for *Plasmodium falciparum* detection. The traditional PCR fragment of the mitochondrial COII gene was positive in five of the randomly selected *Rickettsia*-negative samples; their sequences displayed 97% similarity to the *An. gambiae* voucher JA37 sequence in GenBank (DQ792578) [31]. Therefore, we concluded that these DNA samples are free of *Rickettsia* DNA (Table 1).

The amplified fragments of the *glt*A gene (RKND03 system) from 11 mosquito samples (five *An. gambiae*: N.101731; 101729; 101733; 101722; 101728 and six *An. melas*: N.10244; 10109; 10251; 10111; 10296; 10110) were successfully sequenced. A 164-bp portion of the *glt*A gene from each of these samples was aligned using the BioEdit program, which indicated identical sequences. A BLAST search against all known bacterial genomes revealed that the closest match to a validated bacterium was with *R. felis* (CP000053) at 99.39% (164/165) similarity [32]. In addition to this bacterium, the sequence that was amplified from these mosquito samples demonstrated the same level of similarity to five uncultured *Rickettsia* spp. detected in *Ctenocephalides felis* (cat fleas) from Kenya (JN315974) [33], *Glossina morsitans submorsitans* (tsetse flies) from Senegal (GQ255903) [21], *Pediobius rotundatus* from Iran (FJ666771) [34], *Aulogymnus balani/skianeuros* (gall wasps) from Hungary (FJ666770) [34], and *C. canis* (dog fleas) from Thailand (AF516333) [35].

Rickettsia Felis Detection in Mosquito Samples

Only one mosquito sample (1/848, 0.1%) was tested positive for both the *bio*B and *orf*B genes, according to the *Rickettsia*-specific real-time PCR and the *R. felis*-specific real-time PCR (Table 1). This sample (N.101761) was an *An. gambiae* molecular form S mosquito that had been collected from Kahin, Côte d'Ivoire (1/77, 1.3%). The Ct value for *R. felis* DNA in this sample for the *bio*B and *orfB* real-time PCR systems was 34.27 (4×10^3 copies/mosquito) and 31.61 (2×10^3 copies/mosquito), respectively. For this sample, the *orfB* real-time PCR product exhibited 100% (150/150) sequence similarity with the *orfB* gene of *R. felis* URRWX-Cal2 (GenBank, CP000053) [32].

Molecular Characterization of the New *Rickettsia* Species Identified in the Mosquito Samples

Five samples (4 *An. gambiae* from Côte d'Ivoire: N.101731; 101729; 101733; 101722 and 1 *An. melas* 10244) were amplified and sequenced with the *ompA* primer pair [25]. Each of these sequences was identical when they were aligned and compared using the BioEdit program. The closest validated bacterium was *R. felis* (CP000053) [32], and this species demonstrated 95.9% (562/586) similarity. Moreover, these sequences exhibited 96.06% (562/585) similarity to the *R. felis* DNA detected previously in *C. felis* samples from the USA (AF191026) [36] and *Liposcelis bostrychophila* samples (HM636635) from Louisiana, USA [37].

Two samples (1 *An. gambiae* from Côte d'Ivoire: N.101731 and 1 *An. melas* from Gabon: N.10244) were previously amplified and sequenced with the *gltA* primer set [26], and the resulting two sequences were identical. A sequence analysis of the *Rickettsia* sp. *gltA* gene fragment (1022 bp) indicated a 98.05% (1009/1029) similarity to *Rickettsia felis* URRWXCal2 (CP000053) [32] and a 98.25% (1014/1032 similarity to *R. hoogstraalii* (FJ767737) detected in *Haemaphysalis sulcata* and *Carios capensis* ticks [38], respectively. In addition, a BLAST search indicated that the *Rickettsia* sp. detected in the mosquito samples shared high levels of sequence similarity with the following *Rickettsia* isolates: 99.12% similarity to *Rickettsia* sp. Rf31 (AF516331), which was previously detected in a *C. canis* flea from Thailand [35]; 98.74% similarity to *Rickettsia* sp. SGL01 (GQ255903), which was detected in tsetse flies from Senegal [21]; and 98.25% similarity to *Rickettsia* sp. F82 (JN315974), which was detected in fleas from Asembo, Kenya [33]. In a neighbor-joining analysis based on the alignment of 1022 bp of the *gltA* gene, the *Rickettsia* species detected in the Côte d'Ivoire and Gabon mosquitoes clustered with *R. felis*-like organisms and demonstrated large bootstrap values (Figure 1).

Seven molecular systems were used to PCR amplify and sequence the complete rickettsial *ompB* gene in one Côte d'Ivoire mosquito DNA sample: N.101731 [27]. Only the 6th fragment of the *ompB* gene was successfully amplified with the primer pair 120–3462 and 120–4346. The closest sequence match in the GenBank database was for *Rickettsia felis* URRWXCal2, which demonstrated a 95.74% (809/845) similarity (CP000053) [32]. A fragment of *sca4*, the intracytoplasmic protein-encoding gene, located between bases 21 and 3050 was amplified and sequenced using five molecular systems [28]. Using the D1219f and D1876r primers, the 3rd fragment was successfully aligned and analyzed using ChromasPro. A sequence analysis of this fragment (N.101731) indicated 97.12% (608/626) similarity to *R. felis* URRWXCal2 (CP000053) [32] and *R. felis* (GQ329878), which were detected in the common household insect pest *Liposcelis bostrychophila* [37]. Attempts to amplify one fragment of the 16S rRNA gene [29] with the primer pair Rick_16S.F and Rick_16S.R were unsuccessful.

Finally, because this novel *Rickettsia* species possesses the *ompA* gene, we were able to conclude that it is a member of the spotted fever group [30]. Furthermore, in accordance with the guidelines for the identification of new *Rickettsia* species [30], our molecular analysis of the nearly complete *gltA* gene and the partial sequences of the *ompA*, *ompB*, and *sca4* genes strongly supports the claim that this *Rickettsia* sp. detected in these mosquito samples constitutes a putative novel species (Table 2). To better characterize this *Rickettsia* species, it will be necessary to isolate this organism in cell culture from the mosquito samples and amplify and sequence the complete genes, as described previously.

New Nucleotide Sequence Accession Numbers in GenBank

The *gltA*, *ompA*, *ompB*, and *sca4* gene fragment sequences of the novel *Rickettsia* species detected in the *An. gambiae* molecular form S mosquito from Côte d'Ivoire (N.101731) were deposited in GenBank under the accession numbers JN620082, JN620079, JN620080, and JN620081, respectively. The gltA and ompA gene fragments of the *Rickettsia* species detected in the *An. melas* sample from Gabon (N.10244) were deposited under the accession numbers JQ354961 and JQ354962, respectively.

Discussion

In this work, we used molecular tools to detect the presence of *Rickettsia* spp. in mosquitoes of the *An. gambiae* complex, including the molecular form S of *An. gambiae* and *An. melas*. We believe that our results are reliable. The validity of the data reported herein is based on strict experimental procedures and controls, including rigorous positive and negative controls to validate the test. In addition, each positive PCR result was confirmed by the successful amplification of an additional DNA sequence. We exclude the possibility of cross-contamination between *Wolbachia* spp. and *Rickettsia* spp. after the analysis of primers and probes of qPCR specific for *Rickettsia* spp. (gltA and RCO338) and *R. felis*-specific qPCR(orfB and bioB) in silico and in vitro, experimental assays, on several *Wolbachia* spp. positive samples. Unhappiness, *Rickettsia* culture could not be realized in this study because all mosquito specimens were initially extracted for malaria studies.

R. felis was detected in 1.3% (1/77) of *An. gambiae* molecular form S samples from Kahin, Côte d'Ivoire. *R. felis* belongs to the spotted fever group *Rickettsia* (SFGR) and has been detected at high a prevalence in several species of fleas, ticks, and mites [39]. Recently, *R. felis* was isolated from the non-hematophagous arthropod *Liposcelis bostrychophila* (common booklice) [37]. *R. felis* is the only *Rickettsia* species associated with such a diverse range of invertebrate hosts, and it possesses a mosaic structure genome (size 1.48 Mb) with a high coding capacity (83%) that is indicative of symbiotic bacteria [40]. In Côte d'Ivoire, *R. felis* was previously detected in one specimen of *C. canis* collected from a dog [41]. In Africa, *R. felis* has been detected in fleas from Ethiopia [20], Algeria [42], Congo [43], Côte d'Ivoire [41], and Morocco [23]. Additionally, human cases have been described only in Tunisia, Kenya, Algeria, Lybia, Mali, Gabon and Senegal [9,12,44,45]. The reservoir of *R. felis* has not yet been elucidated [46,47]. Bacteria in the genus *Rickettsia*, have been detected usually in blood-feeding arthropods, but can also be detected in phytophagous insects [48]. *R. felis* PCR-positive blood samples have been reported in opossums (*Didelphis virginiana*) from the USA and dogs from Spain and Australia [49–51]. Recently, the plant-mediated transmission route of endosymbiotic *Rickettsia* had been reported [52]. Further epidemiological studies are warranted to determine the reservoir of *Rickettsia* species in Africa.

We described the presence of a putative novel *Rickettsia* species in 6.5% (5/77) and 1.1% (1/88) of *An. gambiae* molecular form S mosquitoes from Côte d'Ivoire and Gabon, respectively, and in 9% (6/67) of *An. melas* mosquitoes from Gabon. This putative novel *Rickettsia* sp. was shown to be closely related to *R. felis* and *R. felis*-like organisms detected in several arthropods (fleas, tsetse flies, soft ticks and hard ticks) with a global distribution. Both of the *R. felis*-specific real-time PCRs used in our study demonstrated negative results for these samples. In Africa, an *R. felis*-like

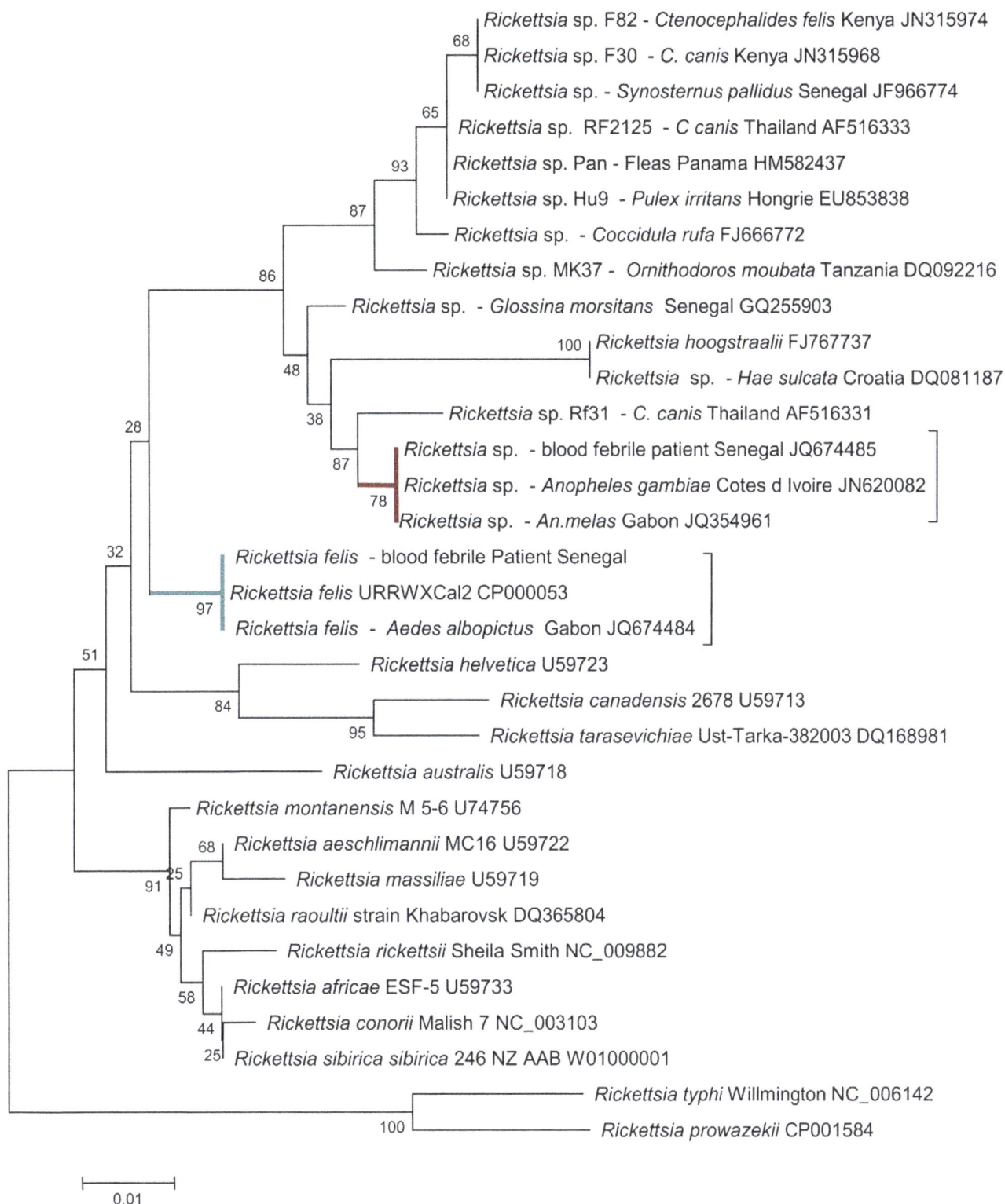

Figure 1. Minimum evolutionary tree using a bootstrap analysis for the putative novel *Rickettsia* species. The nearest GenBank sequences (showed at the end of the *Rickettsia* name) were aligned using the multi-sequence alignment ClustalX and BioEdit programs. The phylogenetic tree was constructed using parsimony and maximum-likelihood methods.

organism was detected in *Archaeopsylla erinacei* fleas in Algeria [42], *C. canis* in Gabon [53], in *Echidnophaga gallinacea* fleas in Egypt [54], *Synosternus pallidus* fleas in Senegal [13], *C. felis* and *C. canis* fleas in

Kenya [33], *Ornithodoros moubata* soft ticks in Tanzania [55], and *Glossina morsitans* tsetse flies in Senegal [21]. In 2005, Rolain et al. [53] suggested that nonhuman primates may represent a reservoir

Table 2. Sequence similarity between the sequenced *Rickettsia* species detected in mosquitoes and *R. felis* URRWXCal2 (CP000053) [32].

	Matching nucleotides	Similarity
Citrate synthase gene (gltA) [26]	1009/1029	98.05%
Outer-membrane protein A gene (ompA) [25]	562/586	95.9%
Outer-membrane protein B gene (ompB) [27]	809/845	95.74%
PS120-protein- (sca 4, gene D) [28,30]	608/626	97.12%

of *R. felis*-like organism, as they detected this bacterium in fleas collected from monkey in Gabon. This hypothesis needs to be further investigated.

Previous quantitative analyses of *R. felis* load in naturally infected cat fleas demonstrated large variability in numbers of rickettsiae present in individual cat fleas, ranging from 1.3×10^3 to 1.6×10^7 [56] and around 12×10^2 to 5×10^7 copies (*bio*B gene) in hedgehogs fleas [22]. Greater *R. felis* burden had been reported in booklice compared to cat fleas [37]. Thus, we found a high load of *Rickettsia* in mosquitoes comparable with those obtained in naturally infected cat fleas. The prevalence of *Rickettsia* spp. in mosquito hosts is comparable to that determined in the soft ticks from Tanzania [55]. However, the prevalence is lower than in other arthropods, as *R. felis* was detected in 10.72% to 100% fleas collected in African countries [20,41–43] and *Rickettsia felis*-like in 91.4% to 100% in fleas and tsetse flies [13,21].

The molecular S form of *An. gambiae* is dispersed across West and East Africa [57] (Figure 2). In a Kenyan and Senegalese study

on fevers of unknown origin, most *R. felis*-infected patients were detected in the rainy season [9,11], and a significant rate of co-infection with malaria and *R. felis* was detected (79.2% in patients with *R. felis*-positive PCR results in Kenya and 10.5% in Senegal) [9,12]. We suspect that only mosquitoes, the malaria vectors, are the prime suspect on *R. felis* transmission. Considering the biting rates of each mosquito species, their rates of infection by *R. felis*, and this new strain of *Rickettsia* in Kahin (Côte d'Ivoire), Libreville and Port Gentil (Gabon), the level of transmission could be high if *Anopheles* mosquitoes can competently transmit *Rickettsia*. In Kahin, individuals without mosquito protection can be bitten by as many as three *R. felis*-infected mosquitoes and 18 *Rickettsia* sp.-infected *An. gambiae* molecular form S mosquitoes in two weeks [2]. In Port Gentil, an individual without mosquito protection can be bitten by a *Rickettsia* sp.-infected *An. melas* mosquito every three days [14]. According to these statistics, the vectorial competence of *An. gambiae* molecular form S and *An. melas* mosquitoes is likely low, although the extent of rickettsial infections is likely underestimated

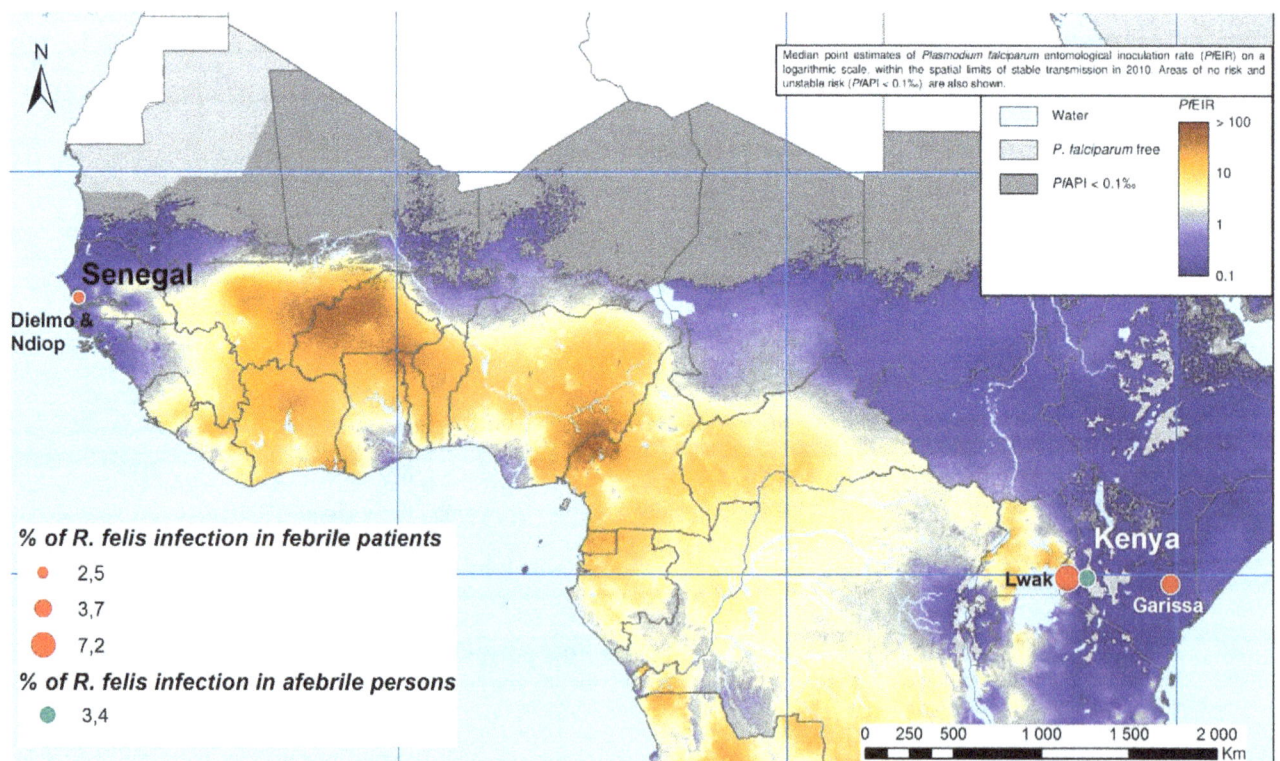

Figure 2. The spatial distribution of *Plasmodium falciparum* entomological inoculation rate (PfEIR) and *Rickettsia felis* infection incidence. 2010 Malaria Atlas Project, available under the Creative Commons Attribution 3.0 Unported License [57].

in Africa. Unfed mosquitoes were tested in our study, but knowing that the time between two bloodmeals for *An.gambiae* s.l. is in average of 2–3 days, the probability that rickettsial DNA from a previous blood meal could not be excluded.

The *glt*A sequence of the new *Rickettsia* sp. detected in *Anopheles* mosquitoes in the current study exhibited a 99.7% (706/708) sequence similarity to that detected in a blood sample of a patient from the Kedougou region of the Bandafassi village in Senegal who had a fever of unexplained origin (GenBank JQ674485) [9]. Two differences had been detected between these *glt*A sequences: 35G-A and 69T-C that led to two amino acids change G12E and L23P, respectively (JQ674485) to *Rickettsia* sp. detected in *An. gambiae* (JN620082 numbering). In addition, in the present study, less of 1% of febrile patients were likely infected with this novel *Rickettsia* sp. Moreover, a specific molecular system by real-time PCR targeting a fragment *glt*A gene of new genotype of *Rickettsia* sp. detected in Senegalese febrile patients was designed [9] and applied on positive *Anopheles* mosquito samples of this study (data not shown). Seven mosquito samples from 11 were tested positive. Thus, we consider this new *Rickettsia* species a potential human pathogen because it was detected in a blood sample from a patient

using molecular methods. Although the isolation of this new species in cell culture from clinical blood or tissue samples and mosquito tissue specimens should be performed. Given the basic attributes of mosquito population abundance and their tendency for multiple human blood meals, we have hypothesized that mosquitoes could play a significant role in rickettsial epidemiology. The detection of *Rickettsia* DNA in mosquitoes is the first step on the vectorial capacity study [8] and other researchers are ongoing in our laboratory to confirm this hypothesis.

Acknowledgments

We would like to thank the technicians from URMITE, Marseille, namely Annick Bernard, Veronique Brice and Stephanie Junoy, for their technical support.

Author Contributions

Conceived and designed the experiments: DR. Performed the experiments: CS FP MON. Analyzed the data: CS FP. Contributed reagents/materials/analysis tools: DR FP. Wrote the paper: CS FP DR. Design of Figure 2: PR.

References

1. Service MW (1993) Mosquitoes (Culicidae). In: Lane RP, Crosskey RW, editors. Medical Insects and Arachnids. London: Chapman & Hall. 120–240.
2. Orlandi-Pradines E, Rogier C, Koffi B, Jarjaval F, Bell M, et al. (2009) Major variations in malaria exposure of travellers in rural areas: an entomological cohort study in western Cote d'Ivoire. Malar J 8: 171. 1475-2875-8-171 [pii];10.1186/1475-2875-8-171 [doi].
3. Girod R, Orlandi-Pradines E, Rogier C, Pages F (2006) Malaria transmission and insecticide resistance of *Anopheles gambiae* (Diptera: Culicidae) in the French military camp of Port-Bouet, Abidjan (Cote d'Ivoire): implications for vector control. J Med Entomol 43: 1082–1087.
4. Yen JH (1975) Transovarial transmission of Rickettsia-like microorganisms in mosquitoes. Ann N Y Acad Sci 266: 152–161.
5. Walker T, Johnson PH, Moreira LA, Iturbe-Ormaetxe I, Frentiu FD, et al. (2011) The wMel *Wolbachia* strain blocks dengue and invades caged *Aedes aegypti* populations. Nature 476: 450–453. nature10355 [pii];10.1038/nature10355 [doi].
6. Almeida FD, Moura AS, Cardoso AF, Winter CE, Bijovsky AT, et al. (2011) Effects of *Wolbachia* on fitness of *Culex quinquefasciatus* (Diptera; Culicidae). Infect Genet Evol S1567–1348(11)00302-9 [pii];10.1016/j.meegid.2011.08.022 [doi].
7. Hertig M, Wolbach SB (1924) Studies on rickettsia-like micro-organisms in insects. J Med Res 44: 329–374.
8. Socolovschi C, Pages F, Raoult D (2012) *Rickettsia felis* in *Aedes albopictus*, the Asian tiger mosquito. Emerg Infect Dis In press.
9. Mediannikov O, Socolovschi C, Edouard S, Fenollar F, Ratmanov P, et al. (2012) Vector borne bacterial infections as leading causes of fever in Africa. Lancet Inf Dis Submitted.
10. Socolovschi C, Mediannikov O, Sokhna C, Tall A, Diatta G, et al. (2010) *Rickettsia felis*-associated uneruptive fever, Senegal. Emerg Infect Dis 16: 1140–1142.
11. Richards AL, Jiang J, Omulo S, Dare R, Abdirahman K, et al. (2010) Human infection with *Rickettsia felis*, Kenya. Emerg Infect Dis 16: 1081–1086.
12. Maina AN, Knobel DL, Jiang J, Halliday J, Feikin DR, et al. (2012) *Rickettsia felis* infection in febrile patients, Western Kenya, 2007–2010. Emerg Infect Dis 18: 328–331. 10.3201/eid1802.111372 [doi].
13. Roucher C, Mediannikov O, Diatta G, Trape JF, Raoult D (2012) A new *Rickettsia* species found in fleas collected from human dwellings and from domestic cats and dogs in Senegal. Vector Borne Zoonotic Dis 12: 360–5.
14. Mourou JR, Coffinet T, Jarjaval F, Pradines B, Amalvict R, et al. (2010) Malaria transmission and insecticide resistance of *Anopheles gambiae* in Libreville and Port-Gentil, Gabon. Malar J 9: 321. 1475-2875-9-321 [pii];10.1186/1475-2875-9-321 [doi].
15. Pages F, Texier G, Pradines B, Gadiaga L, Machault V, et al. (2008) Malaria transmission in Dakar: a two-year survey. Malar J 7: 178. 1475-2875-7-178 [pii];10.1186/1475-2875-7-178 [doi].
16. Machault V, Gadiaga L, Vignolles C, Jarjaval F, Bouzid S, et al. (2009) Highly focused anopheline breeding sites and malaria transmission in Dakar. Malar J 8: 138. 1475-2875-8-138 [pii];10.1186/1475-2875-8-138 [doi].
17. Gillies MT, Coetzee M (1987) A supplement to the anophelinae of Africa south of the Sahara (Afrotropical region). Johannesburg, South Africa: The South African Institut for medical research.
18. Fanello C, Santolamazza F, Della Torre A (2002) Simultaneous identification of species and molecular forms of the *Anopheles gambiae* complex by PCR-RFLP. Med Vet Entomol 16: 461–4.

19. Whiting MF (2002) Mecoptera is paraphyletic: multiple genes and phylogeny of Mecoptera and Siphonaptera. Zoologica Scripta 31: 93–104.
20. Mediannikov O, Abdissa A, Diatta G, Trape JF, Raoult D (2012) *Rickettsia felis* in fleas from Southern Ethiopia. Emerg Infect Dis 18: 1385–6.
21. Mediannikov O, Audoly G, Diatta G, Trape JF, Raoult D (2012) New Rickettsia sp. in tsetse flies from Senegal. Comp Immunol Microbiol Infect Dis 35: 145–50.
22. Khaldi M, Socolovschi C, Benyettou M, Barech G, Biche M, et al. (2012) Rickettsiae in arthropods collected from the North African Hedgehog (*Atelerix algirus*) and the desert hedgehog (*Paraechinus aethiopicus*) in Algeria. Comp Immunol Microbiol Infect Dis 35: 117–122. S0147–9571(11)00108-1 [pii];10.1016/j.cimid.2011.11.007 [doi].
23. Boudebouch N, Sarih M, Beaucournu JC, Amarouch H, Raoult D, et al. (2011) *Bartonella clarridgeiae, B. henselae* and *Rickettsia felis* in fleas from Morocco. Ann Trop Med Parasitol 105: 493–498.
24. Sunish IP, Rajendran R, Paramasivan R, Dhananjeyan KJ, Tyagi BK (2011) *Wolbachia* endobacteria in a natural population of *Culex quinquefasciatus* from filariasis endemic villages of south India and its phylogenetic implication. Trop Biomed 28: 569–576.
25. Fournier PE, Roux V, Raoult D (1998) Phylogenetic analysis of spotted fever group rickettsiae by study of the outer surface protein rOmpA. Int J Syst Bacteriol 48: 839–849.
26. Roux V, Rydkina E, Eremeeva M, Raoult D (1997) Citrate synthase gene comparison, a new tool for phylogenetic analysis, and its application for the rickettsiae. Int J Syst Bacteriol 47: 252–261.
27. Roux V, Raoult D (2000) Phylogenetic analysis of members of the genus *Rickettsia* using the gene encoding the outer-membrane protein rOmpB (ompB). Int J Syst Evol Microbiol 50: 1449–1455.
28. Sekeyova Z, Roux V, Raoult D (2001) Phylogeny of *Rickettsia* spp. inferred by comparing sequences of 'gene D', which encodes an intracytoplasmic protein. Int J Syst Evol Microbiol 51: 1353–1360.
29. Roux V, Raoult D (1995) Phylogenetic analysis of the genus *Rickettsia* by 16S rDNA sequencing. Res Microbiol 146: 385–396.
30. Fournier PE, Dumler JS, Greub G, Zhang J, Wu Y, et al. (2003) Gene sequence-based criteria for identification of new rickettsial isolates and description of *Rickettsia heilongjiangensis* sp. nov. J Clin Microbiol 41: 5456–5465.
31. Roe AD, Sperling FA (2007) Patterns of evolution of mitochondrial cytochrome c oxidase I and II DNA and implications for DNA barcoding. Mol Phylogenet Evol 44: 325–345. S1055–7903(06)00497-0 [pii];10.1016/j.ympev.2006.12.005 [doi].
32. Ogata H, Renesto P, Audic S, Robert C, Blanc G, et al. (2005) The genome sequence of *Rickettsia felis* identifies the first putative conjugative plasmid in an obligate intracellular parasite. PLoS Biol 3: e248.
33. Jiang J, Maina AN, Knobel DL, Cleaveland S, Laudisoit A, et al. (2012) Detection of a Unique *Rickettsia* in Fleas from Asembo, Kenya. submitted.
34. Weinert LA, Werren JH, Aebi A, Stone GN, Jiggins FM (2009) Evolution and diversity of *Rickettsia* bacteria. BMC Biol 7: 6. 1741-7007-7-6 [pii];10.1186/1741-7007-7-6 [doi].
35. Parola P, Sanogo OY, Lerdthusnee K, Zeaiter Z, Chauvancy G, et al. (2003) Identification of *Rickettsia* spp. and *Bartonella* spp. in from the Thai-Myanmar border. Ann N Y Acad Sci 990: 173–181.
36. Bouyer DH, Stenos J, Crocquet-Valdes P, Moron C, Vsevolod P, et al. (2001) *Rickettsia felis*: molecular characterization of a new member of the spotted fever group. Int J Syst Evol Microbiol 51: 339–347.

37. Thepparit C, Sunyakumthorn P, Guillotte ML, Popov VL, Foil LD, et al. (2011) Isolation of a rickettsial pathogen from a non-hematophagous arthropod. PLoS ONE 6: e16396. 10.1371/journal.pone.0016396 [doi].

38. Duh D, Punda-polic V, Avsic-Zupanc T, Bouyer D, Walker DH, et al. (2010) *Rickettsia hoogstraalii* sp. nov., isolated from hard- and soft-bodied ticks. Int J Syst Evol Microbiol 60: 977–84. ijs.0.011049-0 [pii];10.1099/ijs.0.011049-0 [doi].

39. Parola P (2011) *Rickettsia felis*: from a rare disease in the USA to a common cause of fever in sub-Saharan Africa. Clin Microbiol Infect 17: 996–1000. 10.1111/j.1469-0691.2011.03516.x [doi].

40. Merhej V, Raoult D (2011) Rickettsial evolution in the light of comparative genomics. Biol Rev Camb Philos Soc 86: 379–405. BRV151 [pii];10.1111/j.1469-185X.2010.00151.x [doi].

41. Berrelha J, Briolant S, Muller F, Rolain JM, Marie JL, et al. (2009) *Rickettsia felis* and *Rickettsia massiliae* in Ivory Coast, Africa. Clin Microbiol Infect 15 Suppl 2: 251–252.

42. Bitam I, Parola P, De La Cruz KD, Matsumoto K, Baziz B, et al. (2006) First molecular detection of *Rickettsia felis* in fleas from Algeria. Am J Trop Med Hyg 74: 532–535.

43. Sackal C, Laudisoit A, Kosoy M, Massung R, Eremeeva ME, et al. (2008) *Bartonella* spp. and *Rickettsia felis* in fleas, Democratic Republic of Congo. Emerg Infect Dis 14: 1972–1974.

44. Znazen A, Rolain JM, Hammami A, Jemaa MB, Raoult D (2006) *Rickettsia felis* infection, Tunisia. Emerg Infect Dis 12: 138–140.

45. Mokrani K, Tebbal S, Raoult D, Fournier PE (2012) Spotted fever rickettsioses Batna, Easteran Algeria. Ticks Tick Borne Dis In press.

46. Reif KE, Macaluso KR (2009) Ecology of Rickettsia felis: a review. J Med Entomol 46: 723–736.

47. Hii SF, Kopp SR, Abdad MY, Thompson MF, O'Leary CA, et al. (2011) Molecular Evidence Supports the Role of Dogs as Potential Reservoirs for *Rickettsia felis*. Vector Borne Zoonotic Dis. 10.1089/vbz.2010.0270 [doi].

48. Perlman SJ, Hunter MS, Zchori-Fein E (2006) The emerging diversity of Rickettsia. Proc Biol Sci 273: 2097–2106.

49. Oteo JA, Portillo A, Santibanez S, Blanco JR, Perez-Martinez L, et al. (2006) Cluster of cases of human *Rickettsia felis* infection from Southern Europe (Spain) diagnosed by PCR. J Clin Microbiol 44: 2669–2671.

50. Schriefer ME, Sacci JB Jr, Taylor JP, Higgins JA, Azad AF (1994) Murine typhus: Updated roles of multiple urban components and a second typhuslike rickettsia. J Med Entomol 31: 681–685.

51. Hii SF, Kopp SR, Thompson MF, O'Leary CA, Rees RL, et al. (2011) Molecular evidence of *Rickettsia felis* infection in dogs from northern territory, Australia. Parasit Vectors 4: 198. 1756-3305-4-198 [pii];10.1186/1756-3305-4-198 [doi].

52. Caspi-Fluger A, Inbar M, Mozes-Daube N, Katzir N, Portnoy V, et al. (2012) Horizontal transmission of the insect symbiont *Rickettsia* is plant-mediated. Proc Biol Sci 279: 1791–1796. rspb.2011.2095 [pii];10.1098/rspb.2011.2095 [doi].

53. Rolain JM, Bourry O, Davoust B, Raoult D (2005) *Bartonella quintana* and *Rickettsia felis* in Gabon. Emerg Infect Dis 11: 1742–1744.

54. Loftis AD, Reeves WK, Szumlas DE, Abbassy MM, Helmy IM, et al. (2006) Surveillance of Egyptian fleas for agents of public health significance: *Anaplasma, Bartonella, Coxiella, Ehrlichia, Rickettsia*, and *Yersinia pestis*. Am J Trop Med Hyg 75: 41–48. 75/1/41 [pii].

55. Cutler SJ, Browning P, Scott JC (2006) *Ornithodoros moubata*, a soft tick vector for *Rickettsia* in east Africa? Ann N Y Acad Sci 1078: 373–377. 1078/1/373 [pii];10.1196/annals.1374.074 [doi].

56. Reif KE, Stout RW, Henry GC, Foil LD, Macaluso KR (2008) Prevalence and infection load dynamics of *Rickettsia felis* in actively feeding cat fleas. PloS ONE 3: e805.

57. Gething PW, Patil AP, Smith DL, Guerra CA, Elyazar IR, et al. (2011) A new world malaria map: *Plasmodium falciparum* endemicity in 2010. Malar J 10: 378. 1475-2875-10-378 [pii];10.1186/1475-2875-10-378 [doi].

21

A Wide Range of 3243A>G/tRNALeu(UUR) (MELAS) Mutation Loads May Segregate in Offspring through the Female Germline Bottleneck

Francesco Pallotti[1,2], Giorgio Binelli[3], Raffaella Fabbri[4,5], Maria L. Valentino[6,7], Rossella Vicenti[4,5], Maria Macciocca[4,5], Sabina Cevoli[6,7], Agostino Baruzzi[6,7], Salvatore DiMauro[1], Valerio Carelli[6,7]*

1 Department of Neurology, Columbia University, New York City, New York, United States of America, 2 Dipartimento di Scienze Chirurgiche e Morfologiche, University of Insubria, Varese, Italy, 3 Dipartimento di Scienze Teoriche e Applicate, University of Insubria, Varese, Italy, 4 Unità Operativa di Ginecologia e Fisiopatologia della Riproduzione Umana, Ospedale S.Orsola-Malpighi, University of Bologna, Bologna, Italy, 5 Dipartimento di Scienze Mediche e Chirurgiche (DIMEC), University of Bologna, Bologna, Italy, 6 IRCCS Istituto delle Scienze Neurologiche di Bologna, Ospedale Bellaria, Bologna, Italy, 7 Dipartimento di Scienze Biomediche e Neuromotorie (DIBINEM), University of Bologna, Bologna, Italy

Abstract

Segregation of mutant mtDNA in human tissues and through the germline is debated, with no consensus about the nature and size of the bottleneck hypothesized to explain rapid generational shifts in mutant loads. We investigated two maternal lineages with an apparently different inheritance pattern of the same pathogenic mtDNA 3243A>G/tRNA$^{Leu(UUR)}$ (MELAS) mutation. We collected blood cells, muscle biopsies, urinary epithelium and hair follicles from 20 individuals, as well as oocytes and an ovarian biopsy from one female mutation carrier, all belonging to the two maternal lineages to assess mutant mtDNA load, and calculated the theoretical germline bottleneck size (number of segregating units). We also evaluated "mother-to-offspring" segregations from the literature, for which heteroplasmy assessment was available in at least three siblings besides the proband. Our results showed that mutation load was prevalent in skeletal muscle and urinary epithelium, whereas in blood cells there was an inverse correlation with age, as previously reported. The histoenzymatic staining of the ovarian biopsy failed to show any cytochrome-c-oxidase defective oocyte. Analysis of four oocytes and one offspring from the same unaffected mother of the first family showed intermediate heteroplasmic mutant loads (10% to 75%), whereas very skewed loads of mutant mtDNA (0% or 81%) were detected in five offspring of another unaffected mother from the second family. Bottleneck size was 89 segregating units for the first mother and 84 for the second. This was remarkably close to 88, the number of "segregating units" in the "mother-to-offspring" segregations retrieved from literature. In conclusion, a wide range of mutant loads may be found in offspring tissues and oocytes, resulting from a similar theoretical bottleneck size.

Editor: David C. Samuels, Vanderbilt University Medical Center, United States of America

Funding: This study was supported by FAR (Fondo di Ateneo per la Ricerca) from University of Bologna and from University of Insubria. The funders had no role in study design, data collection and analysis, decision to publish, or preparation of the manuscript.

Competing Interests: VC is currently receiving funding for the following clinical trials: clinical trial with EPI-743 (α-tocotrienol quinone) in Leber's hereditary optic neuropathy, Edison Pharmaceuticals, USA, and clinical trial with l-acetyl carnitine in Leber's hereditary optic neuropathy, Sigma-tau, Italy.

* E-mail: valerio.carelli@unibo.it

Introduction

Human mitochondrial DNA (mtDNA) is assumed to be a clonal multi-copy genome of 16,5 kb that is strictly maternally inherited. In each cell, mtDNA may be present either as identical copies (homoplasmy) or as a mixed population of two or more different sequences (heteroplasmy or polyplasmy) [1]. Heteroplasmic mtDNA nucleotide changes, including those causing mitochondrial encephalomyopathies [2], segregate in tissues of the developing embryo as well as in germline cells. Somatic segregation of pathogenic mutations is relevant for clinical expression of mitochondrial diseases by affecting energy-dependent tissues that accumulate high, supra-threshold mutant loads [2,3]. Germline segregation is crucial for maternal transmission of variable mutant loads to the offspring [3].

Heteroplasmy may be theoretically due to coexistence of individual organelles containing either exclusively mutant or exclusively wild-type genomes (inter-mitochondrial heteroplasmy) or to the coexistence in each mitochondrion of both mutant and wild-type genomes in different proportions (intra-mitochondrial heteroplasmy) [4]. The mtDNA molecules are associated with specific coating proteins in discrete nucleoids, physically attached to the inner mitochondrial membrane [5], which may themselves be either homoplasmic or heteroplasmic [6]. Admixture and complementation of heteroplasmic mtDNA genomes may be accomplished by mitochondrial fusion events and exchange of mtDNA between nucleoids [7]. Variable efficiency in complementation has been observed in cellular models harboring different mtDNA mutations [8,9] but inter-mitochondrial complementation has been documented in a mito-mouse model carrying an mtDNA deletion [10]. Recent evidence suggests that nucleoids do not exchange genetic material frequently and are probably homoplasmic [11,12], and may contain up to only one mtDNA molecule [13].

The load of mutant mtDNA may vary markedly between a mother and each of her children and a bottleneck mechanism has been postulated during the germline segregation of mutant mtDNA to explain rapid shifts of heteroplasmy observed within one generation [14–16]. However, the nature of the bottleneck mechanism in humans is still under intense debate. Recent studies led to several potential mechanisms that are not necessarily mutually exclusive. These include i) a marked reduction in the number of mtDNA molecules during the early stages of germline development [17]; ii) aggregation of identical segregating units without a reduction of mtDNA copy number, leading to rapid segregation due to sampling effect [18,19]; iii) preferential replication of a subpopulation of genomes, implying an active selection [20]; iv) rapid mtDNA segregation in preimplantation embryos [21]. Most of the data collected so far have been obtained by studying animal models segregating clusters of mtDNA polymorphic variants [22]. The experimental models provided by animals carrying pathogenic mtDNA mutations ("mutator" mouse) suggested a purifying selection for the most severe mtDNA mutations [23,24]. In humans, the bottleneck model has been tested only in a few studies, using both neutral polymorphisms and pathogenic mtDNA mutations segregating in relatively small pedigrees [25–30]. Apparently, different segregation patterns may operate depending on the mtDNA pathogenic mutation: the 8993T>G mutation associated with neuropathy, ataxia, retinitis pigmentosa (NARP) was characterized by skewed segregation in offspring or oocytes [27], whereas the 3243A>G/tRNA$^{Leu(UUR)}$ mutation associated with mitochondrial encephalomyopathy, lactic acidosis, stroke-like episodes (MELAS) followed a random genetic drift model of segregation in a large sample of oocytes from a single woman [30].

We combined quantitative analysis of mtDNA heteroplasmy in both oocytes and somatic tissues to study the germline and somatic segregation of the 3243A>G/tRNA$^{Leu(UUR)}$ pathogenic mutation [31] in two Italian pedigrees.

Materials and Methods

Patients

We studied two previously reported [32] Italian maternal lineages (Family A in Figure 1 and Family B in Figure 2) carrying the heteroplasmic 3243A>G/tRNA$^{Leu(UUR)}$ mutation. Briefly, the proband from Family A (II-2, Figure 1) was affected with chronic progressive external ophthalmoplegia (CPEO), whereas the proband from Family B (II-4, Figure 2) had the typical MELAS syndrome. Both probands had ragged-red-fibers (RRF) and/or cytochrome c oxidase (COX)-negative fibers in skeletal muscle with different mutation loads.

In family A, the proband's only daughter (III-2) was asymptomatic excepted for frequent migraine attacks and she lacked RRF in muscle biopsy. Her son (IV-1) has been treated with growth hormone for short stature.

In family B, the proband's mother (I-2) was clinically asymptomatic, whereas the proband's only son (III-3) recently developed the full-blown MELAS syndrome.

After approval by the internal review board (1996–1998, Institute of Neurological Clinic, University of Bologna, Director Prof. Elio Lugaresi) and signed informed consent, 20 maternally related individuals from both families agreed to be enrolled in the study aimed at assessing the MELAS mutation loads in somatic tissues. In most cases, we have been able to collect blood samples

(leukocytes- and platelet-enriched pellets or whole blood), muscle biopsies, urinary epithelium, and hair follicles. The proband's only daughter in Family A (III-2), also underwent ovarian stimulation to allow collection of oocytes for genetic analysis and gave informed consent for an ovarian biopsy at the time of oocytes collection. Moreover, two of the proband's sisters in Family B (II-5 and II-7) became pregnant during the time of our investigation and consented to prenatal diagnosis on cells recovered from amniotic fluid.

mtDNA Analysis

Total DNA has been extracted by standard phenol/chlorophorm methods from somatic tissues, including amniocytes. Total oocyte DNA was recovered from single oocytes. Briefly, each oocyte was placed in an Eppendorf tube with one drop PBS and 1.5 µL proteinase K 10 mg/ml in ice, and centrifuged 30 sec 3000 rpm in an Eppendorf table-top centrifuge. After adding 50 µL sterile mineral oil, the mixture was centrifuged 30 sec as before, then digested at 37°C for one hour; digestion was blocked by boiling at 95°C for 15 minutes, followed by 80°C for 20 minutes. Each sample was then frozen and maintained at −80°C until the PCR amplification.

Heteroplasmy was determined by restriction fragment length polymorphism (RFLP) analysis after hot-last cycle PCR amplification as previously described [32]. The sensitivity of this method allowed detection of heteroplasmy as low as 1%.

Estimation of Bottleneck Size in Our Families and Review of Previous Reports

We assessed the bottleneck size in two germline segregations from unaffected females carriers of the MELAS mutation to their offspring or oocytes. For the first segregation (Family A; female III-2 in Figure 1), we were able to estimate the proportion p of mutant mtDNA from the heteroplasmic load found in four primary oocytes collected from this woman and in the somatic tissues available from her only son. For the second segregation (Family B; female I-2 in Figure 2), the same estimate was obtained by averaging the loads of mutant mtDNA found in somatic tissues of five offspring. In both cases, p was taken as an estimate of π, the true proportion in the sample population. Under the binomial distribution, the variance was estimated by $p(1-p)/n$, whereas confidence intervals for p were estimated solving for the equation $z = (p-\pi)/\sqrt{\pi(1-\pi)/n}$. The binomial distribution applies if the levels of mutant mtDNA are solely determined by a sampling error such as may occur during a bottleneck. Confidence intervals were used, in both pedigrees, to test whether the mutant load in a given progeny was compatible with a random sampling event (i.e. the bottleneck in the mother).

The number of "units" undergoing the bottleneck was estimated according to equation (1) in Brown et al. [30] under the assumption that 24 cell divisions are needed to produce the full set of primary oocytes. Each segregating "unit" could be an mtDNA molecule or a nucleoid. We also applied the same statistical approach to a set of "mother-to-offspring" segregations reported in the literature, updating the series reviewed by Chinnery and colleagues [33], and evaluating tissue heteroplasmy in families in which there were at least three siblings besides the proband [34–39].

Oocytes and Ovarian Biopsy

The proband's unaffected daughter in Family A (III-2) underwent surgical laparoscopy during which oocytes were retrieved from both ovaries and a biopsy was taken from the

FAMILY A (CPEO)

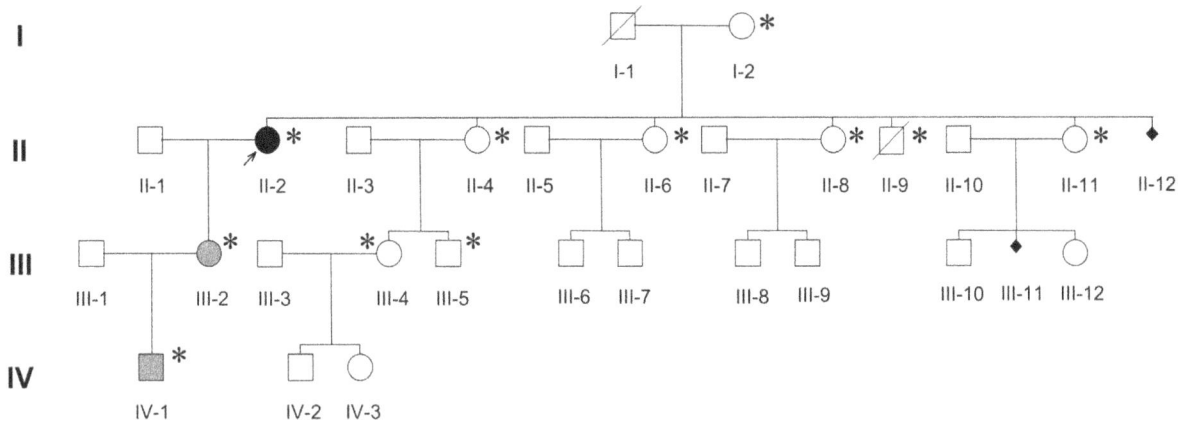

% MUTANT mtDNA (3243tRNA^{Leu}) IN SOMATIC TISSUES FROM FAMILY A

INDIVIDUALS	WHOLE BLOOD	URINE EPITHELIUM	SKELETAL MUSCLE	LEUKOCYTE ENRICHED PELLET	PLATELET ENRICHED PELLET	HAIR FOLLICLES
I-2	0	0	-	-	-	-
II-2	5	32	39	5	7	-
II-4	-	-	0	-	-	-
II-6	-	0	-	-	-	-
II-8	-	0	0	-	-	-
II-9	-	0	0	-	-	-
II-11	-	0	0	-	-	-
III-2	13 – 10*	29 – 46*	44	14	13 – 15*	-
III-4	-	-	0	-	-	-
III-5	-	-	0	-	-	-
IV-1	27	75	-	23	27	-

Figure 1. Pedigree of Family A. Filled symbol indicates the proband (II-2). Shaded symbols indicate asymptomatic individuals carrying the MELAS mutation. Asterisk indicate all the individuals who underwent molecular investigation. Individual III-2 underwent double samplings for some tissues (asterisk, in the table).

right ovary. The oocytes were obtained after ovarian stimulation using a combination of a gonodotrophin-releasing hormone analogue (Triptoreline, Decapeptyl 3.75; Ipsen Biotec, Paris, France) and menotrophins (Metrodin HP, 75 IU; Serono, Milan, Italy) and immediately frozen in liquid nitrogen for DNA analysis [40].

The ovarian biopsy specimen was frozen in liquid nitrogen-cooled isopentane for histological and histoenzymatic staining, following the standard procedure used for muscle biopsies [41]. Ten μM sections were processed for hematoxylin/eosin standard staining and cytochrome c oxidase/succinate dehydrogenase

(COX/SDH) double histoenzymatic staining. One age-matched control ovarian biopsy was used for comparison.

Results

The heteroplasmic load of MELAS mutation assessed in various somatic tissues of maternally related individuals from Families A and B is summarized in Figures 1 and 2. The mutant mtDNA segregated only in some individuals along the maternal line of both families, as previously reported [32].

In Family A, the mutational event most likely occurred between individual I-2 and the CPEO proband (II-2 in Figure 1), considering that mutant mtDNA was absent in all other siblings

FAMILY B (MELAS)

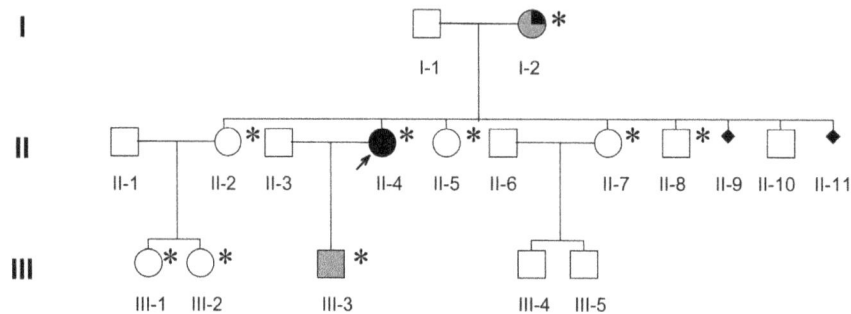

% MUTANT mtDNA (3243tRNA^{Leu}) IN SOMATIC TISSUES FROM FAMILY B

INDIVIDUALS	WHOLE BLOOD	URINE EPITHELIUM	SKELETAL MUSCLE	LEUKOCYTE ENRICHED PELLET	PLATELET ENRICHED PELLET	HAIR FOLLICLES
I-2	0	1	40	0	0	-
II-2	0	0	0	-	-	-
II-4	6	53 – 62*	81	5	4	43
II-5	0	0	0	-	-	-
II-7	0	0	0	-	-	-
II-8	0	0	-	-	-	-
III-1	0	0	0	-	-	-
III-2	-	0	-	-	-	-
III-3	22	86	-	-	-	62

Figure 2. Pedigree of Family B. Filled symbol indicates the proband (II-4). Individual II-4 underwent double samplings for some tissues (asterisk, in the table).

of II-2, as well as in two maternal descendants in the third generation (individuals III-4 and III-5). We relied on the results in mtDNA from muscle and urinary epithelium, or at least one of the two tissues. The MELAS mutation was transmitted to the proband's daughter, individual III-2 and to her son (IV-1), both currently unaffected. The mutant load slowly increased through these three generations, as shown by all tissues tested. In all individuals, the mutant loads in urinary epithelium and skeletal muscle were remarkably similar, whereas in blood-derived cells they were inversely correlated with age, as reported by others [42–44].

Four MII oocytes were retrieved from the proband's daughter (III-2 in Figure 1). Under inverted microscope, the ooplasm had normal size and perivitelline space. Ultrastructurally, the oocytes had normally shaped nuclei with finely dispersed chromatin. The normal morphology of follicles and stromal cells was confirmed by ultrastructural analysis (data not shown).

On double histoenzymatic staining for cytochrome-c-oxidase (COX) and succinate dehydrogenase (SDH) activities, oocytes within follicles were very intensely stained, whereas granulose cells had a less intense stain (Figure 3). This is compatible with the great amount of mtDNA copy number and mitochondria in oocytes.

Remarkably, we failed to detect any sign of COX deficiency, neither in the oocyte cytoplasm nor in the other cell types (i.e.granulosa cells of the ovarian follicle and other stromal cells). Figure 4 shows the RFLP analysis in the four oocytes from individual III-2, which revealed mutant loads ranging from 10% to 67%.

In Family B, the female founder (I-2 in Figure 2) showed mutant mtDNA in skeletal muscle and urinary epithelium. This woman segregated mutant mtDNA only in one of her offspring, the proband affected with MELAS (II-4). None of the proband's siblings had mutant mtDNA in any of the tissues investigated, nor did two maternal descendants in the third generation (III-1 and III-2). Furthermore, amniocytes collected during pregnancies of individuals II-5 and II-7 were also negative for the MELAS mutation (data not shown). Mutant mtDNA was transmitted from the proband to her only son, who is affected with MELAS like his mother. The tissue distribution pattern of somatic mutant loads was similar to that described for Family A, except that the female founder of this pedigree had undetectable mutant mtDNA in blood, only traces in urinary epithelium but a relatively high amount in skeletal muscle. Remarkably, this woman had had two

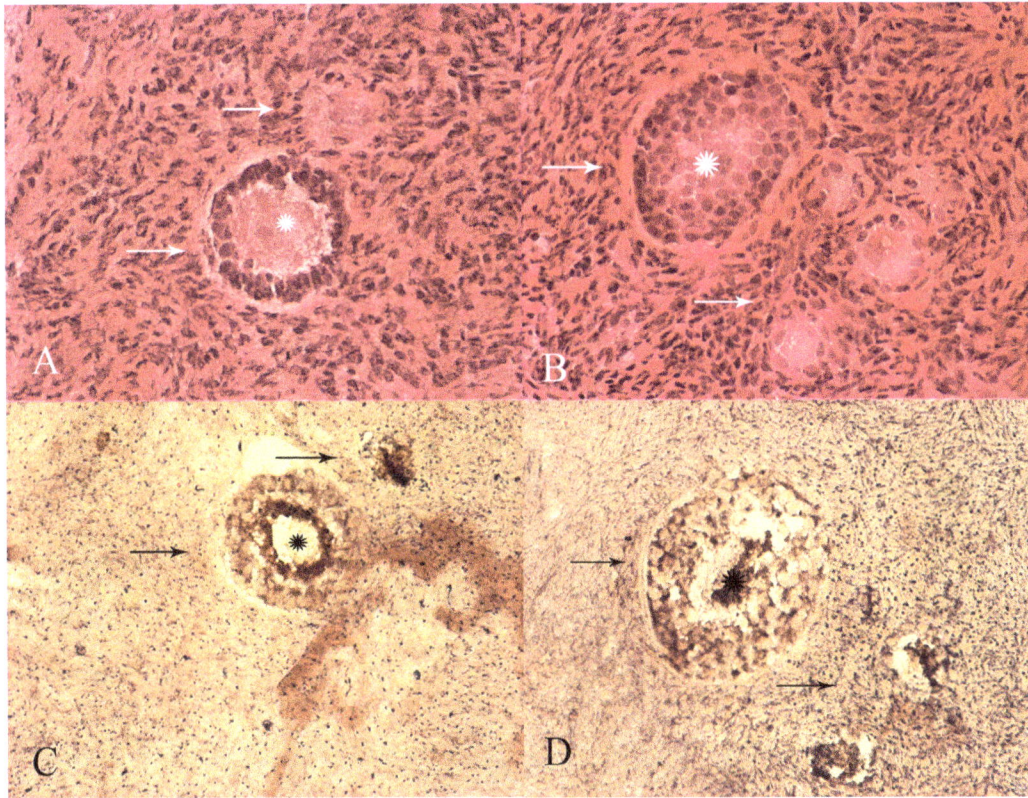

Figure 3. Ovarian follicles. A and C show two ovarian follicles (arrows) of individual III-2 (Family A), stained, respectively, with HE and COX/SDH; B and D, similarly, show three ovarian follicles (arrows), at different stages of maturation, of a control individual (magnification 20x). No evidence of reduced COX stain was observed in any of the tissues from the ovarian biopsy of the individual III-2, in particular the oocytes, as compared to the control (asterisks).

miscarriages besides the five healthy offspring and the daughter with MELAS.

To investigate the "mother-to-offspring" germ line segregation of the MELAS mutation in these two maternal lineages (from individual III-2 in Family A and from individual I-2 in Family B),

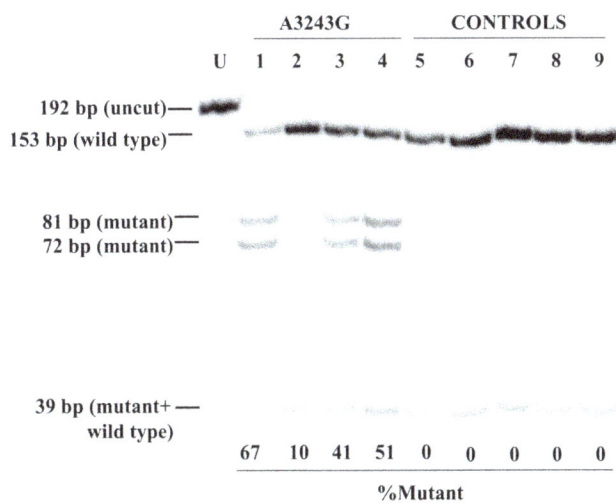

Figure 4. Quantification of the 3243A>G/tRNALeu mutation loads in four primary oocytes from individual III-2 (Family A) and from five control oocytes.

we estimated the percentage of mutant mtDNA in somatic tissues of each offspring in Families A and B, and in each oocyte in Family A. The germline segregation was compatible with a bottleneck event in the mother, according to the binomial distribution. Thus, different mutation loads in the progeny have to be ascribed to chance alone. The bottleneck size, based on the assumption that 24 cell divisions are needed to produce primary oocytes, consisted of 89 segregating units for Family A and 84 for Family B, if we consider only the mutant load in skeletal muscle (Table 1). If we take into account the mtDNA heteroplasmy of urinary epithelium in both Family A and B, the segregation units were 108 (Family A, oocytes from subject III-2 plus urinary epithelium from the only son) and 110 (Family B, urinary epithelium from all offspring) (Table 1).

We reviewed previously reported families segregating the MELAS mutation [33–39] and selected those in which the p of mutant mtDNA was reported for both mother and progeny and included, besides the proband, at least three siblings. We then subjected these "mother-to-offspring" segregations retrieved from the literature to the same test for the binomial distribution that we have used for the analysis of our Italian families. In all included cases (see Table I) the p of mutant mtDNA in the progeny was compatible with a random segregation event in the mother. The number N of "segregating units" was in the range of 59–120, with an average number of $N=88$ (confidence interval at the 0.95 level was $75 \leq N \leq 101$), remarkably close to the values estimated in our study, $N=89$ for Family A and $N=84$ for Family B. These segregations were calculated using different somatic tissues, such as

Table 1. Estimate of bottleneck sizes for the MELAS mutation from a review of the literature.

Source	Ref.	Clinical phenotype mother	Clinical phenotype offspring	Proband's phenotype	Tissue analyzed	p	C.I.	N
Martinuzzi et al (1992)	34	Unaffected	Four, unaffected	MELAS	Skeletal muscle	0.693	0.262–0.935	84
Liou et al (1994)	35	Headache, episodic vomiting	Four, one MELAS	MELAS	Hair follicles	0.237	0.030–0.740	120
De Vries et al (1994)	36	Unaffected	Five, two MELAS and one deafness	MELAS	Fibroblasts	0.282	0.065–0.688	108
De Vries et al (1994)	36	Unaffected	Four, two MELAS and one deafness	MELAS	Skeletal muscle	0.500	0.150–0.850	83
Huang et al (1996)	37	Unaffected	Four, one MELAS	MELAS	Skeletal muscle	0.175	0.024–0.644	84
Koga et al (2000)	38	Muscle weakness	Four, one Leigh syndrome	Leigh syndrome	Hair follicles	0.548	0.175–0.873	84
Dubeau et al (2000)	39	Deafness, cardio-myopathy, short stature	Eight, two MELAS and one migraine and ptosis	MELAS	Urinary epithelium	0.283	0.082–0.443	59
Family A (this work)	–	Unaffected	Four oocytes	CPEO	Oocytes	0.423	0.113–0.808	89
Family A (this work)	–	Unaffected	Four oocytes+one son	CPEO	Oocytes+urinary epithelium from IV-1	0.488	0.188–0.793	108
Family B (this work)	–	Unaffected	Four, one MELAS	MELAS	Skeletal muscle	0.203	0.031–0.665	84
Family B (this work)	–	Unaffected	Five, one MELAS	MELAS	Urinary epithelium	0.115	0.014–0.551	110

p = frequency of mutant mtDNA in the progeny; C.I. = lower and upper limits of confidence interval for π at the 0.95 level; N = estimated size of the bottleneck.

skeletal muscle, hair follicles, fibroblasts and urinary epithelium (Table 1).

Overall, these cumulative data show a close relationship between the tissues analyzed and the relative calculation for bottleneck size (N): for both a postmitotic tissue, such as skeletal muscle and oocytes, N resulted similar, despite the resulting mutation load in offspring was largely distributed in Family A and skewed to the extremes in Family B. Our literature revision revealed that in most cases the "mother-to-offspring" transmission resembled Family A [34,35,36,38,39], whereas only one family was essentially identical to Family B [37], still with very similar estimated bottleneck sizes. The overview of the relationship between mother and offspring mutant loads from our Families A and B, and those retrieved from literature are graphically represented in Figure 5, including the theoretical bottleneck calculated for each of these segregations.

Discussion

This study shows that germline segregation of the 3243A>G/ tRNA^{Leu} MELAS mutation may lead to a wide range of mutational loads in offspring through a similar bottleneck size. Its estimation in the two Italian families here investigated was remarkably close to the average number of segregating units calculated for other "mother-to-offspring" germline segregations retrieved from the literature. In Family A, individual III-2 transmitted intermediate, largely distributed loads of heteroplasmic mutant mtDNA (10% to 75% mutant; Figure 5), as measured in four of her oocytes and in her only son. This resembled most of the other segregations retrieved from the literature (Figure 5). In contrast, in Family B we observed a sharply skewed transmission of mutant from individual I-2 to only one of her offspring (81% mutant; Figure 5). All other siblings had only wild-type mtDNA in the tissues analyzed (0% mutant; Figure 5), including amniocytes from two pregnancies of individuals II-5 and II-7. This was paralleled by only one family previously reported by Huang et al. [37], which had an essentially identical distribution of mutant loads in skeletal muscle of offspring (Figure 5).

The number of "segregating units" (bottleneck size), calculated in these two Italian families and in the several cases retrieved from the literature [28–30] was substantially lower than the 173 segregating units estimated by Brown et al. in the only study that sampled a large set of oocytes (N = 82) from a female carrier of the same MELAS mutation [30]. An important limitation of the current study and those retrieved from the literature is the large error associated with the variance estimated from a very low sample number (≥ 4) [45]. This is an obvious drawback by working with living patients from human pedigrees. A recent study [46] on the segregation of the MELAS mutation through the human embryofetal development concluded that random drift drives germline segregation, similar to Brown's and colleagues conclusions [30], but with some appreciable individual-dependent differences in bottleneck size. Interestingly, in a study based on a large cohort of individuals carrying the MELAS mutation, the mothers with a mutation load greater that 50% tended to have offspring with lower or equal heteroplasmy, whereas the opposite was true for mothers with less than or equal to 50% mutation load [47]. These authors concluded that the random genetic drift model could not fully explain the transmission of the MELAS mutation [47]. Ascertainment bias has also to be considered. The recent finding that one in 200 healthy humans harbors a pathogenic mtDNA mutation out of the ten most frequent, indicates that there is a large pool of maternal lineages were probably these mutations segregate silently, and are possibly

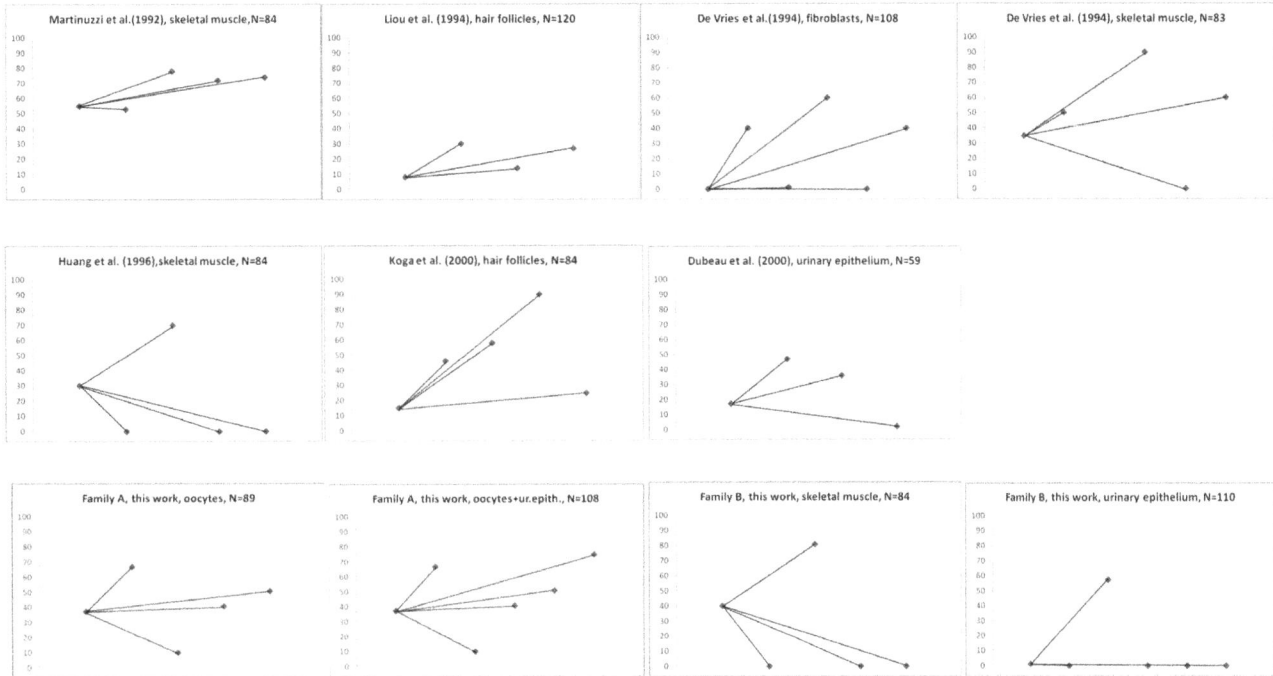

Figure 5. Graphical representation of mother-to-offspring transmission of the MELAS mutation in the two Italian families and the seven other pedigrees retrieved from literature (see Table 1). The mutant load of MELAS mutation (%) is on the y axis. In all panels, the leftmost point is the mother's mutant load, connected to each of the offspring mutant load. The reference, the tissues from which mtDNA mutant load has been assessed and the bottleneck size are indicated.

selected out, missing to express any pathology and not being ascertained at all [48]. Thus, investigation of single pedigrees identified by an affected proband introduces a bias that may be resolved by pooling large cohort of families through multi-centric studies, or by meta-analyses of reported pedigrees.

The analysis of somatic segregation of the MELAS mutation in our two families confirmed that the mutant load is inversely correlated with age in blood cells, whereas skeletal muscle is the tissue of choice, followed by urinary epithelial cells, for detection of the mutation [42–44]. The pattern of mutational load in somatic tissues distinguished the two families, which also differed for the clinical phenotype. In Family A (CPEO), the mutational load in the unaffected female individual III-2 appeared to be similar in skeletal muscle (44%) and urinary epithelium (29%–46%), whereas in the female individual I-2 of Family B (MELAS) the mutational load in skeletal muscle (40%) was much higher than in urinary epithelium (1%). This latter observation might be related to the skewed transmission of mutant mtDNA in the offspring of this woman, resulting in one MELAS patient (81% mutant mtDNAs in skeletal muscle), two miscarriages conceivably due to very high mutant loads, and all remaining unaffected individuals with wild-type mtDNA.

Many recent studies have tried to tackle the issue of mtDNA germline segregation testing the bottleneck hypothesis [17–22]. These studies have employed murine and primate heteroplasmic models and there is no consensus on whether the bottleneck exists, whether there are one or more bottlenecks, and at what stage of development the bottleneck(s) operate. These models do not closely recapitulate the situation of a single mtDNA pathogenic mutation segregating along the maternal line of human pedigrees because most heteroplasmic animals were generated by mixing two mitochondrial genomes that differed for a cluster of polymorphic variants, which may have no or small functional

relevance [49]. This condition is different from the case of a single pathogenic mtDNA mutation arising on a clonal mitochondrial genome, which is typical of humans with mitochondrial disorders. Important differences between the two situations may include the nucleoid composition and the level of mtDNA exchange, if any, between nucleoids. Nucleoids seem to follow the faithful replication model, without consistent genome exchange [6,11,13]. Furthermore, it has been demonstrated that mtDNA molecules may recombine within mitochondria [50–52], a phenomenon that is not relevant when mtDNA is clonal as in most humans, but that may become important in the case of different coexisting genomes with clusters of distinct variants, as in the heteroplasmic animal models or sometimes in humans with multiple heteroplasmies [17–21,53]. No studies address how frequently mtDNA recombination may occur, in which cell type, or during which stage of germ line segregation. Neither heteroplasmic animal models [17–21,49] nor the few available pathologic mito-mouse models [10,23,24] have been fully exploited yet to answer all these questions.

One final question concerns the possible selective pressure on mtDNA pathogenic mutations. The currently available mito-mice clearly indicated that severe mtDNA mutations undergo purifying selection over a few generations [23,24]. The segregation of the MELAS mutation in human tissues has been proposed to be non-random [54], and in vitro studies using cybrids with different nuclear backgrounds showed that segregation of the mutant mtDNA could be driven in opposite directions depending on the nuclear genome [55–57]. Thus, selection of mutant mtDNA may occur differently in different somatic tissues, impinging on the phenotypic expression. Whether such a genotypic selection may also operate during the germ line segregation for "mild" changes, including the MELAS mutation, is currently debated, casting doubts on the random genetic drift mechanism [47]. Staining the ovarian tissue for the histoenzymatic COX/SDH activities failed to reveal any COX-deficient oocyte, nor other cell types. This may indicate that in this particular case there was no oocyte with supra-threshold loads of MELAS mutation or that a very efficient complementation occurs within oocytes, which may escape in the case of MELAS mutation any selection along the germline.

In conclusion, the mechanisms governing the germline segregation and the subsequent somatic distribution of single pathogenic mtDNA mutations in humans remain far from being elucidated. Our study of mother-to-oocytes/offspring tissues transmission of the same pathogenic MELAS mutation shows how wide may be the range of mutant loads segregating through the same bottleneck size.

Acknowledgments

We thank Prof. Eric Schon for supporting this project and for his helpful advice and discussions. We are also indebted with the family members of the two Italian families investigated for their participation to this study.

Author Contributions

Conceived and designed the experiments: FP AB SDM VC. Performed the experiments: FP GB RF MLV RV MM. Analyzed the data: FP GB RF MLV RV MM SDM VC. Contributed reagents/materials/analysis tools: RF MLV SC. Wrote the paper: FP GB RF MLV VC.

References

1. Chinnery PF, Thorburn DR, Samuels DC, White SL, Dahl H-HM, et al.(2000) The inheritance of mitochondrial DNA heteroplasmy: random drift, selection or both? Trends Genet 16: 500–505.
2. Schon EA (2000) Mitochondrial genetics and disease. Trends Biochem Sci 25: 555–560.
3. Carling PJ, Cree LM, Chinnery PF (2011) The implications of mitochondrial DNA copy number regulation during oogenesis. Mitochondrion 11: 686–692.
4. Lightowlers RN, Chinnery PF, Turnbull DM, Howell N (1997) Mammalian mitochondrial genetics: heredity, heteroplasmy and disease. Trends Genet.13: 450–455.
5. Satoh M, Kuroiwa T (1991) Organization of multiple nucleoids and DNA molecules in mitochondria of a human cell. Exp Cell Res 196: 137–140.
6. Jacobs HT, Lehtinen SK, Spelbrink JN (2000) No sex please, we're mitochondria: a hypothesis on the somatic unit of inheritance of mammalian mtDNA. Bioassay 22: 564–572.
7. Legros F, Malka F, Frachon P, Lombes A, Rojo M (2004) Organization and dynamics of human mitochondrial DNA. J Cell Sci 117: 2653–2662.
8. Takai D, Inoue K, Goto YI, Nonaka I, Hayashi JI (1997) The interorganellar interaction between distinct human mitochondria with deletion mutant mtDNA from a patient with mitochondrial disease and with HeLa mtDNA. J Biol Chem 272: 6028–6033.
9. Enriquez JA, Cabezas-Herrera J, Bayona-Bafaluy MP, Attardi G (2000) Very rare complementation between mitochondria carrying different mitochondrial DNA mutations points to intrinsic genetic autonomy of the organelles in cultured human cells. J Biol Chem 275: 11207–11215.
10. Nakada K, Inoue K, Ono T, Isobe K, Ogura A, et al. (2001) Inter-mitochondrial complementation: Mitochondria-specific system preventing mice from expression of disease phenotypes by mutant mtDNA. Nat Med 7: 934–940.
11. Gilkerson RW, Schon EA, Hernandez E, Davidson MM (2008) Mitochondrial nucleoids maintain genetic autonomy but allow for functional complementation. J Cell Biol 181: 1117–1128.
12. Poe BG3rd, Duffy CF, Greminger, MA, Nelson BJ, Arriaga EA (2010) Detection of heteroplasmy in individual mitochondrial particles. Anal Bioanal Chem 397: 3397–3407.
13. Kukat C, Wurm CA, Spåhr H, Falkenberg M, Larsson NG, et al. (2011) Super-resolution microscopy reveals that mammalian mitochondrial nucleoids have a uniform size and frequently contain a single copy of mtDNA. Proc Natl Acad Sci U S A 108: 13534–13539.
14. Olivo P, Van De Walle MJ, Laipis P, Hauswirth WW (1983) Nucleotide sequence evidence for rapid genotypic shifts in the bovine mitochondrial DNA D-loop. Nature 306: 400–402.
15. Ashley MV, Laipis PJ, Hauswirth WW (1989) Rapid segregation of heteroplasmic bovine mitochondria. Nucleic Acids Res 17: 7325–7331.
16. Koehler CM, Lindberg GL, Brown DR, Beitz DC, Freeman AE, et al. (1991) Replacement of bovine mitochondrial DNA by a sequence variant within one generation. Genetics 129: 247–255.
17. Cree LM, Samuels DC, de Sousa Lopez SC, Rajasimha HK, Wonnapinij P, et al. (2008) A reduction of mitochondrial DNA molecules during embryogenesis explains the rapid segregation of genotypes. Nat Genet 40: 249–254.
18. Cao L, Shitara H, Horii T, Nagao Y, Imai H, et al.(2007) The mitochondrial bottleneck occurs without reduction of mtDNA content in female mouse germ cells. Nat Genet 39: 386–390.
19. Cao L, Shitara H, Sugimoto M, Hayashi JI, Abe K, et al. (2009) New evidence confirms that the mitochondrial bottleneck is generated without reduction of mitochondrial DNA content in early primordial germ cells of mice. PLoS Genet 5: e1000756.
20. Wai T, Teoli T, Shoubridge EA (2008) The mitochondrial DNA genetic bottleneck results from replication of a subpopulation of genomes. Nat Genet 40: 1484–1488.
21. Lee HS, Ma H, Juanes RC, Tachibana M, Sparman M, et al. (2012) Rapid mitochondrial DNA segregation in primate preimplantation embryos precedes somatic and germline bottleneck. Cell Rep 1: 506–515.
22. Jenuth JP, Peterson AC, Fu K, Shoubridge EA (1996) Random genetic drift in the female germline explains the rapid segregation of mammalian mitochondrial DNA. Nat Genet 14: 146–151.
23. Stewart JB, Freyer C, Elson JL, Wredenberg A, Cansu Z, et al. (2008) Strong purifying selection in transmission of mammalian mitochondrial DNA. PLoS Biol 6: e10.
24. Fan W, Waymire KG, Narula N, Li P, Rocher C, et al. (2008) A mouse model of mitochondrial disease reveals germ line selection against severe mtDNA mutations. Science 319: 958–962.
25. Larsson NG, Tulinius MH, Holme E, Oldfors A, Andersen O, et al. (1992) Segregation and manifestations of the mtDNA tRNA(Lys) A→G(8344) mutation of myoclonus epilepsy and ragged-red fibers (MERRF) syndrome. Am J Hum Genet 51: 1201–1212.
26. Howell N, Halvorson S, Kubacka I, McCullough DA, Bindoff LA, et al.(1992) Mitochondrial gene segregation in mammals: is the bottleneck always narrow? Hum Genet 90: 117–120.
27. Blok RB, Gook DA, Thorburn DR, Dahl HH (1997) Skewed segregation of the mtDNA nt 8993 (T→G) mutation in human oocytes. Am J Hum Genet 60: 1495–1501.
28. Marchington DR, Hartshorne GM, Barlow D, Poulton J(1997) Homopolymeric tract heteroplasmy in mtDNA from tissues and single oocytes: support for a genetic bottleneck. Am J Hum Genet 60: 408–416.
29. Marchington DR, Macaulay V, Hartshorne GM, Barlow D, Poulton J (1998) Evidence from human oocytes for a genetic bottleneck in an mtDNA disease. Am J Hum Genet 63: 769–775.
30. Brown DT, Samuels DC, Michael EM, Turnbull DM, Chinnery PF (2001) Random genetic drift determines the level of mutant mtDNA in human primary oocytes. Am J Hum Genet 68: 533–536.
31. Goto Y, Nonaka I, Horai S (1990) A mutation in the tRNA(Leu)(UUR) gene associated with the MELAS subgroup of mitochondrial encephalomyopathies. Nature 348: 651–653.
32. Cevoli S, Pallotti F, La Morgia C, Valentino ML, Pierangeli G, et al.(2010) High frequency of migraine-only patients negative for the 3243 A>G tRNALeu mtDNA mutation in two MELAS families. Cephalalgia 30: 919–927.
33. Chinnery PF, Howell N, Lightowlers RN, Turnbull DM (1997) Molecular pathology of MELAS and MERRF. The relationship between mutation load and clinical phenotypes. Brain 120: 1713–1721.
34. Martinuzzi A, Bartolomei L, Carrozzo R, Mostacciuolo M, Carbonin C, et al.(1992) Correlation between clinical and molecular features in two MELAS families. J Neurol Sci.113: 222–229.
35. Liou CW, Huang CC, Chee EC, Jong YJ, Tsai JL, et al. (1994) MELAS syndrome: correlation between clinical features and molecular genetic analysis. Acta Neurol Scand 90: 354–359.
36. de Vries D, de Wijs I, Ruitenbeek W, Begeer J, Smit P, et al. (1994) Extreme variability of clinical symptoms among sibs in a MELAS family correlated with heteroplasmy for the mitochondrial A3243G mutation. J Neurol Sci 124: 77–82.
37. Huang CC, Chen RS, Chu NS, Pang CY, Wei YH (1996) Random mitotic segregation of mitochondrial DNA in MELAS syndrome. Acta Neurol Scand 93: 198–202.
38. Koga Y, Akita Y, Takane N, Sato Y, Kato H (2000) Heterogeneous presentation in A3243G mutation in the mitochondrial tRNA(Leu(UUR)) gene. Arch Dis Child 82: 407–411.
39. Dubeau F, De Stefano N, Zifkin BG, Arnold DL, Shoubridge EA (2000) Oxidative phosphorylation defect in the brains of carriers of the tRNAleu(UUR) A3243G mutation in a MELAS pedigree. Ann Neurol 47: 179–185.
40. Fabbri R, Venturoli S, D'Errico A, Iannascoli C, Gabusi E, et al. (2003) Ovarian tissue banking and fertility preservation in cancer patients: histological and immunohistochemical evaluation. Gynecol Oncol 89: 259–266.
41. Dubowitz V, Sewry CA, Lane RJM (2007) Muscle Biopsy: A practical Approach (3rdEd). Saunders Elsevier, London, UK.
42. Shanske S, Pancrudo J, Kaufmann P, Engelstad K, Jhung S, et al.(2004) Varying loads of the mitochondrial DNA A3243G mutation in different tissues: implications for diagnosis. Am J Med Genet 130A: 134–137.
43. McDonnell MT, Schaefer AM, Blakely EL, McFarland R, Chinnery PF, et al.(2004) Noninvasive diagnosis of the 3243A>G mitochondrial DNA mutation using urinary epithelial cells. Eur J Hum Genet 12: 778–781.

44. Rahman S, Poulton J, Marchington D, Suomalainen A (2001) Decrease of 3243 A->G mtDNA mutation from blood in MELAS syndrome: a longitudinal study. Am J Hum Genet 68: 238–240.

45. Wonnapinij P, Chinnery PF, Samuels DC (2010) Previous estimates of mitochondrial DNA mutation level variance did not account for sampling error: comparing the mtDNA genetic bottleneck in mice and humans. Am J Hum Genet 86: 540–550.

46. Monnot S, Gigarel N, Samuels DC, Burlet P, Hesters L, et al. (2011) Segregation of mtDNA throughout human embryofetal development: m.3243A>G as a model system. Hum Mutat 32: 116–125.

47. Uusimaa J, Moilanen JS, Vainionpää L, Tapanainen P, Lindholm P, et al. (2007) Prevalence, segregation, and phenotype of the mitochondrial DNA 3243A>G mutation in children. Ann Neurol 62: 278–287.

48. Elliott HR, Samuels DC, Eden JA, Relton CL, Chinnery PF (2008) Pathogenic mitochondrial DNA mutations are common in the general population. Am J Hum Genet 83: 254–260.

49. Sharpley MS, Marciniak C, Eckel-Mahan K, McManus M, Crimi M, et al. (2012) Heteroplasmy of mouse mtDNA is genetically unstable and results in altered behavior and cognition. Cell 151: 333–43.

50. Yoneda M, Miyatake T, Attardi G (1994) Complementation of mutant and wild-type human mitochondrial DNAs coexisting since the mutation event and lack of complementation of DNAs introduced separately into a cell within distinct organelles. Mol Cell Biol 14: 2699–2712.

51. Kraytsberg Y, Schwartz M, Brown TA, Ebralidse K, Kunz WS, et al. (2004) Recombination of human mitochondrial DNA. Science 304: 981.

52. D'Aurelio M, Gajewski CD, Lin MT, Mauck WM, Shao LZ, et al. (2004). Heterologous mitochondrial DNA recombination in human cells. Hum Mol Genet 13: 3171–3179.

53. Zsurka G, Hampel KG, Kudina T, Kornblum C, Kraytsberg Y, et al. (2007) Inheritance of mitochondrial DNA recombinants in double-heteroplasmic families: potential implications for phylogenetic analysis. Am J Hum Genet 80: 298–305.

54. Chinnery PF, Zwijnenburg PJ, Walker M, Howell N, Taylor RW, et al. (1999) Nonrandom tissue distribution of mutant mtDNA. Am J Med Genet 85: 498–501.

55. Yoneda M, Chomyn A, Martinuzzi A, Hurko O, Attardi G (1992) Marked replicative advantage of human mtDNA carrying a point mutation that causes the MELAS encephalomyopathy. Proc Natl Acad Sci U S A 89: 11164–11168.

56. Dunbar DR, Moonie PA, Jacobs HT, Holt IJ (1995) Different cellular backgrounds confer a marked advantage to either mutant or wild-type mitochondrial genomes. Proc Natl Acad Sci U S A 92: 6562–6566.

57. Lehtinen SK, Hance N, El Meziane A, Juhola MK, Juhola KM, et al. (2000) Genotypic stability, segregation and selection in heteroplasmic human cell lines containing np 3243 mutant mtDNA. Genetics 154: 363–380.

22

Sodium Bicarbonate Treatment during Transient or Sustained Lactic Acidemia in Normoxic and Normotensive Rats

Franco Valenza[1,4]*, **Marta Pizzocri**[1], **Valentina Salice**[1], **Giorgio Chevallard**[1], **Tommaso Fossali**[1], **Silvia Coppola**[1], **Sara Froio**[1], **Federico Polli**[1], **Stefano Gatti**[2,4], **Francesco Fortunato**[3], **Giacomo P. Comi**[3,4], **Luciano Gattinoni**[1,4]

1 Dipartimento di Anestesia, Rianimazione (Intensiva e Subintensiva) e Terapia del Dolore, Fondazione IRCCS Ca' Granda, Ospedale Maggiore Policlinico, Milan, Italy, 2 Centro di Ricerche Chirurgiche Precliniche, Fondazione IRCCS Ca' Granda, Ospedale Maggiore Policlinico, Milan, Italy, 3 Centro Dino Ferrari, Dipartimento di Scienze Neurologiche, Fondazione IRCCS Ca' Granda, Ospedale Maggiore Policlinico, Milan, Italy, 4 Università degli Studi di Milano, Milan, Italy

Abstract

Introduction: Lactic acidosis is a frequent cause of poor outcome in the intensive care settings. We set up an experimental model of lactic acid infusion in normoxic and normotensive rats to investigate the systemic effects of lactic acidemia per se without the confounding factor of an underlying organic cause of acidosis.

Methodology: Sprague Dawley rats underwent a primed endovenous infusion of L(+) lactic acid during general anesthesia. Normoxic and normotensive animals were then randomized to the following study groups (n = 8 per group): S) sustained infusion of lactic acid, S+B) sustained infusion+sodium bicarbonate, T) transient infusion, T+B transient infusion+sodium bicarbonate. Hemodynamic, respiratory and acid-base parameters were measured over time. Lactate pharmacokinetics and muscle phosphofructokinase enzyme's activity were also measured.

Principal Findings: Following lactic acid infusion blood lactate rose ($P<0.05$), pH ($P<0.05$) and strong ion difference ($P<0.05$) drop. Some rats developed hemodynamic instability during the primed infusion of lactic acid. In the normoxic and normotensive animals bicarbonate treatment normalized pH during sustained infusion of lactic acid (from 7.22 ± 0.02 to 7.36 ± 0.04, $P<0.05$) while overshoot to alkalemic values when the infusion was transient (from 7.24 ± 0.01 to 7.53 ± 0.03, $P<0.05$). When acid load was interrupted bicarbonate infusion affected lactate wash-out kinetics ($P<0.05$) so that blood lactate was higher (2.9 ± 1 mmol/l vs. 1.0 ± 0.2, $P<0.05$, group T vs. T+B respectively). The activity of phosphofructokinase enzyme was correlated with blood pH ($R2=0.475$, $P<0.05$).

Conclusions: pH decreased with acid infusion and rose with bicarbonate administration but the effects of bicarbonate infusion on pH differed under a persistent or transient acid load. Alkalization affected the rate of lactate disposal during the transient acid load.

Editor: Olivier Kocher, Harvard Medical School, United States of America

Funding: The study was funded by Fondazione IRCCS Ca' Granda, Ospedale Maggiore Policlinico, Milan, Italy. The funder had no role in study design, data collection and analysis, decision to publish, or preparation of the manuscript.

Competing Interests: The authors have declared that no competing interests exist.

* E-mail: franco.valenza@unimi.it

Introduction

Lactic acidosis is a frequent cause of acidemia in the intensive care settings, often associated with hemodynamic and/or respiratory impairment [1–9].

Whether it is worth to correct acidemia by infusion of alkaline solutions is a matter of discussion [10–12]. The evidence in favour of pH correction of organic acidemia is poor. Clinical studies are few and inconclusive, particularly with respect to clinical outcome [13;14]. There are a number of evidences against alkalinization therapy [14–23]. International guidelines "recommend against the use of sodium bicarbonate therapy for the purpose of improving hemodynamics or reducing vasopressor requirements in [septic] patients with hypoperfusion-induced lactic acidemia with pH>7.15" [24]. However, the correction of acidemia is common in clinical practice. An on line survey has recently shown that 67% of critical care physicians start to administer alkaline solutions to patients with lactic acidosis when pH is 7.2 [25].

Many experimental models of lactic acidemia do not allow to investigate the effects of a lactic acid load per se, because of confounding factors. Moving from the consideration that in clinical setting lactic acidosis may be transient, as during reperfusion of ischemic regions, or sustained, as in persistent hemodynamic instability, we decided to investigate the effects of bicarbonate infusion in normoxic and normotensive animals subjected to transient or sustained lactic acid load.

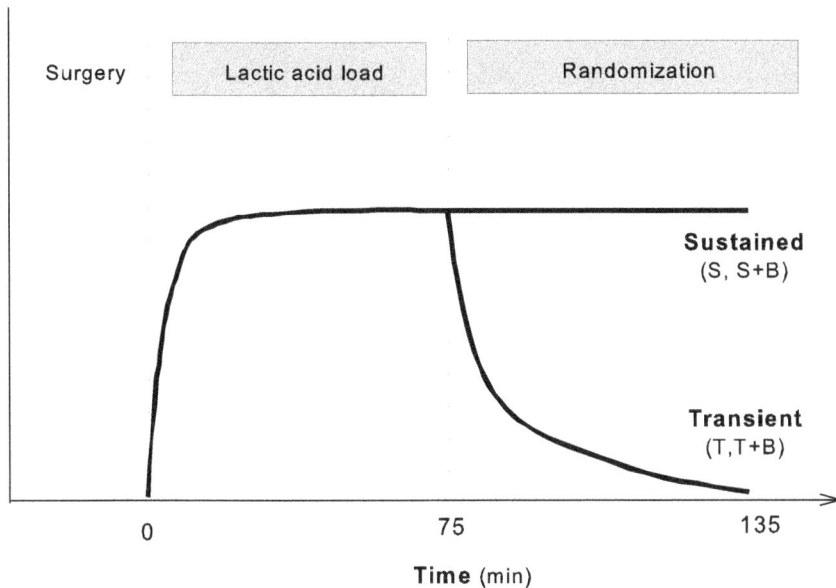

Figure 1. Protocol overview. A schematic overview of the experiment flow is shown in the figure. The investigation consisted of an initial lactic acid load to induce lactic acidemia followed by randomization to sustained (S) or transient (T) lactic acid infusion with or without sodium bicarbonate (B) treatment.

We wish to report here the results of our investigation and discuss the possible underlying mechanisms and clinical implications.

Materials and Methods

This experimental study was performed after the Ethics Committee of our institution and the Italian Ministry of Health approved the protocol (Permit Number: 6/07). All surgery was performed under anesthesia, and all efforts were made to minimize suffering.

Experimental design

A schematic overview of the experiment flow is shown in Figure 1.

The investigation consisted of an initial lactic acid load to induce lactic acidemia followed by randomization to sustained or transient lactic acid infusion with or without sodium bicarbonate treatment.

Anaesthesia and animal preparation

Sprague Dawley rats (weight 250–300 grams) purchased from Charles River, housed in a warmed and humidified ambient with a 12/12 hours day/night shift, received an intraperitoneal injection of 80 mg/kg thiopental. The trachea was cannulated with a 14 gauge tube connected to a pressure transducer (Motorola MPX 2010DP, Phoenix, AZ, USA). Paralysis was obtained with vecuronium bromide 3 mg/kg i.v. Right carotid artery, femoral and subclavian vein were cannulated with 22 gauge catheters. The arterial catheter was connected to a pressure transducer (Bentley Trantec 800, Santa Ana, CA, USA). Blood pressure and airway pressure were continuously monitored and digitally stored (Elekton Colligo, Agliano, AT, Italy) for subsequent analysis.

During the surgical preparation, rats were mechanically ventilated (Harvard-Rodent 683, Harvard Apparatus South Natick, Massachusetts, USA), with a tidal volume of 6 ml/kg, PEEP of 3 cmH$_2$O and respiratory rate set according to mixed expired CO$_2$ (mixCO$_2$), continuously analyzed (Ohmeda 5250 RGM, Ohmeda, Louisville, CO, USA). At the end of the procedure blood was drawn from the arterial line for blood gas analysis (1620 pH/Blood Gas Analyzer and 682 CO-Oxymeter, Instrumentation Laboratory, Lexington, MA, USA). Respiratory rate was set to obtain the desired values of PaCO$_2$ and pH. Inclusion criteria were: pH 7.35–7.45, PaCO$_2$ 35–45 mmHg, lactate <2 mmol/l, hemoglobin >12 g/dl, rectal temperature >36°C, mean arterial pressure (MAP) >90 mmHg. Ventilator parameters remained unchanged throughout the protocol.

If no major problems occurred during surgical preparation and after stabilization time animals were included into the study.

Lactic acid load and randomization process

After confirming inclusion criteria, 14.45 mmol/kg of a 0.55 M solution of L(+) lactic acid (30% in H$_2$O by weight - CH$_3$CH(OH)CO$_2$H- Sigma Aldrich) was infused over 75 minutes through a catheter positioned in a central vein. Animals that met inclusion criteria (pH<7.3, lactate >3 mmol/l and mean arterial pressure >70 mmHg) after the acid load, were randomized by sealed envelopes to one of the following treatments (n = 8 animals per group): S) sustained infusion of lactic acid, S+B) sustained infusion+sodium bicarbonate, T) transient infusion of lactic acid, T+B) transient infusion+sodium bicarbonate. In the sustained groups (group S and S+B), lactic acid was infused throughout the protocol at a rate of 0.20 mmol/kg/min. In the transient groups (groups T and T+B), an equal amount of normal saline was infused. In animals randomized to bicarbonate infusion (groups S+B and T+B) a 1 M solution of sodium bicarbonate was infused at a rate of 0.137 mmol/kg/min; bicarbonate infusion rate was chosen according to pilot studies that suggested a lactate to bicarbonate infusion ratio of 1 M : 0.7 M. If bicarbonate was not infused (groups S and T) an equal volume of normal saline was given to the animals. Experiments were interrupted 60 minutes after randomization (135 minutes after the beginning of the infusion of acid lactic) or if animals developed severe and fatal hypotension.

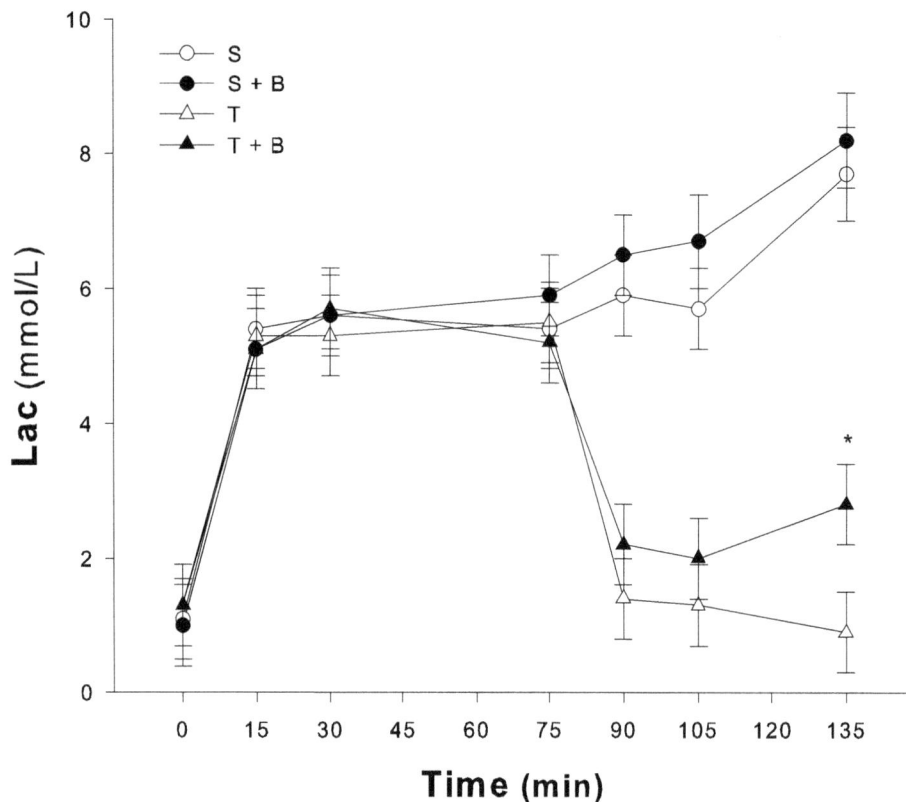

Figure 2. Lactate over time in the four groups. Lactic acid load caused blood lactate to rise in all groups ([#] P<0.05 vs. time 0). After 135 minutes in the sustained groups blood lactate remained high both in the sustained (S) and the sustained+NaHCO₃ (S+B) group. In the transient (T) groups blood lactate levels after 135 minutes were different from values at time 75 minutes (° P<0.05). Animals that received NaHCO₃ (T+B) had higher lactate levels (* P<0.05 vs. transient group).

Outcome measurements

Acid-base parameters. Acid base parameters included measured (pH, pCO₂), and calculated (HCO₃, BE) variables (1620 pH/Blood Gas Analyzer, Instrumentation Laboratory, Lexington, MA, USA). Lactate (Lac), sodium (Na), potassium (K), chloride (Cl) and ionized calcium (iCa) ions were measured (ABL555, Radiometer Danmark) and apparent Strong Ion Difference (SIDa) was calculated as

$$SIDa = (Na + K + iCa) - (Lac + Cl)$$

Glucose and hemoglobin concentration were also measured (ABL555, Radiometer Danmark).

Hemodynamic and respiratory parameters. Hemodynamic parameters (arterial blood pressure and heart rate) and ventilator settings (respiratory rate, tidal volume, positive end-expiratory pressure, mean airway pressure) were recorded throughout the protocol. Oxygenation was studied by arterial blood gas analysis (1620 pH/ Blood Gas Analyzer and 682 CO-Oxymeter, Instrumentation Laboratory, Lexington, MA, USA).

Lactate pharmacokinetics. Lactate wash-out kinetics was studied in the animals where lactate infusion was interrupted after randomization (transient groups: group T and group T+B).

Lactate kinetics was studied using a model previously described [26]. On the base of lactate increase over the first 75 minutes of infusion, clearance of exogenous lactate and basal lactate production were calculated. Lactate clearance (ml/kg/min) was calculated as the ratio between the lactate load (mmol/kg) and the

area under the lactate concentration curve over time (mmol/min/ l). We considered endogenous lactate production constant over the first 75 minutes of lactate infusion and we calculated basal lactate production (μmol/kg/min) as the product of basal lactate concentration (Lacbasal - time 0) and exogenous Lac clearance.

Lactate pharmacokinetics was assessed using the model:

$$y = a + e^{-bx} + cx$$

fitting, animal per animal, lactate concentrations (y) and time (x), where time 0 was considered time 75. The fitting was performed by means of the least squares method using Sigma Stat software (Systat Software, Inc.). From the fitting analysis coefficient b and c were derived animal by animal; using coefficient b, half time decay (T½) was calculated as 1/b. Coefficients and time decay were then compared for statistical significance.

Phosphofructokinase (PFK) activity. After the analysis of the first 32 randomized animals, we conducted a new set of experiments to better interpret our results. Eleven animals were randomized to receive the lactic acid load as previously described. Three animals were sacrificed soon after the acid load; 4 animals received transient infusion of lactic acid+sodium bicarbonate infusion (group T+B) and 4 the acid load without sodium bicarbonate infusion (group T). Oxidative soleus muscle (MS) and glycolytic extensor digitorum longus (ME) were then collected and stored with snap freezing technique for PFK activity analysis. Enzymes' activities were also determined [27]. Protein concentra-

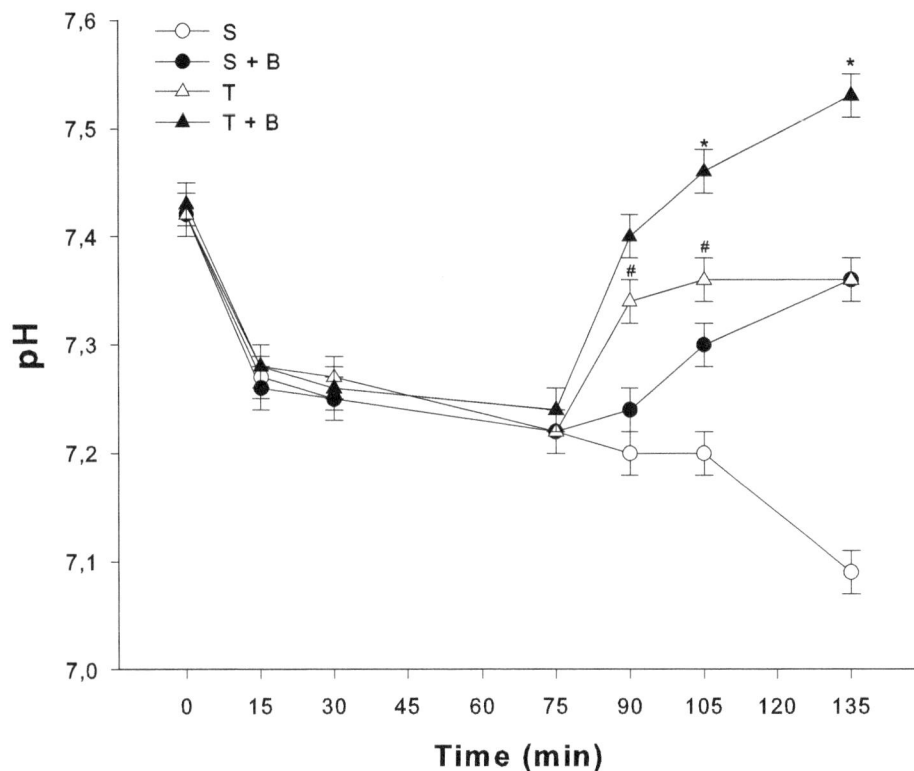

Figure 3. Blood pH over time in the four groups. After 75 minutes of infusion of lactic acid blood pH drop in all groups ($^#$ P<0.05 vs. time 0). At 135 minutes pH normalized in the transient group (T) while overshoot to alkalemic values when animals received NaHCO$_3$ (T+B). In the sustained group (S) pH continued to drop while alkaline infusion (S+B) resulted in correction of acidosis. $^\circ$ P<0.05 vs time 75; * P<0.05 vs. control.

tion was measured according to Lowry [28], and the PFK enzymatic activity was expressed as μmol/min/mg of protein.

Statistical analysis

Results are expressed as mean ± SEM. Analysis of variance was conducted and Bonferroni test was used for all pair-wise comparisons, when indicated. To compare two groups of variables T-test was used or Mann-Whitney Rank Sum Test if normality test failed. Least square linear regression analysis was used to correlate variables. Multiple linear regression was used to correlate base excess and lactate, animal by animal. Statistical significance was accepted as P<0.05. Analysis was performed with the SAS System for Windows version 9.1, unless otherwise specified.

Results

Effects of lactic acid load

Acid-base parameters. The infusion of lactic acid caused lactate to rise (1.2±0.07 mmol/l to 5.5±0.23, P<0.05 time 0 vs. 75, Figure 2) and pH to drop (7.426±0.005 vs. 7.227±0.009, P<0.05, Figure 3). SIDa decreased (31.92±0.54 mEq/l vs. 25.27±0.88, P<0.05) and hemoglobin was significantly lower (13.5±0.3 mg/dl vs. 10.9±0.3, P<0.05). Hyperchloremia (107±0.6 mEq/l vs. 112±0.7, P<0.05) and hypercapnia (40.2±0.6 mmHg vs. 51.2±1.5, P<0.05) also developed. Base excess decreased from 2.08±0.5 mmol/l to −6.3±0.8 (P<0.05). Changes of base excess correlated with changes of lactate (R2 = 0.81, P<0.05, multiple linear regression). Data are presented in Table 1.

Hemodynamic and respiratory parameters. During the primed infusion of lactic acid 11 animals developed severe hemodynamic instability and were excluded. Three animals died soon after randomization (one in group S, two in group S+B) and were replaced in the randomization process so that a total of 32 normoxic and normotensive rats completed the randomization process (n = 8 per group). At baseline, excluded and randomized animals were similar in terms of weight, surgical time, respiratory, acid base and hemodynamic variables except for a trend towards higher values of lactate (1.23±0.07 mmol/l vs. 1.49±0.11, P = 0.056 randomized animals vs. animals who failed lactic acid infusion, respectively), and a significantly higher heart rate (482±17 vs. 431±8 bpm, P<0.05).

Effects of randomization

Acid-base parameters. After the randomization, pH drop over time during the sustained infusion of lactic acid. There was a non significant increase of lactate levels. In the transient groups (T and T+B) 15 minutes after the end of lactic acid infusion, blood lactate concentration, pH and BE values were normal.

When NaHCO$_3$ was infused, pH normalized in the group with sustained infusion (group S+B: from 7.22±0.02 to 7.36±0.04, P<0.05) while rose to alkalemic values in the transient group (group T+B: from 7.24±0.01 to 7.53±0.03, P<0.05). Effects on pH were mainly related to sodium dependent changes of SIDa: Na$^+$ increased from 136.2±3.3 mEq/l to 144.3±1.1 and from 137.5±1.1 to 147.8±1.2 in the sustained group (S+B, P<0.05) and in the transient group (T, P<0.05), respectively.

Hemodynamic and respiratory parameters. As shown in Table 2, through the experimental time, mean arterial pressure

Table 1. Acid base variables and plasma chemistry.

	Min	S	S+B	T	T+B
pH	0	7.42±0.01	7.42±0.01	7.43±0.01	7.43±0.01
	75	7.22±0.02[a]	7.22±0.02[a]	7.23±0.02[a]	7.24±0.01[a]
	135	7.13±0.05[a]	7.36±0.04[bc]	7.36±0.02[b]	7.53±0.03[abc]
pCO₂ (mmHg)	0	40±1.1	39±0.9	42±1.3	40±1.1
	75	55±3[a]	49±2.4	55±2.9	47±3.4
	135	56±4.9[a]	55±4.6[a]	46±2.8	49±4.9
HCO₃ (mmol/l)	0	26.2±0.9	25.3±1	27.5±1	26.9±0.8
	75	22.7±1.6	19.9±1	22.8±1.4	20.0±1.6
	135	19.3±2.6	31.8±4.1[bc]	25.9±1.5	40.5±3[abc]
BE (mmol/l)	0	1.7±1.1	0.8±1.1	3.2±1.1	2.6±0.9
	75	−5±1.9	−7.9±1.1	−4.8±1.6[a]	−7.3±1.7[a]
	135	−10.2±3.5[a]	6.3±4.7[bc]	0.5±1.6	17.4±2.7[abc]
Lac (mmol/l)	0	1.2±0.2	1.1±0.1	1.3±0.1	1.3±0.1
	75	5.4±0.5[a]	6±0.5[a]	5.5±0.4[a]	5±0.5[a]
	135	7.4±1.6[a]	8±1.5[a]	1±0.2[b]	2.9±1[bc]
Na (mEq/l)	0	136.2±3.8	138.8±2.5	137.9±1.3	135±1.5
	75	132.4±2.8	136.2±3.3	138.2±1.5	137.5±1.1
	135	135.3±1.9	144.3±1.1	136.4±1.7	147.8±1.2[abc]
K (mEq/l)	0	4.26±0.16	3.64±0.09	3.94±0.17	3.86±0.17
	75	4.36±0.16	3.75±0.2	4.18±0.25	3.9±0.25
	135	4.73±0.31	3.95±0.45	4.8±0.42	4.36±0.31
Cl (mEq/l)	0	105.3±2.4	109.0±0.7	105.8±0.7	108.0±0.9
	75	110.7±2.3	112.5±1.2	113.2±1.6[a]	112.3±1
	135	110.6±3	112.0±1.5	112.6±0.8[a]	107.3±1.8[c]
SIDa (mEq/l)	0	31.5±1.1	31.5±0.8	33.4±1.1	30.8±1.1
	75	27.1±2.2	23.2±1.4[a]	25.5±2.6[a]	25.7±0.5
	135	29.8±2	30.9±3	32.2±0.8[b]	43.4±1.8[abc]
iCa (mEq/l)	0	0.94±0.13	0.99±0.1	0.98±0.07	0.99±0.07
	75	0.93±0.13	1.07±0.09	1.06±0.06	1.08±0.06
	135	1.02±0.08	0.97±0.11	0.96±0.07	0.85±0.07
Glc (mg/dl)	0	165±18	153±13	149±8	160±17
	75	125±6	116±10	120±7	112±8[a]
	135	116±15	117±12	112±6[a]	79±13[a]
Hb (g/dl)	0	13.4±0.6	14±0.8	13.4±0.5	13.3±0.4
	75	10.9±0.7	11.1±0.8	10.8±0.7[a]	10.8±0.6
	135	7.7±0.5[a]	8.7±1.4[a]	9.9±0.4[a]	9.1±0.5[a]

ANOVA P<0.05:
[a]vs. 0,
[b]vs. 75,
[c]S vs. S+B or T vs. T+B.
BE, base excess; Lac, lactate concentration; Na, sodium concentration; K, potassium concentration; Cl, chloride concentration; SIDa, stron ion difference; iCa, ionized calcium concentration; Glc, glycemia; Hb, hemoglobin concentration.
Data are expressed as mean ± SEM.

and heart rate were similar in sustained and transient lactic acidosis groups. Sodium bicarbonate infusion did not modify hemodynamic parameters.

Ventilator parameters were unchanged and were similar among randomization groups. At the end of the 135 minutes, animals that received sodium bicarbonate infusion were more hypoxemic then their relative controls: 216±36.12 mmHg vs. 269±31.4, group S+B vs group S (P=0.0511) and 272±16.96 mmHg vs. 332±15.87, group T+B vs group T (P<0.05).

Metabolic measurements

Lactate pharmacokinetics. As shown in Figure 2, at the end of the protocol lactate was significantly higher in the T+B group than in the T group.(2.9±1 mmol/l vs. 1±0.2, group T+B vs. group T respectively, P<0.05 – Table 1). Despite similar

Table 2. Hemodynamic and respiratory variables.

	min	S	S+B	T	T+B
Mean arterial pressure (mmHg)	0	134±6.8	132±3.92	134±7.51	133±4.76
	75	140±5.6	131±5.59	134±6.96	139±5.85
	135	108±11.96	103±17.13	119±7.29	113±10.73
Heart rate (beats/min)	0	417±20.77	460±13.55	439±12.21	417±15.88
	75	382±10.84	390±19.82	389±5.9	368±15.18
	135	351±22.03	404±8.7	394±18.73	397±21.99
Tidal Volume (ml)	0	2.81±0.14	3.03±0.19	2.78±0.12	3.03±0.08
	75	2.81±0.14	3.03±0.19	2.78±0.12	3.03±0.08
	135	2.81±0.16	3.03±0.25	2.78±0.12	3.03±0.08
Respiratory rate (breaths/min)	0	72±2.1	64±3.8	70±1.6	69±2.7
	75	71±2.2	64±3.7	71±1.5	69±2.6
	135	71±2.5	64±5.4	70±1.6	70±2.5
Mean airway pressure (cmH$_2$O)	0	6.4±0.2	7.4±0.51	6.5±0.37	6.7±0.4
	75	6.5±0.24	6.9±0.55	6.5±0.27	7.6±0.8
	135	7.1±0.42	6.7±0.27	6.9±0.25	6.8±0.2
Oxygenation (PaO$_2$ - mmHg)	0	300±14.32	314±13.92	328±9.19	295±14.04
	75	277±17.84	281±18.44	298±12.29	273±11.22
	135	269±31.4	216±36.12	332±15.87	272±11.69[c]

ANOVA P<0.05:
[c]S vs. S+B or T vs. T+B.
Data are expressed as mean ± SEM.

endogenous lactate production and clearance, the decay of lactate over time was different when bicarbonate was added (Table 3).

When sodium bicarbonate was infused (group T+B) blood glucose concentration slightly decreases over time (112±8 mg/dl vs. 79±13, time 75 vs. 135 respectively, P = 0.095 – Table 1). Glucose and lactate decay was different in T and T+B groups (Figure 4). Glucose changes over time inversely correlated with changes of lactate (R^2 = 0.582, P<0.05): the higher the changes of lactate, the lower the glucose changes.

PFK activity. The activity of PFK in the oxidative soleus muscle was similar in the studied groups (1.675±0.171 μmol/min/mg of proteins, P = 0.11). Conversely, PFK activity in the glycolytic extensor digitorum longus muscle was higher when bicarbonate was infused (P = 0.067, Figure 5). The higher the blood pH measured before muscle harvest the higher the activity of PFK, as shown by linear regression analysis (R^2 = 0.475, P<0.05).

Discussion

We set up an experimental model of transient versus sustained lactic acid infusion in normoxic and normotensive rats to investigate the systemic effects of lactic acidemia per se without the confounding factor of an underlying organic acidosis. The load of lactic acid caused acidemia of both metabolic and respiratory origin. These effects quickly reversed during the transient infusion. Bicarbonate treatment allowed to normalize acid-base parameters during the sustained infusion of lactic acid, but led to overshoot alkalization during the transient load of acid that affected lactate washout kinetics and glucose metabolism.

A number of animal experiments have been conducted to investigate lactic acidosis. As opposed to other more clinically relevant models such as hypoxia [16–18;29], sepsis [30;31], hemorrhage [20], phenformin intoxication [15;32] or hepatectomy [32], in this study we used an infusion of lactic acid in normoxic and normotensive animals to titrate systemic blood lactate concentrations and pH. While alkali treatment during hypoxia or hemodynamic instability may interfere with the cause and the systemic effects of the underlying acidemia, our model allowed to investigate changes of pH and lactate kinetics without possible confounding variables such as oxygen delivery impairment, mitochondrial defects or abnormalities of lactate clearance.

The effects of lactic acid load in our experiments were straightforward: pH consistently drop down to less than 7.2, while lactate rose to clinically significant levels. The acidemia that

Table 3. Lactate pharmacokinetics.

	T	T+B
Lac$_{basal}$ (mmol/l)	1.3±0.1	1.3±0.1
Lac clearance (ml/kg/min)	13.3±0.8	14.5±1.1
BLP (μmol/kg/min)	17.65±1.2	18.4±1.4
Lac$_{75'}$ (mmol/l)	5.5±0.4	5.2±0.5
b	0.354±0.106	0.19±0.101[a]
T ½ (min)	4.294±0.736	17.983±7.592[a]
c	−0.0589±0.038	0.116±0.058[a]

Mann-Whitney Rank Sum Test P<0.05:
[a]T+B vs. T.
Lac$_{basal}$, lactate concentration at baseline; Lac clearance, clearance of exogenous lactate; BLP, basal lactate production; Lac$_{75'}$, lactate concentration at time 75; b, coefficient b; T ½, half time decay; c, coefficient c.
Data are expressed as mean ± SEM.

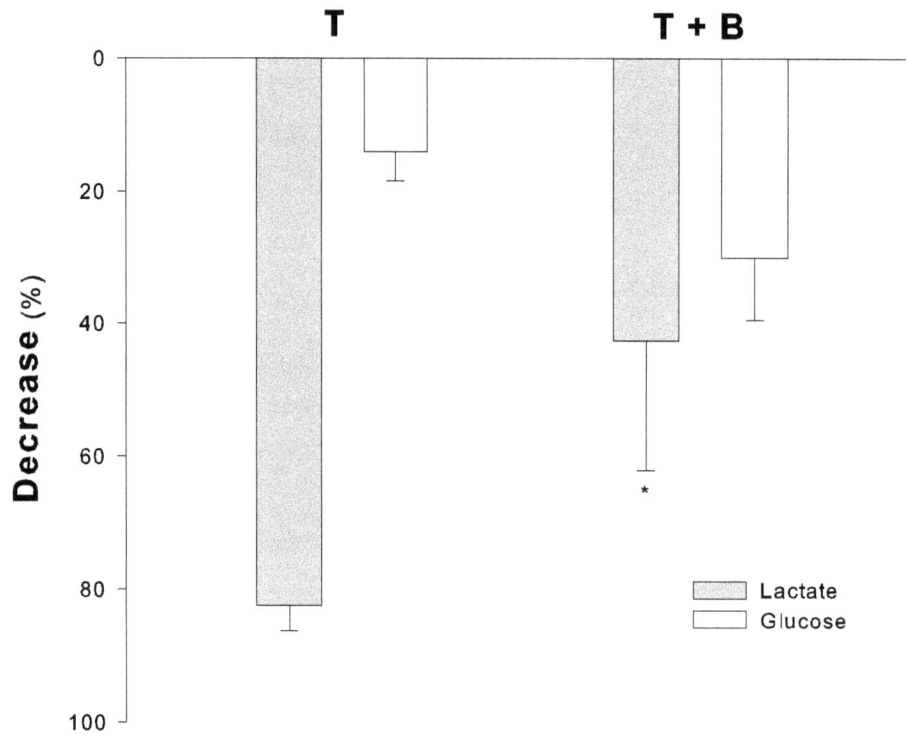

Figure 4. Blood lactate and blood glucose decrease in transient lactic acid infusion group. Decrease over time of blood lactate concentration and glycaemia in the animals with transient lactic acid infusion. Values are expressed as percentage decrease from time 75 to 135 (*P<0.05 vs. transient group).

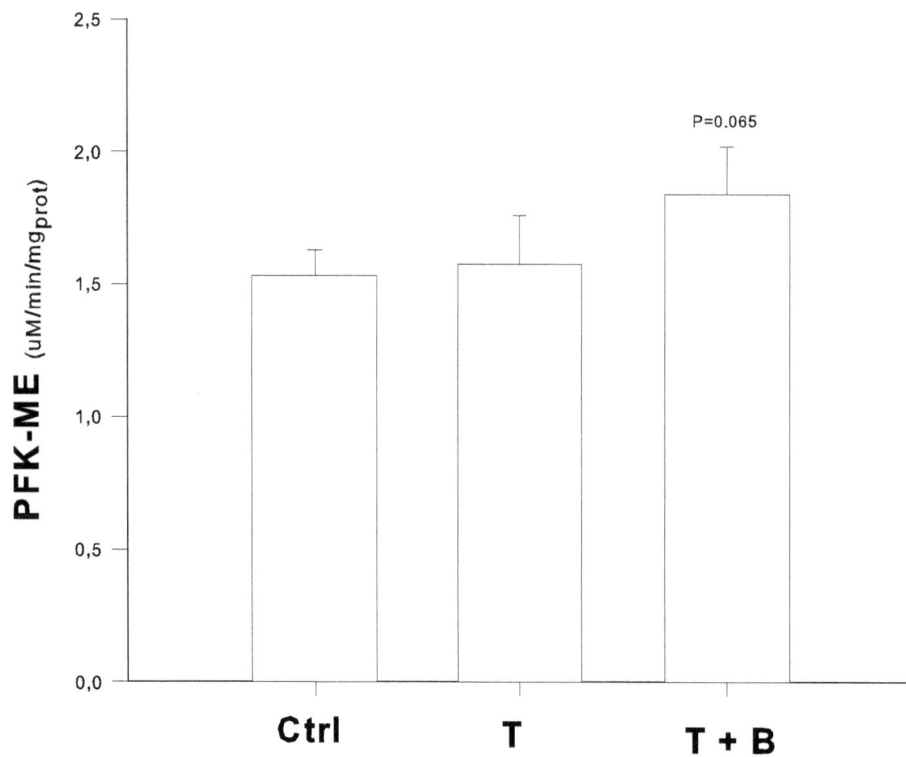

Figure 5. PFK activity. Activity of the glycolytic enzyme phosphofructokinase (PFK) in the glycolitic muscle (ME- extensor digitorum longus) was slightly higher when bicarbonate was infused (P = 0.067). Ctrl = end of lactic acid infusion (i.e 75′ after the start of acid load).

developed was of mixed origin: despite hemodiluition and hyperchloremia, pH changes were mainly due to lactate, as shown by the correlation between base excess drop and lactate rise. However a respiratory contribution to the drop of pH was also evident, whereas minute ventilation was unchanged throughout the protocol. In line with previous experiences [15], the induction of lactic acidemia resulted in a degree of mortality rate. However, at the beginning of randomization animals included in the randomization process were normoxic and normotensive.

After the randomization, pH drop over time during the sustained infusion of lactic acid. Even if not significant, there was a rise in lactate levels. Since $PaCO_2$ and electrolyte concentrations did not change through the randomization, lactate increase may be interpreted as an extra load of organic acid.

Sodium bicarbonate treatment caused pH to rise. Alkalinization mainly occurred because of a sodium dependent change of SIDa, with some possible contribution of the reduction of weak acids due to hemodilution. The role of respiratory alkalosis was negligible, consistent with the fact that the release of CO_2 is known to occur early after the infusion of sodium bicarbonate and depends on both the infusion rate and the concentration of non-bicarbonate buffers [33–35] that was relatively low during the randomization time.

Although the starting concentration of bicarbonate was similar in S+B and T+B groups, pH normalized during sustained infusions of lactic acid (from 7.22 ± 0.02 to 7.36 ± 0.04) while increased up to alkalemic values (from 7.24 ± 0.01 to 7.53 ± 0.03) when acid latic infusion was transient. Re-perfusion of hypoperfused or ischemic territories is characterized by an organic acid washout and a transient acid load, that cause a transient pH decrease. In this case sodium bicarbonate infusion may exceed the desired effect of reversing acidemia. On the contrary, the normalization of pH during sustained lactic acid infusion seems to be relevant, even if we did not find hemodynamic instability at low pH that many physicians advocate to start alkalinization therapy [25].

As expected, sodium significantly increased in both groups treated with bicarbonate. We also observed in these groups an oxygenation decrease probably due to a fluid load.

Bicarbonate infusion affected blood lactate levels differently during sustained or transient acidemia. In fact, lactate slightly rose in the S+B and S groups, but in a similar fashion. On the contrary, when the acid load was transient, at the end of the experiment lactate was significantly higher in the group of animals that received bicarbonate treatment (T+B). The abrupt and wide change of pH that followed bicarbonate infusion in this group possibly affected lactate metabolism, given the modulatory role of pH on blood levels of lactate [15–18;20;31]. Pharmacokinetic results suggest a reduction of the oxidation of lactate after bicarbonate infusion, according to Chiolerò et al. [26]. Lactate kinetics are also in line with those from Druml et al. who found that respiratory alkalosis decreases the clearance of infused lactic acid [36], and Abu Romeh et al. who found in a rat model of hypoxic lactic acidemia that systemic acidosis inhibits net lactic acid production. [29] Because it is known that pH modulates both glycolitic flow [37–40] and lactate cellular uptake [41–44], and because lactate undergoes preferential oxydation when in excess [45], we speculate that lactate was preferentially oxidated at low pH. On the contrary, when bicarbonate was infused, alkalosis favored glucose metabolism so that glucose levels decreased more than lactate and lactate half-life increased. The data on PFK activity seem to confirm this hypothesis.

Provided the effects of bicarbonate infusion on pH differed under a persistent or transient acid load and alkalization affected the rate of lactate disposal during the transient acid load, when deciding to infuse sodium bicarbonate one should take into consideration the metabolic effects of pH on the cell and the possible consequences on adaptation to energy failure [44;46–50].

Acknowledgments

The authors thank Fabio Ambrosetti for valuable technical support.

Author Contributions

Conceived and designed the experiments: FV LG. Performed the experiments: MP VS G. Chevallard TF SC SF SG. Analyzed the data: FP FF G. Comi. Contributed reagents/materials/analysis tools: FF G. Comi. Wrote the paper: FV MP VS SC SF LG.

References

1. Broder G, Weil M (1964) Excess lactate: an index of reversibility in human patients. Science 143(3613):1457–1459.
2. Weil M, Afifi A (1970) Experimental and clinical studies on lactate and pyruvate as indicators of the severity of acute circulatory failure (shock). Circulation 41(6):989–1001.
3. Vitek V, Cowley RA (1971) Blood lactate in the prognosis of various forms of shock. Ann Surg 173(2):308–313.
4. Cady LD, Weil MH, Afifi A, Michaels SF, Liu VY, et al. (1973) Quantitation of severity of critical illness with special reference to blood lactate. Crit Care Med1(2):75–80.
5. Bakker J, Coffernils M, Leon M, Gris P, Vincent JL (1991) Blood lactate levels are superior to oxygen-derived variables in predicting outcome in human septic shock. Chest 99(4):956–962.
6. Gunnerson KJ, Saul M, He S, Kellum JA (2006) Lactate versus non-lactate metabolic acidosis: a retrospective outcome evaluation of critically ill patients. Crit Care 10(1):R22.
7. Jansen TC, van Bommel J, Mulder PG, Rommes JH, Schieveld SJM, et al. (2008) The prognostic value of blood lactate levels relative to that of vital signs in the pre-hospital setting: a pilot study. Crit Care 12(6):R160.
8. Khosravani H, Shahpori R, Stelfox HT, Kirkpatrick AW, Laupland KB (2009) Occurrence and adverse effect on outcome of hyperlactatemia in the critically ill. Crit Care 13(3):R90.
9. Nichol AD, Egi M, Pettila V, Bellomo R, French C, et al (2010) Relative hyperlactatemia and hospital mortality in critically ill patients: a retrospective multi-centre study. Crit Care 14(1):R25.
10. Forsythe SM, Schmidt GA (2000) Sodium bicarbonate for the treatment of lactic acidosis. Chest, 117(1):260–267.
11. Rachoin JS, Weisberg, McFadden CB (2010) Treatment of lactic acidosis: appropriate confusion. J Hosp Med 5(4):E1–E7.
12. Arieff AI (1996) Current concepts in acid-base balance: use of bicarbonate in patients with metabolic acidosis. Current Anaesthesia & Critical Care 7:182–186.
13. Mathieu D, Neviere R, Billard V, Fleyfel M, Wattel F (1991) Effects of bicarbonate therapy on hemodynamics and tissue oxygenation in patients with lactic-acidosis: a prospective, controlled clinical study. Crit Care Med 19(11):1352–1356.
14. Cooper DJ, Walley KR, Wiggs BR, Russell JA (1990) Bicarbonate does not improve hemodynamics in critically ill patients who have lactic acidosis. A prospective, controlled clinical study. Ann Intern Med 112(7):492–498.
15. Arieff AI, Leach W, Park R, Lazarowitz VC (1982) Systemic effects of $NaHCO_3$ in experimental lactic acidosis in dogs. Am J Physiol 242(6):F586–F591.
16. Graf H, Leach W, Arieff AI (1985) Metabolic effects of sodium bicarbonate in hypoxic lactic acidosis in dogs. Am J Physiol 249(5Pt2):F630–F635.
17. Graf H, Leach W, Arieff AI (1985) Evidence for a detrimental effect of bicarbonate therapy in hypoxic lactic acidosis. Science 227(4688):754–756.
18. Rhee KH, Toro LO, McDonald GG, Nunnally RL, Levin DL(1993) Carbicarb, sodium bicarbonate, and sodium chloride in hypoxic lactic acidosis. Effect on arterial blood gases, lactate concentrations, hemodynamic variables, and myocardial intracellular pH. Chest 104(3):913–918.
19. Cooper DJ, Herbertson MJ, Werner HA, Walley KR (1993) Bicarbonate does not increase left ventricular contractility during L-lactic acidemia in pigs. Am Rev Respir Dis 148(2):317–322.
20. Benjamin E, Oropello JM, Abalos AM, Hannon EM, Wang JK, et al. (1994) Effects of acid-base correction on hemodynamics, oxygen dynamics, and resuscitability in severe canine hemorrhagic shock. Crit Care Med 22(10):1616–1623.
21. Tanaka M, Nishikawa T, Mizutani T (1996) Normovolaemic haemodilution attenuates cardiac depression induced by sodium bicarbonate in canine metabolic acidosis. Br J Anaesth 77(3):408–412.

22. Tanaka M, Nishikawa T (1997) Acute haemodynamic effects of sodium bicarbonate administration in respiratory and metabolic acidosis in anaesthetized dogs. Anaesth Intensive Care 25(6):615–620.

23. Boyd JH, Walley KR (2008) Is there a role for sodium bicarbonate in treating lactic acidosis from shock? Curr Opin Crit Care 14(4):379–383.

24. Dellinger RP, Levy MM, Carlet JM, Bion J, Parker MM, et al. (2008) Surviving Sepsis Campaign: international guidelines for management of severe sepsis and septic shock: 2008. Crit Care Med 36(1):296–327

25. Kraut JA, Kurtz I (2006) Use of base in the treatment of acute severe organic acidosis by nephrologists and critical care physicians: results of an online survey. Clin Exp Nephrol 10(2):111–117.

26. Chiolero R, Tappy L, Gillet M, Revelly JP, Roth H, et al. (1999) Effect of major hepatectomy on glucose and lactate metabolism. Ann Surg 229(4):505–513.

27. Ling K H, Byrne W, Lardy H (2010) Phoshoexokinase. In: S.P.. Colowick and N.0.. Kaplan, editors. Methods in enzymology. Academic Press Inc, New York. pp. 306–310.

28. Lowry OH, Rosebrough NJ, Farr AL, Randall RJ (1951) Protein measurement with the Folin phenol reagent. J Biol Chem 193(1):265–275.

29. Abu Romeh S, Tannen RL (1986) Amelioration of hypoxia-induced lactic acidosis by superimposed hypercapnea or hydrochloric acid infusion. Am J Physiol 250(4Pt 2):F702–F709.

30. Chrusch C, Bands C, Bose D, Li X, Jacobs H, et al. (2000) Impaired hepatic extraction and increased splanchnic production contribute to lactic acidosis in canine sepsis. Am J Respir Crit Care Med 161(2Pt 1):517–526.

31. Chrusch C, Bautista E, Jacobs HK, Light RB, Bose D, et al. (2002) Blood pH level modulates organ metabolism of lactate in septic shock in dogs. J Crit Care 17(3):188–202.

32. Park R, Arieff AI (1982) Treatment of lactic acidosis with dichloroacetate in dogs. J Clin Invest 70(4):853–862.

33. Gattinoni L, Taccone P, Carlesso E (2006) Respiratory acidosis: is the correction with bicarbonate worth? Minerva Anestesiol 72(6):551–557.

34. Levraut J, Garcia P, Giunti C, Ichai C, Bouregba M, et al. (2000) The increase in CO_2 production induced by $NaHCO_3$ depends on blood albumin and hemoglobin concentrations. Intensive Care Med 26(5):558–564.

35. Okamoto H, Hoka S, Kawasaki T, Okuyama T, Takahashi S (1995) Changes in end-tidal carbon dioxide tension following sodium bicarbonate administration: correlation with cardiac output and haemoglobin concentration. Acta Anaesthesiol Scand 39(1):79–84.

36. Druml W, Grimm G, Laggner AN, Lenz K, Schneeweiss B (1991) Lactic acid kinetics in respiratory alkalosis. Crit Care Med 19(9):1120–1124.

37. Hood VL, Tannen RL (1998) Protection of acid-base balance by pH regulation of acid production. N Engl J Med 339(12):819–826.

38. Pagliassotti MJ, Donovan CM (1990) Glycogenesis from lactate in rabbit skeletal muscle fiber types. Am J Physiol 258(4Pt 2):R903–R911.

39. Miller BF, Fattor JA, Jacobs KA, Horning MA, Navazio F, et al. (2002) Lactate and glucose interactions during rest and exercise in men: effect of exogenous lactate infusion. J Physiol 544(Pt3):963–975.

40. Hood VL, Tannen RL (1983) Ph control of lactic acid and keto acid production a mechanism of acid-base regulation. Miner Electrolyte Metab 9(4–6):317–325.

41. Sestoft L, Marshall MO (1986) Hepatic lactate uptake is enhanced by low pH at low lactate concentrations in perfused rat liver. Clin Sci Lond 70(1):19–22.

42. Baron PG, Iles RA, Cohen RD (1978) Effect of varying PCO_2 on intracellular pH and lactate consumption in the isolated perfused rat liver. Clin Sci Mol Med 55(2):175–181.

43. Roth DA, Brooks GA (1990) Lactate and pyruvate transport is dominated by a pH gradient-sensitive carrier in rat skeletal muscle sarcolemmal vesicles. Arch Biochem Biophys 279(2):386–394.

44. Halestrap AP, Price NT (1999) The proton-linked monocarboxylate transporter (MCT) family: structure, function and regulation. Biochem J 343(Pt2):281–299.

45. Hollidge-Horvat MG, Parolin ML, Wong D, Jones NL, Heigenhauser GJ (1999) Effect of induced metabolic acidosis on human skeletal muscle metabolism during exercise. Am J Physiol 277(4Pt 1):E647–E658.

46. Valenza F, Aletti G, Fossali T, Chevallard G, Sacconi F, et al. (2005) Lactate as a marker of energy failure in critically ill patients: hypothesis. Crit Care 9(6):588–593.

47. Kitano T, Nisimaru N, Shibata E, Iwasaka H, Noguchi T, et al. (2002) Lactate utilization as an energy substrate in ischemic preconditioned rat brain slices. Life Sci 72(4–5):557–564.

48. Pellerin L (2003) Lactate as a pivotal element in neuron-glia metabolic cooperation. Neurochem Int 43(4–5):331–338.

49. Leverve XM (1999) Energy metabolism in critically ill patients: lactate is a major oxidizable substrate. Curr Opin Clin Nutr Metab Care 2(2):165–169.

50. Leverve XM (2001) Inter-organ substrate exchanges in the critically ill. Curr Opin Clin Nutr Metab Care 4(2):137–142.

23

Selective use of Sequential Digital Dermoscopy Imaging Allows a Cost Reduction in the Melanoma Detection Process: A Belgian Study of Patients with a Single or a Small Number of Atypical Nevi

Isabelle Tromme[1]*, **Brecht Devleesschauwer**[2], **Philippe Beutels**[3], **Pauline Richez**[1], **Nicolas Praet**[4], **Laurine Sacré**[1], **Liliane Marot**[1], **Pascal Van Eeckhout**[1], **Ivan Theate**[1], **Jean-François Baurain**[5], **Julien Lambert**[6], **Catherine Legrand**[7], **Luc Thomas**[8], **Niko Speybroeck**[2]

1 Department of Dermatology, Centre du Cancer, Cliniques Universitaires St Luc, Université catholique de Louvain, Brussels, Belgium, 2 Institute of Health and Society, Faculty of Public Health, Université catholique de Louvain, Brussels, Belgium, 3 Centre for Health Economics Research & Modelling Infectious Diseases, Vaccine & Infectious Disease Institute, Faculty of Medicine & Health Sciences, University of Antwerp, Antwerp, Belgium, 4 Department of Biomedical Sciences, Institute of Tropical Medicine, Antwerp, Belgium, 5 Department of Medical Oncology, Centre du Cancer, Cliniques Universitaires St Luc, Université catholique de Louvain, Brussels, Belgium, 6 Department of Dermatology, Universitair Ziekenhuis, Antwerp, Belgium, 7 Institute of Statistics, Biostatistics and Actuarial Sciences, Université catholique de Louvain, Louvain-la-Neuve, Belgium, 8 Department of Dermatology, Lyon 1 University, Centre Hospitalier Lyon Sud, Pierre Bénite, France

Abstract

Background: Dermoscopy is a technique which improves melanoma detection. Optical dermoscopy uses a handheld optical device to observe the skin lesions without recording the images. Sequential digital dermoscopy imaging (SDDI) allows storage of the pictures and their comparison over time. Few studies have compared optical dermoscopy and SDDI from an economic perspective.

Objective: The present observational study focused on patients with one-to-three atypical melanocytic lesions, i.e. lesions considered as suspicious by optical dermoscopy. It aimed to calculate the "extra-costs" related to the process of melanoma detection. These extra-costs were defined as the costs of excision and pathology of benign lesions and/or the costs of follow-up by SDDI. The objective was to compare these extra-costs when using optical dermoscopy exclusively versus optical dermoscopy with selective use of SDDI.

Methods: In a first group of patients, dermatologists were adequately trained in optical dermoscopy but worked without access to SDDI. They excised all suspicious lesions to rule out melanoma. In a second group, the dermatologists were trained in optical and digital dermoscopy. They had the opportunity of choosing between immediate excision or follow-up by SDDI (with delayed excision if significant change was observed). The comparison of extra-costs in both groups was made possible by a decision tree model and by the division of the extra-costs by the number of melanomas diagnosed in each group. Belgian official tariffs and charges were used.

Results: The extra-costs in the first and in the second group were respectively €1,613 and €1,052 per melanoma excised. The difference was statistically significant.

Conclusions: Using the Belgian official tariffs and charges, we demonstrated that the selective use of SDDI for patients with one-to-three atypical melanocytic lesions resulted in a significant cost reduction.

Editor: Nikolas K. Haass, University of Queensland Diamantina Institute, Australia

Funding: One of the authors (IT) was supported by the Nuovo-Soldati Foundation for Cancer Research. The funders had no role in study design, data collection and analysis, decision to publish, or preparation of the manuscript.

* Email: isabelle.tromme@uclouvain.be

Introduction

Cutaneous melanoma is one of the prime causes of death by cancer in the young Caucasian adult population [1]. Incidence, expressed as lifetime risk, is around 1–2% in Western Europe and the US and is still increasing in many countries [2]. Early detection and immediate surgery is the most effective treatment in reducing mortality. In order to favor this early detection, a technique called "dermoscopy" has been introduced in 1980s.

Optical dermoscopy (OD) is a non-invasive technique that uses a handheld, magnifying, optical device that suppresses light reflection by the stratum corneum either by liquid immersion or by cross-light polarization. It allows the observation of features invisible to the naked eye. Its efficacy to improve diagnostic accuracy for melanoma in a clinical setting has been proven in a meta-analysis [3]. However, this improvement is linked to examiners' training and experience in the technique [4].

Sequential digital dermoscopy imaging (SDDI) allows the storage and retrieval of dermoscopic images, offering a time-lapse comparative analysis of the cutaneous pigmented lesions at different time intervals. The main interest of the technique relates to atypical melanocytic lesions, which are impossible to diagnose by OD as being either benign nevi or very early melanomas. Besides pathological examination, which requires prior excision and diagnoses the nature of the lesions, only the monitoring of the evolution of the lesions helps determining its benign or malignant nature. SDDI has been proven to favor earlier melanoma detection, including melanomas lacking clinical and dermoscopic features for melanoma (so-called "featureless melanomas") [5–8]. The literature about SDDI often focuses on its use in patients with a large number of nevi. Nevertheless, SDDI is also commonly used to monitor a single or a small number of atypical melanocytic lesions [9,10].

Both OD and SDDI have two main objectives: (i) to enhance sensitivity in the melanoma detection, (ii) to increase specificity through reduction of unnecessary excisions of benign lesions.

The present observational study, performed in a clinical setting, focused on patients with one-to-three atypical melanocytic lesions (i.e., lesions considered as suspicious by OD examination) and studied them from a medico-economic point of view. The objective was to compare the costs related to the process of melanoma detection in two situations: (i) the dermatologist, well trained in OD but without access to SDDI, was obliged to excise the lesions to exclude a melanoma, (ii) the dermatologist, well trained in OD and SDDI, had the choice between excision upfront or follow-up by SDDI, leading or not to subsequent excision.

Materials and Methods

Design overview

The present study is a cost comparison of two intervention options for patients presenting to dermatologists because of the patient's concern for melanoma, and having one-to-three atypical/suspicious nevi. The two options were: (i) excision of all suspicious lesions and (ii) excision of highly suspicious and SDDI of slightly or moderately suspicious lesions. It is an observational study of the two options in terms of costs with a common clinical outcome (excisions of benign lesions per patient). We use the observations in a decision tree model to make inferences on the incremental costs between the two patient groups (on a per-patient basis through bootstrapping).

We used the database of the DEPIMELA observational study presented elsewhere [11]. In brief, the inclusion period of the DEPIMELA study ran from 1/10/2009 to 30/9/2010. The present study included all the consecutive patients with one-to-three atypical melanocytic lesions seen during the DEPIMELA study by (i) dermatologists who used OD with adequate training (Group 1) and (ii) dermatologists who used OD and who, in addition, had access to SDDI, with adequate training in both techniques (Group 2). Patients with more than three atypical nevi were excluded from this study. Patients who were already monitored by SDDI for atypical nevi were also excluded. The lesions monitored by SDDI were selected atypical melanocytic lesions. The dermatologists having access to SDDI used the latter only if they considered it helpful in addition to OD (i.e., for difficult lesions). This is referred to as "selective use of SDDI".

The main aim of this study was to compare the costs related to the process of melanoma in Groups 1 and 2. We excluded the costs of melanoma excisions and pathology because these should be the same for each correctly diagnosed melanoma, irrespective of which group they belonged to. Because of this exclusion, the costs were referred as "extra-costs" in this paper. In Group 1, the extra-costs included costs of excision and pathology of benign lesions excised. In Group 2, the extra-costs included costs of SDDI and/or costs of excision and pathology of benign lesions excised.

OD was performed with a Delta 20 Dermoscope (Heine, Herrshing, Germany) or a Dermoscope DermoGenius Basic II (Linos Photonics, Munich, Germany). For SDDI, the dermatologists in our study used the FotoFinder Dermoscope (Teachscreen Software, Bad Birnbach, Germany).

Reference diagnosis was pathological analysis in Group 1, pathological analysis or stability of the SDDI picture after a minimum of three months in Group 2.

The DEPIMELA study was approved on 28 November 2008 by the ethics committee of the Université catholique de Louvain (number B40320085012). Part of the medical file was copied by the dermatologist in a structured document to provide the elements needed by the study. At that time, the patient gave his verbal consent, which was acknowledged by the dermatologist. A written consent was not required in this kind of observational study. Indeed, the subject of the present survey was the practice of the dermatologists and the economical consequences of the technique they used, rather than the patients themselves. The latter freely chose their dermatologist irrespective of the study (and were not randomized). The ethics committee approved this procedure.

Setting and participants

Group 1. Twelve volunteer dermatologists adequately trained in OD were recruited from French-speaking Belgian private and hospital practices without access to SDDI. Populations seen by these dermatologists were not statistically different in terms of age, sex and risk factors for melanoma (p values>0.1). We included the following risk factors: (i) a personal history of melanoma, (ii) a family history of melanoma (at least 2 melanomas in first-degree relatives), (iii) Fitzpatrick's skin phototype I (very fair skin) or (iv) a stay of at least one year in a tropical country before the age of 15. They were a priori not different in terms of social status and access to a dermatologist (approximation assessed according to the fact that all the dermatologists had mixed private/non private facilities). The dermatologists were considered as adequately trained if (i) they had received more than ten hours of initial training in OD and (ii) they maintained self-training. They included all consecutive patients who had one-to-three melanocytic lesions which were excised because of low to high suspicion of melanoma. Patients who had asked for the excision for cosmetic or comfort reasons were excluded, if the dermatologist had no doubt about the benignancy of the lesion.

Group 2. Ten dermatologists from an academic dermatology department (Cliniques Universitaires St Luc, Brussels, Belgium), agreed to refer to the department's pigmented lesion clinic (PLC) all their patients with any melanoma suspicion and any lesion they would have removed to exclude a melanoma. The PLC was run by two dermatologists adequately trained in OD and SDDI. The PLC dermatologist decided either to excise the lesions or to monitor these by SDDI. The reasons for excision were: (i) high suspicion of melanoma in a flat lesion, (ii) any suspicion of melanoma in a raised lesion (in order not to miss an advanced melanoma), and (iii) any suspicion of melanoma if the patient refused the follow-up by SDDI.

The monitoring by SDDI was conducted after three months and after nine additional months. Three months is the commonly accepted interval before the first follow-up [12] and has been shown to detect 93% of *in situ* melanomas of the non-lentigo maligna type and 96% of invasive melanomas [5]. Patients missing the first check-up were called and offered another appointment. A second follow-up after one year is ideal to detect the remaining proportion of so-called "slow-growing" melanomas [13]. This second follow-up was presented as optional for patients with moderately atypical lesions and without any of the aforementioned risk factors for melanoma. In these cases, patients were instructed to observe their lesion and return if any change was observed. Excision was performed if any significant change was observed, according to the literature [7,12].

Outcomes

The present study analysed a part of the DEPIMELA study database from an economic point of view. The aim was to compare the extra-costs in both Groups. In Group 1, the extra-costs included the excision costs of all the benign nevi excised because of having been considered as suspicious by dermatologists well trained in OD: in Group 2, the extra-costs included the SDDI follow-up costs and/or benign lesions excision costs when patients were monitored in a place where SDDI was available. We first computed the observed costs in both groups, then the simulated costs of both groups obtained from a decision-tree model. The latter allowed us to obtain an idea of the uncertainty of our results.

Costs

Unit costs were based on official tariffs and charges in Belgium in 2012 [14] (Table 1). Although the coverage of OD and SDDI by the national Belgian health care system only became effective on 1/3/2014, we used the 2012 figures because we already knew their official reimbursement amounts in November 2012. The SDDI examination official cost includes: (a) total body examination by OD, (b) electronic storage of atypical nevi dermoscopic pictures and (c) localization of these nevi on the body. This cost is added to the cost of the consultation. Currently, the following restrictions for reimbursement of the SDDI examination costs apply in Belgium: (i) SDDI is only reimbursed for patients with a personal history of melanoma, a family history of melanoma (at least two melanomas in first-degree relatives) or patients with Atypical Mole Syndrome (AMS) (simplified from Newton Bishop's definition: ≥ 100 nevi and ≥2 atypical nevi) [15]; (ii) irrespective of the number of OD and/or SDDI examinations per year, only one OD and only one SDDI examinations are reimbursed per year. Nevertheless, in our comparative cost analysis, we applied these unit costs to every unit of associated resource use, as if (i) the reimbursement would be effective for all the patients (irrespective of their history or phenotype) and (ii) the number of SDDI reimbursements in a year would not be limited.

The costs were calculated using the currently prevailing treatment pathways in Belgium. We considered the most common situation which is the following. The patient is examined during a first consultation and the possible decision to excise a lesion is discussed at this time. The excision is performed a few days or weeks thereafter. The stitches are removed and the scar is checked by the general practitioner. If several excisions are performed the same day, the second and the third excision costs are divided by two and the pathology cost remains the same for one or more lesions. We took into account the observed number of patients

with two or three excisions made the same day to calculate the extra-costs. Regarding immunohistochemistry, it is generally admitted that this is useful to exclude melanomas in cases of nevi with severe atypia. These nevi are much more frequent in the second group as demonstrated in the DEPIMELA study [11]. We assumed that two immunostains (HMB 45 and a cocktail of antibodies including gp100, tyrosinase and MelanA) were performed in a number of benign nevi equivalent to the number of melanomas in each group. In accordance with Belgian guidelines [16], personal non-medical costs such as travel fare as well as indirect costs due to absence from work for the consultations or because of scarring were not taken into account.

Classification bias

It cannot be excluded that some lesions followed by SDDI were in fact (very) slow-growing melanomas. Nevertheless, the vast majority of the patients continued to be monitored in our institution. We have, therefore, followed up these patients for more than three years. In addition, it cannot be excluded that some melanomas could have been missed in the first group but would have been correctly diagnosed if included in the second group.

Selection bias

Social status and access to a dermatologist were not measured and can therefore be considered as a potential bias.

Data analysis

Both groups were compared using a cost comparison focused on the costs of unnecessary excision and/or follow-up costs. These costs were defined as "extra-costs" because the costs of melanoma excisions and pathology were not taken into account (these should be the same for each correctly diagnosed melanoma, irrespective of which group they belonged to). The extra-costs were calculated by patient and not by lesion because several lesions were excised or monitored by SDDI at the same time, which reduced the costs per patient in both cases. The extra-costs were then divided by the number of melanomas detected in each group, to obtain an "additional cost per diagnosed melanoma".

Statistical analysis

A decision-tree model was developed to assess the statistical significance of the total extra-cost difference between both groups [17]. A probabilistic sensitivity analysis (PSA) was integrated in the model to express parameter uncertainty [18]. Data derived parameter distributions were defined based on the clinical characteristics of both groups (Table 2), and the unit costs listed in table 1 were attributed on the simulated values drawn from these parameter distributions. All calculations were performed in R 3.0.1 (R Core Team, 2013) [19]. For each of the 10,000 iterations of the model, a value was sampled from each parameter distribution, such that a distribution of 10,000 estimates was obtained from each outcome (with the cost difference between both groups being the primary outcome of interest). We will report the proportion of iterations resulting in OD being more expensive than selective SDDI. To assess which input parameters had the greatest influence on the variability in the overall output, i.e. the cost difference between both groups, we complemented the PSA with a variable importance analysis. We calculated standardized regression coefficients as a measure of variable importance. These were obtained by first standardizing the input parameters and the output (i.e. subtracting the mean and dividing by the standard deviation), and subsequently regressing the standardized input

Table 1. Current unit costs in Belgium (2012), expressed in Euros.

Item	Cost
Dermatologist's consultation cost	28.88
General practitioner's consultation cost	23.67
Cutaneous tumor excision with suture	54.10
Second cutaneous tumor excision with suture	27.05
Cutaneous tumor(s) pathology	62.02
Immunohistochemistry	25.41
Optical dermoscopy	6.39
Sequential digital dermoscopy imaging	23.22

Costs are the same in academic hospitals and non-academic hospitals or private practices.

parameters against the standardized output. R code is available as supplementary file to the manuscript (Code S1).

Results

Patients' progress in Group 1 and 2 are summarized in Figure 1.

Group 1

Of the 7,434 patients examined during one year for melanoma detection, 603 were eligible for this study and underwent surgery. There was no patient with more than three atypical/suspicious nevi who had to be excluded (probably because patients with many atypical nevi were either referred to a PLC or underwent regular excisions of their new atypical/suspicious nevi). The mean age of these 603 patients was 41 years (from 4 to 86 years) and the sex ratio (M:F) was 0.57. Six hundred and forty excisions were performed, leading to the diagnosis of 70 melanomas. The melanoma/non-melanoma ratio (M/NM-R) was 1/8.14. Regarding benign lesions, excision and pathology observed costs were €112,920, which can also be expressed as €1,613 for every melanoma excised.

Group 2

During the same year, 1,926 patients were examined for melanoma detection and 219 were eligible for the present study.

The mean age of these 219 patients was 39 years (from 14 to 88 years) and the sex ratio (M:F) was 0.58. Eighty-eight patients required immediate excision of suspicious lesions, leading to the diagnosis of 29 melanomas. Seven patients underwent excision because they refused the SDDI monitoring; all these lesions were diagnosed as benign by pathology. The 124 remaining patients agreed to be monitored by SDDI for a total of 157 lesions. The short-term follow-up was planned after three months. Six patients missed their appointment and were re-contacted. Finally, all the 124 patients were examined within six months. Eleven lesions had changed after 3 months and were excised, three of these were melanomas. A second check by SDDI after one year was suggested to the 113 remaining patients. The dermatologists insisted on the importance of this examination in patients with very atypical lesions and/or with identified other melanoma risk factors. All these patients came to this one year appointment, as well as many other patients of this group, even if this appointment had been presented to them as optional. Only 23 patients did not show-up after 18 months. They all were clearly informed they had to observe their nevi and to request a visit in case of change. However, none came back for this reason. The second follow-up visit led to the excision of five monitored lesions, which were all diagnosed as benign by pathology. Finally, 32 melanomas and 79 non-melanomas were excised: the total M/NM-R was 1/2.47. The three melanomas excised after the short-term SDDI visit were *in situ* for two of them and very early invasive (Clark level II,

Table 2. Parameter distributions for probabilistic uncertainty analysis.

Parameter	Group 1 Distribution	Group 1 Mean	Group 1 Range	Group 2 Distribution	Group 2 Mean	Group 2 Range
Number of patients with unnecessary excisions	Binomial (7434, 533/7434)	533	490–577	Binomial (1926, 79/1926)	79	62–96
Proportion of patients with >1 unnecessary excision	Beta (33, 500)	0.06	0.04–0.08	0	–	–
Average number of unnecessary excisions per patient	Gamma (570, 533)	1.07	0.98–1.16	1	–	–
Number of excised Melanomas	Poisson (70)	70	54–87	Poisson (32)	32	21–44
Number of patients registered by SDDI at inclusion time	–	–	–	Poisson (124)	124	103–146
Proportion of patients followed up by SDDI at 3–6 months	–	–	–	1	–	–
Proportion of patients followed up by SDDI at 12 months	–	–	–	Beta (90, 34)	0.73	0.64–0.80

SDDI = Sequential Digital Dermoscopy Imaging.
The mean is defined as the mean of the distribution. The range is constructed as the 2.5[th] and 97.5[th] of the concerned distribution. We assumed the different parameters in that table to be independent.

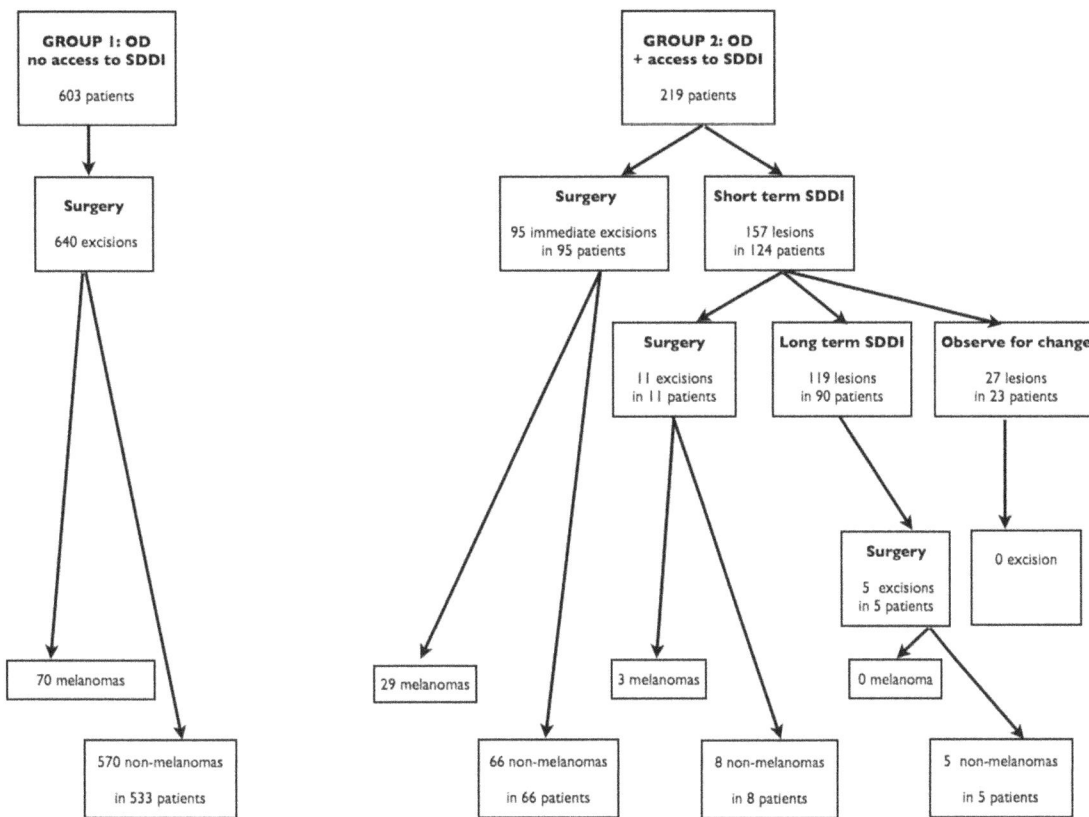

Figure 1. Study flowchart. The evolution of the patients is divided into two groups. In Group 1, patients were examined by dermatologists adequately trained in optical dermoscopy (OD). In Group 2, patients were examined by dermatologists adequately trained in optical dermoscopy and who had access to sequential digital dermoscopy imaging (SDDI).

0.2 mm of Breslow's thickness) for the remaining case. The total observed extra-cost was €33,658 and was nearly equally distributed between excision and pathology costs (€17,233) and SDDI follow-up costs (€16,425). The extra-cost, for each melanoma excised, was €1,052 in Group 2. The follow-up period for the DEPIMELA study was one year. In addition, most patients have been seen in the institution during the following 2.5 years and any melanoma was reported.

Comparison of Group 1 and Group 2

The observed total direct extra-costs in Group 1 versus Group 2 are shown Figure 2. This figure shows also the decision-tree model which was used to simulate the extra-costs resulting from melanoma detection. Parameter distributions for probabilistic uncertainty analysis are presented in Table 2. Through this probabilistic uncertainty analysis we estimated the mean cost difference between Group 2 and Group 1 at €548 (95% credibility interval: 65–1856) (Figure 3, Table 3). The extra-costs per melanoma excised presented in Table 3 (€1,633 in Group 1 and €1,085 in Group 2) and the extra-cost per melanoma excised presented in Figure 2 (€1,613 in Group 1 and €1,052 in Group 2) are different because the first ones were simulated and the second ones were observed. The proportion of iterations, resulting in OD being more expensive than selective SDDI, was equal to 96.5%. At a 5% significance level, this indicates a significant statistical difference between the extra-costs in both groups. Figure 4 shows the tornado graph (i.e., standardized regression coefficients of the different parameters, ranked according to their absolute values). The coefficients reflect how many standard deviations the output

will change per standard deviation increase in an input. The largest source of uncertainty is, logically, the number of excised melanomas in both groups (denoted "Mela OD" and "Mela SDDI"). The R-squared of the variable importance regression model was 0.95.

Discussion

The present observational study, performed in a clinical setting, focused on patients with one-to-three suspicious melanocytic lesions (i.e., lesions considered as suspicious by OD examination) and studied them from a medico-economic point of view. From a sample of 822 patients, we showed that, when a dermatologist well trained in dermoscopy had the choice between excision and follow-up by SDDI (leading or not to subsequent excision), the extra-costs were statistically lower than if he was obliged to excise the lesions in order to rule out melanoma. Extra-costs included costs of SDDI and/or costs of excision and pathology of benign lesions excised.

To the best of our knowledge, this is the first medico-economic study on SDDI. This technique is reimbursed in Belgium and in several other European countries but, in most countries, only for patients at high risk for melanoma (i.e., mainly patients with personal history of melanoma and/or AMS). It has probably been assumed that SDDI is cost-effective in these groups. We studied patients with one-to-three suspicious melanocytic lesions. Most of them were at low risk for melanoma. In the Belgian context, the costs borne by these patients are higher with selective SDDI follow-up (where reimbursement is not covered) than in the case of

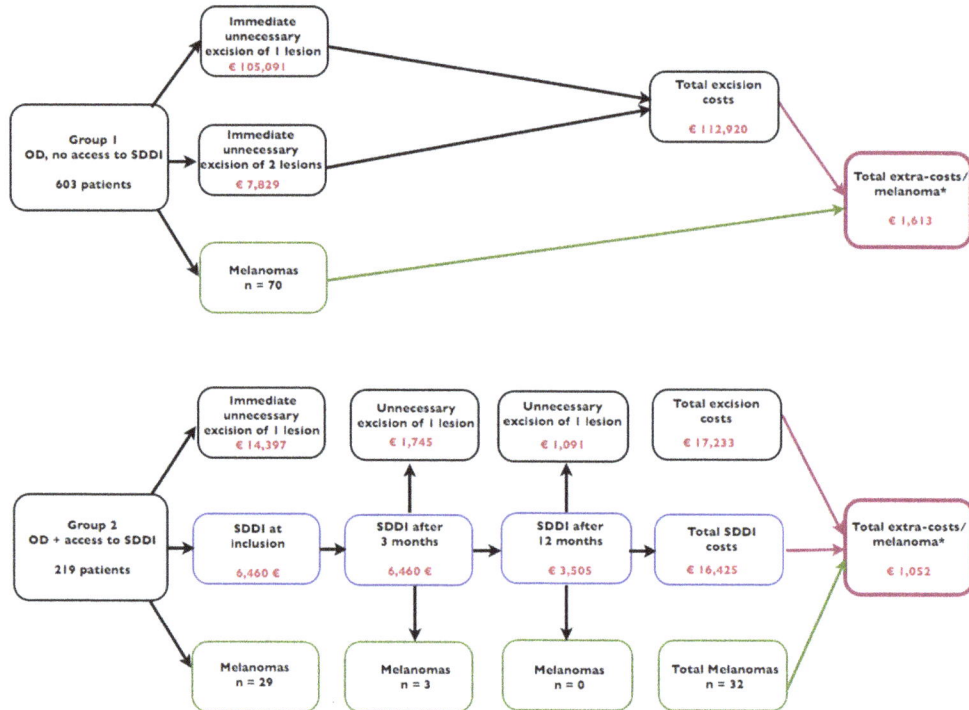

Figure 2. Observed total direct extra-costs distributed in the decision-tree model. This figure shows the observed total direct extra-costs distributed in a decision tree model. In Group 1, patients were examined by dermatologists adequately trained in optical dermoscopy (OD). In Group 2, patients were examined by dermatologists adequately trained in optical dermoscopy and who had access to sequential digital dermoscopy imaging (SDDI). *Melanoma excision costs are not taken into account because these should be the same for each correctly diagnosed melanoma, irrespective of which group they belonged to.

systematic excision (which is completely reimbursed). However, we have shown that the costs borne by the national health care system were higher in the case of systematic excision, including if the SDDI costs are reimbursed without restriction. As a result, we believe that, in Belgium, all patients' SDDI costs should be reimbursed.

We excluded patients with many atypical nevi because most of them are classified in the AMS [15]. This syndrome increases the

melanoma risk, not only because a melanoma can arise on an atypical nevus but, predominantly, because the skin of these patients is at high risk of generating melanomas from isolated melanocytes. Therefore, these patients must, ideally, be monitored by SDDI for many years and the method of analyzing the costs of this follow-up should be different from the method used in the present study.

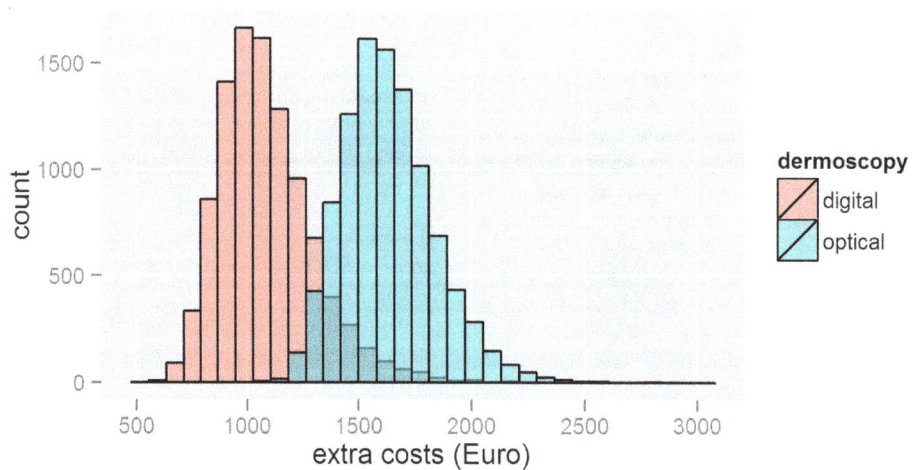

Figure 3. Histogram of the estimated extra costs of sequential digital dermoscopy imaging versus optical dermoscopy. The extra-costs are defined as the costs of excision and pathology of benign lesions and/or the costs of follow-up by sequential digital dermoscopy imaging. These extra-costs are divided by the number of melanomas diagnosed in each group.

Table 3. Simulated costs of excision, pathology and/or follow-up of benign lesions, expressed in Euros (mean+95% credibility interval).

	Group 1[a]	Group 2[a]	Difference[b]
Excisions*	76,536 (70,314–82,850)	10,710 (8403–13,011)	65,82 (60,289–78,320)
Pathology**	36,394 (33,512–39,355)	6529 (5240–7893)	29,86 (27,160–35,586)
Follow-up by SDDI***	-	16,419 (13,510–19,475)	−16,419 (−18,967– −10,971)
Total	112,929 (103,947–121,967)	33,658 (29,052–38,257)	79,271 (70,902–98,963)
Total/melanoma diagnosed	1633 (1289–2091)	1085 (758–1588)	548 (65–1856)

*Includes consultations, optical dermoscopy in Group 1, and surgery.
**Includes classical pathology and immunohistochemistry for very atypical nevi.
***Includes consultations and sequential digital dermoscopy imaging.
[a]Two-sided 95% credibility interval (constructed as the distribution's 2.5[th] and 97.5[th] percentile).
[b]One-sided upper 95% credibility interval (constructed as the distribution's 5th and 100th percentile).

The present study focused on patients with one-to-three suspicious melanocytic lesions, divided into two groups. In Group 1, patients were examined by dermatologists adequately trained in OD. In Group 2, patients were examined by dermatologists adequately trained in OD and having access to SDDI if needed. The extra-costs in the first and in the second group were respectively €1,613 and €1,052 per melanoma diagnosed. The gain linked to SDDI selective use was more than €500 per melanoma diagnosed. Since the acquisition cost of the SDDI equipment was around €20,000 in 2012, its appropriate use in hospitals could win back the excess investment for the health care payer to correctly diagnose melanoma (even when ignoring SDDI's benefits to AMS patients, as we did here). Nevertheless, irrefutable evidence of this would require specific prospective studies.

The cost difference between both groups is closely related to the M/NM-Rs differences. The M/NM-Rs were 1/8.14 in Group 1 and 1/2.47 in Group 2. It could be argued that this difference between both M/NM-Rs was linked to a higher level of experience in OD in Group 2. However, the skill level in OD is limited by the technology itself. Most atypical nevi cannot be differentiated from very early melanomas and their evolution over time is the only way to have more information. It could also be

argued that this difference was partially due to a different population in a University hospital (Group 2). Interestingly, if all the lesions considered as moderately suspicious and monitored by SDDI without final excision had been added to the non-melanoma lesions excised in Group 2, the M/NM-R in Group 2 would be 1/7.78. This number is not statistically different from the 1/8.14 in Group 1 (p value = 0.2).

Even with the availability of SDDI, the number of excised benign lesions will never be reduced to zero for several reasons: (i) raised ambiguous melanocytic lesions should not be monitored because of the risk of missing an advanced melanoma, (ii) excision of Spitz nevi is generally recommended, even if it is controversial for typical lesions in children [20], (iii) some clinically and dermoscopically atypical nevi mimic melanomas and will always be excised.

Kittler et al. found in an experimental study that the possibility of follow-up by SDDI reduced the number of benign excised lesions, but only by very experienced dermoscopists [21]. This allows us to insist on the fact that our results cannot be extrapolated to beginners in dermoscopy: if the excision rate does not decrease thanks to SDDI availability, the costs would probably be higher in the second group. As mentioned by Kittler et al in the same publication [21], compliance is a critical point for the success

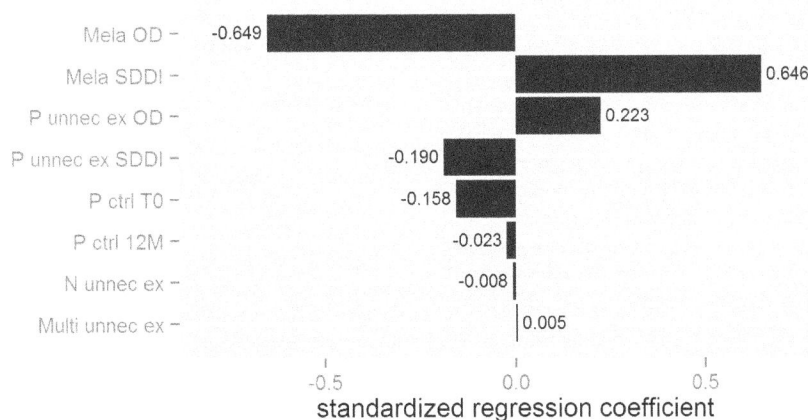

Figure 4. Sensitivity analysis: tornado graph. *Mela OD*: number of excised melanomas in the optical dermoscopy (OD) group; *Mela SDDI*: number of excised melanomas in the sequential digital dermoscopy imaging (SDDI) group; *P unnec ex OD*: number of patients with unnecessary excisions in OD group; *P unnec ex SDDI*: number of patients with unnecessary excisions in SDDI group; *P ctrl T0*: number of patients registered by SDDI at inclusion time; *P ctrl 12 M*: proportion of patients followed-up by SDDI at 12 months; *N unnec ex*: average number of unnecessary excisions per patient; *Multi unnec ex*: proportion of patients with >1 unnecessary excision.

of monitoring. Our rate of compliance was very good, compared to other studies [5,22]. Only 3.6% of patients had to be re-contacted.

This study is not a cost-effectiveness analysis, because only costs were compared between both groups. A further comparison based on cost-effectiveness would require relating cost-differences between the groups to effect-differences. In economic evaluation, these effect-differences typically include improvements in health related quality of life (HRQoL) and survival. HRQoL was expected to be higher in Group 2, because unnecessary surgeries and scars were avoided. Concerning the survival, the three melanomas found by SDDI were *in situ* or very early invasive (Clark level II, Breslow's thickness 0.2 mm). *In situ* melanoma never metastasize. The 10–20 year melanoma specific survival rates for melanomas with Clark II level and Breslow thickness < 0.25 have been reported to be close to 100% (98.3 to 100%) [23,24]. The other melanoma patients, diagnosed with OD in both groups, had a life expectancy not linked to the group they belonged to, but only linked to the stage of their melanoma.

Our analysis provided clear indications that the average per-patient costs were lower in Group 2 than in Group 1. Although no statistical testing has been undertaken in the absence of prospective survival studies, the current consensus in the literature is that, on average, survival is expected to be similar in both groups [23,24]. Furthermore, it seems intuitively highly likely that the HRQoL per average patient was higher in Group 2 than in Group 1, for the reasons we explained above. Therefore, with lower costs, similar survival, and higher HRQoL, Group 2 was likely to dominate Group 1. However, since there is no separate study showing significant effectiveness and since costs and effects are likely to be correlated, a formal economic evaluation alongside a prospective clinical trial would be required to provide irrefutable evidence on this matter [25]. Perhaps our study can serve as a further incentive to set up such a (albeit costly) study. Fundamentally our study is limited by the relatively small sample of patients diagnosed by SDDI plus the lack of any study comparing OD *versus* OD and selective use of SDDI in terms of effectiveness in the general population, let alone in terms of cost-effectiveness.

Regarding SDDI literature, on the one hand, a meta-analysis of 14 SDDI studies concluded on the safety of the technique that among 383 melanomas detected, more than half were *in situ* and the rest were early invasive melanomas (thickness always thinner than 1 mm) [26]. All these melanomas had an excellent prognosis but the thickest ones had a low risk of metastasis. It is, however, unclear whether the slightly later detection of the melanomas excised because of a change on SDDI pictures would have had an impact on melanoma-related mortality. On the other hand, more than half of melanomas detected by SDDI are "featureless melanomas", i.e. melanomas which would perhaps have been missed by OD [7]. Finally, the benefit of very early detection should be weighed against the risk of significant progression of monitored melanomas, which is probably very low but not equal to zero. Nevertheless, regarding the SDDI use in a very large number of PLC in the world, we can conclude that experts in dermoscopy assume SDDI to be safe (when performed by experienced dermoscopists in compliant patients).

Our results can only partially be extrapolated to other countries where SDDI is not reimbursed or where the price and/or the conditions of reimbursement are very different from those chosen in this study. The price of consultations, excisions and pathology vary also from one country to another. Our results should be confirmed by a multicenter randomized study and could be extrapolated to other countries if the same calculations are made using the specific prices of each country.

Our study has some limitations. The excision and pathology of benign lesions are probably not always useless: some very dysplastic nevi and some atypical Spitz nevi, despite a final diagnosis of benignancy, will be treated as melanomas because the pathologist cannot completely exclude a melanoma diagnosis [20,27]. Nevertheless, these cases are rare. This is an observational study and therefore patients were not randomized between the two groups. The potential bias are the following. First, it cannot be excluded that some lesions from Group 2, considered as benign after a three or twelve month follow-up, were slow-growing melanomas and had been lost from our follow-up. The subgroup of so-called "slow-growing melanomas" is diagnosed by SDDI after a median period of 20 months [13]. The prevalence of such melanomas is unknown but seems to be low. Even if very rare cases are diagnosed by SDDI after more than five years, the risk of having missed such melanomas in our study is extremely low. Return to the PLC if any change was observed could be burdensome to patients. If only one melanoma was missed, we must consider two extreme situations. If the melanoma was diagnosed in a very early stage (*in situ* or Clark II), our conclusions are unchanged because the extra-costs per melanoma in Group 2 would be lower. If the melanoma was diagnosed in an advanced stage, the use of SDDI must then be considered as unsafe. Second, it is possible that some featureless melanomas were missed in Group 1 and would have been diagnosed by SDDI. Although SDDI permits an earlier diagnosis due to the identification of the so-called "featureless melanomas" [5–8], melanoma prevalence was probably similar in both groups. In terms of costs, this difference should not influence the detection costs, but perhaps the treatment costs. Third, according to some authors, part of the *in situ* melanomas would be indolent forms without metastatic potential [28]. The proportion of *in situ*/invasive melanomas is not statistically different in both groups (p value>0,1). Nevertheless, as this proportion is high (around 1/1.7), if we had to remove all the *in situ* melanomas from our study, our sample sizes would become smaller and our results may therefore no longer be statistically significant. Fourth, reimbursement driven unit costs from home to hospital were not taken into account. This could perhaps have increased the extra-costs in Group 2. Although reimbursement driven unit costs are generally low in Belgium, this might not be the case in countries with a lower population density and/or a lower dermatologist to patient ratio. Fifth, social status and access to a dermatologist were not measured and can therefore be considered as a potential bias.

Conclusion

Assuming that SDDI would be reimbursed and easily available to all patients with atypical nevi, the present observational study showed that selective SDDI reduces the extra-costs in the process of melanoma detection in patients with one-to-three atypical nevi. It would be interesting to confirm our results, obtained from a non-randomized observational study, by a multicenter randomized study. When practiced by dermoscopy experts, SDDI allows the follow-up of benign atypical lesions, avoiding their systematic excision. The extra-costs, mostly linked to the excision of atypical nevi mimicking early melanomas, will never be reduced to zero, but could be significantly reduced by SDDI in certain conditions, as was described above.

Supporting Information

Code S1 R code for the cost-minimization model and sensitivity analysis.

Author Contributions

Conceived and designed the experiments: I. Tromme BD PB NP LT NS. Performed the experiments: I. Tromme PR LS LM PVE I. Theate JFB. Analyzed the data: BD CL. Contributed reagents/materials/analysis tools: LM PVE I. Theate. Wrote the paper: I. Tromme BD JL LT NS.

References

1. SEER Cancer statistics: Available: http://seer.cancer.gov/csr/1975_2010/ Accessed 10 May 2013.
2. Erdmann F, Lortet-Tieulent J, Schuz J, Zeeb H, Greinert R, et al. (2013) International trends in the incidence of malignant melanoma 1953–2008–are recent generations at higher or lower risk? Int J Cancer 132: 385–400.
3. Vestergaard ME, Macaskill P, Holt PE, Menzies SW (2008) Dermoscopy compared with naked eye examination for the diagnosis of primary melanoma: a meta-analysis of studies performed in a clinical setting. Br J Dermatol 159: 669–676.
4. Kittler H, Pehamberger H, Wolff K, Binder M (2002) Diagnostic accuracy of dermoscopy. The Lancet Oncology 3: 159–165.
5. Altamura D, Avramidis M, Menzies SW (2008) Assessment of the optimal interval for and sensitivity of short-term sequential digital dermoscopy monitoring for the diagnosis of melanoma. Arch Dermatol 144: 502–506.
6. Haenssle HA, Korpas B, Hansen-Hagge C, Buhl T, Kaune KM, et al. (2010) Selection of patients for long-term surveillance with digital dermoscopy by assessment of melanoma risk factors. Arch Dermatol 146: 257–264.
7. Kittler H, Guitera P, Riedl E, Avramidis M, Teban L, et al. (2006) Identification of clinically featureless incipient melanoma using sequential dermoscopy imaging. Arch Dermatol 142: 1113–1119.
8. Menzies SW, Emery J, Staples M, Davies S, McAvoy B, et al. (2009) Impact of dermoscopy and short-term sequential digital dermoscopy imaging for the management of pigmented lesions in primary care: a sequential intervention trial. Br J Dermatol 161: 1270–1277.
9. Carli P, Ghigliotti G, Gnone M, Chiarugi A, Crocetti E, et al. (2006) Baseline factors influencing decisions on digital follow-up of melanocytic lesions in daily practice: an Italian multicenter survey. J Am Acad Dermatol 55: 256–262.
10. Schiffner R, Schiffner-Rohe J, Landthaler M, Stolz W (2003) Long-term dermoscopic follow-up of melanocytic naevi: clinical outcome and patient compliance. Br J Dermatol 149: 79–86.
11. Tromme I, Sacre L, Hammouch F, Legrand C, Marot L, et al. (2012) Availability of digital dermoscopy in daily practice dramatically reduces the number of excised melanocytic lesions: results from an observational study. Br J Dermatol 167: 778–786.
12. Menzies SW, Gutenev A, Avramidis M, Batrac A, McCarthy WH (2001) Short-term digital surface microscopic monitoring of atypical or changing melanocytic lesions. Arch Dermatol 137: 1583–1589.
13. Argenziano G, Kittler H, Ferrara G, Rubegni P, Malvehy J, et al. (2010) Slow-growing melanoma: a dermoscopy follow-up study. Br J Dermatol 162: 267–273.
14. INAMI: honoraires, prix, remboursements. Available: http://www.inami.fgov.be/insurer/fr/rate/index.htm Accessed 19 December 2012.
15. Newton Bishop JA, Bataille V, Pinney E, Bishop DT (1994) Family studies in melanoma: identification of the atypical mole syndrome (AMS) phenotype. Melanoma Res 4: 199–206.
16. Belgian Health Care Knwoledge Center. Report 183C: Belgian guidelines for economic evaluations and budget impact analyses: second edition 2012. Available: https://kce.fgov.be/sites/default/files/page_documents/KCE_183C_economic_evaluations_second_edition_0.pdf Accessed 2 May [13] 2013.
17. Gray AM CP, Wolstenholme JL, Wordsworth S (2011) Decision analytic modelling: decision trees. in: Applied Methods of Cost-effectiveness Analysis in Health Care, Oxford University Press. 179–202.
18. Gray AM CP, Wolstenholme JL, Wordsworth S (2011) Representing uncertainty in decision analytic models. in: Applied Methods of Cost-effectiveness Analysis in Health Care, Oxford University Press. 249–259.
19. R Foundation for Statistical Computing V, Austria. (2013) R: A language and environment for statistical computing. Available: http://www.R-project.org/ Accessed 10 August 2013.
20. Luo S, Sepehr A, Tsao H (2011) Spitz nevi and other Spitzoid lesions part II. Natural history and management. J Am Acad Dermatol 65: 1087–1092.
21. Kittler H, Binder M (2001) Risks and benefits of sequential imaging of melanocytic skin lesions in patients with multiple atypical nevi. Arch Dermatol 137: 1590–1595.
22. Argenziano G, Mordente I, Ferrara G, Sgambato A, Annese P, et al. (2008) Dermoscopic monitoring of melanocytic skin lesions: clinical outcome and patient compliance vary according to follow-up protocols. Br J Dermatol 159: 331–336.
23. Green AC, Baade P, Coory M, Aitken JF, Smithers M (2012) Population-based 20-year survival among people diagnosed with thin melanomas in Queensland, Australia. J Clin Oncol 30: 1462–1467.
24. Gimotty PA, Elder DE, Fraker DL, Botbyl J, Sellers K, et al. (2007) Identification of high-risk patients among those diagnosed with thin cutaneous melanomas. J Clin Oncol 25: 1129–1134.
25. Dakin H, Wordsworth S (2013) Cost-minimisation analysis versus cost-effectiveness analysis, revisited. Health Econ 22: 22–34.
26. Salerni G, Teran T, Puig S, Malvehy J, Zalaudek I, et al. (2013) Meta-analysis of digital dermoscopy follow-up of melanocytic skin lesions: a study on behalf of the International Dermoscopy Society. J Eur Acad Dermatol Venereol 27: 805–814.
27. Duffy K, Grossman D (2012) The dysplastic nevus: from historical perspective to management in the modern era: part I. Historical, histologic, and clinical aspects. J Am Acad Dermatol 67: 1 e1–16; quiz 17–18.
28. Carli P (2007) Identification of incipient tumors by means of sequential dermoscopy imaging: a new way to inflate the "epidemic" of melanoma? Arch Dermatol 143: 805; author reply 805–806.

24

Epithelial-Mesenchymal-Transition-Like and TGFβ Pathways Associated with Autochthonous Inflammatory Melanoma Development in Mice

Maria Wehbe[1,2,3], **Saïdi M. Soudja**[1,2,3], **Amandine Mas**[1,2,3], **Lionel Chasson**[1,2,3], **Rodolphe Guinamard**[1,2,3], **Céline Powis de Tenbossche**[4], **Grégory Verdeil**[1,2,3], **Benoît Van den Eynde**[4], **Anne-Marie Schmitt-Verhulst**[1,2,3]*

1 Centre d'Immunologie de Marseille-Luminy (CIML), Aix-Marseille Université UM2, Marseille, France, **2** Institut National de la Santé et de la Recherche Médicale (INSERM), Marseille, France, **3** Centre National de la Recherche Scientifique (CNRS), Marseille, France, **4** Ludwig Institute for Cancer Research and Cellular Genetics Unit, UCL, Brussels, Belgium

Abstract

We compared gene expression signatures of aggressive amelanotic (Amela) melanomas with those of slowly growing pigmented melanomas (Mela), identifying pathways potentially responsible for the aggressive Amela phenotype. Both tumors develop in mice upon conditional deletion in melanocytes of *Ink4a/Arf* tumor suppressor genes with concomitant expression of oncogene H-Ras^{G12V} and a known tumor antigen. We previously showed that only the aggressive Amela tumors were highly infiltrated by leukocytes concomitant with local and systemic inflammation. We report that Amela tumors present a pattern of de-differentiation with reduced expression of genes involved in pigmentation. This correlates with reduced and enhanced expression, respectively, of microphthalmia-associated (*Mitf*) and *Pou3f2/Brn-2* transcription factors. The reduced expression of Mitf-controlled melanocyte differentiation antigens also observed in some human cutaneous melanoma has important implications for immunotherapy protocols that generally target such antigens. Induced Amela tumors also express Epithelial-Mesenchymal-Transition (EMT)-like and TGFβ-pathway signatures. These are correlated with constitutive Smad3 signaling in Amela tumors and melanoma cell lines. Signatures of infiltrating leukocytes and some chemokines such as chemotactic cytokine ligand 2 (Ccl2) that contribute to leukocyte recruitment further characterize Amela tumors. Inhibition of the mitogen-activated protein kinase (MAPK) activation pathway in Amela tumor lines leads to reduced expression of EMT hallmark genes and inhibits both proinflammatory cytokine Ccl2 gene expression and Ccl2 production by the melanoma cells. These results indicate a link between EMT-like processes and alterations of immune functions, both being controlled by the MAPK pathway. They further suggest that targeting the MAPK pathway within tumor cells will impact tumor-intrinsic oncogenic properties as well as the nature of the tumor microenvironment.

Editor: Bart O. Williams, Van Andel Institute, United States of America

Funding: This work was supported by institutional funding from INSERM and CNRS, and by grants from the "Institut National du Cancer" (INCA) and the INCA PROCAN program (to AMSV), the European Communities (Integrated project "Cancerimmunotherapy" LSHC-CT-2006-518234 to AMSV and to BVdE) and the "Association pour la Recherche sur le Cancer" (to AMSV). MW and SMS were the recipients of doctoral fellowships from the "Association pour la Recherche sur le Cancer." The funders had no role in study design, data collection and analysis, decision to publish, or preparation of the manuscript.

Competing Interests: The authors have declared that no competing interests exist.

* E-mail: verhulst@ciml.univ-mrs.fr.

Introduction

Melanoma tumors arise from neural crest-derived melanocytes, cells specialized in the synthesis of melanin pigments [1]. The transition from normal melanocytes to metastatic melanomas occurs through a multistage process [2]. The acquisition of invasive behavior in cancers of epithelial origin is due in part to a phenotypic switch called epithelial-mesenchymal-transition (EMT). In this process, epithelial cells lose contacts with neighboring cells and assume migratory characteristics. EMT, described as the developmental switch undergone by cells from a polarized epithelial to a motile mesenchymal phenotype during embryonic development, has emerged as a central process of cancer progression [3–5]. It is characterized by decreased epithelial and increased mesenchymal markers [6]. Many EMT inducers such as TGFβ [7] have been identified, and molecular

mechanisms related to the highly invasive characteristics of cancer cells have been intensively investigated [3,6]. In particular, oncogenic Ras or activation of the MAPK pathway and TGFβ have been shown to cooperatively regulate epithelial cell plasticity and invasiveness [5,8,9].

We have described a mouse model of inducible melanoma based on the conditional deletion of the *Ink4a/Arf* tumor suppressor genes with concomitant expression of the H-Ras^{G12V} oncogene and the cancer-germline gene P1A (*Trap1a*), encoding a natural mouse tumor antigen. We previously showed that two types of cutaneous tumors expressing P1A develop in induced mice: pigmented melanomas (Mela) that grow slowly and amelanotic (Amela), more aggressive tumors [10]. Both types of melanomas were deleted at the *Ink4a/Arf* locus and expressed transcripts for H-Ras^{G12V}, albeit expression was higher in the Amela tumors [11]. The more aggressive Amela melanomas were highly infiltrated by leukocytes concomitant with local and systemic inflammation [11]. Neither tumor infiltration by leukocytes nor systemic inflammation was observed in Mela-bearing mice.

Here we compare the gene expression signatures of both tumor types, identifying pathways potentially responsible for the aggressive Amela phenotype. We show (i) a de-differentiated phenotype with reduced expression of Mitf, (ii) expression of genes akin to those defining EMT and (iii) expression of genes encoding chemokines and immuno-modulating cytokines characterizing aggressive (Amela) compared to slow progressor (Mela) melanomas. EMT-like and TGFβ-pathway signatures, correlated with constitutive Smad3 signaling, also characterized Amela tumor cells. Inhibition of the MAPK activation pathway in Amela tumor lines led to reduced Smad3 signaling, affected expression of EMT hallmark genes and inhibited proinflammatory cytokine Ccl2 gene expression and production by the melanoma cells. We conclude that in this model of autochthonous inflammatory melanoma, EMT-like processes and alterations of immune functions are linked, both being controlled by the MAPK pathway.

Results

Segregation of Mela, Amela and Normal Skin Gene Expression Profiles

To characterize the molecular differences between Mela and Amela tumors, we performed gene expression microarrays on 8 whole tumor samples, as well as on a pool of healthy mouse skins (see Methods and Fig. S1). Skin from control mice was chosen for the gene expression studies because it corresponds to the environment in which the tumors develop that may have topical characteristics in terms of stromal cells and leukocytes that are also present in the tumors.

To identify more precisely the genes differentially expressed between Mela and Amela tumors, gene expression array datasets were subjected to the microarray data analysis program Significance Analysis of Microarrays (SAM) [12]. This analysis revealed 1195 genes differentially expressed between the two types of tumors (>2 fold, p value <0.001), 813 of which were down-regulated in Amela versus Mela tumors.

Using hierarchical clustering analysis, three distinct groups were identified based on the similarity of their expression patterns. These segregated Mela from Amela tumors and both tumors from normal skin. Examples of clusters of genes are shown (i) upregulated selectively in Amela-tumors (Fig. S1A), (ii) up- and down-regulated, respectively, in Mela- and Amela-tumors (Fig. S1B), (iii) up-regulated (Fig. S1C) or (iv) down-regulated (Fig. S1D) in both Amela and Mela tumors, as compared to normal skin.

Down-regulation of Transcripts Controlling Melanocyte Differentiation in Amela Tumors is Associated with up-regulation of *Pou3f2/Brn2* Transcripts and Increased Aggressiveness

According to microarray data, transcripts controlling pigmentation, keratinization and epidermis development were down-regulated in Amela versus Mela tumors (Fig. 1A-Table S1). These include (Fig. 1A–E) genes (*Tyrp1*, *Si*, *Mlana*) encoding melanosomal proteins (Tyrosinase related protein 1/gp75, Silver/gp100, Melan-A/Mart-1), as well as genes encoding transcription factors Mitf, Pax3 and Sox10, known to be required for expression of the melanosomal proteins (for review [13]). This pattern of gene expression was verified by quantitative reverse transcriptase-polymerase chain reaction (QRT-PCR) in Amela versus Mela

tumors (Fig. 1B), as well as in the corresponding tumor lines (Fig. 1C). QRT-PCR data also confirmed that the gene encoding the master transcription factor for melanocyte differentiation (*Mitf*), which is highly expressed in Mela tumors, was down-regulated in Amela tumors (Fig. 1D). In man, a correlation between MITF expression in primary melanomas and survival has been described, with de-differentiated melanomas being associated with poor prognosis [14]. Interestingly, the *Pou3f2* gene encoding a transcription factor also called Brn2 showed higher expression in Amela compared to Mela tumors (Fig. 1A, E). This is consistent with data showing *Brn2* expression up-regulation by Ras and MAPK signaling [15] and BRN2 repression of MITF expression in some human melanoma cell lines [16]. These results are in agreement with the reported correlation between the aggressiveness of human melanomas and down-regulation of expression of genes controlling melanocyte differentiation, including *MELANA*, *MC1R*, *PAX3* and *c-KIT* [17,18].

Inflammatory Gene Expression Profile in Amela Tumors

Among the genes with up-regulated expression in Amela tumors, some characterize immune response components or chemotaxis (Tables 1- Table S2). To distinguish signatures of leukocytes infiltrating selectively Amela tumors from those intrinsic to the tumor, we compared gene expression profiles of whole Amela tumors with their *in vitro* derived cell lines (see Methods). This analysis permitted us to identify the transcriptional signatures for the Amela tumor infiltrates (genes down-regulated more than twofold in the Amela tumor lines compared to the whole Amela tumors) (Table S2). Most of these genes were characterized by a myeloid lineage expression, while some pertained to lymphocytes or stromal cells (Table S2), in agreement with our previous cellular analysis. Indeed, the Amela tumor infiltrate was found to be composed mainly of myeloid cells, a majority of which expressed the CD11b and Gr-1 markers, akin to "Myeloid Derived Suppressor Cells (MDSC)", whereas T cells composed about 10% of the hematopoietic cell infiltrate [11].

We also identified Amela tumor-intrinsic expressed genes (Table 1). Some encode factors involved in angiogenesis such as Vegfa, or molecules involved in signaling and controlling proliferation or invasion. Interestingly, among the genes considered as signatures for leukocytes selectively infiltrating Amela tumors (Table S2), some encode receptors (*ccr1*) for chemokines encoded by genes (*ccl2*, *ccl5*, *ccl7*) expressed in Amela tumors (Table 1).

Thus, inflammation, possibly initiated by cytokines produced by Amela tumors (see later section), may be further amplified by myeloid cells recruited by tumors [11].

Gene Set Enrichment Analysis

To identify pathways that might impart the phenotypes described for the two types of melanomas we performed gene set enrichment analyses (GSEA) using gene set 2.0 (http://www.broadinstitute.org/gsea). Specifically, an established collection of more than 100 cancer related, curated gene sets provided by the Molecular Signatures Database (MSigDB, www.broadinstitute.org/gsea/msigdb) as well as those collected from the literature, were used to interrogate the gene expression dataset in order to compare gene set enrichment in each type of melanoma.

We found 40 gene signatures specifically enriched in either the Amela tumors or in the Mela tumors (p $<$ 0.05) (not shown). Notably, a significant number of the gene sets enriched in the Amela versus the Mela tumors were classifiers for either EMT or pathways known to induce EMT, such as TGFβ pathways (Fig. 2A-Fig. S2).

A

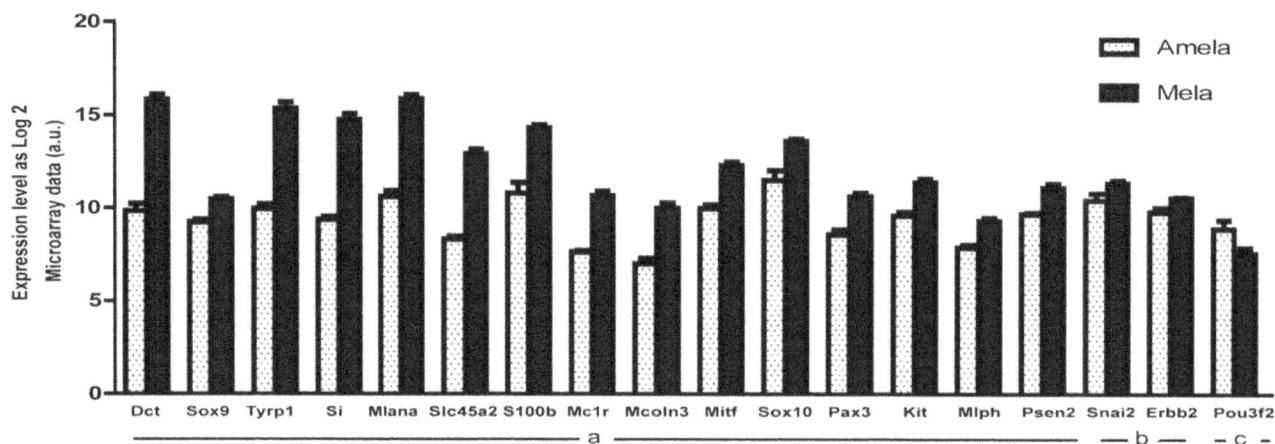

B 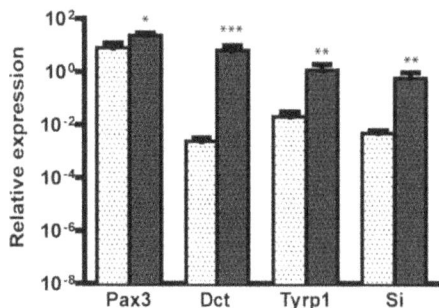   **C**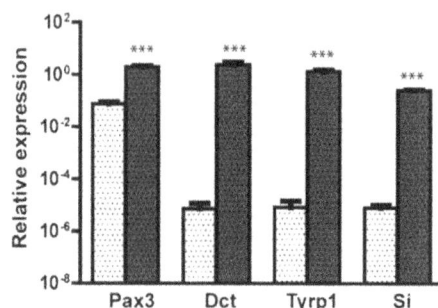

D 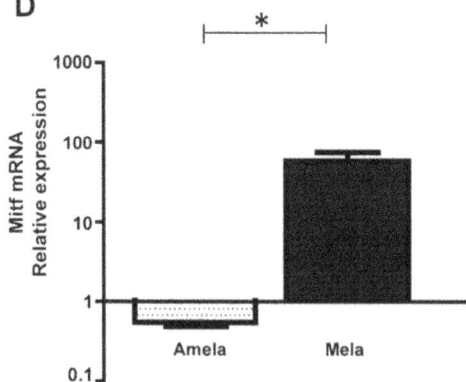   **E**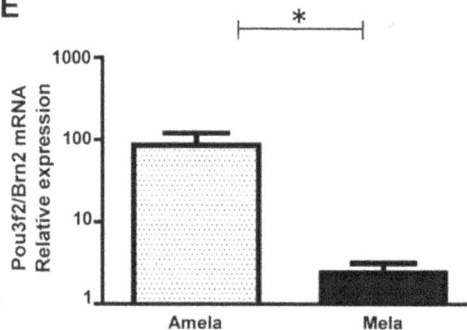

Figure 1. Differential expression in Amela and Mela tumors of genes involved in pigmentation, differentiation and development of melanocytes. A. Microarray data as log2 for Amela and Mela tumors are shown in arbitrary units (a.u.). For these genes, ratio of gene expression as log2 Amela/Mela is < -1 (a) or between -1 and 0 (b) with p values < 0.05; for Pou3f2 (c), ratio of gene expression as log2 Amela/Mela is > 1 with p value < 0.05. B–C. Validation of expression of four genes (from A) by QRT-PCR in Amela and Mela tumors *ex vivo* (B) and of corresponding melanoma lines cultured *in vitro* (C). D–E. Relative expression of transcripts for *Mitf* (D) and for *Brn2/Pou3f2* (E) in induced Mela and Amela tumors *ex vivo*. Amela tumors are represented by white dotted bars and Mela tumors by black dotted bars. For *ex vivo* analysis (B, D, E) values were normalized to those for skins of control mice, 6 samples of each tumor and 4 skin samples were analyzed. For *in vitro* analysis (C), 3 different cDNA preparations from two Mela and 8 Amela tumor lines were used and values were normalized to those for B16F10 cells. ***p value < 0.001; **p value < 0.01; *p value < 0.05 (see methods).

Table 1. Amela tumor-intrinsic expressed genes controlling angiogenesis, invasion and cytokines.

Gene symbol	Gene name	[b]Log2 ratio Amela/Mela	[c]Log2 ratio Amela/Line
[a]*Angiogenesis*			
Vegfa	Vascular endothelial growth factor A	1.45	−1.71
Foxc2	Forkhead box C2	1.36	−0.40
Tnfaip2	Tumor necrosis factor, alpha induced protein 2	1.32	−0.91
Adamts1	a disintegrin-like and metallopeptidase (reprolysin type) with thrombospondin type 1, motif, 1	1.12	0.07
[a]*Proliferation and invasion*			
Igfbp3	Insulin-like growth factor binding protein 3	3.15	0.64
Lox	Lysyl oxidase	2.5	0.33
Tbx3	T-box 3	2.4	−0.4
Stat4	Signal transducer and activator of transcription 4	2.10	−1.62
Igfbp4	Insulin-like growth factor binding protein 4	1.70	1.64
Axl	AXL receptor tyrosine kinase	1.68	0.07
Socs3	Suppressor of cytokine signaling 3	1.31	0.08
Loxl2	Lysyl oxidase-like 2	1.2	0.17
[a]*Immune response and chemotaxis*			
Ccl2	Chemokine (C-C motif) ligand 2	2.25	−2.46
Cxcl5	Chemokine (C-X-C motif) ligand 5	2.19	0.75
IL6	Interleukin 6	1.66	0.72
Ccl5	Chemokine (C-C motif) ligand 5	1.61	−1.57
Ltbp1	Latent transforming growth factor beta binding protein 1	1.86	−0.657
Pla2g7	Phospholipase A2, group VII (platelet-activating factor acethylhydrolase, plasma)	1.55	−0.98
Chst2	Carbohydrate sulfotransferase 2	1.40	0.98
Ccl7	Chemokine (C-C motif) ligand 7	1.38	−1.03
Cxcl10	Chemokine (C-X-C motif) ligand 10	1.23	−0.48
Uaca	Uveal autoantigen with coiled-Coil domains and ankyrin repeats	1.19	0.45
F8	Coagulation factor 8	1.07	−0.11

[a]Genes characterizing angiogenesis, proliferation and invasion, immune response components or chemotaxis that show higher expression in Amela versus Mela primary tumors and are expressed at similar level in Amela primary tumors and Amela lines in culture.
[b]Ratio of gene expression as Log2 primary Amela/primary Mela > 1 with p value < 0.001;
[c]Ratio of gene expression as Log2 primary Amela/cultured Amela line < 1 or with p value n.s.).

Aggressive Amela Tumors are Associated with a Signature Akin to EMT

In agreement with the GSEA analysis, among the genes distinguishing Amela from Mela tumors and qualifying as intrinsically tumor-expressed, we identified genes encoding proteins associated with melanoma progression, akin to those characterizing EMT (Table 2). These include transcriptional regulators Hmga2, Twist1 and Snail1, whose expression is up-regulated, and Id2, whose expression is down-regulated. Changes in adhesion molecule transcripts (down-regulation of E-cadherin/ *Cdh1*, up-regulation of N-cadherin/ *Cdh2* and integrin alpha 5/ *Itgav* transcripts) also characterize EMT.

We next compared the mRNA level of different epithelial and mesenchymal markers on both types of tumors by QRT-PCR. As shown in Fig. 2B, the Amela tumors expressed higher levels of transcripts for mesenchymal markers (Snail1, Twist1 and Hmga2) than Mela tumors and a lower level of E-cadherin/*Cdh1* and *Id2* transcripts. Given recent reports implicating Snail1 in both inflammation and EMT-like processes in the skin [19] or in melanoma cells [20], we analyzed its expression by immunohistology on Amela tumors (Fig. S3). It should be noted that staining

with the commercially available anti-Snail1 antibody revealed mostly cytoplasmic Snail1, although Snail1's function as a repressor of transcription is dependent on its nuclear localization [21]. Snail1 shuttles between the cytoplasm and the nucleus in a regulated manner that is not fully understood. Post-translational modifications including phosphorylation on serine and threonine residues, ubiquitination and lysine oxidation affect Snail1 protein stability, subcellular localization and activity [21–24]. Thus, although Snail1 appears to be expressed in Amela tumors, further biochemical analyses would be required to analyze post-translational modifications of the protein and their influence on its localization and function.

Genes Involved in the TGFβ Pathway in Amela Lines

Since the GSEA analysis showed a significant enrichment of genes involved in TGFβ pathways, we identified the genes upregulated in the Amela tumors known to take part in the TGFβ pathways based on the literature (Table 3). In particular, transcripts encoding components of the TGFβ pathway (Ltbp1, Igfbp3) are upregulated in Amela tumors, although no active TGFβ appeared to be secreted (see next section).

A

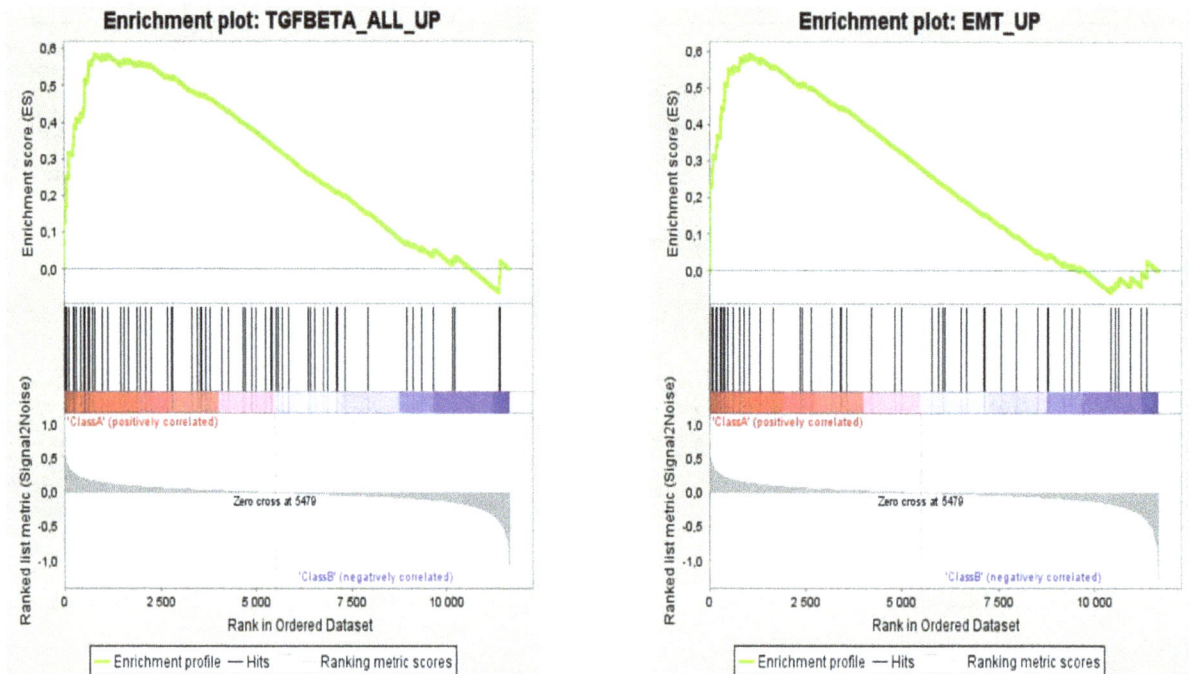

B

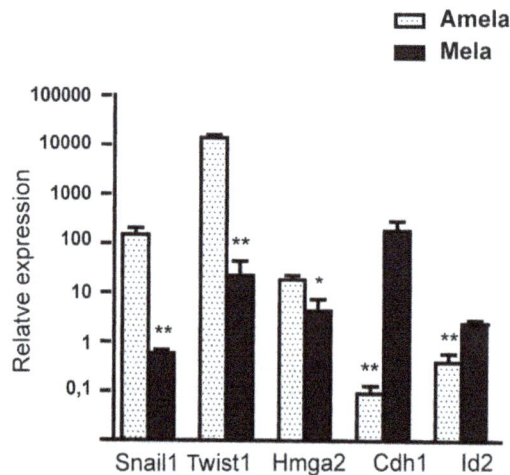

Figure 2. EMT and TGFβ pathway signatures in Amela melanomas. A. Representative gene set enrichment analysis (GSEA) plots of EMT (right graph) and TGFβ pathway (left graph) gene signatures. Each plot is divided into two sections. The first section (class A) shows results for gene sets that have a positive enrichment score (gene sets that show enrichment at the top of the ranked list here associated with Amela samples). The second section (class B) shows the results for gene sets that have a negative enrichment score (gene sets that show enrichment at the bottom of the ranked list here associated with Mela samples). Data provided as in Fig. S2. **B.** QRT-PCR analysis for expression of transcripts encoding mesenchymal and epithelial markers in Amela (white dotted bars) and Mela (black dotted bars) tumors. Values were normalized to those for skin from control mice. Data are represented as mean ± s.e.m of three independent experiments in which 7 samples of Amela and 7 samples of Mela tumors were analyzed. **p value < 0.01; *p value < 0.05.

TGFβ acts as tumor suppressor in early cancer. In later stages of cancer, however, TGFβ can promote tumors toward invasive and metastatic phenotypes [25,26]. TGFβ binding to its receptor induces the formation of a heteromericcomplex composed of TGFβ receptor type II (TβRII) and I (TβRI). The latter transmits the signal through phosphorylation of receptor-regulated Smads such as Smad2 and Smad3. Both of those Smads form heteromeric complexes with Smad4 and are then translocated into the nucleus, where they regulate expression of target genes both by direct DNA

Table 2. Genes up-regulated or down-regulated in Amela tumors involved in EMT.

Gene symbol	Gene name	[b]Log2 ratio Amela/Mela	[c]Log2 ratio Amela/Lines
[a]Cell adhesion/ECM matrix/Cytoskeleton			
Itgbl1	Integrin beta like 1	2.18	0.20
Lamb1-1	Laminin beta 1, subunit 1	1.47	−0.76
Sdc2	Syndecan-1	1.36	0.36
Cdh2	N-cadherin	1.25	−0.33
Col4a1	Collagen, type IV, alpha 1	0.99*	0.87
Col11a1	Collagen, type XI, alpha 1	0.81*	−0.54
Itgav	Integrin alpha 5	0.62*	−0.30
Col6a1	Collagen, type VI, alpha 1	0.57*	0.96
Itga3	Integrin alpha 3	0.46*	−1.90
[a]Proteases . Protease linhibitors			
Mmp10	Metallopeptidase 10	2.67	1.26
Pcolce	Procollagen C-endopeptidase enhancer protein	1.03	−0.93
Mmp19	Metallopeptidase 19	0.92*	0.20
Serpinb9	Serine peptidase inhibitor, Clade B, member9	0.72*	0.75
[a]PDGF/PDGF receptor pathway			
Ccl2	Chemokine CC motif ligand 2	2.23	−2.46
Pdgfc	Platelet dervied growth factor, C polypeptide	1.59	−0.31
Cmkor1	Chemokine CXC motif receptor 7 (CXCR7)	1.46	−0.52
Pdgfa	Platelet dervied growth factor, alpha	0.67	0.39
Pdgfd	Platelet dervied growth factor, D polypeptide	0.47	0.26
[a]Hypoxia			
Upp1	Uridine phosphorylase	1.74	−0.75
Il11	Interleukin 11	1.69	−0.97
Hif1a	hypoxia inducible factor 1, alpha subunit	0.59*	−1.46
[a]Transcription factors			
Hmga2	high mobility group alpha 2	3.71	−1.05
Twist1	Twist homolog 1 (Drosophila)	2.07	−0.78
Foxc2	Forkhead box c2	1.36	−0.40
Snai1	Snail homolog 1 (Drosophila)/Snail1	1.16	−0.07
[d] Down-regulated in Amela			
Cdh1	E-Cadherin	−3.62	2.28
Id2	Inhibitor of DNA binding 2	−0.83*	0.6

[a]Genes known to be involved in EMT that show higher expression in Amela versus Mela primary tumors and are expressed at similar level in Amela primary tumors and Amela lines in culture.
[b]Ratio of gene expression as log2 primary Amela/primary Mela > 1 with p values < 0.05;
*Ratio of gene expression as log2 primary Amela/primary Mela between 0 and 1 with p values < 0.05;
[c]Ratio of gene expression as Log2 (primary Amela-/cultured Amela line) < 1 and/or with p value > 0.05 (ns). Log2 (primary Amela /cultured Amela line) < - 1 corresponds to higher expression in cultured Amela line than in primary Amela.
[d]Genes known to be involved in EMT that show lower expression in primary Amela versus Mela tumors.

binding and through interaction with other transcription factors, coactivators, and corepressors.

We used computational methods to test the hypothesis that some of the genes within the Amela up-regulated cluster are coordinately regulated by the Smad3 transcription factor. Using the Clover program, we found a significant statistical enrichment for conserved Smad binding sites in the promoters of genes highly expressed in Amela tumors as compared to background sequences. Analysis of promoter sequences identified many genes with multiple, conserved Smad binding sites (Table S3).

Evidence for Constitutive Activation of the TGFβ Pathway in Amela cell lines and tumors

To measure TGFβ bioactivity from Amela cell culture supernatants with high sensitivity we used the SBE-SEAP reporter line MFBF11 [27] (see methods). Samples that were not activated with acid did not induce reporter activity. After activation with acid, all samples were able to strongly induce reporter activity, showing that Amela tumor cells express the latent form of TGFβ (Fig. 3A).

We transduced Amela as well as B16F10 melanoma cell lines with the lentivirus-based Smad3-reporter vector expressing green fluorescent protein (SBE-GFP) [28]. Surprisingly, even in the

Table 3. Representative TGFβ Related Genes expressed in Amela tumors and cultured cell lines.

TGFβ related genes

[a]Gene symbol	Gene name	[b]log2 ratio Amela/Mela	[c]log2 ratio Amela /Lines	[d]References
Igfbp3	Insulin-like growth factor binding protein 3	3.15	0.64	[1]
Cspg2	Versican	2.55	0.04	[2–4]
Itgbl1	Integrin beta-like 1	2.18	0.20	[4]
Cald1	Caldesmon 1	1.93	−0.08	[5–7]
Ltbp1	Latent transforming growth factor beta binding protein 1	1.78	−0.66	[8]
Nid1	Nidogen	1.72	0.66	[9]
Igfbp4	Insulin-like growth factor binding protein 4	1.60	1.64	[10]
Lamb1-1	Laminin B1 subunit 1	1.47	−0.76	[4,7,11–12]
Cmkor1	Chemokine CXC motif receptor 7 (RDC1, CXCR7)	1.46	−0.52	[2,6,12–14]
Fhl2	Four and a half LIM domains 2	1.43	−0.40	[2,6–7,12–13]
Lrp1	Low density lipoprotein receptor-related protein 1	1.40	0.88	[15]
Plat	Plasminogen activator, tissue	1.40	0.99	[16]
Bmp1	Bone morphogenetic protein 1	1.30	0.54	[6–7,12]
Smad3	MAD homolog 3 (Drosophila)	1.19	−0.23	[17]
Slc29a1	Solute carrier family 29 (nucleoside transporters), member 1	1.18	1.00	[5,7,12]
Cdh6	Cadherin 6	1.18	0.28	
Rdh10	Retinol dehydrogenase 10 (all-trans)	1.11	0.29	[6–7,13]
Col4a1	Collagen type IV, alpha 1	0.99*	0.87	[7,11–13]
Wnt2	Wingless-related MMTV integration site 2	0.97*	0.48	[18]
Tgfbr2	Transforming growth factor receptor 2	0.96*	0.01	[19]
Marcksl1	MARCKS-like 1	0.94*	0.88	[20]
Rhoq	Ras homolog gene family, member Q	0.90*	0.37	[20]
Ext1	Extososes multiple 1	0.85*	0.43	[2,6–7]
Ier3	Immediate early response 3	0.84*	−0.43	[5,7,12–13]
Tgfb3	Transforming growth factor 3	0.82*	0.23	[19]
Pdgfa	Platelet derived growth factor, alpha	0.67*	0.39	[2,5–7,21]
Col6a1	Collagen type VI, alpha 1	0.57*	0.96	[4,7,22]
Itga3	Integrin alpha 3	0.46*	−1.90	[4,7,23]
Cd44	CD44 antigen	0.41*	−1.47	[24]
Skil	SKI-like	0.40*	0.49	[2,7,13]
Igf2r	Insulin-like growth factor 2 receptor	0.38*	0.10	
Tgfbr3	Transforming growth factor receptor 3	0.20*	−0.23	[19]

[a]Genes known to be TGFβ responsive that show higher expression in Amela versus Mela primary tumors and are expressed at similar level in Amela primary tumors and in Amela lines in culture.
[b]Ratio of gene expression as log2 primary Amela/primary Mela > 1 with p values < 0.05;
*Ratio of gene expression as log2 primary Amela/primary Mela between 0 and 1 with p values < 0.05;
[c]Ratio of gene expression as Log2 (primary Amela/cultured Amela line) < 1 and/or with p value > 0.05 (ns). Log2 (primary Amela/cultured Amela line) < - 1 corresponds to higher expression in cultured Amela lines than in primary tumor.
[d]Numbered references can be found in Text S1.

absence of TGFβ, we detected GFP-fluorescent Amela tumor cells, but no fluorescent B16F10 cells (Fig. 3B), although all cell populations responded to TGFβ induction. A heterogeneous constitutive GFP expression was observed in all tested Amela lines. Based on GFP expression in these cells in the presence or absence of added TGFβ, Amela cells were sorted by FACS. Amela cells expressing GFP constitutively are called Amela[C] and Amela cells expressing GFP after TGFβ-induction are called Amela[I]. QRT-PCR analysis showed higher expression of 3 selected Smad3-regulated genes in Amela[C] compared to Amela[I] cells (Fig. 3C).

To explain the constitutive activation of Smad3 in Amela[C] cells, we wondered if this population expressed active TGFβ, which was not detected when analyzing supernatants from the whole population. To test this hypothesis, supernatants of Amela[C] and Amela[I] cells were tested in the SBE-GFP-reporter assay. Only acid-treated supernatants from both cell types induced reporter activity, showing that the basal activation of Smad3 in Amela[C] cells did not result from autocrine TGFβ (Fig. 3, Fig. S4A).

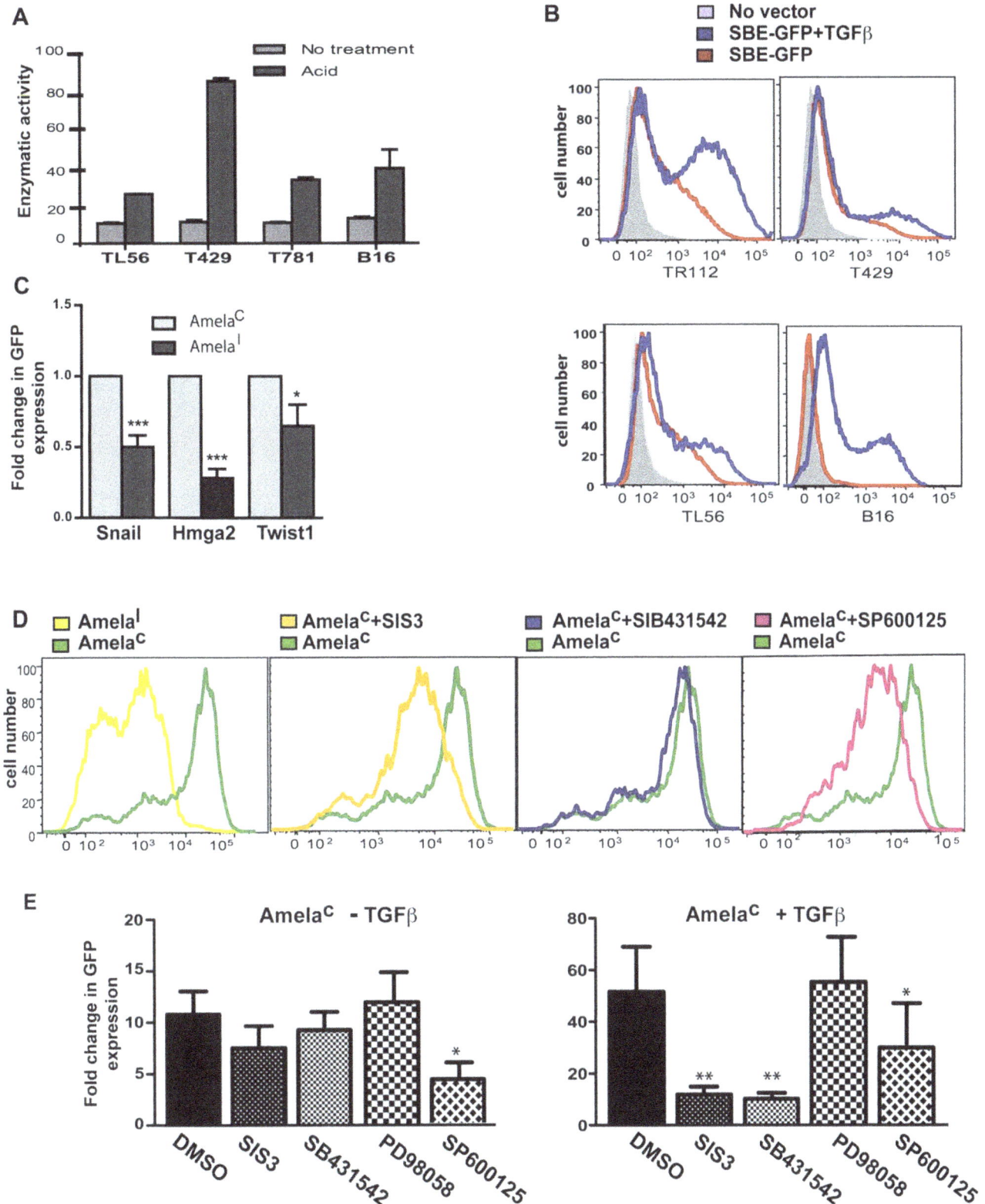

Figure 3. Analysis of the TGFβ pathway in melanoma lines and tumors. A. Supernatants from Amela cell lines incubated in serum-free DMEM were either acid treated (acid) or not (no treatment) and were tested for TGFβ content using reporter line MFBF11 (see Methods). Bars represent means ± s.d. of triplicate wells in one representative experiment. Serum-free DMEM (no TGFβ) was used for baseline measurement. B. Flow cytometry analysis of GFP expression in SBE-GFP-transduced Amela and B16F10 cell lines preincubated in serum-free DMEM without addition (red lines) or in the presence of TGFβ (blue lines). Non-transduced Amela cell lines were used as control (gray filled). C. Comparison of the expression of 3 genes associated with EMT by Amela^C and Amela^I cell lines by QRT-PCR (see text). Results are represented as fold change in relative expression where the value for Amela^C is set to 1 for each gene. Data are represented as mean ± s.e.m of two independent experiments in which 4 different lines of each type were tested. D-E. Flow cytometry analysis of GFP expression in SBE-GFP-transduced Amela^C cell lines as in (B). The effect of various

inhibitors was assessed on Amela^C cells during the incubation in serum-free DMEM without (-) or with addition (+) of TGFβ. GFP expression in one Amela^C line before and after treatment with various inhibitors in the absence of TGFβ is shown in (D). In (E)results show fold change of mean GFP fluorescence intensity in Amela^C without (panel at left) or with (panel at right) addition of TGFβ. The value for Amela^I in the absence of TGFβ is set to 1. Data are represented as mean ± s.e.m of four independent experiments. ***p value < 0.001; **p value < 0.01; *p value < 0.05.

Involvement of Ras Signaling Pathways in Smad Activation in Amela Tumors

Smads are modular proteins with conserved Mad Homology 1 (MH1), intermediate linker and MH2 domains. TβRI phosphorylates the COOH-terminal serine residues of Smads (pSmad3C). The linker domain may be phosphorylated (pSmad3L) by Ras-dependent kinases such as extracellular signal-regulated kinase (ERK) and c-Jun NH2-terminal kinase (JNK) [29]. We investigated the role of the Ras signaling pathways in Smad3 constitutive activity in Amela^C cells (Fig. 3D). Constitutive expression of GFP in the Amela^C cells was significantly inhibited only by JNK inhibitor, SP600125 (Fig. 3D–E). It was not inhibited by either SIS3, a specific inhibitor of TGFβ-induced Smad3 phosphorylation, or by SB431542, an inhibitor of TβRI kinase activity (Fig. 3D–E). In contrast, both SIS3 and SB431542 were efficient at inhibiting TGFβ-induced GFP expression in Amela^C lines. This result suggests that Ras signaling may be involved in inducing Smad3 activity in Amela^C cells via activation of JNK.

EMT in Amela Tumor Cells is Controlled by MAPK Signaling Pathways

If the active Ras/MAPK pathway is responsible for activation of the transcriptional acivity of Smad3 leading to expression of an EMT-like transcriptional program, it was expected that inhibition of that pathway would lead to down-regulation of the expression of genes characterizing EMT. To test this possibility, we analyzed the effects of JNK and ERK inhibitors on the expression of various genes by QRT-PCR (Fig. 4A). The JNK inhibitor (SP600125) led to downregulation of Snail/Snail1, Fn1, Cdh2 and upregulation of Cdh1 transcripts. Hmga2 and Vim transcripts were decreased in the presence of the ERK (PD 98059), but not the JNK inhibitor. These data are concordant with previous results in other tumor types for Hmga2 [30]. When combining JNK and ERK inhibitors, however, a further inhibition of Hmga2 transcripts was observed.

Amela Tumors Express High Levels of Phosphor-Smad3L and Phosphor-JNK in vivo

Given the enrichment in genes involved in the TGFβ pathway detected in the Amela tumors, we tested whether pSmad3L could be detected by immunohistology on tumor sections (Fig. 5A). Antibody to CD45 was used to identify tumor-infiltrating leukocytes together with anti-pSmad3L antibody. In the Amela tumors a high frequency of tumor cells were labeled with anti-pSmad3L antibody, whereas most infiltrating leukocytes were not labeled. In Mela tumors, few infiltrating leukocytes were detected and most tumor cells were negative or very weakly stained with anti-pSmad3L antibodies. When analyzing expression of phosphorylated JNK (pJNK), we similarly observed strong staining in Amela tumors and very weak staining in the Mela tumors (Fig. 5B). These data show a correlation between JNK activation revealed by pJNK and Smad3 phosphorylation in its linker domain, and suggest that Smad3 is constitutively active in the Amela tumors as it is in the corresponding cell lines.

Proinflammatory Ccl2 Cytokine Production in Amela Tumor Cells is Controlled by MAPK Signaling Pathways

We further analyzed the control of production of the proinflammatory cytokine Ccl2 and confirmed by QRT-PCR data the differential expression of its transcript between Amela and Mela tumors (Fig. 6A), as well as by cultured Amela and Mela tumor cell lines (Fig. 6B). Cytokine production was readily detected in 24 h supernatants of Amela, but not of Mela, nor of B16.F10 lines (Fig. 6C). We next addressed whether production of the proinflammatory cytokine was under the control of the MAPK pathway by testing the effect of the inhibitors on Ccl2 gene expression (Fig. 6D) and cytokine production (Fig. 6E) by the Amela tumor cells. Data indicate a significant inhibition of Ccl2 transcripts and cytokine production when cells were incubated in the presence of the JNK inhibitor or the ERK and JNK inhibitors (Fig. 6).

These resuts suggest that oncogenic Ras expression coordinately controls expression of an EMT and a proinflammatory gene expression program via activation of the MAPK pathway.

Discussion

We sought to understand the molecular bases of tumor cell heterogeneity in the autochthonous TiRP mouse melanoma model. To do this, we compared gene expression profiles of the slowly progressing pigmented Mela and fast growing amelanotic Amela tumors. These tumors arise as a result of Cre-mediated deletion of the Ink4a/Arf genes in melanocytes together with expression of H-ras^{G12V} and P1A encoding a mouse tumor antigen. These events were observed in both types of tumors although higher levels of H-ras^{G12V} and P1A transcripts were detected in Amela tumors [10,11]. A threshold level of H-ras^{G12V} may be required for oncogenic H-ras to signal to any of the several downstream pathways, which it can activate. These include the MAPK pathways involving notably ERK and JNK, as well as phosphoinositide-3-kinase/Akt and NF-κB pathways [31,32]. Combined with absence of p16/Arf tumor suppressors, the level of H-ras^{G12V} may thus control key factors determining differentiation (Brn2, Mitf), EMT (JNK, Smad3, TGFβ signaling) and Ccl2 production (MAPK, JNK) during melanoma development as discussed hereafter.

Mice developing Amela melanomas presented a systemic Th2-profile of cytokines [11] associated with high expression of Vegfa by the tumors (Table 1), a situation analogous to that found in patients with metastatic melanoma [33]. Il6 was also up-regulated selectively in the Amela melanomas (Table 1), in agreement with high level detection of Il-6 in Amela tumor supernatant and serum of Amela-bearing mice [11] and with previous reports on its induction by oncogenic Ras in different cell types [34], including melanomas in a distinct model of H-ras^{G12V}-induced melanoma in mice [35].

Other cytokine genes expressed selectively by Amela tumors include those encoding Ccl2, Ccl5, and Ccl7 (Table 1), all 3 of which can contribute to the recruitment of Ccr1-expressing myeloid leukocytes (Table S2). This pattern of cytokine gene expression is thus consistent with the identified immune cell gene expression signature in the Amela tumors (Table S2) and myeloid

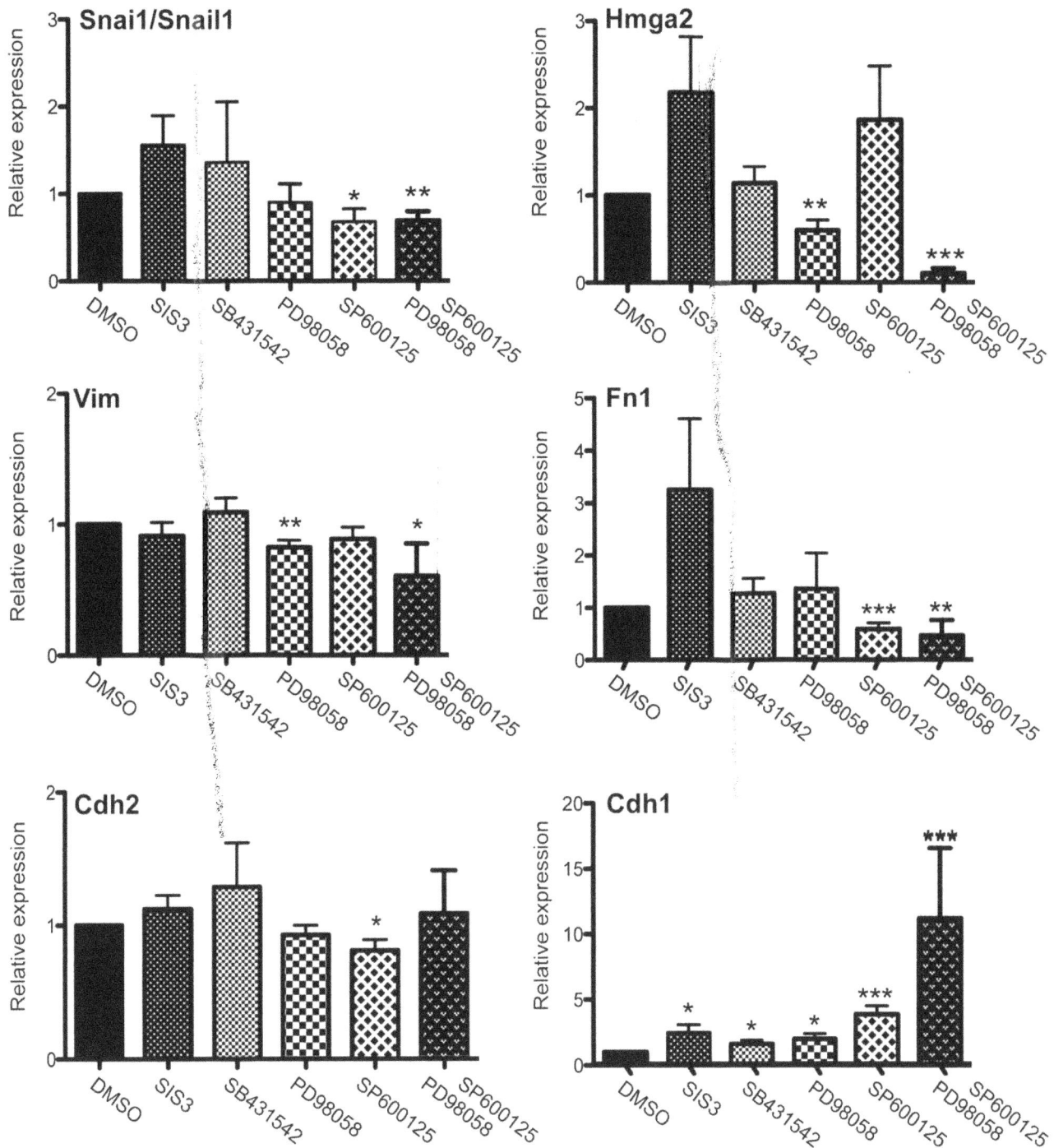

Figure 4. Effect of MAPK pathway inhibitors on the expression of EMT hallmark genes in Amela tumor lines. QRT-PCR analysis for expression of 6 transcripts encoding mesenchymal and epithelial markers in Amela tumor cells in the absence (value set to 1) or presence of inhibitors, as indicated. Data are represented as mean ± s.e.m of three independent experiments in which 5 samples were analyzed. ***p value < 0.001; **p value < 0.01; *p value < 0.05.

cell infiltrate detected in the Amela tumors [11]. The latter may in turn amplify inflammation in the tumor microenvironment [11].

Tumor expression of the proinflammatory cytokine Ccl2, also called monocyte chemoattractant protein 1 (MCP1), has been associated with macrophage migration to the tumor and promotion of tumor growth in transplanted tumor models [36] and human melanoma xenografts [37]. More recently, Ccl2 has also been implicated in recruitment of MDSC to transplanted tumors [38] and to an autochthonous glioma [39] in mice. These data are in line with our observation of a strong myeloid infiltrate in Amela tumors [11] and a gene expression signature for Amela-infiltrating myeloid cells producing additional inflammatory cytokines (Table S2).

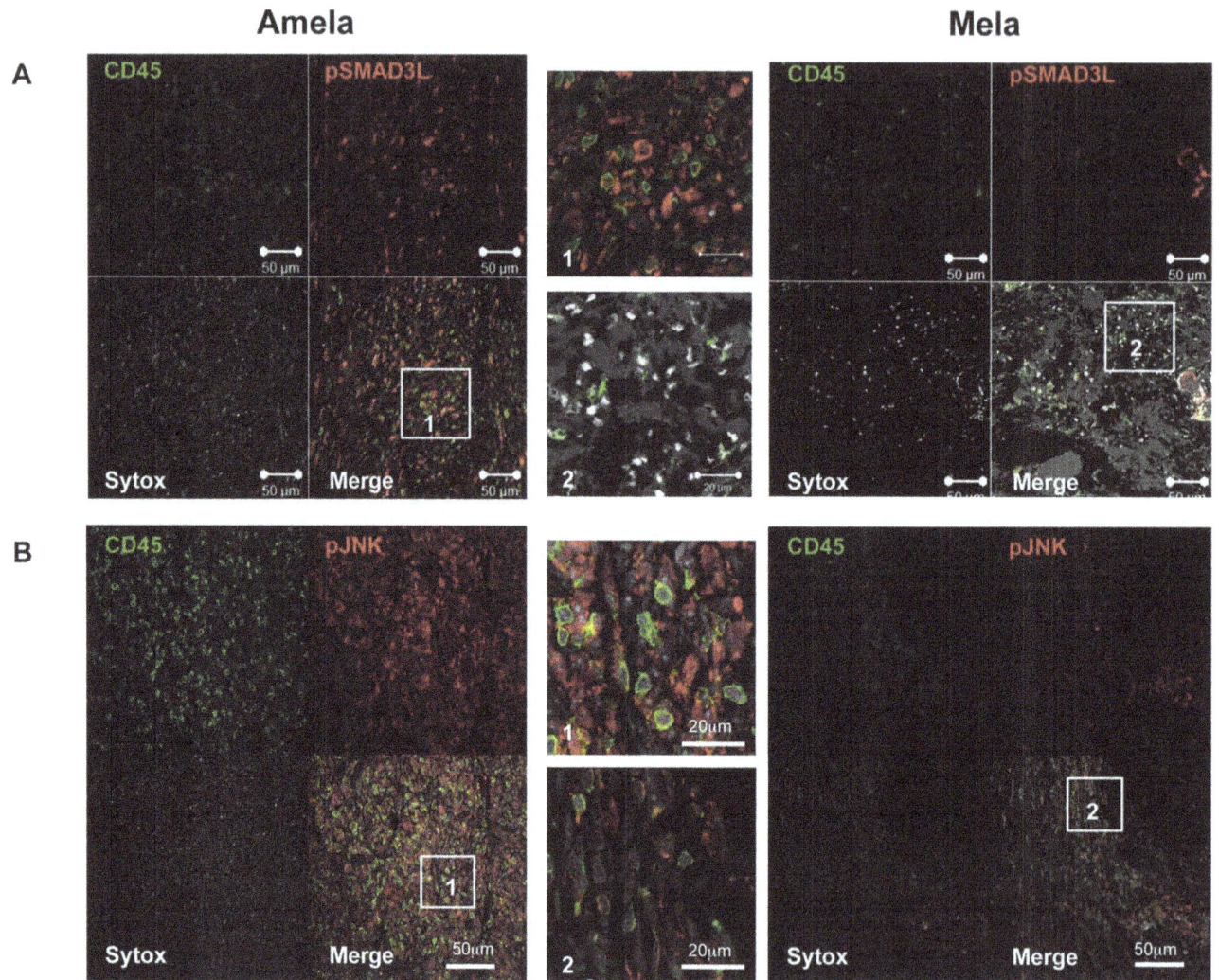

Figure 5. Analysis of phosphorylated Smad3 and JNK in melanoma tumors. Sections of Amela and Mela tumors were analyzed by immunohistology after staining with anti-CD45 mAb (green) and with anti-Phospho-Smad3L (pSmad3L) (A) or with anti-Phospho-JNK (pJNK) (B) (red). Sytox blue stains nuclei (white). Bars correspond to 50 μm in the 4 quadrant-figures and to 20 μm in the magnifications of the highlighted fields (labeled 1 and 2). In A, the brightfield image is superimposed on the "merge" image. Images are representative of 3 tumors of each type. Immunofluorescence was quantified using NIH ImageJ software for the determination of relative densities of expression of given markers within fixed section areas (fraction area). Values were, respectively (A) 1.95 ± 0.73 for Mela and 13.78 ± 1.55 for Amela tumor Phospho-Smad3L staining (unpaired t test p < 0.0001) and (B) 5.39 ± 1.05 for Mela and 26.36 ± 3.26 for Amela Phospho-JNK staining (unpaired t test p < 0.0005).

Evidence for the role of local inflammation in the promotion of melanoma progression has recently accumulated although the initiating events and the nature of the infiltrating cells may differ. For instance, ultraviolet B radiation (UVB), a major contributor to skin carcinogenesis, was shown to promote melanomagenesis in neonatal mice transgenic for hepatocyte growth factor (HGF) via recruitment of IFNγ-producing macrophages to neonatal skin by UVB-induced ligands to the chemokine receptor Ccr2 [40,41], a process which does not occur in adult mice. Interestingly, HGF has been shown to induce epithelial scattering through MAPK-mediated upregulation of Snail1 [42].

In addition to this proinflammatory circuit in Amela tumors, we observed a gene expression signature characterizing an EMT-like process, which was not expressed by Mela tumors. Therefore a signaling link may exist between inflammatory cytokine gene expression and an EMT-like gene expression profile.

Amela melanomas showed a decrease in E-cadherin/*Cdh1* transcripts compared to Mela tumors. E-cadherin expression was decreased in melanoma cell lines compared to normal human epidermal melanocytes [43]. In contrast, transcripts for N-cadherin/*Cdh2*, another member of the cadherin family, were up-regulated in Amela cells. Loss of E-cadherin and gain of N-cadherin expression is known as "cadherin switching" [44]. It can promote motility and invasion of cancer cells and is usually observed in EMT, especially in melanoma [45].

Amela cells also expressed zinc-finger transcription factor Snail1, a transcriptional repressor of E-cadherin expression [46]. Expressed in many cancers, Snail1 was reported to regulate genes involved in EMT-like processes during malignant melanoma development [47]. TGFβ is a major inducer of Snail1 expression [48], associated with EMT [25,49]. Our microarray results showed a higher expression of genes associated with TGFβ signaling in Amela compared to Mela tumors. Although not

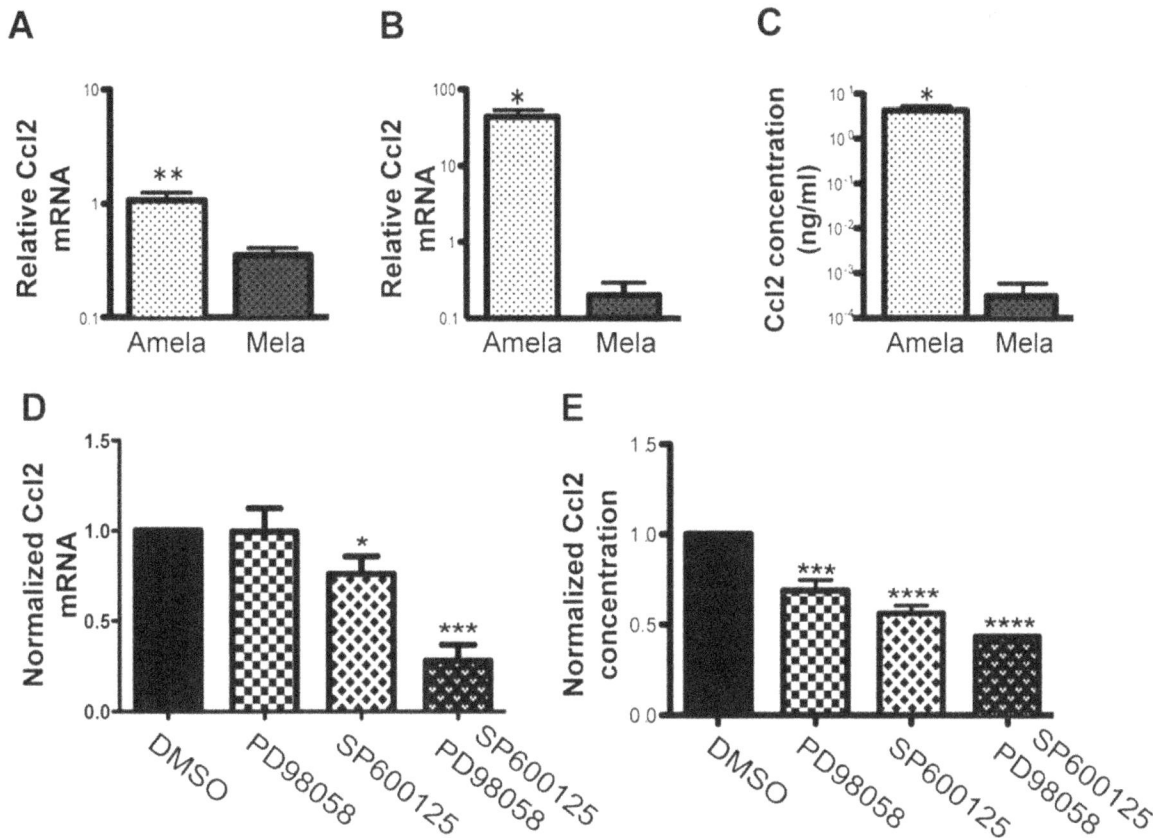

Figure 6. Specific expression of Ccl2 in Amela tumors is controlled by Ras signalling pathways. (A-B) QRT-PCR analysis of Ccl2 transcript expression in induced Mela and Amela primary tumors (A) and in the corresponding cell lines in vitro (B). (C) Concentration of secreted Ccl2 in the supernatant of 24 h cultures of Amela and Mela cell lines as measured by ELISA. (D) Expression of Ccl2 transcript by QRT-PCR and (E) concentration of secreted protein by ELISA, in the absence (value set to 1) or presence of inhibitors in 24 h cultures, as indicated. (A–C) Amela tumors are represented by white dotted bars and Mela tumors by black dotted bars. For primary tumor analysis (A) 6 samples of each tumor were analyzed. For in vitro analysis (B), values were normalized to those for B16F10 cells. In (C), supernatants from 24 h cell cultures were tested and values are expressed as ng/ml. In D–E, culture conditions were as described in Methods. Experiments involved 10 Amela lines in (D) and 4 in (E). ****p value < 0.0001; ***p value < 0.001; **p value < 0.01; *p value < 0.05.

secreting active TGFβ, Amela cells appear to secrete the inactive form of TGFβ, which can be activated by different factors. We observed a constitutive activity of the TGFβ signaling pathway in Amela lines in the absence of exogenous TGFβ, which did not result from autocrine stimulation through TβRI (Fig. 3, Fig. S4A). Rather, it may depend on JNK activity which probably resulted from the activation of the Ras pathway in the Amela tumor lines, in agreement with studies on H-Ras^{G12V} transformed epithelial lines [7,50] and patient colorectal tumors [50,51]. The higher expression of H-Ras^{G12V} in the Amela as compared to the Mela tumors may thus contribute to activation of the Smad pathway leading to an EMT-like gene expression signature. Accordingly, expression of hallmark EMT genes such as *Snai1/Snail1* and *Fn1* was downregulated in the presence of a JNK inhibitor in conditions that increased expression of the *Cdh1* gene in Amela tumor lines (Fig. 4).

In melanoma, both the Ras-Raf-MEK-ERK (MAPK) and the PI3K-AKT (AKT) signaling pathways are constitutively activated through multiple mechanisms, and thus exert several key functions in melanoma development and progression [52]. In human melanomas expressing the BRAF mutation V600E, up-regulation of Snail1 was found to be inversely correlated with progression-free and overall survival of patients [53]. Its up-regulation

appeared to depend mostly on ERK, but not on JNK activation in those melanomas. However, evidence for constitutive phosphor-JNK expression was also found in human melanoma lines expressing BRAF or NRAS activating mutations [54]. In the Amela tumors, JNK appeared to induce smad-3 activity and to contribute, together with activated ERK to expression of Snail1 and repression of Cdh1 gene expression. Constitutive production of the myeloid cell recruiting chemokine Ccl2 by the Amela cells also appeared dependent on both the JNK and the ERK activation pathways.

Of note, expression of another transcriptional regulator of the Snail-family, Slug a master regulator of neural crest cell specification and migration in many species [55,56] encoded by the snai2 gene, was found to be down-modulated in the more aggressive Amela as compared to the Mela tumors (Fig. 1A – Tables S1). This observation is in line with data reporting higher expression of Slug in human benign melanocytic lesions prior to neoplastic transformation [55,57] than in primary or metastatic melanomas in a manner that correlated with the level of expression of transcription factor Mitf [57] . Indeed, down-regulation of the pigmentation program in Amela tumor cells was associated with down- and up-regulation of Mitf and Brn2 transcription factors, respectively. In a recent study visualizing simultaneously increase of Brn2 promoter activity and decrease in pigmentation of melanoma cells, Brn2 expression was associated with a de-differentiated, invasive phenotype [58]. In a Braf mutant melanoma model in mice, increased Brn2 expression also led to increased invasiveness [59]. Among Brn2 target genes previously described in a melanoma line [60], some were up-regulated in Amela tumors and are known to play a role in invasiveness (*Hmga2*, *Twist1*, *Fn1*). Interestingly many potential Brn2 target genes significantly up-regulated in Amela tumors are involved in the development of the nervous system linking the melanomas to their neural crest cell origin (data not shown).

For the Amela tumors the observation that more rapidly growing amelanotic tumors develop in some cases at the site where pigmented melanomas initially developed [10,11] is in favor of a process of de-differentiation. *In vivo* transfer of primary melanotic tumors in immunodeficient mice also led to "outgrowth" of amelanotic tumors. Analysis at the clonal level should be performed to establish whether de-differentiation in pigmented cells gives rise to amelanotic cells or whether pre-existing amelanotic cells outgrew the pigmented cells. Since we generally observed only one tumor developing per mouse, the probability that two independent transformation events would be at the origin of the pigmented and amelanotic tumors at the same site is small. Therefore, a unique transformation event may have taken place in a precursor common to pigmented and non-pigmented cells of neuroectodermal origin, possibly at the level of a Schwann cell precursor [61]. Whether a non-pigmented cell constitutes the melanoma-initiating cell, as recently suggested [62], will require further studies. It is worth mentioning the potential importance of the notion that non-pigmented as well as pigmented cells may need to be targeted by therapeutic treatments. Indeed, immunotherapy protocols have often been directed at melanocyte differentiation antigens, which may not be expressed in non-pigmented tumor-precursor/-initiating/de-differentiated cells. In this respect the TiRP mouse melanoma model presents the advantage of being designed to express a known antigen concomitantly with the transforming oncogene. Ongoing pre-clinical immunotherapy protocols are testing the efficiency of treatments directed at such a model antigen [63].

Materials and Methods

Mice

Ethics statement. All procedures were approved by the Regional "Provence-Alpes-Cote d'Azur" Committee on Ethics for Animal Experimentation (authorization: #13.21, date: 11/02/2000) and were in accordance with French and European directives. All efforts were made to minimize animal suffering.

TiRP (*Tyr-iRas-P1A-transgenic Ink4a/Arf^flox/flox*) mice [10], kept on the B10.D2 background [11] were treated as described [10,11] for melanoma induction (Supplemental Information -SI- for details). Non-transgenic *Ink4a/Arf^flox/flox* mice, used as controls, never develop melanomas.

Mouse Melanoma Cell Lines

B16 mouse melanoma line B16F10 (ATCC number CRL-6475), originally derived by I. Fidler (M.D. Anderson Cancer Center, Houston, Tx), was received from Dr. AF Tilkin-Mariamé (INSERM-U563, Toulouse, France). Mela and Amela mouse melanoma cell lines were established in culture from, respectively, homogeneously melanotic and amelanotic induced melanomas in TiRP mice, as described [10] and were further cultured in DMEM (GibcoRL) with 10% FCS (see Text S1).

Microarrays Analysis

Gene expression profiles were analyzed by two-color micro arrays on: (i) - induced Amela and Mela tumors (4 independent tumors of each type, being either homogeneously amelanotic (Amela) or homogeneously melanotic (Mela)) compared to each other or to control mice skin (pool from two control mice); (ii) - induced Amela tumors versus cultured lines established from induced Amela tumors (4 independent tumors). For each experimental sample, two technical replicates (dye-swaps) were examined.

Isolation of RNA from Melanoma Tumors and Tumor Cell Lines

Total RNA was isolated from melanoma frozen tissues or skin (conserved at -80°C in RNA later) using RNeasy Mini Kit column purification and digestion with RNase free DNaseI according to the manufacturer's protocols (Qiagen). Total RNA from cultured melanoma lines was extracted using Trizol reagent (Invitrogen life technologies Inc.) and resuspended in RNase-free water. RNA quality and quantity were determined using a bioanalyzer (Agilent technologies) and a Nanodrop spectrophotometer ND-1000 (Nanodrop technology), respectively.

RNA Labeling and Hybridization

These steps were performed by the "Plate-Forme Transcriptome, Nice-Sophia Antipolis" as described [64] (see Text S1). Probe sequences are available on the MEDIANTE web site (http://www.microarray.fr:8080/merge/index).

Data Analysis

Fluorescence intensity measurements and data analyses were as described (see Text S1). Microarray data have been submitted to NCBI GEO database: http://www.ncbi.nlm.nih.gov/geo/query/acc.cgi?acc=GSE29304.

Quantitative Reverse Transcriptase Chain-reaction

cDNA was generated using the superscript first-strand synthesis system for RT-PCR according to the manufacturer's instruction (Invitrogen). Quantitative real time PCR was performed with a Prism 7500 fast real time PCR system using Sybr green PCR Master Mix (Applied Biosystem). Thermal cycle conditions and primers are detailed (see Text S1).

Active TGFβ Measurement

The MFBF11 TGF-reporter cells expressing a plasmid containing SMAD-binding elements driving the expression of secreted alkaline phosphatase (SEAP), kindly provided by Ina Tesseur (Stanford University School of Medicine, Stanford, CA), were treated as described [27]. Amela cells and reporter cells (MFBF11) were incubated overnight in 1 ml serum-free DMEM. 500 μl of the Amela cell supernatants were either acid-activated followed by neutralization to pH 7.4 or non-activated by addition of 100 μl NaCl 0.5 M (see Text S1). Treated supernatants were added to reporter cells. SEAP activity was measured using Great EscAPe SEAP Reporter system 3 (BD Biosciences, San Jose, CA) with a Lmax plate photometer (Molecular Devices, Sunnyvale, CA). The same assay was performed using reporter cell lines expressing the green fluorescent protein (SBE-GFP) [28]. Expression of GFP was measured by flow cytometry (CANTO II-BD Biosciences) and data were analyzed using FlowJo^TM software (Tree Star).

Cell Transduction with Lentiviral Reporter Constructs for Fluorescence Tracking of Smad3 Signaling

Amela and B16F10 cell lines were transduced with Lentiviral vectors encoding the reporter SBE-GFP [28] (see Text S1). Infected cells were selected on the basis of GFP expression in the presence of TGFβ using a FACS.

Flow Cytometry

SBE-GFP-transduced melanoma cells, incubated overnight at 1×10^5 cells/well in 24-well flat-bottom tissue culture plates (BD Falcon, San Jose,CA), were washed twice with PBS and incubated in 1 ml serum-free DMEM/P/S for 24 h. After a further overnight incubation in the same medium or with TGFβ 10 ng/ml (recombinant human TGFβ; R&D), GFP expression was analyzed by flow cytometry (CANTO II-BD Biosciences) and data were analyzed using FlowJo™ software (Tree Star).

Kinase Inhibitors

SBE-GFP-transduced melanoma cells were treated as above except for the addition of inhibitors during the overnight incubation in the presence or absence of TGFβ 5 ng/ml. Inhibitors were Smad3 inhibitor SIS3 10 μM (Calbiochem), TGFβRI kinase inhibitor SB431542 10 μM, JNK inhibitor SP600125 10 μM (Calbiochem) and ERK inhibitor PD 98059 (10 μM). When testing the effect of kinase inhibitors on EMT or Ccl2 transcripts, Amela cells were plated at 10^5 cells in 1 ml FCS containing medium for 24 h, followed by 24 h in medium without FCS and 24 h in the same medium in the presence of control DMSO or inhibitors as above. For each tumor line, cells from 4 wells were pooled and processed for QRT-PCR analysis.

Immunofluorescence

Snap-frozen tumors in tissue-Tek (Sakura Finetek) were fixed in 4% paraformaldehyde, permeabilized with methanol and stained with a polyclonal rabbit anti-pSmad3L(Ser208/213) antibody (28029, IBL) or rabbit anti-pJNK antibody (ab4821, Abcam) and with anti-CD45 monoclonal antibody. Confocal microscopy was performed with a Zeiss LSM510 microscope. Image processing was performed with Zeiss LSM software and Adobe Photoshop.

Detection of Ccl2 Transcripts by QRT-PCR and Secreted Protein by ELISA

Amela cell lines were cultured as indicated above in the absence or presence of kinase inhibitors. Culture supernatants were collected and kept frozen for detection of secreted Ccl2 by ELISA. The cell pellets were treated for detection of Ccl2 transcripts by QRT-PCR, as described above. Mouse Ccl2 (MCP-1) ELISA ready-SET-Go! (eBioscience) was used for quantification of Ccl2 production by Amela tumor lines.

Statistical Analyses

Statistical analyses were performed with the Student's unpaired t test using GraphPad and two-tailed P values are given as follows: (*) $P < 0.05$; (**) $P < 0.01$; and (***) $P < 0.001$.

Supporting Information

Figure S1   Unsupervised Hierarchical Clustering of melanoma tumors and healthy skin samples. Each row represents a gene, and each column represents a sample. Each experimental sample is represented by 2 or 3 values associated to 2 or 3 different hybridizations. The expression level of each gene in a single tumor is relative to its median abundance across all tumors and is depicted according to a color scale in which red and green expression levels are, respectively, above and below the median. The magnitude of deviation from the median is represented by the color saturation. The dendrogram of samples (matrix on top) represents overall similarities in gene expression profiles. Four clusters are shown: - clusters of genes highly expressed selectively in Amela (A) or in Mela (B) tumors; - clusters of genes which expression is up-regulated (C) or down-regulated (D) in both tumors as compared to healthy skin.

Figure S2   Heatmap output for the 80 most differentially expressed transcripts between Amela and Mela tumors. Each row represents a gene and each column represents a sample. Each experimental sample is represented by 2 or 3 values associated to 2 or 3 different hybridizations. Expression values are represented as colors, where the range of colors (red, pink, light blue, dark blue) shows the range of expression values (high, moderate, low, lowest). These genes were provided in the GSEA plots shown in Fig. 2.

Figure S3   EMT signature gene expression in Amela tumors. Snail expression in Amela (A–C) and Mela (D–F) tumors was analyzed by immunohistology on tumor sections. It shows Dapi staining for nuclei (white), anti-CD45 antibody staining for leukocytes (green) and anti-Snail antibody staining (red). Scale bars: 50-μm (A, C, D, F) and 20-μm (B, E). In C and F, the anti-Snail antibody was pre-incubated with the immunizing peptide (see Supplemental Methods). Data are representative of 3 tumors of each type.

Figure S4   Analysis of the TGFβ3 pathway in melanoma lines and tumors. A. Supernatants from Amela[C] and Amela[I] cell lines incubated in serum-free DMEM were either acid treated (acid) or not (no treatment) and were tested for TGFβ using a reporter line expressing SBE-GFP (see Methods). The mean of GFP fluorescence intensity is represented. Bars represent means ± s.e.m. of triplicate wells for 4 samples in one representative experiment. Serum-free DMEM (no TGFβ) was used for baseline measurement. B. Control staining of Amela and Mela tumors analyzed by immunohistology in Fig. 4A in the presence of secondary goat anti-Rat fluorescent (Alexa546) antibody, but in the absence of Rat anti-Phospho-Smad3L antibody. Anti-CD45 mAb and Sytox blue staining are as in Fig. 4A.

Table S1   Genes involved in pigmentation, differentiation and development of melanocytes down-regulated or up-regulated in Amela versus Mela tumors as shown in Figure 1A.

Table S2   Genes characterizing immune response components or chemotaxis that show higher expression in Amela vs Mela tumors but are expressed at lower level in Amela lines in culture than in Amela tumors.

Table S3   Table representing the genes highly expressed in Amela tumors having one or multiple conserved Smad binding sites in their promoter (in silico analysis). For each gene, the conserved Smad binding sites (CAGA), their number and their p values are represented.

Acknowledgments

We thank Pascal Barbry and Kevin Lebrigand (CNRS, Sophia-Antipolis, Nice, France) for guidance on micro array analysis, Lee Leserman for suggestions on the manuscript and the CIML imaging and animal facilities personnel for assistance.

Author Contributions

Conceived and designed the experiments: MW AMSV SMS BVdE. Performed the experiments: MW AM LC SMS RG CPdT GV. Analyzed the data: MW AM LC RG GV AMSV. Wrote the paper: MW AMSV.

References

1. Busca R, Ballotti R (2000) Cyclic AMP a key messenger in the regulation of skin pigmentation. Pigment Cell Res 13: 60–69.

2. Herlyn M, Berking C, Li G, Satyamoorthy K (2000) Lessons from melanocyte development for understanding the biological events in naevus and melanoma formation. Melanoma Res 10: 303–312.

3. Huber MA, Kraut N, Beug H (2005) Molecular requirements for epithelial-mesenchymal transition during tumor progression. Curr Opin Cell Biol 17: 548–558.

4. Thiery JP, Sleeman JP (2006) Complex networks orchestrate epithelial-mesenchymal transitions. Nat Rev Mol Cell Biol 7: 131–142.

5. Kalluri R, Weinberg RA (2009) The basics of epithelial-mesenchymal transition. J Clin Invest 119: 1420–1428.

6. Radisky DC (2005) Epithelial-mesenchymal transition. J Cell Sci 118: 4325–4326.

7. Peinado H, Quintanilla M, Cano A (2003) Transforming growth factor beta-1 induces snail transcription factor in epithelial cell lines: mechanisms for epithelial mesenchymal transitions. J Biol Chem 278: 21113–21123.

8. Gotzmann J, Huber H, Thallinger C, Wolschek M, Jansen B, et al. (2002) Hepatocytes convert to a fibroblastoid phenotype through the cooperation of TGF-beta1 and Ha-Ras: steps towards invasiveness. J Cell Sci 115: 1189–1202.

9. Janda E, Lehmann K, Killisch I, Jechlinger M, Herzig M, et al. (2002) Ras and TGF[beta] cooperatively regulate epithelial cell plasticity and metastasis: dissection of Ras signaling pathways. J Cell Biol 156: 299–313.

10. Huijbers IJ, Krimpenfort P, Chomez P, van der Valk MA, Song JY, et al. (2006) An inducible mouse model of melanoma expressing a defined tumor antigen. Cancer Res 66: 3278–3286.

11. Soudja SM, Wehbe M, Mas A, Chasson L, Powis de Tenbossche C, et al. (2010) Tumor-initiated inflammation overrides protective adaptive immunity in an induced melanoma model in mice. Cancer Res 70: 3515–3525.

12. Tusher VG, Tibshirani R, Chu G (2001) Significance analysis of microarrays applied to the ionizing radiation response. Proc Natl Acad Sci U S A 98: 5116–5121.

13. Cheli Y, Ohanna M, Ballotti R, Bertolotto C (2010) Fifteen-year quest for microphthalmia-associated transcription factor target genes. Pigment Cell Melanoma Res 23: 27–40.

14. Salti GI, Manougian T, Farolan M, Shilkaitis A, Majumdar D, et al. (2000) Micropthalmia transcription factor: a new prognostic marker in intermediate-thickness cutaneous malignant melanoma. Cancer Res 60: 5012–5016.

15. Goodall J, Wellbrock C, Dexter TJ, Roberts K, Marais R, et al. (2004) The Brn-2 transcription factor links activated BRAF to melanoma proliferation. Mol Cell Biol 24: 2923–2931.

16. Goodall J, Carreira S, Denat L, Kobi D, Davidson I, et al. (2008) Brn-2 represses microphthalmia-associated transcription factor expression and marks a distinct subpopulation of microphthalmia-associated transcription factor-negative melanoma cells. Cancer Res 68: 7788–7794.

17. Ryu B, Kim DS, Deluca AM, Alani RM (2007) Comprehensive expression profiling of tumor cell lines identifies molecular signatures of melanoma progression. PLoS One 2: e594.

18. Kamaraju AK, Bertolotto C, Chebath J, Revel M (2002) Pax3 down-regulation and shut-off of melanogenesis in melanoma B16/F10.9 by interleukin-6 receptor signaling. J Biol Chem 277: 15132–15141.

19. Du F, Nakamura Y, Tan TL, Lee P, Lee R, et al. (2010) Expression of snail in epidermal keratinocytes promotes cutaneous inflammation and hyperplasia conducive to tumor formation. Cancer Res 70: 10080–10089.

20. Kudo-Saito C, Shirako H, Takeuchi T, Kawakami Y (2009) Cancer metastasis is accelerated through immunosuppression during Snail-induced EMT of cancer cells. Cancer Cell 15: 195–206.

21. Dominguez D, Montserrat-Sentis B, Virgos-Soler A, Guaita S, Grueso J, et al. (2003) Phosphorylation regulates the subcellular location and activity of the snail transcriptional repressor. Mol Cell Biol 23: 5078–5089.

22. Zhou BP, Deng J, Xia W, Xu J, Li YM, et al. (2004) Dual regulation of Snail by GSK-3beta-mediated phosphorylation in control of epithelial-mesenchymal transition. Nat Cell Biol 6: 931–940.

23. Peinado H, Del Carmen Iglesias-de la Cruz M, Olmeda D, Csiszar K, Fong KS, et al. (2005) A molecular role for lysyl oxidase-like 2 enzyme in snail regulation and tumor progression. EMBO J 24: 3446–3458.

24. Zhang K, Rodriguez-Aznar E, Yabuta N, Owen RJ, Mingot JM, et al. (2012) Lats2 kinase potentiates Snail1 activity by promoting nuclear retention upon phosphorylation. Embo J 31: 29–43.

25. Massague J (2008) TGFbeta in Cancer. Cell 134: 215–230.

26. Xu J, Lamouille S, Derynck R (2009) TGF-beta-induced epithelial to mesenchymal transition. Cell Res 19: 156–172.

27. Tesseur I, Zou K, Berber E, Zhang H, Wyss-Coray T (2006) Highly sensitive and specific bioassay for measuring bioactive TGF-beta. BMC Cell Biol 7: 15.

28. Stuelten CH, Kamaraju AK, Wakefield LM, Roberts AB (2007) Lentiviral reporter constructs for fluorescence tracking of the temporospatial pattern of Smad3 signaling. Biotechniques 43: 289–290, 292, 294.

29. Yamagata H, Matsuzaki K, Mori S, Yoshida K, Tahashi Y, et al. (2005) Acceleration of Smad2 and Smad3 phosphorylation via c-Jun NH(2)-terminal kinase during human colorectal carcinogenesis. Cancer Res 65: 157–165.

30. Li D, Lin HH, McMahon M, Ma H, Ann DK (1997) Oncogenic raf-1 induces the expression of non-histone chromosomal architectural protein HMGI-C via a p44/p42 mitogen-activated protein kinase-dependent pathway in salivary epithelial cells. The Journal of biological chemistry 272: 25062–25070.

31. Nielsen C, Thastrup J, Bottzauw T, Jaattela M, Kallunki T (2007) c-Jun NH2-terminal kinase 2 is required for Ras transformation independently of activator protein 1. Cancer Res 67: 178–185.

32. Choi BY, Choi HS, Ko K, Cho YY, Zhu F, et al. (2005) The tumor suppressor p16(INK4a) prevents cell transformation through inhibition of c-Jun phosphorylation and AP-1 activity. Nature structural & molecular biology 12: 699–707.

33. Nevala WK, Vachon CM, Leontovich AA, Scott CG, Thompson MA, et al. (2009) Evidence of systemic Th2-driven chronic inflammation in patients with metastatic melanoma. Clin Cancer Res 15: 1931–1939.

34. Ancrile B, Lim KH, Counter CM (2007) Oncogenic Ras-induced secretion of IL6 is required for tumorigenesis. Genes Dev 21: 1714–1719.

35. Yang J, Splittgerber R, Yull FE, Kantrow S, Ayers GD, et al. (2010) Conditional ablation of Ikkb inhibits melanoma tumor development in mice. J Clin Invest 120: 2563–2574.

36. Walter S, Bottazzi B, Govoni D, Colotta F, Mantovani A (1991) Macrophage infiltration and growth of sarcoma clones expressing different amounts of monocyte chemotactic protein/JE. International journal of cancer Journal international du cancer 49: 431–435.

37. Gazzaniga S, Bravo AI, Guglielmotti A, van Rooijen N, Maschi F, et al. (2007) Targeting tumor-associated macrophages and inhibition of MCP-1 reduce angiogenesis and tumor growth in a human melanoma xenograft. The Journal of investigative dermatology 127: 2031–2041.

38. Huang B, Lei Z, Zhao J, Gong W, Liu J, et al. (2007) CCL2/CCR2 pathway mediates recruitment of myeloid suppressor cells to cancers. Cancer Lett 252: 86–92.

39. Fujita M, Kohanbash G, Fellows-Mayle W, Hamilton RL, Komohara Y, et al. (2011) COX-2 blockade suppresses gliomagenesis by inhibiting myeloid-derived suppressor cells. Cancer Res 71: 2664–2674.

40. Zaidi MR, De Fabo EC, Noonan FP, Merlino G (2012) Shedding light on melanocyte pathobiology in vivo. Cancer Res 72: 1591–1595.

41. Zaidi MR, Davis S, Noonan FP, Graff-Cherry C, Hawley TS, et al. (2011) Interferon-gamma links ultraviolet radiation to melanomagenesis in mice. Nature 469: 548–553.

42. Grotegut S, von Schweinitz D, Christofori G, Lehembre F (2006) Hepatocyte growth factor induces cell scattering through MAPK/Egr-1-mediated upregulation of Snail. Embo J 25: 3534–3545.

43. Poser I, Dominguez D, de Herreros AG, Varnai A, Buettner R, et al. (2001) Loss of E-cadherin expression in melanoma cells involves up-regulation of the transcriptional repressor Snail. J Biol Chem 276: 24661–24666.

44. Wheelock MJ, Shintani Y, Maeda M, Fukumoto Y, Johnson KR (2008) Cadherin switching. J Cell Sci 121: 727–735.

45. Li G, Satyamoorthy K, Herlyn M (2001) N-cadherin-mediated intercellular interactions promote survival and migration of melanoma cells. Cancer Res 61: 3819–3825.

46. Cano A, Perez-Moreno MA, Rodrigo I, Locascio A, Blanco MJ, et al. (2000) The transcription factor snail controls epithelial-mesenchymal transitions by repressing E-cadherin expression. Nat Cell Biol 2: 76–83.

47. Kuphal S, Palm HG, Poser I, Bosserhoff AK (2005) Snail-regulated genes in malignant melanoma. Melanoma Res 15: 305–313.

48. Nieto MA (2002) The snail superfamily of zinc-finger transcription factors. Nat Rev Mol Cell Biol 3: 155–166.

49. Moustakas A, Heldin CH (2007) Signaling networks guiding epithelial-mesenchymal transitions during embryogenesis and cancer progression. Cancer Sci 98: 1512–1520.

50. Sekimoto G, Matsuzaki K, Yoshida K, Mori S, Murata M, et al. (2007) Reversible Smad-dependent signaling between tumor suppression and oncogenesis. Cancer Res 67: 5090–5096.

51. Matsuzaki K, Kitano C, Murata M, Sekimoto G, Yoshida K, et al. (2009) Smad2 and Smad3 phosphorylated at both linker and COOH-terminal regions transmit malignant TGF-beta signal in later stages of human colorectal cancer. Cancer Res 69: 5321–5330.

52. Meier F, Schittek B, Busch S, Garbe C, Smalley K, et al. (2005) The RAS/RAF/MEK/ERK and PI3K/AKT signaling pathways present molecular

targets for the effective treatment of advanced melanoma. Front Biosci 10: 2986–3001.

53. Massoumi R, Kuphal S, Hellerbrand C, Haas B, Wild P, et al. (2009) Down-regulation of CYLD expression by Snail promotes tumor progression in malignant melanoma. J Exp Med 206: 221–232.

54. Lopez-Bergami P, Huang C, Goydos JS, Yip D, Bar-Eli M, et al. (2007) Rewired ERK-JNK signaling pathways in melanoma. Cancer Cell 11: 447–460.

55. Gupta PB, Kuperwasser C, Brunet JP, Ramaswamy S, Kuo WL, et al. (2005) The melanocyte differentiation program predisposes to metastasis after neoplastic transformation. Nature genetics 37: 1047–1054.

56. LaBonne C, Bronner-Fraser M (2000) Snail-related transcriptional repressors are required in Xenopus for both the induction of the neural crest and its subsequent migration. Developmental biology 221: 195–205.

57. Shirley SH, Greene VR, Duncan LM, Torres Cabala CA, Grimm EA, et al. (2012) Slug expression during melanoma progression. The American journal of pathology 180: 2479–2489.

58. Pinner S, Jordan P, Sharrock K, Bazley L, Collinson L, et al. (2009) Intravital imaging reveals transient changes in pigment production and Brn2 expression during metastatic melanoma dissemination. Cancer Res 69: 7969–7977.

59. Arozarena I, Sanchez-Laorden B, Packer L, Hidalgo-Carcedo C, Hayward R, et al. (2011) Oncogenic BRAF induces melanoma cell invasion by downregulating the cGMP-specific phosphodiesterase PDE5A. Cancer Cell 19: 45–57.

60. Kobi D, Steunou AL, Dembele D, Legras S, Larue L, et al. (2010) Genome-wide analysis of POU3F2/BRN2 promoter occupancy in human melanoma cells reveals Kitl as a novel regulated target gene. Pigment Cell Melanoma Res 23: 404–418.

61. Adameyko I, Lallemend F, Aquino JB, Pereira JA, Topilko P, et al. (2009) Schwann cell precursors from nerve innervation are a cellular origin of melanocytes in skin. Cell 139: 366–379.

62. Boiko AD, Razorenova OV, van de Rijn M, Swetter SM, Johnson DL, et al. (2010) Human melanoma-initiating cells express neural crest nerve growth factor receptor CD271. Nature 466: 133–137.

63. Grange M, Buferne M, Verdeil G, Leserman L, Schmitt-Verhulst AM, et al. (2012) Activated STAT5 promotes long-lived cytotoxic CD8+ T cells that induce regression of autochthonous melanoma. Cancer Res 72: 76–87.

64. Le Brigand K, Russell R, Moreilhon C, Rouillard JM, Jost B, et al. (2006) An open-access long oligonucleotide microarray resource for analysis of the human and mouse transcriptomes. Nucleic Acids Res 34: e87.

Permissions

All chapters in this book were first published in PLOS ONE, by The Public Library of Science; hereby published with permission under the Creative Commons Attribution License or equivalent. Every chapter published in this book has been scrutinized by our experts. Their significance has been extensively debated. The topics covered herein carry significant findings which will fuel the growth of the discipline. They may even be implemented as practical applications or may be referred to as a beginning point for another development.

The contributors of this book come from diverse backgrounds, making this book a truly international effort. This book will bring forth new frontiers with its revolutionizing research information and detailed analysis of the nascent developments around the world.

We would like to thank all the contributing authors for lending their expertise to make the book truly unique. They have played a crucial role in the development of this book. Without their invaluable contributions this book wouldn't have been possible. They have made vital efforts to compile up to date information on the varied aspects of this subject to make this book a valuable addition to the collection of many professionals and students.

This book was conceptualized with the vision of imparting up-to-date information and advanced data in this field. To ensure the same, a matchless editorial board was set up. Every individual on the board went through rigorous rounds of assessment to prove their worth. After which they invested a large part of their time researching and compiling the most relevant data for our readers.

The editorial board has been involved in producing this book since its inception. They have spent rigorous hours researching and exploring the diverse topics which have resulted in the successful publishing of this book. They have passed on their knowledge of decades through this book. To expedite this challenging task, the publisher supported the team at every step. A small team of assistant editors was also appointed to further simplify the editing procedure and attain best results for the readers.

Apart from the editorial board, the designing team has also invested a significant amount of their time in understanding the subject and creating the most relevant covers. They scrutinized every image to scout for the most suitable representation of the subject and create an appropriate cover for the book.

The publishing team has been an ardent support to the editorial, designing and production team. Their endless efforts to recruit the best for this project, has resulted in the accomplishment of this book. They are a veteran in the field of academics and their pool of knowledge is as vast as their experience in printing. Their expertise and guidance has proved useful at every step. Their uncompromising quality standards have made this book an exceptional effort. Their encouragement from time to time has been an inspiration for everyone.

The publisher and the editorial board hope that this book will prove to be a valuable piece of knowledge for researchers, students, practitioners and scholars across the globe.

List of Contributors

Gregory M. Enns, Monisha K. Shah, Kristina Cusmano-Ozog and Anna-Kaisa Niemi
Department of Pediatrics, Division of Medical Genetics, Lucile Packard Children's Hospital, Stanford University, Stanford, California, United States of America

Tereza Moore, Anthony Le and Tina M. Cowan
Department of Pathology, Stanford University, Stanford, California, United States of America

Kondala Atkuri
Department of Genetics, Stanford University, Stanford, California, United States of America

Pedro Cahn, Patricia Patterson and Alejandro Krolewiecki
Fundacion Huesped, Buenos Aires, Argentin

Julio Montaner
University of British Columbia, Vancouver, Canada

Patrice Junod
Clinique Médicale du Quartier Latin, Montréal, Canada

Jaime Andrade-Villanueva
Antiguo Hospital Civil de Guadalajara "Fray Antonio Alcalde", CUCS, Universidad de Guadalajara, Guadalajara, Jalisco, Mexico

Isabel Cassetti
Helios Salud, Buenos Aires, Argentina

Juan Sierra-Madero
Instituto Nacional de Ciencias Medicas y Nutricion, Mexico, Mexico

Arnaldo David Casiro
Hospital General de Agudos Teodoro Alvarez, Buenos Aires, Argentina

Raul Bortolozzi
División Estudios Clínicos, Centro Diagnó stico Médico de Alta Complejidad S.A. (CIBIC), Santa F é, Argentina

Sergio Horacio Lupo
Instituto CAICI, Santa Fé, Argentina

Nadia Longo, Emmanouil Rampakakis and John S. Sampalis
JSS Medical Research, Westmount, Canada

Nabil Ackad
Abbott Laboratories, Montréal, Canada

John S. Sampalis
McGill University, Montréal, Canada

Anja Brinckmann, Claudia Weiss, Friederike Wilbert, Angelika Zwirner and Markus Schuelke
Department of Neuropediatrics, Charité University Medical School, Berlin, Germany

Arpad von Moers
DRK-Kliniken Westend, Berlin, Germany,

Gisela Stoltenburg-Didinger
Department of Neuropathology, Charité University Medical School, Berlin, Germany

Ekkehard Wilichowski
Department of Pediatrics and Pediatric Neurology, Georg August University, Göttingen, Germany

Friederike Wilbert and Markus Schuelke
NeuroCure Clinical Research Center, Charité University Medical School, Berlin, Germany

Roman H. Haefeli, Michael Erb, Dimitri Robay, Corinne Anklin and Nuri Guevens
Santhera Pharmaceuticals, Liestal, Switzerland

Roman H. Haefeli
Biozentrum, University of Basel, Basel, Switzerland

Anja C. Gemperli
Institut Straumann AG, Basel, Switzerland

Isabelle Courdier Fruh
Novartis Pharma AG, Basel, Switzerland

Robert Dallmann
Institute of Pharmacology and Toxicology, University of Zürich, Zürich, Switzerland

Shehnaz Apabhai, Grainne S. Gorman, Joanna L. Elson, Douglass M. Turnbull and Michael I. Trenell
Mitochondrial Research Group, Newcastle University, Newcastle upon Tyne, United Kingdom,,

Grainne S. Gorman, Douglass M. Turnbull and Michael I. Trenell
NIHR Biomedical Research Centre for Ageing and Age-related Disease, Newcastle University, Newcastle upon Tyne, United Kingdom

Grainne S. Gorman, Laura Sutton, Douglass M. Turn bull and Michael I. Trenell
Newcastle Centre for Brain Ageing and Vitality, Newcastle University, Newcastle upon Tyne, United Kingdom

Thomas Plötz
School of Computing, Newcastle University, Newcastle upon Tyne, United Kingdom

Steven J. Reynolds, Claire W. Hallahan, Marybeth Daucher, Richard T. Davey Jr., Anthony S. Fauci and Thomas C. Quinn
National Institute of Allergy and Infectious Diseases, National Institutes of Health, Bethesda, Maryland, United States of America

Steven J. Reynolds and Thomas C. Quinn
Johns Hopkins University School of Medicine, Baltimore, Maryland, United States of America

Cissy Kityo, Geoffrey Kabuye, Diana Atwiine, Frank Mbamanya, Francis Ssali and Peter Mugyenyi
Joint Clinical Research Center, Kampala, Uganda

Robin Dewar
SAIC-Frederick, Inc., National Cancer Institute, National Institutes of Health, Bethesda, Maryland, United States of America

Mark R. Dybul
O'Neill Institute for National and Global Health Law, Georgetown University Law Center, Washington, D. C., United States of America
George W. Bush Institute, Dallas, Texas, United States of America

Alicia M. Celotto, Wai Kan Chiu and Michael J. Palladino
Department of Pharmacology and Chemical Biology, University of Pittsburgh School of Medicine, Pittsburgh, Pennsylvania, United States of America
Pittsburgh Institute for Neurodegenerative Diseases, University of Pittsburgh School of Medicine, Pennsylvania, United States of America

Wayne Van Voorhies
Molecular Biology Program, New Mexico State University, Las Cruces, New Mexico, United States of America

Lynn T. Matthews
Division of Infectious Disease, Beth Israel Deaconess Medical Center, Boston, Massachusetts, United States of America

Janet Giddy and Jane Hampton
HIV Program, McCord Hospital, Durban, South Africa

Musie Ghebremichael, Karen Axten, Rajesh T. Gandhi and David R. Bangsberg
Ragon Institute of Massachusetts General Hospital, Massachusetts Institute of Technology, and Harvard University, Boston, Massachusetts, United States of America

Anthony J. Guarino
Institute of Health Professions, Massachusetts General Hospital, Boston, Massachusetts, United States of America

Aba Ewusi
Division of Internal Medicine, Harvard Vanguard Medical Associates, Boston, Massachusetts, United States of America

Emma Carver
Department of Emergency Medicine, University Hospital of Wales, Cardiff, Wales

Meghan C. Geary
Albany Medical College, Albany, New York, United States of America

Rajesh T. Gandhi
Division of Infectious Disease, Massachusetts General Hospital, Boston, Massachusetts, United States of America

David R. Bangsberg
Mbarara University of Science and Technology, Mbarara, Uganda
Center for Global Health, Massachusetts General Hospital, Boston, Massachusetts, United States of America

Anna Golubitzky, Phyllis Dan, Sarah Weissman, Gabriela Link and Ann Saada
Monique and Jacques Roboh Department of Genetic Research, Department of Genetics and Metabolic Diseases, Hadassah, Hebrew University Medical Center, Jerusalem, Israel

Jakob D. Wikstrom
Department of Endocrinology and Metabolism, Hadassah, Hebrew University Medical Center, Jerusalem, Israel

Joseph E. Reiner, Rani B. Kishore and Kristian Helmerson
Physical Measurement Laboratory, National Institute of Standards and Technology, Gaithersburg, Maryland, United States of America

Barbara C. Levin
Material Measurement Laboratory, National Institute of Standards and Technology, Gaithersburg, Maryland, United States of America

Thomas Albanetti, Nicholas Boire, Ashley Knipe and Koren Holland Deckman
Department of Chemistry, Gettysburg College, Gettysburg, Pennsylvania, United States of America

Aristeidis Parmakelis and Marina Moustaka
Department of Ecology and Taxonomy, Faculty of Biology, National and Kapodistrian University of Athens, Panepistimioupoli Zografou, Athens, Greece

Aristeidis Parmakelis, Nikolaos Poulakakis and Christos Louis
Department of Biology, University of Crete, Heraklion, Crete, Greece

Aristeidis Parmakelis, Nikolaos Poulakakis, Jonathon C. Marshall, Adalgisa Caccone and Jeffrey R. Powell
Department of Ecology and Evolutionary Biology, Yale University, New Haven, Connecticut, United States of America

Christos Louis
Institute of Molecular Biology and Biotechnology, Foundation of Research and Technology Heraklion, Vassilika Vouton, Heraklion, Crete, Greece

Michel A. Slotman
Department of Entomology, Texas A&M University, College Station, Texas, United States of America

Jonathon C. Marshall
Department of Zoology, Weber State University, Ogden, Utah, United States of America

Parfait H. Awono-Ambene, Christophe Antonio-Nkondjio and Frederic Simard
Organisation de Coordination pour la Lutte Contre les Endémies en Afrique Centrale (OCEAC), Yaoundé, Cameroon

Frederic Simard
Institut de Recherche pour le Développement (IRD), Bobo Dioulasso, Burkina Faso

Vichet Phan, Sopheak Thai, Kimcheng Choun and Johan van Griensven
Sihanouk Hospital Center of HOPE, Phnom Penh, Cambodia

Lutgarde Lynen and Johan van Griensven
Institute of Tropical Medicine, Antwerp, Belgium

Maria A. Rocca, Paola Valsasina, Elisabetta Pagani and Massimo Filippi
Neuroimaging Research Unit, Scientific Institute and University Ospedale San Raffaele, Milan, Italy

Maria A. Rocca, Paola Valsasina, Elisabetta Pagani, Giancarlo Comi and Massimo Filippi
Division of Neuroscience, Department of Neurology, Institute of Experimental Neurology, Scientific Institute and University Ospedale San Raffaele, Milan, Italy

Stefania Bianchi-Marzoli and Jacopo Milesi
Department of Ophthalmology, Scientific Institute and University Ospedale San Raffaele, Milan, Italy

Andrea Falini
Department of Neuroradiology, Scientific Institute and University Ospedale San Raffaele, Milan, Italy

Caroline Aspord, Julie Charles, Marie-Therese Leccia, David Laurin, Marie-Jeanne Richard, Laurence Chaperot and Joel Plumas
Etablissement Français du Sang Rhone-Alpes, R&D Laboratory, La Tronche, France
University Joseph Fourier, Grenoble, France
INSERM, U823, Immunobiology & Immunotherapy of Cancers, La Tronche, France

Julie Charles and Marie-Therese Leccia
Centre Hospitalier Universitaire Grenoble, Michallon Hospital, Dermatology, pole pluridisciplinaire de medecine, Grenoble, France

Marie-Jeanne Richard
Centre Hospitalier Universitaire Grenoble, Michallon Hospital, Cancerology and Biotherapy, Grenoble, France

Geoffray Keller, Martin Cour, Romain Hernu, Julien Illinger, Dominique Robert and Laurent Argaud
Hospices Civils de Lyon, Groupement Hospitalier Edouard Herriot, Service de Réanimation Mé dicale, Lyon, France

Geoffray Keller, Martin Cour, Dominique Robert and Laurent Argaud
Université de Lyon, Université Lyon 1, Faculté de médecine Lyon-Est, Lyon, France

Michael V. Zaragoza
Genetics & Metabolism Division, Pediatrics Department and Center for Mitochondrial and Molecular Medicine and Genetics (MAMMAG), University of California Irvine,Irvine, California, United States of America

Joseph Fass and Dawei Lin
Bioinformatics Core, UC Davis Genome Center, University of California Davis, Davis, California, United States of America

Marta Diegoli and Eloisa Arbustini
Centre for Inherited Cardiovascular Diseases, IRCCS Foundation Policlinico San Mateo, Pavia, Italy

Cristina Mazzaccara, Rosario Liguori, Domenico Vitale and Lucia Sacchetti
CEINGE – Advanced Biotechnologies S. C. a R. L., Naples, Italy

Cristina Mazzaccara, Rosario Liguori and Lucia Sacchetti
Department of Biochemistry and Medical Biotechnologies, University of Naples Federico II, Naples, Italys

Dario Iafusco, Alfonso Galderisi and Francesco Prisco
Department of Pediatrics, Second University of Naples, Naples, Italy

Maddalena Ferrigno
SDN Foundation, Naples, Italy

Francesca Simonelli and Paolo Landolfo
Department of Ophthalmology, Second University of Naples, Naples, Italy

Mariorosario Masullo
Department of Study of the Institutions and Territorial Systems, University of Naples 'Parthenope'', Naples, Italy

Elisa Boschetti, Francesca Bianco, Antonio D. Pinna, Massimo Del Gaudio, Vincenzo Stanghellini, Loris Pironi, Kerry Rhoden and Roberto De Giorgio
Department of Surgical and Medical Sciences, University of Bologna, Bologna, Italy

Elisa Boschetti, Valerio Carelli, Giovanna Cenacchi and Vitaliano Tugnoli
Department of Biomedical and Neuromotor Sciences, University of Bologna, Bologna, Italy

Roberto D'Alessandro
Institute of Neurological Sciences, University of Bologna, Bologna, Italy

Rita Rinaldi
Neurology Unit, St. Orsola-Malpighi Hospital, Bologna, Italy

Carlo Casali
Department of Medico-Surgical Sciences and Biotechnologies, University 'La Sapienza', Rome, Italy

Shruti Tewari and Narayanan Srinivasan
Centre of Behavioural and Cognitive Sciences, University of Allahabad, Allahabad, Uttar Pradesh, India

Sammyh Khan and Nick Hopkins
School of Psychology, University of Dundee, Dundee, Scotland, United Kingdom

Stephen Reicher
School of Psychology, University of St Andrews, St Andrews, Scotland, United Kingdom

Cristina Socolovschi, Pavel Ratmanov and Didier Raoult
Aix Marseille Université, URMITE, UM63, CNRS 7278, IRD 198, Inserm 1095, Marseille, France

Frédéric Pages
CIRE/ARS Océan Indien, La Réunion, France

Mamadou O. Ndiath
IRD, Laboratoire de Paludologie, UMR 198 URMITE, Dakar, Sénégal

Francesco Pallotti
Department of Neurology, Columbia University, New York City, New York, United States of America
Dipartimento di Scienze Chirurgiche e Morfologiche, University of Insubria, Varese, Italy

Giorgio Binelli
Dipartimento di Scienze Teoriche e Applicate, University of Insubria, Varese, Italy

Rossella Vicenti and Maria Macciocca
Unità Operativa di Ginecologia e Fisiopatologia della Riproduzione Umana, Ospedale S.Orsola-Malpighi, University of Bologna, Bologna, Italy

Raffaella Fabbri, Rossella Vicenti and Maria Macciocca
Dipartimento di Scienze Mediche e Chirurgiche (DIMEC), University of Bologna, Bologna, Italy

Maria L. Valentino, Sabina Cevoli, Agostino Baruzzi and Valerio Carelli
IRCCS Istituto delle Scienze Neurologiche di Bologna, Ospedale Bellaria, Bologna, Italy
Dipartimento di Scienze Biomediche e Neuromotorie (DIBINEM), University of Bologna,Bologna, Italy

Franco Valenza, Marta Pizzocri, Valentina Salice, Giorgio Chevallard, Tommaso Fossali, Silvia Coppola, Sara Froio, Federico Polli and Luciano Gattinoni
Dipartimento di Anestesia, Rianimazione (Intensiva e Subintensiva) e Terapia del Dolore, Fondazione IRCCS CáGranda, Ospedale Maggiore Policlinico, Milan, Italy

Stefano Gatti
Centro di Ricerche Chirurgiche Precliniche, Fondazione IRCCS CáGranda, Ospedale Maggiore Policlinico, Milan, Italy

Francesco Fortunato and Giacomo P. Comi
Centro Dino Ferrari, Dipartimento di Scienze Neurologiche, Fondazione IRCCS CáGranda, Ospedale Maggiore Policlinico, Milan, Italy

Franco Valenza, Stefano Gatti, Giacomo P. Comi and Luciano Gattinoni
Università degli Studi di Milano, Milan, Italy

Isabelle Tromme, Pauline Richez, Laurine Sacré, Liliane Marot, Pascal Van Eeckhout and Ivan Theate
Department of Dermatology, Centre du Cancer, Cliniques Universitaires St Luc, Université catholique de Louvain, Brussels, Belgium

Brecht Devleesschauwer and Niko Speybroeck
Institute of Health and Society, Faculty of Public Health, Universite´ catholique de Louvain, Brussels, Belgium

Philippe Beutels
Centre for Health Economics Research & Modelling Infectious Diseases, Vaccine & Infectious Disease Institute, Faculty of Medicine & Health Sciences, University of Antwerp, Antwerp, Belgium

Nicolas Praet
Department of Biomedical Sciences, Institute of Tropical Medicine, Antwerp, Belgium

Jean-François Baurain
Department of Medical Oncology, Centre du Cancer, Cliniques Universitaires St Luc, Université catholique de Louvain, Brussels, Belgium

Julien Lamberts
Department of Dermatology, Universitair Ziekenhuis, Antwerp, Belgium

Catherine Legrand
Institute of Statistics, Biostatistics and Actuarial Sciences, Université catholique de Louvain, Louvain-la-Neuve, Belgium

Luc Thomas
Department of Dermatology, Lyon 1 University, Centre Hospitalier Lyon Sud, Pierre Be´ nite, France

Maria Wehbe, Saïdi M. Soudja, Amandine Mas, Lionel Chasson, Rodolphe Guinamard, Grégory Verdeil and Anne-Marie Schmitt-Verhulst
Centre d'Immunologie de Marseille-Luminy (CIML), Aix-Marseille Université UM2, Marseille, France
Institut National de la Santé et de la Recherche Médicale (INSERM), Marseille, France
Centre National de la Recherche Scientifique (CNRS), Marseille, France

Céline Powis de Tenbossche and Benoît Van den Eynde
Ludwig Institute for Cancer Research and Cellular Genetics Unit, UCL, Brussels, Belgium

Index

www.ingramcontent.com/pod-product-compliance
Lightning Source LLC
Chambersburg PA
CBHW080536200326
41458CB00012B/4449